Ward Rounds in
Obstetrics and Gynecology

Ward Rounds in Obstetrics and Gynecology

Editors
Sunanda R Kulkarni
MD PGD (Sexual Science and Mental Health)

Ex-Professor and Head
Department of Obstetrics and Gynecology
Bangalore Medical College and Research Institute
DNB Coordinator
Chinmaya Mission Hospital
Bengaluru, Karnataka, India

K Srinivas
MS DGO DNB MNAMS PGDMLE FICOG MA

Associate Professor
Department of Obstetrics and Gynecology
Bangalore Medical College and Research Institute
Bengaluru, Karnataka, India

Foreword
Sir Sabaratnam Arulkumaran

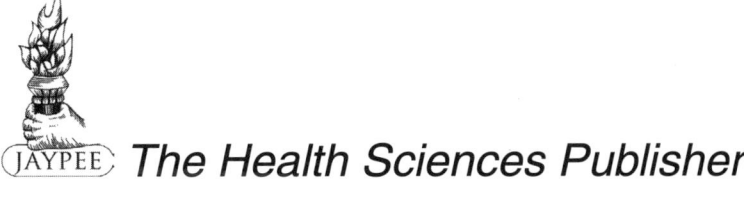

JAYPEE *The Health Sciences Publisher*

New Delhi | London | Panama

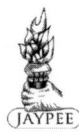 **Jaypee Brothers Medical Publishers (P) Ltd**

Headquarters
Jaypee Brothers Medical Publishers (P) Ltd
4838/24, Ansari Road, Daryaganj
New Delhi 110 002, India
Phone: +91-11-43574357
Fax: +91-11-43574314
Email: jaypee@jaypeebrothers.com

Overseas Offices

J.P. Medical Ltd
83 Victoria Street, London
SW1H 0HW (UK)
Phone: +44 20 3170 8910
Fax: +44 (0)20 3008 6180
Email: info@jpmedpub.com

Jaypee-Highlights Medical Publishers Inc
City of Knowledge, Bld. 235, 2nd Floor, Clayton
Panama City, Panama
Phone: +1 507-301-0496
Fax: +1 507-301-0499
Email: cservice@jphmedical.com

Jaypee Brothers Medical Publishers (P) Ltd
17/1-B Babar Road, Block-B, Shyamoli
Mohammadpur, Dhaka-1207
Bangladesh
Mobile: +08801912003485
Email: jaypeedhaka@gmail.com

Jaypee Brothers Medical Publishers (P) Ltd
Bhotahity, Kathmandu, Nepal
Phone: +977-9741283608
Email: kathmandu@jaypeebrothers.com

Website: www.jaypeebrothers.com
Website: www.jaypeedigital.com

© 2018, Jaypee Brothers Medical Publishers

The views and opinions expressed in this book are solely those of the original contributor(s)/author(s) and do not necessarily represent those of editor(s) of the book.

All rights reserved. No part of this publication may be reproduced, stored or transmitted in any form or by any means, electronic, mechanical, photocopying, recording or otherwise, without the prior permission in writing of the publishers.

All brand names and product names used in this book are trade names, service marks, trademarks or registered trademarks of their respective owners. The publisher is not associated with any product or vendor mentioned in this book.

Medical knowledge and practice change constantly. This book is designed to provide accurate, authoritative information about the subject matter in question. However, readers are advised to check the most current information available on procedures included and check information from the manufacturer of each product to be administered, to verify the recommended dose, formula, method and duration of administration, adverse effects and contraindications. It is the responsibility of the practitioner to take all appropriate safety precautions. Neither the publisher nor the author(s)/editor(s) assume any liability for any injury and/or damage to persons or property arising from or related to use of material in this book.

This book is sold on the understanding that the publisher is not engaged in providing professional medical services. If such advice or services are required, the services of a competent medical professional should be sought.

Every effort has been made where necessary to contact holders of copyright to obtain permission to reproduce copyright material. If any have been inadvertently overlooked, the publisher will be pleased to make the necessary arrangements at the first opportunity. The **CD/DVD-ROM** (if any) provided in the sealed envelope with this book is complimentary and free of cost. **Not meant for sale.**

Inquiries for bulk sales may be solicited at: jaypee@jaypeebrothers.com

Ward Rounds in Obstetrics and Gynecology

First Edition: **2018**

ISBN: 978-93-5270-239-8

Printed at Sanat Printers

Dedicated to

My parents
Late Dr RH Kulkarni
Late Ms Vimala Kulkarni
My mentors who made me what I am professionally
Dr Sunanda R Kulkarni and Dr Damayanthi HR
My parents who made me what I am as a human
Dr K Krishna Jois and Ms K Shantha
My family who always supported unconditionally
Ms Radhika Srinivas and Rahul Niranjan Srinivas
K Sridhar (Brother) and his family
My inspirers who continue to teach me
Students and Patients

Sunanda R Kulkarni
K Srinivas

Contributors

Anupama Hari MD DGO DNB PhD
Professor
Department of Obstetrics and Gynecology
Gandhi Medical College and Hospital
Hyderabad, Telangana, India

BS Rama Murthy MBBS MD
Consultant Sonologist
Srinivasa Ultrasound Scanning Centre
Bengaluru, Karnataka, India

D Leela MD DGO DNB FRCOG
DNB Coordinator
Vishakhapatnam, Andhra Pradesh, India

Haresh U Doshi MD (Gynec) PhD FICOG Diploma (USG)
PGDMLS PGDCR PGCML PGDHHM
Professor and Head
Department of Obstetrics and Gynecology
Gujarat Cancer Society Medical College, Hospital and Research Centre
Ahmedabad, Gujarat, India

Hemant Deshpande MBBS MD
Professor and Head
Department of Obstetrics and Gynecology
Dr D Y Patil Medical College and Hospital
Pune, Maharashtra, India

HR Damayanthi MD DGO
Ex-Professor and Superintendent
Cheluvamba Hospital
Mysore Medical College and Research Institute
Mysuru, Karnataka, India

IB Vijayalakshmi
MD DM (Card) FICC FIAMS FIAE FICP FCSI FAMS DSc
Ex-Professor
Department of Pediatric Cardiology
Sri Jayadeva Institute of Cardiovascular Sciences and Research
Bengaluru, Karnataka, India

K Srinivas MS DGO DNB MNAMS PGDMLE FICOG MA
Associate Professor
Department of Obstetrics and Gynecology
Bangalore Medical College and Research Institute
Bengaluru, Karnataka, India

Korula George MBBS MD DGO MRACOG
Professor and Head
Department of Reproductive Medicine
Baptist Hospital
Bengaluru, Karnataka, India

KV Malini MD DGO FICOG PGDMLE
Ex-Professor and Head
Department of Obstetrics and Gynecology
Bangalore Medical College and Research Institute
Bengaluru, Karnataka, India

Lalithambica Karunakaran MDDGO
Professor
Department of Obstetrics and Gynecology
Government TD Medical College
Alappuzha, Kerala, India

Michael George Muto MD
Associate Professor
Department of Obstetrics and Gynecology and Reproductive Biology
Harvard Medical School
Program Director, Gynecologic Oncology Fellowship
Brigham and Women's Hospital and the Dana Farber Cancer Institute
Boston, Massachusetts, USA

Muralidhar V Pai MBBS DGO MD FICOG
Professor and Head
Department of Obstetrics and Gynecology
Kasturba Medical College
Manipal, Karnataka, India

Nagesh CM MD DM (Cardio)
Associate Professor
Deapartment of Cardiology
Sri Jayadeva Institute of Cardiovascular Sciences and Research
Bengaluru, Karnataka, India

Padma Balasubramanian
Board Certified in Endocrinology, Diabetes and Metabolism
Endocrinologist
Beth Israel Specialty Group, BID-Plymouth, MA
Active Staff of the Division of Endocrinology and Diabetes
Beth Israel Deaconess Medical Center (BIDMC)
Boston, Massachusetts, USA

Radhakrishnan P MRCOG
Bangalore Fetal Medicine Centre
Bengaluru, Karnataka, India

Ratnamala Desai MD DGO
Professor and Head
Department of Obstetrics and Gynecology
SDM College of Medical Sciences and Hospital
Dharwad, Karnataka, India

Ravindra S Pukale MD DGO
Associate Professor
Department of Obstetrics and Gynecology
Adichunchanagiri Institute of Medical Sciences
Bellur, Karnataka, India

S Habeebullah MBBS MD MNAMS
Professor
Department of Obstetrics and Gynecology
Mahatma Gandhi Medical College and Research Institute
Ex-Professor and Head
Department of Obstetrics and Gynecology
Jawaharlal Institute of Postgraduate Medical Education and Research
Puducherry, India

S Rathnakumar BSc MD DGO
Ex-Professor
Department of Obstetrics and Gynecology
Madras Medical College and
Institute of Social Obstetrics & Government Kasturba Gandhi Hospital for Women and Children
Chennai, Tamil Nadu, India

Sunanda R Kulkarni
MD PGD (Sexual Science and Mental Health)
Ex-Professor and Head
Department of Obstetrics and Gynecology
Bangalore Medical College and Research Institute
DNB Coordinator
Chinmaya Mission Hospital
Bengaluru, Karnataka, India

Sunil Karanth MD FNB EDIC FCICM
Chairman, Critical Care Services
Consultant and Head
Department of Critical Care Medicine
Manipal Hospital
Bengaluru, Karnataka, India

UD Bafna MD
Professor and Head
Department of Gynec-Oncology
Kidwai Memorial Institute of Oncology
Bengaluru, Karnataka, India

Umadevi MD
Ex-Professor
Department of Gynec-Oncology
Kidwai Memorial Institute of Oncology
Bengaluru, Karnataka, India

S Vijayalakshmi MD DGO
Professor and Head
Department of Obstetrics and Gynecology
Adichunchanagiri Institute of Medical Sciences
Bellur, Karnataka, India

Foreword

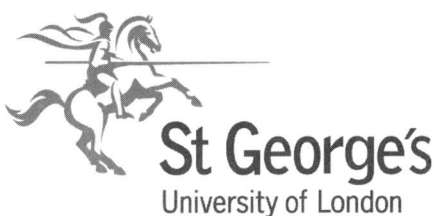

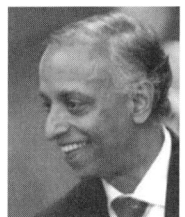

It was rather refreshing to read a book which has adapted a problem-based learning approach with case-based discussions. The modern undergraduate and postgraduate curriculum is increasingly adapting this methodology of learning. The learning would also suit mini clinical examination, which is used for assessment.

The approach to the chapters with a clinical history, examination findings followed by investigations is what we do on a daily basis. However, the thinking for possible differential diagnosis and management may differ based on the knowledge and experience of the individual caring for the patient. Each chapter addresses this issue by starting with the case history, examination and investigations. Pertinent questions follow with appropriate answers. The answers are practical approach to the case and are enhanced by detail medication tables, suitable illustrations and flowcharts followed by references for further knowledge enhancement.

I would strongly recommend this 'New Refreshing Approach' book with 18 chapters in obstetrics and 16 in gynecology for medical students, postgraduates and practicing clinicians. My sincere congratulations to the editors and the authors for bringing out this excellent book.

Sir Sabaratnam Arulkumaran
PhD DSc FRCS FRCOG
Emeritus Professor
Department of Obstetrics and Gynecology
St George's University
London, UK

Preface

Two year's effort has at last come to the stage of harvesting, yes this book, a dream come true for us, has seen the light of the day because of the efforts and wishes of a huge team of our friends, well wishers and great teachers of obstetrics and gynecology (OBG) and who have directly or indirectly contributed to this book. We fail in our duty if we do not acknowledge their help and support in bringing out this book on time.

Dr Sabaratnam Arulkumar, a great name in the field of OBG was kind enough to write a foreword to this work of ours which has increased the weight of this book tremendously for which we express our sincere thanks to him.

We would like to thank all the contributors of the various chapters who at a phone call or a mail of ours happily and positively responded and did the work to our satisfaction, some of them in a very short period of notice given by us.

We should not forget the support given by our office people and colleagues, especially Dr Trishula Joshi who helped in scrutinizing the work, some of our postgraduate students like Dr Shruthi Nagabhushan and Dr Sukanya Suresh who helped in preparing the document on time and we extend our gratitude to them.

Dr Raja Muni Reddy, Fetal Medicine Consultant; Dr SK Sithayyan, Cardiologist; Dr Chitra Narasimhan, Pediatrician; Dr Sangeetha Keskar, Pathologist; Dr Suvarna Jyothi, Consultant, and Registrar in Department of Obstetrics and Gynecology at Chinmaya Mission Hospital, Bengaluru, Karnataka have given their suggestions and inputs in their concerned fields.

We would like to thank Shri Jitendar P Vij (Group Chairman), Mr Ankit Vij (Group President), Ms Ritu Sharma (Director–Content Strategy), Ms Sunita Katla (PA to Group Chairman and Publishing Manager), Mr Manish Pahuja (General Manager–Production), Mr Venugopal V (Associate Director–South), Ms Samina Khan (Executive Assistant Director–Content Strategy), and Mr Rajesh Sharma (Production Coordinator), for all their support to bring this work in the form of a book which we hope would be of immense help to the undergraduate and postgraduate students and also consultants.

We are extremely thankful to the patients of our hospital from whom we have learnt the art and science of obstetrics and are in a position to put them all including some of the rare photographs in the form of a chapter in this book.

The unconditional support given by our family members [Radhika and Rahul Niranjan (wife and son of Dr K Srinivas)] cannot be acknowledged by words of thanks alone. Still we express our thanks to them also.

We would be delighted to know if there are any suggestions by the experts in the field, students and every user of this book which would help us to improve the further editions of the book.

Sunanda R Kulkarni
Sunanda28@yahoo.com
K Srinivas
srinivaskjois@gmail.com

Contents

Chapter 1:	**History Taking and Examination** *Ravindra S Pukale*	1
Chapter 2:	**Antepartum Hemorrhage** *Haresh U Doshi*	15
Chapter 3:	**Breech Presentation** *KV Malini*	26
Chapter 4A:	**Congenital Cardiac Disease in Pregnancy** *Sunanda R Kulkarni*	41
Chapter 4B:	**Heart Diseases and Pregnancy: Cardiologist's Perspective** *Nagesh CM*	54
Chapter 4C:	**Pregnancy with Mitral Stenosis and Mitral Regurgitation and Cardiac Failure** *IB Vijayalakshmi*	71
Chapter 5:	**Diabetes in Pregnancy** *Lalithambica Karunakaran*	86
Chapter 6:	**Fever in Pregnancy** *D Leela*	101
Chapter 7:	**Anemia in Pregnancy** *Sunanda R Kulkarni*	113
Chapter 8:	**Hypertensive Disorders of Pregnancy** *Muralidhar V Pai*	131
Chapter 9:	**ICU Rounds for Obstetricians** *Sunil Karanth*	139
Chapter 10:	**Fetal Growth Restriction** *Sunanda R Kulkarni*	168
Chapter 11:	**Liver Diseases in Pregnancy** *Hemant Deshpande*	178
Chapter 12:	**Multiple Pregnancy** *S Habeebullah*	190
Chapter 13:	**Preterm Labor** *S Vijayalakshmi*	201

Chapter 14:	Case with Previous Aneuploidy K Srinivas	215
Chapter 15:	Case with Previous Cesarean Delivery K Srinivas	223
Chapter 16:	Retropositive Pregnancy K Srinivas	234
Chapter 17:	Recurrent Pregnancy Loss Ratnamala Desai	246
Chapter 18:	Case-based Approach to Thyroid Disorders in Pregnancy Padma Balasubramanyam	257
Chapter 19:	Abnormal Uterine Bleeding Sunanda R Kulkarni	265
Chapter 20:	Benign Ovarian Tumors: A Clinical Approach HR Damayanthi	279
Chapter 21:	Cervical Cancer Michael George Muto	292
Chapter 22:	Epithelial Ovarian Cancer UD Bafna	304
Chapter 23:	Invasive Procedures in Obstetrics and Gynecology Practice Radhakrishnan P	314
Chapter 24:	Fibroid Uterus Sunanda R Kulkarni	326
Chapter 25:	Genital Prolapse K Srinivas	342
Chapter 26:	Infertility Korula George	360
Chapter 27:	Carcinoma Endometrium Umadevi	367
Chapter 28:	Postoperative Rounds K Srinivas	380
Chapter 29:	Primary Amenorrhea S Ratnakumar	391
Chapter 30:	Secondary Amenorrhea Anupama Hari	397
Chapter 31:	Examination of a Sexual Assault Victim K Srinivas	409

Chapter 32:	Bedside Ultrasonography in Obstetrics *BS Rama Murthy*	420
Chapter 33:	Vulval Hematoma *Sunanda R Kulkarni*	426
Chapter 34:	Rare Photo Gallery *Sunanda R Kulkarni, K Srinivas*	432

Index   *447*

1

CHAPTER

History Taking and Examination

Ravindra S Pukale

History taking of a patient who has come to your OPD plays a very important role. Detailed history taking and thorough clinical examination and relevant investigations will give the accurate diagnosis and helps in the management of cases.

OBSTETRICS

Problems with teenage pregnancy
- *Medical:* Anemia, malnutrition, preeclampsia
- *Obstetrics:* Fetal malpresentation, cephalopelvic disproportion, preterm delivery.

Problems in pregnancies in women
Above 35 years age
- Increased incidence of chromosomal anomalies and fetal anomalies
- Increased incidence of obesity, hypertension, APH, IUGR, GDM, postdatism, cervical dystocia, incordinate uterine contractions, malpositions (OP), prolonged labor due to reduced elasticity of soft tissues and impaired mobility of joints, increased operative vaginal deliveries and its associated maternal and fetal complications and higher incidence of lactation failure.

History

- To assess the health status of the mother and the fetus.
- To assess fetal gestational age and to obtain baseline investigations.
- To organize continued obstetric care and risk assessment.
  - Name: Identification of the patient
  - Wife of:
  - Marital status:
  - Date of first examination:
  - Address (along with contact number):
  - Age: Extremes of age, i.e. teenage and elderly (30 or above) are obstetric risk factors
  - *Gravida*: Pregnant state, both present and past, irrespective of gestational age.
  - *Parity*: State of previous pregnancy beyond the period of viability
  - Gravida and para both refer to pregnancies and not live babies
  - Duration of marriage: Relevant to note the fecundity or fertility
  - Religion
  - Occupation: For interpreting the social status
  - Occupation of the husband.

Incidence of Down's syndrome is said to increase from **1:350** at **35** years to **1:109** at the age of **40** years and further to **1:32** at the age of **45** years.

- To assess the socioeconomic condition. to anticipate complications associated with low socioeconomic status like preeclampsia, anemia, prematurity

- To obtain an idea regarding affordability of the treatment provided
- To give proper antenatal advice regarding family planning.
  - Period of gestation in the diagnosis—to be expressed in terms of completed weeks.

Calculation

In early weeks of gestation, counting is done from first day of last menstrual period and in later weeks, it is done from the expected date of delivery.

Start the presentation noting her gravida, para status and duration of amenorrhea in months as presentation and never as complaint, e.g. A G2P1L1 presenting with amenorrhea of 8 months.......

If a pregnant lady has no complaints, it can be presented as admitted for safe confinement, if with complaints the nature and duration of complaints may be mentioned.

In a term pregnant lady, pain abdomen, features suggestive of preeclampsia, symptoms suggestive of labor need to be enquired like, leak per vaginum (PV), bleeding PV, headache, blurring of vision, etc. Perception of fetal movements can assure to some extent about the fetal well-being.

Chief Complaints

Categorically, the genesis of complaints are to be noted. If there are no complaints, general enquiry about her well-being has to be made, e.g. history of leak PV, bleed PV; history of pain abdomen.

History of Presenting Illness

Elaboration of the chief complaints has to be done regarding the onset, duration, severity, progression and use of any medications. History of pain abdomen (details need to be taken to differentiate between true and false labor pains, UTI, etc.).

Obstetric History

Married life and query about consanguinity has to be made (infertility, precious pregnancy, causes for congenital anomalies, etc.).

Parity Index

Mention about gravidity, parity, living issues, abortions (GPLA).

Complications associated with grand multipara (women who has given birth to at least 4 viable children): (1) Pendulous abdomen that leads to malpresentation; (2) Pronounced lordosis leads to increase in pelvic inclination and nonengagement of fetal head at term; (3) Medical problems like anemia, hypertension, GDM; (4) Multiple pregnancy. (5) Placenta praevia; (6) Contracted pelvis and osteomalacic changes in pelvis due to calcium deficiency; (7) Rupture uterus; (8) PPH.

It is summed up as: status of gravida, parity, number of deliveries, abortions (including MTPs) and living issue (Table 1).

Table 1: Details of obstetric history

No.	Year and date	Pregnancy events	Labor events	Methods of delivery	Puerperium	Baby with breastfeeding and immunization details
1						
2						

For example, G3P1L1A1
- List out the significant events during each trimester based on the duration of pregnancy.

Pregnancy events: History of hyperemesis, fever with rashes, HDP, GDM, thyroid and other medical disorders
Labor events: Ask about spontaneous/induced, duration of each pregnancy (to rule out previous preterm birth). Outcome, history of blood transfusion
Mode of delivery: Vaginal/by instrumentation, Cesearean section.
Baby: Age/sex, birth weight, admission in NICU, breastfeeding, duration of breastfeeding, milestones.

- Enquire about the duration from last pregnancy/last abortion.
- History of any contraceptive usage between last childbirth/abortion and present pregnancy.
- Rh-negative pregnancy—history of previous pregnancies and administration of anti-D immunoglobulin previously.

Rh-isoimmunization
Anti-D Ig is given prophylactically to all D negative women at 28 weeks of pregnancy and a second dose is given after delivery, preferably within 72 hours, if the infant is D positive. The second dose is required because the half-life of Ig is only 6 weeks.

History of Present Pregnancy

*Number of antenatal visits (booking status) and immunization status has to be noted.

Women with at least 3 antenatal visits, who have received 2 doses of injection TT and taken 100 tablets of iron and folic acid (with ultrasound desirable but not mandatory) are said to be booked.
- Number of antenatal visits
  - *Ideal:* Once every four weeks in the first 28 weeks, every 2 weeks till 36 weeks and weekly after 36 weeks.

RCH has agencies like JrHA(F), SrHA(F)/LHV, *Anganwadi* workers, ASHA workers, VHGs to take care of the ANCs and they are not deprived of routine antenatal care, but the minimum prescribed visits are given by doctor and the rest by the above said agencies, to make them convenient. In simple terms, *Instead of they going to, healthcare providers, the care provider goes to their doors.*

- To decrease the load in antenatal clinics, RCH program has advised 3 antenatal visits in an uncomplicated pregnancy at least once in each trimester with an additional visit in the 3rd trimester:
  - As soon as she becomes pregnant
  - Once in 2nd trimester
  - At 32 weeks.
  - At 36 weeks or once in the last trimester.

  WHO Recommendation—minimun 4 visits 1 at 16 weeks, 28 weeks, 32 and 36 weeks.

However, in case of high-risk pregnancies, the number of visits can be increased/individualized based on the patient's condition.

Iron supplementation (WHO)—60 mg elemental iron and 250 µg folic acid once or twice daily for 6 months in pregnancy and 3 months postpartum.
Ministry of Health, Government of India, now recommends 100 mg elemental iron with 500 µg folic acid in the second half of pregnancy for a period of at least 100 days.

For example:

Effects of UTI in pregnancy:
- Preterm delivery
- Low birth weight
- Preeclampsia
- Anemia

1st Trimester

Symptoms of hyperemesis, threatened abortion, etc. Any medication or radiation exposure, fever with rashes (congenital rubella syndrome), UTI during first trimester has to be enquired along

---
*Certain symptoms commonly seen in particular trimesters have to be ruled out by taking negative history.

Table 2: True labor pain vs false labor pain

Feature	True labor pains	False labor pains
Duration of gestation	Usually happens at term	Any duration of gestation in T3
Nature of pain	Intermittent, increasing in severity and frequency	No specific pattern
Location	Low back	Abdomen
Radiation	Lower abdomen and thighs	No radiation
Relieving factors	None	Enema and sedation
Association	Vaginal discharge/leak/blood	Constipation/UTI symptoms
Examination	Uterus acting and cervical changes	None

with any medical or surgical events during pregnancy.

2nd Trimester

Date of quickening needs to be asked for symptoms of UTI, GDM, etc.

> Quickening—first perception of fetal movements by the mother.

3rd Trimester

- Symptoms of anemia, preeclampsia.
- History of leaking PV, pedal edema, pain abdomen—to differentiate between true and false labor pains (Table 2).

Menstrual History

Previous cycles: Duration and amount of flow.
LMP: First day of last normal menstrual period
EDD: Expected date of delivery.
Calculation: As per Naegele's formula it is obtained as follows (in regular cycles):
EDD = LMP + (9 months) + 7 days.

High-quality ultrasound measurement of the embryo or fetus during the first trimester of pregnancy is the most accurate method of establishing or confirming gestational age.

If the pregnancy is the result of assisted reproductive technology (ART), the clinician should use the ART-derived gestational age to assign the EDD. For example, for a pregnancy that results from *in vitro* fertilization, the clinician should use the age of the embryo and the date of the transfer to establish the EDD.

As soon as the clinician has data from the last menstrual period, the first accurate ultrasound examination, or both, the gestational age and the EDD should be calculated, discussed with the patient, and recorded clearly in the patient's medical record.

For research and surveillance purposes, the clinician should use the best obstetric estimate, rather than calculations based only on the last menstrual period, to determine gestational age.

Subsequent changes to the EDD should only be made in rare circumstances, should be discussed with the patient, and should be recorded clearly in the patient's medical record.

Past History

Medical

TB, asthma, hypertension, DM, epilepsy, cardiac disorders, thyroid disorders.

Surgical

General/gynecological.

Family History

Hypertension, DM, TB, blood dyscrasias, multiple pregnancies, congenital anomalies, etc.

Personal History

Enquire about diet, appetite, sleep, bowel and bladder habits and any health affecting habits. Previous history of blood transfusion, steroid therapy, drug allergy.

Diet recommendations in pregnancy
- Extra 300 kcal/day, 10 g protein/day
- RDA of iron in pregnancy is 30 mg.

Importance

- Anemia in pregnancy (advice is to be given to have food rich in iron, folate, vitamin B_{12})
- Diabetes in pregnancy—diet for maintainance of sugar levels and for decision regarding insulin dosage.

Summary

Mrs X aged _____ years, w/o _____ with socioecomic status _____ with _____ period of gestation has come with complaints of _____

Provisional Diagnosis

Examination

General Physical Examination

- *Build*—obese/average/thin.
- *Nutrition*—good/average/poor.
- *Height*—short stature is likely to be associated with a small pelvis (4.7 feet or lesser is considered to be short stature in India).
- *Weight*—for adequate weight gain during pregnancy (Table 3).

Table 3: Recommended weight gain in pregnancy

	BMI (pre-pregnancy)	Recommended weight gain (kg)
Low	<19.8	12.5–18
Normal	19.8–26	11.5–16

Contd...

Contd...

| High | 26–29 | 7–11.5 |
| Obese | >29 | 7 |

Range of weight gain
- Women carrying twins—16–20 kg
- Young adolescents—weight gain at upper end of the range
- Short women—weight gain at the lower end of the range

Rate of weight gain in the second half of pregnancy is 500 g/week.
(BMI becomes important or is of value only when prepregnancy weight is known)

- *Pallor, icterus, cyanosis, clubbing, lymphadenopathy* or *edema*
- *Tongue, gums, teeth* and *tonsils*—for evidence of infections, malnutrition (glossitis, cheilosis, bald tongue, etc.)
- *Neck*—neck veins, lymph nodes and thyroid examination.
- *Edema of legs*—pitting type.

Physiological edema subsides after 12 hours of recumbent posture/rest and is usually more by evening. It is limited to below ankle.

It could be physiological or pathological due to preeclampsia, anemia with hypoproteinemia, cardiac failure or nephrotic syndrome or hepatic failure.

Vitals

Pulse Rate

- BP—disappearance of sounds (Korotkoff 5) is taken as the representation of DBP in pregnancy (because of presence of large fistula at the placental site)
- Temperature if relevant/required
- Respiratory rate and type of respiration.

Systemic Examination

In pregnancy systolic murmurs more than grade II, any diastolic murmur is considered to be pathological. Sometimes cardiac diseases are diagnosed only during pregnancy.

- CVS—S1S2 + presence/absence of murmurs
- RS—bilateral NVBS heard, no added sounds
- CNS—within normal limits.
- Breasts—to be examined for presence of any lesions/growth/mass.

See for normal pregnancy changes—increase in size of breast, montgomery tubercles, secondary areola.

Nipples size and shape need to be assessed for breastfeeding postpartum.

Positions

- Arms by the sides (A)
  - *Arms raised above the head (B)*
  - *Hands pressing against waist (to contract pectoral muscles) (C)*
- Abdomen—for any palpable organs.

Obstetric Examination

A verbal consent is taken for the examination and the abdomen is fully exposed.

Position

Dorsal with thighs slightly flexed.

The examiner stands on the right side of the patient.

Inspection

To note:
- Whether the uterine ovoid is longitudinal, transverse or oblique
- The contour of the uterus—fundal notching, convex or flattened anterior wall, cylindrical or spherical shape
- Any undue enlargement of uterus
- Any skin changes over the abdomen or scar marks over the abdomen
- Fundus of the uterus is just palpable over the symphysis pubis at 12 weeks.

Palpation

- Height of the uterus—uterus is centralized if it is deviated. The ulnar border of the left hand is placed at the uppermost level of the fundus and an approximate duration of pregnancy is ascertained in terms of weeks of gestation
- SFH can be measured with a tape.

Obstetric Grips (Leopolds Maneuver) (Fig. 1)

1. *Fundal grip:* Palpation is done facing the patient's face. The whole fundal area is palpated using both hands laid flat on it to find out which pole of the fetus is in the fundus.
   - Broad, soft, irregular mass: Breech
   - Smooth, hard, globular mass: Head
   - Neither of the poles palpated in the fundus: Transverse Lie
2. *Lateral or umbilical grips:* Palpation is done facing the patient's face.

   Hands are placed flat on either side of the umbilicus to palpate one after the other, the sides of the uterus to find out the position of back, limbs and anterior shoulder from above downwards.
   - Smooth, curved, uniformly resistant feel—back
   - Irregular knob like structures—limbs
3. *First pelvic grip (Leopold's third maneuver):*

   Done by facing the patients face to ascertain presenting part, attitude, ballotabilty.

   The outstretched thumb and four fingers of the right hand are placed over the lower pole of the uterus, keeping the ulnar border of the palm over pubic symphysis to ascertain the presenting part and engagement. The unengaged head can move freely from side to side and both the poles remain at the same level.
4. *Second pelvic grip (Pawlik's grip or Leopold's fourth maneuver):*

   It is done facing the patient's feet.

   Four fingers of both the hands are placed on either side of the midline in the lower pole of the uterus and parallel to inguinal ligament. The fingers are pressed

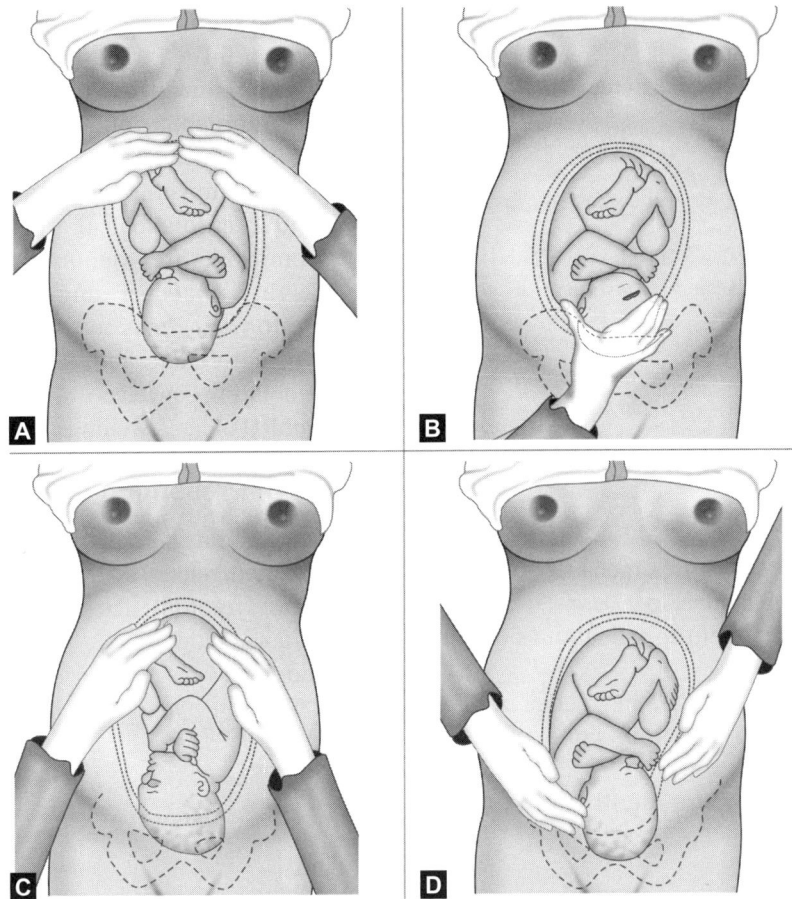

Fig. 1: Obstetric palpation—Leopold's maneuvers

downwards and backwards in a manner of approximation of finger tips to palpate the part occupying the lower pole of uterus.
Engagement of head: Head is engaged when the greatest horizontal plane, the biparietal diameter, has passed the plane of pelvic brim.

Per Speculum Examination

Look for any:
- Leak PV (in cases of PROM)
- OS open/closed (preterm, incomplete/inevitable abortion)
- Cervical length (preterm).

Per Vaginal Examination

- Cervix—position, consistency, effacement in cm, dilatation of cervical os presenting part—station, position
- Presence/absence of membranes
- Pelvic assessment (done in primigravidas by 38 weeks in multigravida previous uncomplicated vaginal delivery itself is a proof of adequacy of pelvis)
- Points to be noted in pelvic assessment
  - Sacral promontory
  - Sacral curvature
  - Sacrosciatic notch
  - Pelvic side walls

- Ischial spines (prominent/not)
- Subpubic angle
- Intertuberous diameter.

- Sacral promontory is usually not felt—pelvis adequate
- Sacral curvature—convex/concave/flat (based on the type of pelvis)
- Sacrosciatic notch should admit min 2 fingers
- Pelvic side walls can be convergent/divergent/straight
- Subpubic angle can be acute/obtuse
- Intertuberous diameter should admit minimum four knuckles.

GYNECOLOGY

History

- Importance toward maintenance of patient—physician relationship
- Allow the patient to talk about her chief symptoms
- After that, ask the patient series of direct and detailed questions concerning her symptoms
  - Name—for the identification of the patient
  - Wife of
  - Age—some disorders are common in certain age groups; helpful in narrowing down the differential diagnosis.
    ◊ Childhood—foreign body, vaginitis, ovarian tumors
    ◊ Adolescence—menstrual disorders, uterovaginal anomalies, PCOS, precocious/delayed puberty, germ cell tumors
    ◊ Reproductive age group—menstrual disorders, infections, benign lesions of genital tract, pregnancy related problems
    ◊ Older age—menopause related problems, malignancies.
  - Address (along with contact No.)
  - Social status
    ◊ Anemia is known to be more common in lower social strata
    ◊ Affordability of treatment becomes an influential factor in management.
  - Chief complaints—to be taken in detail and in chronological order. Common complaints are amenorrhea, abnormal vaginal bleed, dysmenorrhea, pain abdomen, mass felt per abdomen, vaginal discharge, mass per vagina, inability to conceive, urinary symptoms, genital ulcers/swellings.

History of Presenting Illness

- Elaborate chief complaints
- Associated/related symptoms
- General symptoms like recent weight loss/gain/fever/fatigue
- Bladder/bowel symptoms.

Pain Abdomen

SOCRATES

S-site
O-onset
C-character
R-radiation
A-associations
T-time
E-exacerbating factors
S-severity.

Normal menstruation
- Cycle length: 21–35 days
- Mean blood loss: Up to 70–80 mL
- If associated with clots—pathological
- Duration: 2–7 days

Menstrual History

- Age of menarche
- Regularity of cycles

- Duration of a period
- Length of cycle
- Intermenstrual bleeding (always pathological).

If present conditions like cancer cervix, cancer endometrium, intrauterine device, foreign bodies, fibroid polyp need to be ruled out.

- Dysmenorrhea—enquire if it occurs before, during or after the cycles.
- Amount of bleeding:
  - If excess
  - Pictorial blood loss assessment chart.

Pads	Factor	1	2	3	4	5	6	7
	X 1	II	I	I				
	X 5	III	II	II				
	X 20	III	I					
Total			87	31	11			

- Pads:
  - Lightly soaked—multiply by factor 1
  - Moderately soaked—multiply by factor 5
  - Heavily soaked—multiply by factor 20.

In case of usage of tampons, multiply by 1, 5 and 15.

Total score >100

Heavy Menstrual Bleeding

- In case of menopause ask regarding
  - Menarche
  - Postmenopausal bleed (importance is to rule out malignancies like cancer cervix or cancer endometrium)
  - Menopausal symptoms—vasomotor, mood, urinary symptoms, etc.
  - Calcium intake.

Obstetric History

- Marital status
- Consanguinity
- Parity
- Details of each pregnancy
  - Years and events
  - Pregnancy related events
  - Mode of delivery
  - Puerperal events
  - Baby details
  - Duration of breastfeeding
  - Duration of contraceptive usage
  - Number of miscarriages/molar pregnancies
    ◊ Nulliparous—most common: Endometriosis, endometrial cancer, breast cancer
    ◊ Multiparous—most common: Adenomyosis, cervical cancer, pelvic organ prolapse
    ◊ Recent delivery or miscarriage—sepsis, RPOC.

Contraceptive History

- *Combined OCPs—protective against ovarian and endometrial cancer*
- *IUCD—can cause HMB, dysmenorrhea*
- *LNG-IUS—can cause amenorrhea.*

Sexual History (in Case of Infertility)

- History of cohabitation (gaining importance these days due to changing trends in lifestyle)
- Vaginismus
- Sexual satisfaction or orgasm
- Dyspareunia
- Vaginal dryness
- In husband, premature ejaculation, erectile dysfunction.

Past History

Medical

Diabetes, thyroid disorders, epilepsy, TB, cardiac disease and others (influential in the management of cases).

Surgical

- Breast surgery (fibroadenoma), pelvic surgery (for adhesions), surgery for inguinal hernia in childhood (androgen insensitivity).
- Any hospital admission.

Family History

- Familial cancers—ovarian, endometrial, breast
- Any medical disorders
- Any infectious diseases.

Summary

Miss/Mrs X aged ___ years belonging to socioeconomic status _____ has come with complaints of _____

Provisional Diagnosis

Examination

General Physical Examination

- Built—obese/thin—to rule out endocrinopathy, menstrual abnormality.
- Obesity can lead to CAD, hypertension, diabetes, etc. which are risk factors for endometrial cancers.
- Nutrition—average/normal.
- Development of secondary sexual characters—breast, axillary hair, pubic hair.
- Height, weight, BMI
- Evidence of pallor, icterus, cyanosis, lymphadenopathy (cervical, left supraclavicular, axillary and inguinal) or edema.
- Examination of neck—thyroid enlargement, lymphadenopathy.
- Teeth, gums, tonsils—for septic foci, important before general anaesthesia is being given.
- PR, BP, RR.
- Examination of spine (important while performing surgeries during spinal anesthesia).

Breast Examination

- To be done in all women aged more than 40 years, as breast carcinoma is the second most common malignancy in females.

Positions

- Arms by the sides (A)
- Arms raised above the head (B)
- Hands pressing against waist (to contract pectoral muscles) (C).

Inspection
Look for dimpling of skin, erythema, edema, nipple retractions, nipple eczema.

Palpation
Look for nipple discharge, palpable mass/nodes (E).

Systemic Examination

- Cardiovascular system
- Respiratory system
- Central nervous system

> Tanner's staging of pubic hair, breast needs to be done in case of delayed menarche.

> - Bloody nipple discharge—suspect papilloma/sometimes breast cancer
> - Greenish—breast cyst
> - Clear—sign of abnormal cells (including cancer cells).

> - CVS—to rule out cardiac diseases like RHD and CHD
> - RS—to rule out any lung pathology—BA, TB.

Abdominal Examination

Inspection

- Distension/ascites
- Any mass

History Taking and Examination

- Umbilical position
- Presence of scars
- Presence of dilated veins/sinuses/visible peristalsis
- Discoloration over umbilical area/flanks
- Presence of hernia or divarication of recti.

Palpation
- Areas of tenderness
- Organomegaly
- Mass—size, shape, surface, site, extent, margins, mobility, consistency (mass arising from pelvis—cannot get below the mass, lower border cannot be made out because of the presence of symphysis pubis).

Percussion
- Presence of fluid thrill, shifting dullness—to look for evidence of free fluid
- In ascites—fluid thrill and shifting dullness will be present
- In an encysted/a large ovarian cyst—no shifting dullness.

Encysted ascites is seen most commonly in tuberculosis.

Auscultation
Presence of hypoactive/hyperactive bowel sounds.

Pelvic Examination

Instruct the patient to empty her bladder before performing pelvic examination.

Various positions
Dorsal, lithotomy, Sims' lateral (Figs 2 to 5)
- Dorsal—patient lying supine with legs flexed at hip and knee with feet resting on examination couch
- Lithotomy—supine with patient's legs in stirrups
- Sims'—left lateral position with left leg extended and right leg flexed at knee and hip and left arm by the side of patient
- Lateral position.

Prerequisites
- Patient should have emptied the bladder
- Female attendant should be present (in case of male examiner)

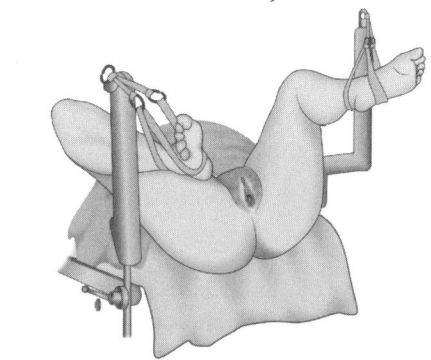

Fig. 3: Lithotomy position

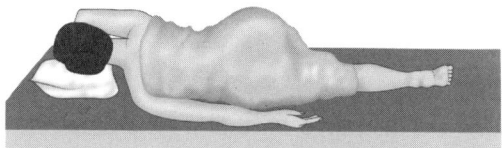

Fig. 4: Sims' position

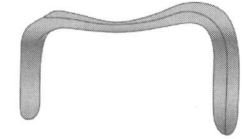

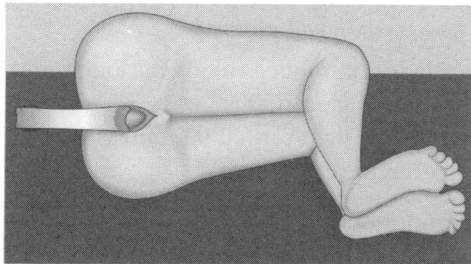

Fig. 5: Sims' speculum and examination in left lateral position

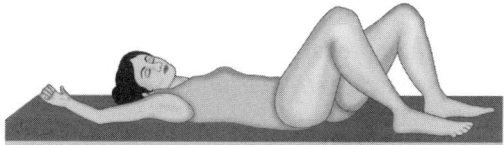

Fig. 2: Dorsal position

- A good light source
- Sterile gloves, sterile lubricants and instruments
- Consent from parent or guardian in case of examination of a minor or unmarried.

(In case of minor, it is better not to do digital vaginal examination if there is no absolute indication).

Vulvovaginal Examination

Inspection
- Vulva
  - Pubic hair distribution
  - Skin lesions—color changes, ulcer, swelling, growth
- Introitus
- Clitoris
- Hymen
- Descent of uterus or cervix—ask to strain to elicit stress incontinence, genital prolapse, perineal tears, hemorrhoids, anal fissures or anal fistula
- Perineal body
- Anus.

Palpation
Urethral discharge, Bartholin's glands, levator ani tear.

> Stress incontinence: Only condition where examination should be done with full bladder.

Speculum Examination

Labia minora are separated first and then Cusco's or Sims' speculum is introduced as follows (Figs 6 and 7):
- Blade is introduced along the longitudinal axis of vagina, firstly.
- Blade is then turned 90° and vagina and cervix are examined.

Vagina
- Presence of blood
- Discharge to be collected to detect monilial, trichomonal, chlamydial and gonococcal infections

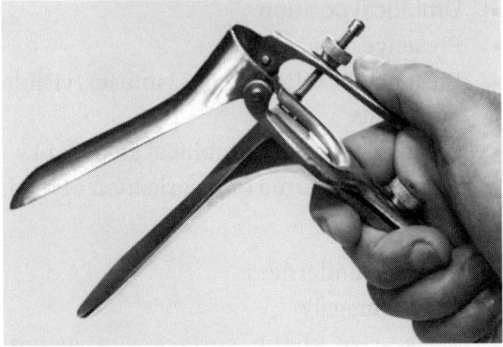

Fig. 6: Cusco's speculum

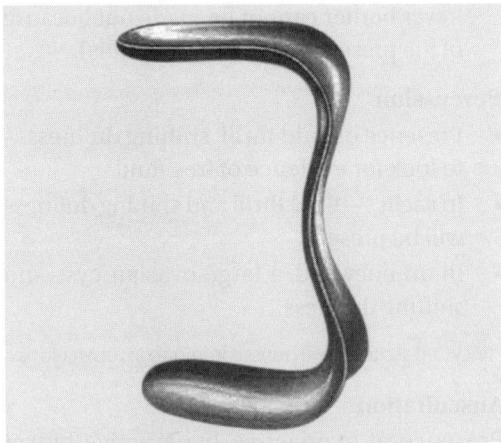

Fig. 7: Sims' speculum

- Dryness
- Mucosal characteristics—color, vascularity, edema, etc.
- Growth
- Structural abnormalities (anterior vaginal wall cysts, vaginal septum).

Cervix
- Color—normally pink
- External os—round in nulliparous, transversely slit in multiparous
- Position—posterior/mid position, anterior
- Discharge—s/o infections
- Bleeding through os
- Tears and lacerations
- Nabothian follicles or cysts
- Polyps/growths

- Erosions
- Bleeding on touch.

Bimanual Examination (Abdominopelvic Examination)

- Introduce well lubricated gloved index and middle fingers into the vagina
- Place the other hand over the infraumbilical region of abdomen and gently press while sweeping the pelvic structures towards the fingers palpating the abdomen
- Coordinate the activity of two hands to evaluate the following.

Uterus
- Position—anteverted/retroverted/mid-position
- Size—normal/enlarged
- Shape—regular/irregular
- Consistency—soft/firm
- Mobility—mobile/fixed/restricted
- Tenderness—absent/present
- Tumors if found, size, location, number, shape, consistency, tenderness, mobility, relation with uterus, transmitted mobility.

Cervix
Position, consistency, os open or closed.

Adnexa (Table 4)
- Presence of mass
- Normally tubes are not palpable and rarely normal ovaries are palpable.
- Adnexal mass has to be evaluated for, size, shape, consistency, tenderness, mobility, nodularity relation with uterus and cervix, transmitted mobility.

Table 4: Differentiating features of uterine and adnexal masses

Characteristics	Uterine	Adnexal
Location	Central	Lateral
Uterus	Not palpable	Palpable
Groove between uterus and mass	Absent	Present
Transmitted mobility	Present	Absent

Contd...

Bimanual Examination of Uterus (Fig. 8)

Consistency
- Soft—pregnancy, pyometra
- Hard—malignancy, calcfied myomas.

Enlargement
- Regular—pregnancy, adenomyosis, pyometra, hematometra, etc.
- Irregular—myoma, endometriosis.

Mobility
- Mobile—myoma, adenomyosis, pregnancy
- Fixed/restricted—PID, endometriosis, malignancy.

Per Rectal Examination

This is commonly not done.

It is done when Ca cervix, Ca endometrium, Ca ovary or endometriosis are being suspected clinically.

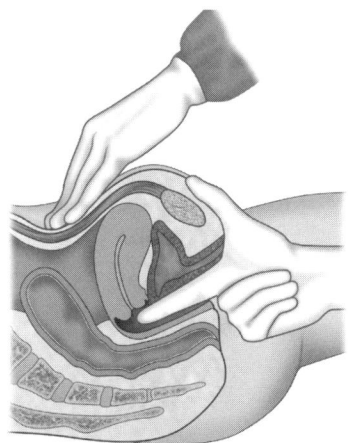

Fig. 8: Bimanual examination

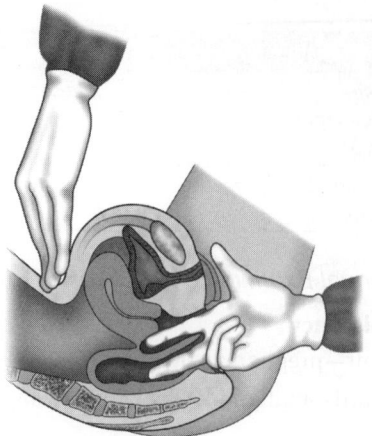

Fig. 9: Rectovaginal examination

To look for any abnormalities in:
- Rectal mucosa.
- Parametrium.
- Uterosacral ligaments (endometriosis).

> Best done after a course of antibiotics.

Examination under anesthesia

It is done for the examination of carcinoma cervix and endometrium.

Other modern, advanced modes of diagnosis have replaced this examination.

Rectovaginal Examination (Fig. 9)

It is done in case of suspicion of fistulae and cancers.

Bibliography

Obstetrics
1. Bedside Obstetrics and gynaecology by Richa Saxena, 2nd edition.
2. DC Dutta Textbook of Obstetrics.
3. Practical Manual of Obstetrics and Gynaecology for PG Examination (Jaypee Publications).
4. Practical Obstetrics and Gynaecology by Parulekar.
5. Williams Obstetrics, 24th edition.

Gynecology
1. Berek and Novak's Gynaecology.
2. DC Dutta Textbook of Gynaecology.
3. Jeffcoates Principles of Gynaecology.
4. Lakshmi Sheshadri Textbook of Gynaecology.
5. Practical Manual of Obstetrics and Gynaecology for PG Examination (Jaypee Publications).
6. Shaws Textbook of Gynaecology.

2 CHAPTER

Antepartum Hemorrhage

Haresh U Doshi

CASE 1

Patient Mrs M, wife of Mr N, Resident of Karnataka, aged 34 years belonging to lower socioeconomic class fourth gravida para 2, abortion 1 with 2 living issues was admitted in emergency 3 days back with complaint of:
- Amenorrhea since 7 months
- Bleeding per vaginal (PV) for 2 hours
- No history of leaking per vaginal (PV)
- No history of pain in abdomen.

Patient is having 7 months amenorrhea. She suddenly developed bleeding PV 3 days back which was moderate in amount and not associated with pain in abdomen or backache. There was no history of leaking PV. She was feeling fetal movements well. She immediately rushed to the hospital and was admitted after examination. She was given intravenous (IV) fluid. Blood investigations were sent and crossmatching was asked. Ultrasonography (USG) was carried out. Bleeding stopped after one hour of admission and as her vitals were stable, she was sent to ward after 6 hours.

Trimester History

First Trimester
- Natural conception
- No history of any drug intake or radiation exposure
- No history of bleeding per vaginum
- No antenatal visits taken.

Second Trimester
- She perceived quickening in 4th month
- She received one injection tetanus toxoid (TT) by health worker
- She was given iron folic acid (IFA) tablets by health worker but took it irregularly
- No blood investigations or USG was done.

Menstrual History
- Past menstrual cycles (PaMP)—3–5/30 days regular cycles with normal flow
- Last menstrual period (LMP)
- Estimated date of delivery (EDD).

Obstetric History

She is gravida 4 para 2, live 2, abortion 1. Her 2 deliveries were full term normal deliveries at home without any complications. In 3rd pregnancy she had spontaneous incomplete abortion at 2 months gestation, for which D and E was done in hospital.

Past History

There is no past history of any major disease or surgery.

Personal History
- My patient is a homemaker. She does not smoke and has any addiction

- She is taking mixed diet and takes approximately 2,000 k calories per day.

Family History
Nothing significant.

Socioeconomic History
She belongs to lower middle class according to modified Kuppuswamy scale.

On Examination
My patient is conscious and well oriented to time, place and person. She is fairly built and fairly nourished. Her height is 5 feet and weight is 54 kg. There is mild pallor. Sclera, teeth and gums normal. No neck veins and no thyroid swelling. There is mild pedal edema.

Vitals
- Her pulse is 92/min
- Her BP is 116/70 mm Hg
- Her RR is 18/min
- Her temperature is normal.

Breast Examination
Breast shows normal changes of pregnancy.

Systemic Examination
Cardiovascular system (CVS), respiratory system (RS), and central nervous system (CNS): No abnormality detected.

Abdominal Examination
Inspection
- Abdomen uniformly distended
- Linea nigra and striae gravidarum present
- No scar on abdomen.

Palpation
- Uterus relaxed
- Fundal height is around 30 weeks
- Symphysiofundal height is 27 cm
- Abdominal girth is 30 inches

- *Fundal grip:* Regular hard mass felt symptom of fetal head
- *Lateral grips:* Back felt on right side and limbs on left side
- *Pelvic grip:* Broad irregular nonballotable mass felt symptom of breech.

Auscultation

Fetal heart rate is 136/min heard on right side above umbilicus.

Final Diagnosis
A 34-year-old G4P2L2A1 with 30 weeks period of gestation with single live fetus in breech presentation with history of APH due to placenta previa confirmed by USG.

Her investigations:
- Hb 9.4 g% and blood group B +ve
- USG by TVS showed anterior placenta previa reaching up to os.

Q. 1. How do you define antepartum hemorrhage (APH). What is its incidence? What are the causes of APH?

Bleeding from or into the genital tract after 28 weeks of pregnancy till delivery of fetus is considered APH. Some western authorities consider starting limit 24 weeks of pregnancy. As there is no special entity like intrapartum hemorrhage bleeding up to delivery of fetus, i.e. 2nd stage is included in APH and 3rd stage hemorrhage is grouped under PPH.

APH complicates 3–5% of pregnancies and is a leading cause of perinatal and maternal mortality worldwide.[1]

The two major causes are placenta previa (part or whole of the placenta implanted in lower uterine segment) and abruptio placentae (premature separation of normally situated placenta) and accounts for more than 2/3rd cases. In 5–10% cases, local lower genital tract causes are responsible. They include cervical polyp, ectropion, carcinoma cervix, vaginal varicosities, vaginal trauma. In remaining 20-25% cases, cause may be unexplained. In this last group excessive show, marginal sinus rupture, circumvallate placenta might be the causes.

Q. 2. How will you clinically differentiate between placenta previa and abruptio placentae?

Clinically placenta previa and abruption placenta may be differentiated as follows:

	Placenta previa	Abruptio placentae
1.	Painless bleeding	Painful bleeding/backache
2.	Bleeding bright red	Dark red in color, may be absent in concealed
3.	Hypertension—normal incidence	HT associated in >1/3rd cases
4.	Uterus normal—soft	Uterus hard-tense
5.	Uterus nontender	Uterus tender on palpation
6.	Fundal height as per gestational age	More than gestational age in concealed variety
7.	Malpresentation and/or high presenting part	Normal presentation
8.	FHS usually normal	Fetal distress or death possible
9.	General condition and/or anemia proportionate to visible blood loss	Out of proportion
10.	DIC uncommon	DIC common

Q. 3. What are the risk factors for placenta previa?

Risk factors for placenta previa are as follows:
- Increased age >35 years—fourfold increased risk
- Increased parity
- Past history of placenta previa—six-eight-fold increased risk
- Multiple pregnancy
- Previous LSCS—3-4 times increased risk, increases linearly with number of CS[2]
- Previous history of MTP, MRP, curettage
- Smoking—twofold increased risk
- Residence at high altitude
- Race—higher in Asians
- First trimester bleeding.

Q. 4. What are the risk factors for abruptio placentae?

Risk factors for abruptio placentae are as follows:
- Increased age
- Increased parity
- Hypertension in pregnancy—in preeclampsia and chronic HT fivefold increased risk[3]
- Prior abruption—5-17% with one abruption, up to 25% in >1 abruption[4]
- Multiple gestation—threefold increased risk
- Premature rupture of membranes (PROM)—threefold increased risk
- Smoking—twofold increased risk
- Cicaine use, alcohol use
- Uterine leiomyoma
- External trauma—vehicular accidents, forceful external cephalic version (ECV)
- Thrombophilia—factor V Leiden mutation and prothrombin gene mutation
- Pregnancy following ART
- First trimester bleeding
- Race—African, Americans, Caucasians
- Familial association—hereditary.

Q. 5. How will you classify placenta previa?

Originally placenta previa was classified into four types:
1. *Low-lying:* Placenta is implanted in the lower uterine segment but it has not reached up to internal os of cervix
2. *Marginal:* Placenta edge reaches up to os but does not cover it. It can be anterior or posterior.
3. *Incomplete:* Placenta covers the internal os but does not cover it when it is dilated.

4. *Complete (central):* Placenta covers the internal os even when it is fully dilated.

Type II posterior is called **dangerous placenta previa** because by covering the sacrum it decreases the available AP diameter of the inlet and comes in the way of engagement which leads to nonengagement of the fetal presenting part which can otherwise effectively compress the placenta to stop bleeding and secondly even little compression leads to fetal distress and even death.

Now USG classification is much used:
- Placental edge >2 cm from os wherein vaginal delivery may be tried.
- Placental edge <2 cm from os where cesarean section is the rule.

Q. 6. What is McAfee Johnson expectant treatment for placenta previa? On what observations it was started?

McAfee Johnson expectant treatment is continuation of pregnancy after bleeding stops. It includes hospitalization and bed rest. After bleeding stops gentle speculum examination is carried out to exclude vaginal and cervical bleeding and USG-TVS confirms the diagnosis of placenta previa. Close daily observation of patient's vitals and daily fetal well-being assessment is done. Blood is kept crossmatched and ready and pregnancy is continued till term. In Rh-negative patient with spouse Rh-positive injection anti-D 300 µg should be given. In pregnancy less than 34 weeks steroids are administered to prevent RDS in newborn.

This expectant treatment was based on three observations:
1. First, bleeding is never dangerous for mother or baby.
2. Bleeding stops on its own.
3. When first bleeding occurs fetus is usually premature.

Q. 7. When will you terminate expectant line of treatment?

In following conditions expectant treatment is terminated:
- Repeated bouts of heavy bleeding—usually after 3rd bout nobody waits
- When 37 weeks are reached
- If there is fetal distress or fetal death
- If PROM has occurred
- If active labor starts.

Q. 8. In which patient you will give outpatient treatment?

Patient who are reliable, stable, staying nearby the hospital or have adequate emergency transport facility available can be managed as outpatient in expectant management. Cochrane review for 'interventions for placenta previa' showed that outcome of such patients is no different from indoor patients.[5]

Q. 9. How will you diagnose placenta previa by USG ?

Placenta previa can be easily diagnosed by USG by checking its relation to internal cervical os. Transvaginal sonography (TVS) is better than transabdominal sonography (TAS). TAS may be less accurate when there is—(1) posterior placenta previa and fetal head is inbetween, (2) in obese patients, and (3) with underfilling or overfilling of bladder.

During a myometrial contraction, the wall of the uterus may thicken and imitate placental tissue. Secondly, the lower uterine segment may shorten and bring the inferior edge of the placenta into contact with the internal cervical os, creating a condition that mimics placenta previa. To avoid this pitfall, a contraction is suspected if the myometrium is thicker than 1.5 cm and repeat imaging is performed after 30 minutes.

Transvaginal sonography, done gently is not harmful, can be safely done and its sensitivity is 87.5%, specificity is 98.5%, PPV is 93.3% and NPV is 97.6%.[6] Currently the sensitivity of TVS for diagnosis of placenta previa is almost 100%. In actively bleeding, patient if one wants to avoid TVS, transperineal (translabial) USG with abdominal probe is equally sensitive.

In TVS distance from the internal os is measured and documented.

Q. 10. When you see placenta previa on USG what other things you will note in the same examination?

When placenta previa is confirmed on TVS examination, one should look for placenta accreta whether it is present or not and also check for vasa previa if necessary by applying color Doppler. One should also note on which side—above, below, right or left placental edge is nearby so that at cesarean section hand can be passed in that direction to reach the membranes and deliver the baby by rupturing it. This avoids cutting through the placenta to deliver the baby.

Q. 11. What do you know about placental migration?

At 18 weeks anomaly scan as high as 26% placenta may be seen low lying. Out of them more than 95% resolve by the third trimester, i.e. placenta relocates away from the cervical os in the upper segment. This is called placental migration.

If placental edge is 2 cm away from os at 18 weeks almost 100% will migrate.

If placenta crosses the os by 2 cm almost 100% sensitivity for placenta previa at term.

Placental migration is misnomer because decidual invasion of either side of os by chorionic villi persists. It probably results from differential growth of lower and upper myometrial segments as pregnancy progresses. Second theory is it is degeneration of the peripheral placental tissue that receives a suboptimal vascular supply and growth in better perfused area of upper segment so called placental trophotropism.

Q. 12. What is the role of double set-up examination in placenta previa in present times?

With sonography widely available placenta previa and its type, i.e. relation with internal os is already known before term. So, double set-up examination has no role in modern obstetrics. It was done in past to decide for vaginal delivery or cesarean section by doing per vaginam in occupational therapy and checking the placental edge to differentiate between major degree and minor degree placenta previa.

In practice once diagnosed cesarean section is preferred for all cases of placenta previa.

Q. 13. How will you deliver the baby at cesarean section in placenta previa?

As already discussed above one should be knowing from prior USG that on which side of the placenta membranes are nearest. Hand should be passed in that direction by separating the placenta from uterine wall. Once membranes are reached they are ruptured and bay is delivered by catching the head in cephalic presentation and by catching the leg and delivering as breech in all other presentations.

If placenta is all around the site of incision and membranes appear to be far on USG, or there is difficulty in the method described above to reach the membranes, one can readily cut through the placenta to reach the fetal presenting part. One should be quick as in cutting through the placenta fetal blood is also lost. However, one should not be panicky after cutting through the placenta as only few cotyledons are cut and not excessive fetal blood is lost in few seconds.

Q. 14. How will you control PPH at cesarean section?

Postpartum hemorrhage at cesarean section in case of placenta previa is controlled by drugs, manipulative methods and surgical techniques.

Drugs include oxytocin, ergometrine and prostaglandins. Direct intramyometrial injection PGF2 alpha 250 µg may be given if patient is in shock and peripheral circulation is poor or when arterial ligation is already done.

Manipulative methods include uterine massage, bimanual compression directly or by hot mops, uterine tamponade by Bakri balloon or Sengstaken-Blakemore tube or uterine packing (Druzin's).[7]

Surgical methods include oversewing the defect, understitching, Brace sutures, Cho suture, uterine artery ligation, internal iliac ligation, stepwise devascularization and hysterectomy. Complications are more likely to arise from delay in making the decision to proceed with hysterectomy.

Q. 15. What is morbidly adherent placenta? What are its different types and incidence?

When decidua basalis is deficient and Nitabuch's layer is absent, placenta gets directly implanted to the myometrial wall. It is called morbidly adherent placenta or placenta accreta. When chorionic villi invades the myometrium it is called placenta increta and when it reaches the serosal surface or invades the bladder or bowel, it is called placenta percreta.

Its incidence has increased by tenfold in last few years, and at present, it is 1 in 2,500 pregnancies. Out of all cases of morbidly adherent placenta accreta is 79%, increta is 14% and percreta is 7%.[8]

In the presence of placenta previa, risk of accreta rises to 5% and with placenta previa and prior cesarean section, it rises up to 20% and increases manyfold with number of cesarean sections.

Q. 16. How will you diagnose placenta accreta?

Ultrasonography criteria for diagnosis of placenta accreta are as follows:
- Loss of normal hypoechoic retroplacental myometrial zone
- Thinning and disruption of uterine serosa-bladder interface
- Focal exophytic masses within the placenta
- Numerous intraplacental vascular lacunae.

Use of color Doppler and 3D power Doppler further confirms the diagnosis. On color Doppler features are hypervascularity, markedly dilated vessels, lacunar flow and vascular lakes with increased peak systolic velocity.

Magnetic resonance imaging (MRI) is helpful when ultrasound findings are inconclusive and for diagnosis of placenta percreta.

MRI features of placenta accreta include uterine bulging, heterogeneous signal intensity within the placenta and dark intraplacental bands on T2-weighted images. Gadolinium-enhanced MRI adds to the specificity and more clearly distinguishes placenta accreta from percreta.

Q. 17. How will you manage a case of placenta accreta?

In a confirmed case of placenta accreta, "planned preterm cesarean hysterectomy" after 34 weeks with placenta left in situ is advocated.[9] For placenta percreta, surgeon or urologist should be involved during surgery. Preoperative arterial catheterization and embolization or balloon occlusion of uterine vessels after delivery of fetus decreases the blood loss at operation and hysterectomy may also be avoided.

Placenta accreta diagnosed on table is very difficult to manage. Any attempt to remove the placenta should be avoided as it can lead to torrential bleeding. Hysterectomy straight away with placenta in situ is lifesaving.

Conservative management by cutting the cord flush to placenta and leaving the placenta and closing the uterus is another option. Segmental resection of the involved lower segment and suturing the defect and injection of dilute vasopressin subendothelially are also reported. When placenta is left behind, close observation is required. Spontaneous placental resorption is reported in 75% of cases.[10] Postoperative methotrexate is not always helpful. Potential complications of conservative treatment include delayed hemorrhage requiring surgery, infection, fistula formation and even uterine necrosis. Women who conceive after conservative management have more chances of abortion, preterm labor and recurrent placenta previa.[11]

Q. 18. What is vasa previa? How it is diagnosed? How it is managed?

Literal meaning of vasa previa is vessels previous to the presenting part. It is associated with placenta previa, velamentous insertion of cord, succenturiate lobe and bipartite placenta. It is also reported more in pregnancy resulting from IVF-ET. Incidence varies from 0.08% to 0.002%. Here, the vessels are running free in membranes and as they are not protected by Wharton's jelly, they are fragile and prone to rupture and compression. There are of two types—type I occurs with single-lobed placenta with velamentous insertion of cord and type II occurs when vessels join the placenta to an accessory lobe.

Vasa previa can be effectively diagnosed by transvaginal sonography with color Doppler. Clinically, rarely it can be diagnosed by feeling pulsations in membranes during PV examination. It can be accidentally diagnosed by brisk hemorrhage on rupture of membranes with acute fetal distress.

In diagnosed cases, treatment is cesarean section at 36 weeks.

Q. 19. What do you mean by massive hemorrhage? How will you manage a case of massive antepartum hemorrhage?

When there is >1,000 mL blood loss and/or signs of clinical shock, it is called massive hemorrhage. In massive hemorrhage, resuscitation is done first. Two IV lines are secured with wide bore cannulae preferably No. 16. Blood is sent for cross matching and urgent demand is put. Call for help is made. Blood investigations, including coagulation panel (if abruption is suspected) are ordered. Crystalloid, i.e. Ringer lactate or normal saline is pushed fast. Initial 1 liter should go in 15–20 min, give at least 2 liters in first two hours and then fluid is replaced for ongoing losses. Cochrane review has shown that for resuscitation crystalloids are as effective as colloids in critically ill patients.[12] PCV is started as soon as available. Self-retaining catheter is kept. Oxygen is given by mask and vasopressors are used as necessary. Intensivists and anesthetists are involved, central venous pressure catheter may be kept and definitive treatment to stop the bleeding, e.g. cesarean section is carried out.

Proper documentation and proper communication with the patient and her family is must for dealing with any critically ill patients.

Obstetric hemorrhage is one of the major causes of maternal mortality in developing countries and is the cause of up to 50% of the estimated 50,000 maternal deaths that occur globally each year.[13] Every hospital should have a set protocol for dealing with massive hemorrhage.

Q. 20. What are the different grades of placental abruption?

There are two grading systems for abruptio placentae.

Page classification

- *Grade 0:* Clinically unrecognized before delivery (diagnosis based on examination of placenta postpartum)
- *Grade I:* External bleeding slight or mild uterine tetany, tenderness may or may not be present, FHS are good and no evidence of maternal shock
- *Grade II:* External bleeding present and there is uterine tetany, usually with uterine tenderness, fetal distress or death but no evidence of shock
- *Grade III:* There is evidence of maternal shock or coagulation defect. There is intrauterine fetal death (IUFD).

Sher and Statland classification

- *Grade I:* Not recognized clinically before delivery, usually recognized by presence of retroplacental clot
- *Grade II:* Clinical signs of abruption are present, but the fetus is still alive
- *Grade III:* The fetus is dead, IIIa—without coagulopathy, IIIb—with coagulopathy.

Q. 21. How will you confirm the diagnosis of placental abruption? What is the role of USG?

Diagnosis of placental abruption is mainly clinical which is supported by laboratory and pathologic studies. Unlike placenta previa, USG is less helpful. Sonographic appearance of retroplacental hemorrhage is variable. Initially, it is hyperechoic than myometrium, after 48 hours it becomes isoechoic and after few days it becomes hypoechoic.

Sensitivity and specificity of USG for diagnosis of placental abruption 24% and 96%, respectively. Thus, USH will fail to detect three-quarter of cases of abruption. However when ultrasound suggests an abruption likelihood that there is an abruption is high.[14]

MRI can help but it is not a practical modality for an acute problem, such as abruption.

Q. 22. How will you manage a case of placental abruption?

Usual treatment of clinically recognized abruption is by rapid IV fluids administration in the form of crystalloids, colloids packed cell volume (PCVs) and rapid termination of pregnancy. Delivery may be achieved by vaginal route by doing artificial rupture of membranes (ARM) and giving oxytocin drip. Usually the labor progresses rapidly. If vaginal delivery is not expected in few hours or there is obstetric indication cesarean section should be readily done. In cases of severe fetal distress with significant abruption, decision to delivery time of less than 20 minutes in cesarean section saves the baby.[1] Cesarean section in presence of disseminated intravascular coagulation (DIC) should be done with prior or simultaneous correction of the coagulation defect.

Q. 23. Why termination is the usual treatment of placental abruption?

Because unlike placenta previa there are other risks apart from hemorrhagic shock like acute renal failure and DIC which are lethal complications. In placenta previa, first bleeding usually stops on its own while in abruption bleeding continues till it kills fetus first and then mother.

Q. 24. In which case of placental abruption you will give expectant treatment?

In an exceptional case when separation is small, not increasing, patient is stable and fetus is premature, expectant treatment may be employed.

Q. 25. Why ARM is done in case of placental abruption?

ARM is done in proved case of placenta abruption for the following advantages:

- It increases uterine contractions and thus causes rapid delivery and control of blood loss.

- It decreases bleeding from placental site as with drainage of amniotic fluid uterine size is decreased leading to compression of spiral arterioles.
- Reduces entry of thromboplastin in the circulation and thus decreases DIC.

Q. 26. Why DIC is common in abruption and not in placenta previa? How will you manage DIC?

Disseminated intravascular coagulation (DIC) is common in placental abruption because thromboplastin released from damaged decidua and myometrium readily enters general circulation to bring about widespread microcoagulation in the body. Also good amount is consumed in retroplacental clot. Fetal death further aggravates this situation.

In placenta previa, all bleeding is external so thromboplastin does not enter the circulation.

Disseminated intravascular coagulation is treated by blood products, i.e. FFP, cryoprecipitate and platelet transfusions. One unit of FFP raises fibrinogen by 10 mg/dL. 10–15 mL/kg (3–4 units) raises all factors levels by 20%. Cryoprecipitate also raises fibrinogen by 10 mg/dL/unit. It is rich in factors VII and XIII which it raises by 2%/unit. Platelets transfusions raises platelet count by 5,000–10,000/unit. Associated anemia is treated by PCVs and simultaneous treatment of the cause of DIC is must. Availability of blood products in present times has changed the scenario and mortality due to DIC is decreasing. Once the crisis is over, liver soon starts generating adequate coagulation factors.

Q. 27. What is Couvelaire uterus? Why it is named so? What is the treatment?

Couvelaire uterus, also known as uteroplacental apoplexy, was first described by Couvelaire in 1912. In severe concealed hemorrhage, there is widespread extravasation of blood into the uterine musculature and beneath the uteine serosa giving a mottled black appearance. Blood is also seen occasionally between leaves of the broad ligament, under the tubal serosa, in the substance of the ovaries and free in the peritoneal cavity. It is treated by uterotonic agents. Myometrial hemorrhages seldom interfere with uterine contractions sufficiently to produce severe postpartum hemorrhage (PPH) and usually not an indication for hysterectomy.

Q. 28. What are the causes of unexplained APH? What are the maternal and perinatal consequences of unexplained APH?

In some cases of APH, no identifiable cause is found and it is called unexplained APH. Here, the causes may be excessive show, marked decidual reaction on endocervix, marginal sinus rupture or rarely due to circumvallate placenta. Pregnancies complicated by unexplained APH are at a greater risk of preterm delivery and induced labor.[15]

Q. 29. What is the relation of MSAFP estimation to APH?

Maternal serum alpha fetoprotein (MSAFP) estimation when done as a part of triple marker or quadruple marker test in second trimester is found elevated in cases of APH, both due to placenta previa and placental abruption. Its cause is not found but it is elevated by >2 MoM.

Q. 30. What is bedside clot test for detection of coagulation defect?

Take 2 mL of venous blood in clean plain test tube. After 4 minutes, tilt the tube slowly to see if clot has formed. Tilt the tube again every minute until the blood clots and tube can be turned upside down.

Failure of a clot to form after 8 minutes suggests hypofibrinogenemia.

If there is no retraction of clot in 1 hour, it suggests thrombocytopenia.

If clot breaks down easily or dissolves in 1 hour it suggests increased fibrinolysis.

Q. 31. What is modified Apt test?

It is test to detect fetal Hb and thus fetal blood. Add small amount of tap water to bloody vaginal fluid. Shake the sample and then add 1 cc of 1% sodium hydroxide. Read after 2 minutes. Pink color suggests fetal Hb while yellow to brown color suggest adult Hb. This test is carried out for diagnosis of vasa previa when bleeding occurs after rupture of membranes.

Q. 32. What is the role of tocolysis in cases of APH?

Tocolysis is generally contraindicated in any type of APH. In mild cases of APH use of tocolysis is reported so as to have effects of steroids administration. Betamimetics are contraindicated due to side effects of tachycardia and hypotension. Calcium channel blockers are not used because of risk of hypotension. The drug of choice for tocolysis when used is magnesium sulfate.

Magnesium sulfate is also recommended for neuroprotection of very premature (<30 weeks) fetus when delivery has to be done or delivery is expected within 24 hours.[16]

Q. 33. What is the role of cervical suture in placenta previa to prevent bleeding?

There is no scientific support for prophylactic use of cervical suture to prevent bleeding. It was tried with the logic that it might prevent stretching of lower segment and thereby prevent placental separation and prevent bleeding.

Q. 34. How will you manage third stage of labor in case of APH?

For both major types of APH, i.e. placenta previa and abruptio placentae, active management of third stage is must, because both are likely to be followed by PPH.

In placenta previa, causes of PPH are poorly contracting lower segment, large placenta, fragile and soft lower segment and cervix causing traumatic PPH and rarely morbidly adherent placenta.

In placental abruption, uterine atony, coagulation defect and hypertension in some of the cases cause PPH.

In both the conditions, blood already lost before delivery puts the patient in precarious situation and even moderate amount of loss after delivery is dangerous.

Q. 35. What anesthesia is used for cesarean section in APH?

Regional anesthesia is usually now preferred. It leads to less bleeding than general anesthesia which causes uterine relaxation. When patient is in shock or has severe hypertension or when surgery is expected to be prolonged general anesthesia is preferred.

Points to Remember

1. Barring few common risk factors, for placenta previa risk factors are more related to past pregnancy while risk factors for placental abruption are found in current pregnancy
2. Autologus blood donation (if Hb is 11.0g%) before scheduled cesarean section and intraoperative cell salvage strategy are quite helpful in managing placenta previa
3. Availability of blood products has changed the scenario for the management of DIC. They should be readily used
4. Placenta accreta should always be managed at tertiary care level institute by multidisciplinary approach
5. Most important cause of death in APH is PPH
6. Cesarean section remains the safest option in all types of moderate to severe APH.

References

1. Calleja-Agius J, Custo R, Brincat MP. Placental abruption and placenta praevia. Eur Clin Obstet Gynaecol. 2006;2:121-7.

2. Silver RM, Landon MB, Rouse DJ, et al. Maternal morbidity associated with multiple repeat cesarean deliveries. Obstet Gynecol. 2006;197:1226-32.
3. Ananath CV, Peltier MR, Kinzler WL, et al. Chronic hypertension and risk of placental abruption. Am J Obstet Gynecol. 2007;197:273.
4. Tikkanen M. Etiology, clinical manifestations, and prediction of placental abruption. Acta Obstet Gynecol Scand. 2010;89:732-40.
5. Neilson JP. Interventions for suspected placenta praevia: Cochrane review updated 31 Dec 2002, published 20 Jan 2010.
6. Leerentveld RA, Gilberts EC, Arnold MJ, et al. Accuracy and safety of transvaginal sonographic placental localization. Obstet Gynecol. 1990;76:759-62.
7. Druzin ML. Packing of lower uterine segment for control of post-cesarean bleeding in instances of placenta previa. Surg Gyneclo Obstet. 1989; 169:543.
8. Wu S, Kocherginsky M, Hibbard JU. Abnormal placentation: Twenty-year analysis. Am J Obstet Gynecol. 2005;192:1458.
9. Eller A, Porter T, Soisson P, et al. Optimal management strategies for placenta accreta. BJOG. 2009;116:648-54.
10. Sentilhes L, Ambroselli C, et al. Maternal Outcome After Conservative Treatment of Placenta Accreta. Obstetrics and Gynecology. 2010;115(3):526-34.
11. Provonsal M, Courbiere B, Agostini A, et al. Fertlity and obstetric outcome after conservative management of placenta accreta. Int J Gynecol Obstet. 2010;109:147.
12. Perel P, Roberts I, Pearson M. Colloids versus crystalloids for fluid resuscitation in critically ill patients. Cochrane Database of Systematic Reviews. 2007;4. Art. No.: CD000567.
13. Khan KS, Wojdyla D, Say L, et al. WHO analysis of causes of maternal death: a systematic review. Lancet. 2006;367: 1066-74.
14. Glantz C, Purnell L. Clinical utility of sonography in the diagnosis and treatment of placental abruption. J Ultrasound Med. 2002;21:837-40.
15. Bhandari S, Raja EA, Shetty A, et al. Maternal and perinatal consequences of antepartum haemorrhage of unknown origin. BJOG. 2014; 121(1):44-50.
16. NHMRC. Antenatal Magnesium Sulphate Prior to Preterm Birth for Neuroprotection of the Fetus, Infant and Child: National Clinical Practice Guidelines 2010. Available at: *www.adelaide.edu.au/arch/antenatalMagnesium_SulphateGuidelines.pdf*

3

Breech Presentation

KV Malini

CASE 1

A 24-year-old, primigravida comes with history of amenorrhea of 8 months for regular antenatal care (ANC).

Obstetric History

- She is primigravida, booked and immunized elsewhere
- Married life: 2 years, nonconsanguineous.

First Trimester

- Pregnancy was confirmed at 1½ months by home pregnancy test
- NT scan at 12th week was normal.

Second Trimester

No complaints, second trimester scan showed no fetal anomalies, placenta fundal, posterior grade 0.

Third Trimester

- No complaints.
- Has come for routine antenatal check up.
- On examination, general physical examination was normal.

Obstetric Examination

Inspection

Abdomen is uniformly stretched, longitudinal.

Palpation

SFH = 33 cm, abdominal girth 34 inches uterus relaxed, liquor normal.

Leopold's first maneuver: Round, hard globular, ballottable and independently mobile structure symptom of head felt at fundus.

Second maneuver: Back on left side, limbs on right side.

Third maneuver: Broad, firm, irregular, non-ballottable mass symptom of breech felt at lower pole.

Auscultation

FHS heard on left upper quadrant, 140/min, regular.

Final Diagnosis

Primigravida, 34 weeks of gestation with uncomplicated breech presentation.

> When buttocks of the fetus enters the pelvis before head, it is called breech presentation. The term 'Breech' is derived from ' britches' – a cloth covering the loin and thighs!

Q. 1. What is the incidence[1] of breech presentation?

It depends on the gestational age:
- At term—3–4%
- At 32 weeks—7%
- Before 28 weeks—25%

Q. 2. What are the varieties[2] of breech presentation?

Broadly there are two varieties: Complete and incomplete.
- Complete breech (5-10%)—Flexed attitude maintained, polarity changed (cannonball position) (Fig. 1A)
- Frank breech (50-70%)—hips flexed, knees extended (pike position) (Fig. 1B)
- Footling or kneeling (10-30%)—one or both hips extended, foot presenting/knee presenting (Fig. 1C).

Q. 3. What is the etiology[3-5] of breech presentation?

- Prematurity is the mostcommon cause
- Fetal abnormalities—hydrocephalus (50%), myelomeningocele, Prader-Willi syndrome, trisomy
- Intrauterine growth restriction (IUGR)
- Poly- or oligohydramnios
- Short umbilical cord
- Nulliparous women
- Uterine anomalies—bicornuate/septate
- Placenta previa/cornual placentation
- Contracted pelvis
- Multiple pregnancy
- Maternal anticonvulsant medications
- Alcohol/substance abuse.

Q. 4. How do you diagnose breech presentation?

Clinical: During antenatal period.[6,7]
The presence of hard ballotable mass suggestive of fetal head at fundus gives the suspicion which can be confirmed by scan.

During labor: Soft and irregular presenting part which can be mistaken for face is felt through dilated cervix. If it is complete breech-feet can be felt. Foot is identified by the presence of heel and the big toe which is shorter and not vey mobile.

Differentiating points between frank breech and face

- *In frank breech:* The anal opening and two ischial tuberosities are in same straight line
- *In face presentation:* The mouth and the malar eminences form a triangle.

Table 1: Differentiation during PV examination

Breech	Face
Soft parts felt	Soft parts felt
Orifice felt which grips the finger and meconeum staining	Orifice with alveolar prominence and suckling
Ischial tuberosities and orifice lie in a straight line	Zygoma and oral orifice form a triangle
Genitals may be felt, especially in a male baby, may be mistaken for nose	

Q. 5. What is the role of USG in diagnosis of breech?

- It confirms the diagnosis and gives the idea about the variety of breech (Fig. 2)
- Congenital abnormalities of the fetus/uterus/position of placenta which could be the etiological factors, can be ruled out

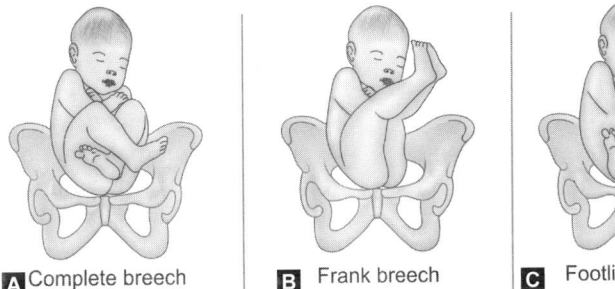

Figs 1A to C: Different varieties of breech presentation

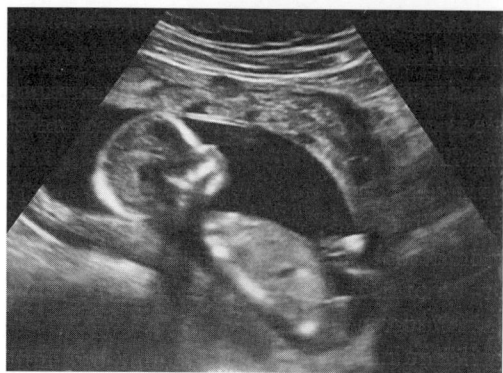

Fig. 2: USG showing breech presentation

- Estimated fetal weight. Attitude of the fetal head and amniotic fluid volume can be made out which will help in deciding for external cephalic version.

Q. 6. What is the role of other imaging modalities like CT scan and MRI?

Computed tomography scan and MRI[9] will give additional information about the pelvic capacity. During pregnancy, it is better to avoid CT scan.

Q. 7. In the diagnosis mention was made about uncomplicated breech presentation. What is complicated breech? Is it same as complications of breech?

When breech presentation is associated with any maternal risk factors, it is called complicated breech, e.g. mother having gestational diabetes mellitus (GDM)/hypertension with breech presentation.

Complications of breech are inherent to breech presentation, e.g. premature rupture of membranes (PROM), cord prolapse, difficulty in after coming shoulders/head.

Q. 8. What is the mechanism by which breech delivers?

In mechanism of breech delivery,[10] the cardinal movements take place at three levels: (a) The buttocks and the lower limbs, (b) the shoulders and the arms, and (c) the head. The sacrum could be either anterior or posterior.

Mechanism when the sacrum is anterior (Figs 3A to G)

Buttocks and Lower Limbs

Engagement: Bitrochanteric diameter which is 10 cm is the diameter of engagement. The engagement occurs in one of the oblique diameters of the pelvis. We will discuss the mechanism in right sacrum anterior (RSA) which is the most favorable.

Descent: In RSA position the sacrum is in right anterior quadrant and bitrochanteric diameter is in right oblique diameter of the pelvis. Descent occurs until the buttocks reach the pelvic floor and is delayed in breech presentation.

Flexion: Lateral flexion takes place at the waist and anterior hip becomes the leading point. This takes place along with descent.

Internal rotation of breech: When the buttocks reach the pelvic floor, the bitrochanteric diameter rotates through 1/8th of a circle (45°) and comes to anteroposterior diameter of pelvis.

Delivery of the buttocks: If occurs by lateral flexion. The anterior hip hitches against the pubic symphysis, lateral flexion occurs and the posterior hip is born over the perineum and then the anterior hip slips out under the pubic symphysis.

Delivery of the trunk follows: Restitution occurs and buttocks will occupy the same position as when engagement occurred.

Shoulder and Arms

Descent and engagement: Bisacromial diameter (12 cm) is the diameter of engagement and shoulder engages in the same oblique diameter as the buttocks, i.e. right oblique diameter.

Internal rotation: The bisacromial diameter rotates through 1/8th of a circle (45°) and the anterior shoulder hitches under the pubic symphysis.

The delivery of the shoulders: The posterior shoulder is then born by lateral flexion. This is followed by delivery of the anterior shoulder under the pubic symphysis.

Restitution: Once the shoulders are delivered restitution occurs with untwisting of the trunk.

Head
Descent and engagement: The head enters the pelvis in the opposite oblique diameter and gets engaged in the left oblique diameter, the diameter of engagement being suboccipito-frontal which is 10 cm.

Flexion: Flexion of the head takes place with further descent.

Internal rotation: The head strikes the pelvic floor and rotates through 1/8th of a circle (45°) in the opposite direction to that of the buttocks and shoulder and occiput comes under the pubic symphysis. There is external rotation of the trunk simultaneously and the back remains anterior.

Birth of the head by flexion: The occiput hitches under the pubic symphysis and the chin, mouth, nose, forehead, vertex and occiput are born over the perineum in succession.

Q. 9. What is the mechanism if the sacrum is posterior?

It is important that the back remains anterior in breech delivery.

Rarely, back routes posteriorly bringing sacrum and occiput posterior.[10] If the head is flexed, the glabella comes under the pubic symphysis; the nape of the neck, occiput, and vertex roll over the perineum. The face finally emerges under the pubis. This delivery is facilitated by lifting baby's body up.

If head is extended, the chin hitches under the pubic symphysis and the submental area of the neck is in the pubic angle. For delivery to take place the obstetrician has to lift the baby's body up so that the occiput, vertex and head can pass over the perineum.

Q. 10. Is it safe to have vaginal breech delivery?

Vaginal breech delivery is associated with slightly increased maternal morbidity and perinatal morbidity and mortality are three times that of cephalic presentation.

With spontaneous delivery and in case of frank breech presentation maternal morbidity is not so high.

Q. 11. What are risks for the fetus?

Prolapse of the umbilical cord, fetal asphyxia and birth injuries are the main risks.[11-13] Associated prematurity and congenital malformations add to the risks. Fetal mortality is least in frank breech presentation and maximum in footling presentation.

Birth asphyxia: It is due to cord compression after the buttocks are born and also during delivery of after-coming head. Cord prolapse also can cause birth asphyxia. Other causes are aspiration of amniotic fluid during premature attempt at respiration even before the head is born and delayed delivery of the head.

Injury to the brain: The after-coming head in breech presentation passes though the pelvis rapidly and there is compression followed by decompression resulting in tearing of the tentorium cerebelli and intracranial hemorrhage. Risk is more when there is preterm delivery, delivery through incompletely dilated cervix and undiagnosed fetopelvic disproportion.

Other injuries caused as a result of manipulations during delivery include:
- Fractures of the femur, humerus, clavicle, odontoid process and skull
- Hematoma—of sternomastoid or thighs
- Visceral injuries—rupture of liver, adrenal glands, kidneys and hemorrhage into

testicles; injury to testicles may be severe enough to cause anorchia
- Trauma to pharynx while delivering aftercoming head by putting finger into the mouth
- Nerve injury—cervical and brachial plexus paralyses, injury to spinal cord
- Dislocation of hip joint, temporomandibular joint.

Q. 12. Are there any long-term morbidity?

Minimal brain dysfunction could be there. One study reported increased frequency of learning and motor defects in infants delivered by breech vaginally.[14] It could be related to asphyxia or trauma.

Q. 13. What is the incidence of cord prolapse in breech presentation?

Incidence of cord prolapse in breech presentation is 3.5%[15] which is much higher than in cephalic presentation (0.25%). In frank breech, it is same as in cephalic presentation and highest in footling (16–19%).

Q. 14. Can we prevent these fetal hazards?

- External cephalic version can be done to decrease the incidence of breech presentation
- Careful selection of the cases for vaginal delivery and conduct of delivery by skilled obstetricians along with team of neonatologist and anesthesiologist
- Judicious decisions for elective cesarean delivery.

All these will prevent fetal hazards.

Q. 15. Is it safer to deliver all breech presentations by cesarean?

Outcomes for children at 2-year follow-up from Multicenter International Trial showed that there was no difference in planned cesarean delivery and the planned vaginal delivery group. American College of Obstetricians and Gynecologists (ACOG) committee opinion no. 340[16] states that "with proper selection of cases and meticulous management during labor with a liberal decision for cesarean delivery in case need arises, many term breeches can be delivered vaginally safely."

Q. 16. What is term breech trial? What are the shortcomings of this trial?

In term breech trial,[17] 2088 patients from 121 centers from 26 countries were enrolled in the study, with random assignment to either planned cesarean delivery or planned vaginal delivery. In October 2000, the first results of term breech trial were published (Lancet). Perinatal mortality or serious neonatal morbidity was significantly lower in cesarean group. There was no difference in maternal morbidity or in 2-year follow-up of the neonates.

A number of questions were raised following publication of the term breech trial, largely about selection criteria and the conduct of labor.

Inconsistencies in the care of women in the term breech trial have also been criticized.

Q. 17. How do you manage breech presentation in the above case? Would you like to do any intervention?

In the above case, it is uncomplicated breech presentation without any anomalies at 34 weeks. Though the success rate for external cephalic version is higher at this gestational period, it is not recommended as recurrence rate is high,[18] and there is risk of preterm delivery. We can wait for spontaneous version.

Q. 18. What is external cephalic version? When it is done?

External cephalic version is a procedure in which breech presentation is converted into cephalic presentation by manipulations performed through the abdominal wall. It is done at or after 36 weeks as the chance of recurrence is less after 36 weeks. And also if need arises to deliver the woman because of complications of the procedure, then complications of preterm delivery are not so severe. In multiparous women, it can be done after 37 weeks.[19,20] It can also be done at the time of early labor and sometimes even during active labor. With expert hands, it is successful.

Q. 19. Why external cephalic version is done?

With breech presentation the perinatal mortality is 2-3 times more as compared to cephalic presentation. Benefits for fetus also include elimination of pulmonary hypertension of the newborn associated with cesarean delivery. Studies have shown that external cephalic version (ECV) reduces the breech presentation by 60% and rate of cesaraen delivery by 50%.[21]

Q. 20. Are there any contraindications for external cephalic version?

Attempts at external cephalic version should be done in all breech presentations seen at 36 weeks in nulliparous and at 37 weeks in parous women provided some contraindications are ruled out.[22] There is a mnemonic for contraindications for ECV:

> Mnemonic—PPP THAMASA
> P–Pelvis should be adequate
> P–Pregnancy-induced hypertension
> P–Precious pregnancy—better avoid in case of BOH
> T–Tumors in pelvis
> H–Hydramnios/oligoamnios
> A–Anomalies of the uterus
> M–Multiple pregnancy
> A–Anomalies of the fetus/anomalies of growth (IUGR and macrosomia)
> S–Scar on the uterus
> A–Antepartum hemorrhage

Q. 21. Can you explain the procedure? How it is done?

Prerequisites for ECV

- Gestational age at >36 weeks
- Recent ultrasound examination—for amniotic fluid volume estimation
- Reassuring fetal heart pattern
- Informed consent regarding risks associated with ECV
- Facilities to perform emergency cesarean operation when the need arises.

It may be performed either in labor room or in the ward.

The woman is counseled about the procedure and the slight discomfort it can cause.

An ultrasound examination is done to know the position of the back, the attitude of the fetus, position of placenta, liquor volume and fetal heart rate.

A forward or backward some rsault can be performed. Forward roll is preferred to backward flip. Woman is placed in supine position with the thighs semiflexed and slight left lateral tilt. If the breech is engaged, it must be pushed out of the pelvis abdominally. If the head is caught under the costal margin and prevents the disengagement of breech, the head should be manipulated sideways prior to the disengagement. Both the poles are held with the hands and head is brought to the lower pole gently. No extra pressure is exerted. The fetal heart is monitored either continuously or every 2 minutes. If there is any fetal heart irregularities, immediately the fetus is repositioned and NST is performed.

> Breech presentation—ECV in labor room, counseling, disimpaction, version—backward roll and head at lower pole

ECV is successful in 65–70% of the cases. At the end of the successful procedure, CTG is performed. US examination is repeated to rule out any abruption. PROM is ruled out. The woman can be sent home after the procedure. If she is already in labor then monitored for progress of labor.[22]

Q. 22. Do we need anesthesia for this procedure?

Though the procedure can be easily done under regional anesthesia, its use is controversial and is not recommended.[23]

Q. 23. Do we need tocolytics, if so which one and what is the dose?

If there are uterine contractions then tocolytics may be needed.[24] Earlier terbutaline was used but now it carries a FDA black box warning and is not used. Nifedipine 10–20 mg orally 30 minutes prior to the procedure may be used.

Q. 24. Is it a safe procedure? Are there any complications of ECV?

Complications of ECV[21,25] are:
- Placental abruption
- Cord entanglement and fetal heart abnormalities
- Fetal death
- Rupture of the membranes with/without cord prolapse
- Preterm labor
- Rarely rupture of uterus
- Very rarely amniotic fluid embolism and maternal death.

So ECV should be performed with utmost care and gentleness and by an experienced person with careful monitoring of the fetus as well as the mother throughout the procedure.

Q. 25. Can we perform this procedure in women who are Rh negative?

It can be performed in Rh negative mothers. But anti-D should be given immediately after the procedure. Risk of fetomaternal hemorrhage is 6%. It is safer to do Kleihauer-Betke test to know the amount of fetomaternal hemorrhage before administering the immunoglobulin.[26]

Q. 26. Which are the factors unfavorable for vaginal delivery?

Factors regarded as unfavorable for vaginal breech birth include the following:[27]
- Other contraindications to vaginal birth (e.g. placenta previa, compromised fetal condition, BOH)
- Clinically inadequate pelvis
- Footling or kneeling breech presentation
- Prelabor rupture of membranes
- Large baby (usually defined as larger than 4,000 g)
- Growth-restricted baby (usually defined as smaller than 2,000 g)
- Hyperextended fetal neck in labor (diagnosed with ultrasound or X-ray where ultrasound is not available)
- Lack of presence of a clinician trained in vaginal breech delivery
- Previous cesarean section.

Q. 27. Which are the factors favorable[27] for vaginal breech delivery?

- Frank or complete breech
- Gestational age 36–42 weeks
- Estimated fetal weight between 2,500 g–4,000 g
- Flexed fetal head
- Adequate maternal pelvis
- Spontaneous labor
- Zatuchni-Andros score >4.

Q. 28. What is Zatuchni-Andros score?

In 1964, Zatuchni and Andros devised a score[28] based on 6 clinical variables at admission to ascertain likelihood of successful vaginal delivery.

Factor	0	1	2
Parity	Nullipara	Multipara	Multipara
Gestational age	39	38	37
Estimated fetal weight	8 lb	7–8 lb	7 lb
Previous breech	Nil	One	Two
Dilatation	2 cm	3 cm	4 cm or more
Station	– 3 or greater	– 2	– 1 or less

Zatuchni-Andros score of less than 4 predicted poor outcome for women with breech presentation.

Breech risk scoring by Westin[29] includes all the parameters of the pelvis at inlet, cavity and outlet apart from type of breech presentation, estimated fetal weight, cervical condition and history of previous deliveries. Score of 12 or more constitutes a safe level for vaginal delivery. It is too elaborated and not used in contemporary practice.

Q. 29. What are the methods of vaginal breech delivery?

Spontaneous: It is not recommended except in cases of IUFD. Happens rarely when the baby is too small or if the maternal pelvis is too large.

Assisted-breech delivery: Here spontaneous delivery is awaited up to the umbilicus and simple maneuvers are used by the assistant for delivery of the arms and after-coming head with minimal analgesic or anesthetic requirements.

Breech extraction: This is used when delivery of the baby is urgent because of fetal distress and emergency cesarean delivery facilities are not available as happens in case of cord prolapse with full dilation of cervix in breech presentation. It can also be used for the second of twin with breech presentation. Here, the obstetrician delivers the fetus by traction using the relevant maneuvers for delivery of the legs, arms and after-coming head. General anesthesia or major nerve blocking procedures are required.

Q. 30. How do you manage vaginal breech delivery?

In breech presentation, the most yielding part, i.e. breech comes first and successively the larger and less yielding parts come later, the head being the largest and the last. That is why fetopelvic disproportion should be ruled out carefully while contemplating vaginal delivery.

Management in first stage of labor[10,30]
- The woman is counseled about the mode of delivery and consent is taken for vaginal breech delivery after explaining the risks associated
- The woman can be ambulant provided breech is engaged and well applied to cervix
- Avoid too frequent vaginal examinations. Per vaginal examination is indicated at the onset of labor and after rupture of membranes to rule out cord prolapse
- Start IV line and infuse crystalloids. Better to keep her nil by mouth or on oral liquids
- Fetal heart rate is monitored throughout labor preferably by continuous electronic monitoring
- Progress of labor is monitored using partograph and well documented. When progress is slow because of inadequate uterine contractions, oxytocin augmentation should be used with caution. If there is poor progress of less than 0.5 cm/h cervical dilation or if there is no progress in 2 hours despite contractions, then cesarean delivery should be performed.

Keep ready the following things: Inform the anesthetist and neonatologist. Keep one assistant to give push during delivery. Keep set ready for episiotomy, an extra-dry towel to wrap the baby. Newborn resuscitation kit and a pair of obstetric forceps, preferably Piper's, if not available low forceps for the after-coming head.

Q. 31. How do you manage the second stage?[10,30]

With good progress, when the breech begins to distend the perineum, bring the woman to the edge of the table. Paint with antiseptics and drape. Make sure that the bladder is empty. Woman is encouraged to bear down during contractions. Remember not to intervene until the fetus is born up to the umbilicus except for episiotomy. Episiotomy is preferred for all breech deliveries unless the perineum is very lax. Premature traction on the baby is to be avoided as it can lead to deflexion of the head and extension of the arms above or behind the head.

Maneuvers should be gentle and unhurried. Suprapubic pressure by the assistant helps to aid delivery and keep the head in flexion.

It is important that the woman bears down during each contraction once the body has been born because when the head is out of contracting upper segment, the delivery has to be done by the voluntary action of abdominal muscles and assistance by suprapubic pressure.

After full cervical dilatation, if delivery is not imminent after active pushing for 60 minutes, caesarean delivery has to be performed.

Delivery of breech: Usually legs deliver spontaneously in flexed breech presentation. In case of extended breech, once the body is delivered up to the umbilicus, the legs may have to be delivered by pressure on popliteal fossa causing abduction of the thighs away from midline (breech decomposition by Pinard's maneuver).

Baby's back is kept anterior and the body is wrapped in a warm towel to prevent any premature attempt at respiration and amniotic fluid aspiration.

The fetal pelvis is now grasped with fingers resting on the iliac crests and thumb on the sacrum (femoropelvic grip) to prevent damage to internal organs.

A loop of the umbilical cord is pulled down to minimize compression. Feel for pulsations.

Once the baby is born up to the umbilicus, the delivery is expedited gently and skillfully within 5–10 minutes so as to prevent anoxic brain damage.

Delivery of shoulders and arms: The assistant keeps the hand over the fundus and exerts steady pressure to keep the head flexed and prevent extension of arms.

Mother is asked to push and gentle downward traction is applied till the axilla is under the pubic symphysis. Gentle downward traction with initial 90° rotation through one arc to deliver the left scapula and then a 180° rotation to the other will affect delivery of the right scapula and arm. Simultaneously flexing the elbow once the axilla is under the pubic symphysis will facilitate the delivery of arms.

Delivery of the after-coming head: In almost all cases, the back rotates anteriorly spontaneously. But sometimes, it may rotate posteriorly which should be avoided by the obstetrician. Baby's body is lowered till the nape of the neck is seen under the pubic symphysis. The suprapubic pressure exerted by the assistant (Kristellar's maneuver) will guide the head into pelvis and keeps the head in flexion. With continued suprapubic pressure, the head is delivered in flexion by gently raising the body. The speed of the delivery of after-coming head should be slow enough (>1 minute) to prevent injury to the brain and sufficiently rapid to avoid asphyxia.

After-coming head can also be delivered by **Burns-Marshall method** where the baby is allowed to hang by its own weight. Suprapubic pressure is applied and when the nape of the neck is visible, the baby is grasped at the ankles with fingers in-between. Then steady traction is applied and the trunk is swung upward in a wide arc over the mother's abdomen. Simultaneous slipping of the perineum facilitates the delivery of the face, sinciput and occiput in succession over the perineum.

Q. 32. Is there a mnemonic for assisted-breech delivery?

Mnemonic for assisted-breech delivery is "BRUSH ASIDE".

- **B**–Breech on perineum, empty the bladder, bring mother to edge of the table, and consider episiotomy

- R–Rotate thighs and flex knees—to decompose the breech
- U–Umbilicus visible—pull a loop of cord and push aside
- S–Sacrum anterior
- H–Hold on, delivery till this stage is spontaneous
- A–Avoid traction
- S–Scapulae visible, get ready to deliver arms
- I–Initiate arm rotation to anterior
- D–Deliver the head
- E–Explain and document to prevent any medicolegal problems.

Q. 33. What is the role of oxytocin in labor management?

Oxytocin induction or augmentation is not contraindicated in breech presentation.[31] However, it should be used with caution. If the cervix is not favorable, induction of labor should not be considered unless there are some other associated factors, e.g. anomalous fetus/IUFD or very preterm fetus.

Oxytocin augmentation should not be considered unless the clinician is very sure that the cause for failure to progress is inefficient uterine action and not an undiagnosed fetopelvic disproportion.

Q. 34. Do you need anesthesia for assisted-breech delivery?

Epidural anesthesia[32,33] is preferred for assisted-breech delivery. If it is not given, then pudendal block or perineal infiltration may have to be used.

Q. 35. How do you manage if there is arrest of breech?

If there is failure of descent of breech in spite of good uterine contractions then fetopelvic disproportion has to be suspected and cesarean section should be performed. If this cannot be done, delivery can be facilitated by reducing the bulk of the breech, a procedure called decomposition.[10,30] This is accomplished by bringing down the legs.

In flexed breech, the hand is introduced into the vagina, the foot is identified by the presence of heal and the small toes and then it is brought down. Procedure is repeated for the other foot. Labor is allowed to progress.

In extended breech, decomposition is accomplished by Pinard's maneuver as the legs are high up and may be impossible to reach.

Q. 36. How do you manage if there is difficulty in delivering the shoulders?

It could be because of the extended arms which is indicated by winging of the scapula.

Cardinal rule is to wait for the axilla to be seen below the pubic symphysis.

There are two methods of delivering the shoulders and arms.

Lovset's maneuver:[30,34] The fetus is grasped with femoropelvic grip using a dry towel and rotated through 180° so that posterior arm (which enters the pelvis first and is below the sacral promontory) comes below the pubic symphysis and delivers. This maneuver is repeated in reverse direction to deliver the other arm.

If the trunk cannot be rotated then induce deep ansthesia, grasp the feet of the baby and move the feet up. Then introduce fingers along the humerus till elbow is reached. The fingers are placed parallel to the humerus and used to splint the arm, which is swept downward and delivered through vulva. Then the anterior arm is delivered by depressing the fetus toward mother's perineum and delivering the arm in the same manner as that of posterior arm. This maneuver is also called as **classical method.**

Q. 37. How do you manage nuchal arm?

Sometimes, one or both the arms may be at the back of the neck and impacted at brim of the pelvis. It can be managed by modified Lovset's maneuver by rotating the back through 180° in the direction of the arm that is trapped. If this fails then the nuchal arm has to be extracted by hooking the fingers over it and forcing the arm over the shoulder and down the ventral surface, which may fracture the clavicle or humerus.[10,30]

Q. 38. How do you manage if there is difficulty in after-coming head?

It could be due to deflexion of the head, undiagnosed hydrocephalus, or contracted pelvis.[10,30,35]

If it is due to deflexion and arrest is at the midpelvis or the outlet, Mauriceau-Smellie-Veit maneuver can be used. Here, the index and middle fingers of one hand are applied over the maxilla while the fetal body rests over the palm and forearm. The forearm is straddled by the fetal legs. Two fingers of the other hand are hooked behind the shoulders. Downward traction is exerted till the suboccipital region appears below the pubic symphysis while the assistant continues to give suprapubic pressure. The body is then lifted up toward maternal abdomen and the chin, mouth, nose, sinciput and finally the occiput deliver successively over the perineum.

McRobert's maneuver can be used if the arrest is at the inlet and Mauriceau-Smellie-Veit maneuver fails or alternatively Piper's forceps or Simpson's forceps can be applied.

> Bracht's simple, efficient, and effective method: The breech is allowed to deliver spontaneously to the umbilicus without push or pull. The knee-extended legs of the flexed breech were not brought down. The body and extended legs were then grasped in both hands, with the fingers around the lower back and the thumbs around the posterior aspect of the thighs, while the upward and anterior rotation of the body was maintained. When the anterior rotation was nearly complete the baby's body was held, not pressed, against the mother's symphysis using only a force equivalent to the weight of that portion of the baby already born. The mere maintenance of this position, added to the uterine contractions and, if necessary, gentle suprapubic pressure by an assistant, allowed the baby's head to deliver spontaneously in full extension.

Q. 39. What is Wigand-Martin's maneuver[30]?

It is same as Mauriceau-Smellie-Veit maneuver except for the fact that the fingers of one hand are used to apply suprapubic pressure instead of hooking behind the shoulders.

Q. 40. Can you describe Piper's forceps and its application?

Piper's forceps[10,30] are preferred by some obstetricians if simple suprapubic pressure fails to deliver the after-coming head. Piper's forceps are special forceps designed to deliver the after-coming head in breech presentation. It has minimal pelvic curve, long and curved shanks and handles are depressed below the arch of the shanks. Because of these special features, it can be introduced over the perineum, directly over the head. Hence, the traction over the neck and damage to structures of the neck is avoided.

The orientation of the forceps is concave edges towards the occiput and convex edge towards the face. The cephalic application is biparietal and mento-occipital.

Application of Forceps

The baby's feet are grasped and the body is lifted up slightly using a dry towel wrapped around the body to avoid extension of the head. The left blade is applied first. Like in conventional forceps application, the right hand is introduced between the head and the left lateral wall of vagina. The left blade is introduced between fingers and the head. The fingers are removed, handle is steadied by an assistant. Then the right blade is held with right hand and similarly introduced into the vagina. The forceps blades are locked and episiotomy is given now or before the application of forceps. Traction is applied outward and posterior until the nape of the neck is seen under the subpubic angle. Then the direction is changed to outward and anterior until the face, sinciput and occiput are born over the perineum in flexion.

Q. 41. How do you deliver the baby if back turns posterior?

Back turning posterior or chin to pubis rotation is rare.[10,30] If this happens the preferred management is to:
- Institute anesthesia
- Cease traction
- Dislodge the chin from behind the pubis
- Rotate the face posteriorly and back anteriorly
- Apply suprapubic pressure and flex the head
- Deliver the head by Piper's forceps.

If this technique fails, the modified Prague maneuver may be used. In this, two fingers of one hand are placed below the shoulders grasping it, while the other hand is used to drag the feet up over mother's abdomen.

Q. 42. How do you mange if there is entrapment of the after-coming head?

Very rarely the incompletely dilated cervix will constrict around the neck and prevent delivery of the after-coming head. It is common with preterm fetus. If this happens, gentle traction is applied over the fetal body and cervix is manually slipped over the occiput.

If this fails then Duhressen incision[10] can be given at 4 and 8 o'clock or 2 and 10 o'clock position to deliver the entrapped head.

Alternatively, IV nitroglycerine[36] 100 µg, or general anesthesia to relax the cervix can be given. Some have described Zavanelli maneuver[37] and cesarean delivery after replacing the head high into the uterus.

Q. 43. Is there any role for symphysiotomy? How do you do it?

If there is difficulty in delivery of after-coming head and cephalopelvic disproportion is suspected and cesarean delivery is not possible then symphysiotomy can be performed.[38]

Procedure: The suprapubic skin painted with antiseptic lotion and infiltrated with 0.5% lignocaine. Indwelling catheter is placed into the bladder. The index fingers are placed in the vagina and lateral pressure is exerted to displace the urethra from midline, vertical stab incision is made over the pubic symphysis deep down cutting the cartilage joining the two pubic bones. Then the delivery of head is accomplished. After delivery there is no need to close the incision, but to reduce the postoperative pain, elastic strapping is applied from one iliac crest to the other. Antibiotics and analgesics are given. Catheter is left in situ for 5 days.

Q. 44. How do you deliver breech while doing cesarean section?

Lower segment transverse incision is made to deliver the baby. The method of delivery is same as that for vaginal breech delivery. The after-coming head can be entrapped by lower segment, and the incision may have to be enlarged in 'J' shaped manner. Some prefer to use forceps for delivering the after-coming head.

Q. 45. What is breech extraction?

Breech extraction means immediate extraction of the baby vaginally when signs of fetal distress demands delivery without any delay and emergency cesarean delivery is not possible. This is done under general anesthesia by a skilled obstetrician. Cervix should be fully dilated and bladder and rectum should be empty. Pelvis should be adequate.

Procedure: The breech is decomposed and feet are bought down in complete breech and Pinard's maneuver is used for extended breech. After this spontaneous delivery is not awaited and delivery of the arms and shoulders and after-coming head are accomplished using the maneuvers described for management of arrest cases. Traction from below and fundal pressure are substituted for uterine contractions to facilitate the delivery.

Q. 46. Any other method to reduce breech presentation other than external cephalic version (ECV)?

There are some recent trials employing moxibustion of acupoint BL 67 which is beside the outer corner of fifth toenail with or without acupuncture applied to the same acupoint. Moxibustion[39,40] is the traditional Chinese method of application of heat generated by combustion of herbs like *Artemisia vulgaris*, to provide stimulation of the acupoints. This will work by stimulating the fetal movements. There are many randomized control trials supporting the use of moxibustion. When acupuncture is used with moxibustion the rate of cephalic version is more. Even yogic postures like inverted asanas (e.g. Shirsasana) are said to be used to promote version. Though use of all these alternative medicines and traditional methods are being realized, these need to be examined further.

Q. 47. What is star gazing fetus? How do you manage it?

Deflexion of fetal head in breech presentation has been described by Ballas and colleagues.[41] There are four grades:

- Grade 0: Complete flexion
- Grade 1: Deflexion (military attitude)
- Grade 2: Extension-deflexion angle of 90° or less
- Grade 3: Hyperextension-deflexion angle of 90° or more.

The deflexion angle is measured[42] in the X-ray between main axis of cervical vertebrae and upward extension of main axis of thoracic vertebrae.

Simple deflexion carries no excess risk. Hyperextension of the fetal head has been described as "Star gazing fetus". It is a serious problem and occurs in about 5% of breech presentations.

It may be caused as a result of spasm or congenital shortening of the extensor muscles of neck, congenital tumors of the neck or umbilical cord around the neck, uterine anomalies, fetal anomalies, or tumors in the placental site.

The diagnosis is by ultrasound examination (earlier by plain X-ray abdomen).

When there is star gazing fetus ECV cannot be done and there is a definite risk of injury to the lower cervical spinal cord (21%) during vaginal delivery. Because of excessive stretching of the spinal cord, extreme flexion of the neck during delivery and marked torsion, there could be partial or complete laceration of the cervical spinal cord, occasional tears in the dura and epidural hemorage. There is varying degrees of damage to the cord, brainstem, nerve roots and meninges. All these injuries are caused usually at the time of delivery when there is sudden flexion of the head as it passes through the vagina. But sometimes the injury may occur during pregnancy. Mode of delivery in hyperextension is by cesarean section.

References

1. Collea JV. Current management of breech presentation. Clin Obstet Gynecol. 1980; 23:525.
2. Fischer R, Rossue RM. Emedicine.medscape.com/article/26215-overview visited on 24-12-2015.
3. Hill L. Prevalence of breech presentation by gestational age. Am J Perinatol. 2008;7:92-3.
4. Sekulick SR, Mikov A, Petrovic DS, et al. Probability of Breech Presentation and its significance. J Mater Fet Neonat Med. 2010; 23(10):1160-4.
5. Barun FH, Jones KL, Smith DW. Breech presentation as an indicator of fetal abnormality. J Paed. 1975;86:419-21.
6. Nassar N, Roberts CL, Cameron CA, et al. Diagnostic accuracy of clinical examination for detection of noncephalic presentation in late pregnancy: cross sectional analytical study. Br J Med. 2006;333:578.
7. Lydon-Rochelle M, Albers L, Gorwada J, et al. Accuracy of Leopolad maneuvers in screening

for malpresentations: a prospective study. Birth. 1993;20:132.
8. Rojansky N, Tanos V, Lewin A, et al. Sonographic evaluation of fetal head extension and maternal pelvis in breech presentation. Acta Obstet Gynecol Scand. 1994;73:607.
9. Van Loon AJ, Mantingh A, Serlier EK, et al. Randomized controlled trial of magnetic resonance pelvimetry in breech presentation at term. Lancet. 1997;350:1799.
10. Cunningham, Leveno, Bloom, et al. Breech presentation and delivery: Williams Obstetrics, 23rd edition, New York: Mc Graw Hill; 2009.
11. Geutjens G, Gilbert A, Helsen K. Obstetric brachial plexus palsy associated with breech delivery. J Bone Joint Surgery (Br). 1996;78;303.
12. Gifford GS, Morton SC, et al. A meta-analysis of infant outcome after breech delivery. Obstet Gynecol. 1995;85:1047.
13. Tiwary CM. Testicular injury in breech delivery. Urology. 1989;34:210.
14. Faber Nijholt R, Huisjes JH, Towen CL, et al. Neurological follow up of 281 children born in breech presentation—a controlled study. BMJ. 1983;286:9.
15. Lore M. Umbilical cord prolapse and other cord emergencies. Glob Libr Womens Med; 2008. DOI: 10.3843/GLOWM.10136.
16. American College of Obstetricians and Gynecologists: Mode of term in singleton breech delivery. Committeee Opinion No 340, July 2006.
17. Hannah ME, Hannah WJ, Hewson SA, et al. Planned caesarean section versus planned vaginal birth for breech presentation at term: a randomized multicenter trial. Lancet. 2000;356:1375.
18. Westgren M, Edvall H, Nordstrom L, et al. Spontaneous cephalic version of breech presentation in the last trimester. Br J Obstet Gynecol. 1985;92:19.
19. American College of Obstetricians and Gynecologists: External Cephalic Version: Practice Bulletin No 13, February 2000.
20. Collaris RJ, Oei SG. External cephalic version: a safe procedure—a systematic review of version related risks. Acta Obstet Gynecol Scand. 2004;83:511.
21. Zhang J, Bowes WA, Fortsey JA, et al. Efficacy of external cephalic version: a review. Obstet Gynecol. 1993;82:306.
22. Hofmeyr GJ. Eexternal cephalic version facilitation for breech presentation at term. Cochrane Database Systematic Review 2:CD000184,2000.
23. Macathur AJ, Gagnon S, Tureanu LM, Downey KN. Anaesthesia facilitation of external cephalic version: a meta-analysis. Am J Obstet Gynecol. 2004;191:1219.
24. Van Dorsten JP, Schifrin BS, Wallace RL. Randomized control trial of external cephalic version with tocolysis in late pregnancy. Am J Obstet Gynecol. 1981;141:417.
25. Chan LY, Tang JL, Tsoi KF, et al. Intrapartum caesarean delivery after successful external cephalic version: a meta-analysis. Obstet Gynecol. 2004;104:155.
26. Marcus RG, Crewe Brown H, Krawitz S, et al. Fetomaternal haemorrhage following successful and unsuccessful attempts at external cephalic version. Br J Obstet Gynaecol. 1975;82:578.
27. Albrechten S, Rasmussen S, Reigstad H, et al. Evaluation of a protocol for selecting fetuses in breech presentation for vaginal delivery or caesarean section. Am J Obstet Gynecol. 1997;177:586.
28. Zatuchni GP, Andros GJ. Prognostic index for vaginal delivery in breech presentation at term. Prospective study. Am J Obstet Gynecol. 1967;98(6):854-7.
29. Westin B. Acta Obstet Gynecol. Scand. 1977; 56:505.
30. Posner GD, Dy J, Black AY, Jones GD. Breech Presentation in Oxorn Foote—Human Labor and Birth, 6th Edition. McGraw Hill Education; 2013.
31. Fait G, Daniel Y, Lessing JB, et al. Can labor with breech presentation be induced? Gynecol Obstet Investig. 1998;469:181.
32. Chadha YC, Mahmood TA, Dick MJ, et al. Breech delivery and epidural anaesthesia. Br J Obstet Gynecol. 1992;99:96.
33. Confino E, Ismajovich B, Rudick V, et al. Extradural analgesia in the management

of singleton breech delivery. Br J Anaesth. 1985;57:892.
34. Lovset. J Obstet Gynec Br Emp. 1937;55:295.
35. Green Top Guideline No 20b: management of breech presentation, RCOG, December 2006.
36. Dufour PH, Vinatier D, Orazi G, et al. The use of intravenous nitroglycerine for emergency cervicouterine relaxation. Acta Obstet Gynecol Scand. 1997;76:287,
37. Styeyn W, Piper C. Favorable neonatal outcome after fetal entrapment and partially successful Zavanelli maneuver in a case of breech presentation. Am J Perinatol. 1994;11:348.
38. Sunday-Adeoye IM, Okonta PT, Womey D. Symphysiotomy at the Mater Misericordiae Hospital Afikpo Nigeria: A review of 1013 cases. J Obstet Gynecol. 2004;24(5):525.
39. Cardini F, Weixin H. Moxibustionfor correction of breech presentation: A Randomized Contolled Trial. JAMA. 1998;280:1580.
40. Cardini F, Lombardo P, Regalia, et al. A randomized controlled trial of moxibustion for breech presentation. Br J Obstet Gynecol. 2005;112(6):743.
41. Ballas S, Toaff R, Jaffa AJ. Deflexion of fetal head in breech presentation, incidence, management and outcome. Obstet Gynecol. 1978;52(6):653-5.
42. Ballas S, Toaff R. Br J Obstet Gynecol. 1976;83: 201-4.

CHAPTER 4A

Congenital Cardiac Disease in Pregnancy

Sunanda R Kulkarni

Patient by name X wife of Mr Y aged 29 years, Gravida III para 1, abortion 1 Living 1 with the following history.
- Amenorrhea—8 months
- Breathlessness—30 days
- Palpitation—30 days.

Patient c/o of easy fatigability and weakness and breathlessness, gets tired while doing household activities. Since last 30 days, she gets breathlessness. She gets exertional palpitation regularly.

No history of orthopnea, paroxysmal nocturnal dyspnea.

No history of pedal edema, chest pain, syncope attack.

No history of blood loss by any route.

She had gone to a nearby primary health care (PHC) only once in this pregnancy and was told that she has to go higher institution for further investigation as she had a cardiac lesion. As she was asymptomatic and previous pregnancies were uneventful she did not bother and thought that it was a passing phase.

Trimester History

1st Trimester
- Spontaneous conception
- No history of radiation or exposure to teratogen
- No history of bleeding, fever or any drug intake
- No history of hyperemesis.

2nd Trimester
- Perceived quickening in 4th month
- Had only one ANC
- She was taking iron and folic acid (IFA) prophylaxis
- 2nd trimester scan was normal
- Had taken one doses of TT.

Menstrual History

Menstrual cycle = 3/28–30 days, regular. Last mentrual period (LMP), estimated date of delivery (EDD).

Obstetric History

ML 15 years, non-consanguineous marriage

1st—full-term normal delivery (FTND) delivered at home and was uneventful. She delivered a male baby, alive and healthy and he is 5 years old.

2nd pregnancy—spontaneous abortion at home.

Past History
- There was history of upper respiratory tract infection on and off in her childhood
- There was no history suggestive of rheumatic fever.

Personal History

- She was the offspring of non consanguineous marriage
- She had studied up to standard 7th
- She was home maker
- Her bowel and bladder habits were normal
- Appetite was good
- No habits of chewing tobacco.

Socioeconomic History

She belonged to low socioeconomic class II according to BG Prasad classification.

Dietary History

Total caloric intake is about 1800 Kcal and protein intake 30–40 g/day.

Summary

Patient by name X coming from low socioeconomic class, with history of amenorrhea 8 months, palpitation and breathlessness since 30 days, G3P1L1A1 with suspected cardiac lesion.

On Examination

- Patient is conscious and cooperative. She is thin built, moderately nourished. Her height 5' and weight 50 kg, BMI 22.2 kg/m^2. Gait was normal, but she was anxious.
- No cyanosis, clubbing, pallor or icterus. She was breathless.
- Afebrile
  - Pulse rate 106/m. Regular, volume good, equal on both sides.
  - BP—120/70 mm Hg, pallor +
  - Jugular venous pressure (JVP)—not raised
  - Chorionic villus sampling (CVS)—inspection
  - Apex beat half an inch lateral to mid clavicular line, in 5th intercostal space.
  - No precordial bulge.
  - Palpation—parasternal lift present
  - Auscultation—S1, S2 heard
    ◊ Fixed splitting S2 heard
    ◊ Soft ejection systolic murmur 2/6 grade heard.
- Respiratory rate 20/m, thoracoabdominal type
- Lungs—clear.

Abdominal Examination

Inspection

- Abdomen uniformly enlarged
- Linea nigra and striae gravidarum seen
- All hernial sites were intact
- No scar marks.

Palpation

- Fundal height around 32 weeks
- Symphysiofundal height 31.5 cm
- Abdominal girth—31 inches
- No organomegaly or ascites
- Fundal grip—broad soft irregular mass suggestive of breach
- Lateral grip—back felt on right side and limbs on the opposite side
- Pelvic grip—hard round mass suggestive of head
- Liquor appeared normal
- Auscultation—Fetal heart rate (FHS) 150/m regular.

Provisional Diagnosis

- 30-year-old lady G3P1L1A1 with 32 weeks of gestation with single live fetus in cephalic presentation with anemia, ASD without congestive cardiac failure in sinus rhythm
- ASD is suspected for the following reasons:
  - She had repeated respiratory infection in childhood
  - Ejection systolic murmur 2/6 grade heard in pulmonary area
  - Fixed slitting S2 heard s/o ASD
  - Loud P2 heard s/o pulmonary hypertension.

Q. 1. What are the investigation findings?

General Investigations

- Hb—8 g% peripheral smear- microcytic hypochromic anemia.
- Urine
  - Albumin—nil
  - Sugar—nil
- Serology—HbsAg, HIV 1 and 2, VDRL—negative
- TSH—2.15 µ IU/mL
- RBS—90 mg%
- Scan—2nd trimester normal
- Fetal Echo—showed normal heart

Normally fetal echo is done at 22 weeks, since patient came at 32 weeks it was done at 32 weeks—to clarify the doubt and to relieve the anxiety of patient.

Specific Investigations

Electrocardiography—sinus tachycardia, incomplete right bundle branch block (RBBB)
Echo:
- Ostium secundum ASD
- Left to right shunt
- LV EF—65%
- Pulmonary hypertension (mild).

Final Diagnosis

Patient by name X, a home maker from socioeconomic class 2, G2P1L1A1 of 32 weeks gestation with cephalic presentation in ROA position with anemia, ASD in sinus rhythm and mild pulmonary hypertension admitted for safe confinement.

Q. 2. How will you manage this patient?

Admission is needed in this case to evaluate further and also for observation and correction of anemia. Maximum cardiac load also will be at this juncture:

- As the patient appears to be non-compliant I want to give iron sucrose injections and folic acid supplementation
- Intake output chart will be maintained as increased fluid over load can lead to failure of right heart
- Patient will be encouraged to be ambulatory
- Steroids 12 mg 12 hours apart 2 doses will be given IM for pulmonary maturity for fetal lung maturity as these patients are more prone for premature labor
- ASD patients can go for supraventricular tachycardia hence precautionary measures will be taken like regular monitoring of pulse, if irregular:
  - ECG
  - Oxygen mask
  - Medications like verapamil, quinidine, lanolin which are safe in pregnancy will kept ready.

I will follow up the patient daily to evaluate cardiac and pulmonary function and also do the fetal monitoring with scan and Doppler.

Scan every 2 weeks. NST twice weekly and Doppler once a week.

In this case as there is mild pulmonary hypertension with pregnancy, I will wait for spontaneous labor. Delivery should be in left lateral position. Prophylactic vacuum and forceps will be kept ready.

Q. 3. How will you manage this patient in OT if cesarean is needed?

- Lateral tilt on OT table, to avoid supine hypotensive syndrome
- Fluid balance to be monitored
- General anesthesia is safer as spinal can cause sudden hypotension
- Pulse oximeter and NIBP (non-invasive blood pressure recording) to monitor the vitals of the patient during surgery
- Prophylactic antibiotics.

Q. 4. How will you manage in postoperative period?

- Pulse, BP, intake output chart, temperature to be maintained and O_2 saturation monitored
- Patient to be ambulated early along with compression stockings to avoid thrombosis.

- Encourage early breastfeeding
- In this case thromboprophylaxis is not indicated as there is arrhythmias.

Q. 5. What advise will you give the patient at the time of discharge?

- To come for follow up after one week
- Continue calcium and iron tablets
- To consult cardiologist for evaluation of ASD after puerperium
- To avoid lifting heavy weight
- Contraception.

Baby

- Consultation with the pediatrician.
- ECHO.

Q. 6. What are the hemodynamic changes in pregnancy which mimic cardiac disease?

Pregnancy mimics heart disease—increased pulse rate, edema, dyspnea, shifting of heart beat, ECG changes and murmurs.

Signs	Comments
Signs—edema	Compression of IVC and pelvic veins
Distended jugular veins	Hypervolemia may mimic CCF
Collapsing pulse	Increased stroke volume and decreased vascular resistance
Shifted apical beat	Hypervolemia and elevated diaphragm
Heart sounds S3 and occasional S4	Hyperdynamic
Systolic murmur at the base of heart	Increased flow across the semilunar valve. Grade 3 murmurs heard at aortic and pulmonary area
Continuous murmur due to venous hum at neck and mammary region	Hyperdynamic circulation, disappears after pressing or upright position

Q. 7. What are the radiological and echocardiac changes which mimic cardiac disease?

- *Chest X-ray—apparent cardiomegaly, and increased vascular markings:* Upward displacement of enlarging uterus. hyperdynamic circulation.
- *ECG—Axis deviation, ST segment depression, T wave inversion:* Rotation of the heart due to enlarged uterus.
- *Echo—Tricuspid and mitral regurgitation:* Hyperdynamic circulation, hypervolemia, functional.

Q. 8. What are the cardiovascular changes in normal pregnancy?

- Heart rate increased 20%
- Stroke volume increased 30%
- Cardiac output increased 30–50%
- Systemic vascular resistance decreased 20% (Only thing to decrease)
- Oxygen consumption increased 30%
- Heart is pushed to left side
- A normal heart can adapt to the changes of pregnancy but cardiac diseased patient may not be able to compensate for the changes.

Q. 9. How do you diagnose a case of cardiac disease in pregnancy?

Even though physiological changes in pregnancy mimic as cardiac disease, underlying are the few points which will help to clinch the diagnosis

They are 3 generations family history, diastolic murmur, systolic murmur with thrill, dyspnea at rest history of rheumatic carditis, etc. ECG and echo will confirm the diagnosis.

Q. 10. What are the maternal risk factor for CHD?

- Lithium
- Alcohol
- *Antiepileptic drugs:* Phenytoin, carbamazepine, valproic acid

- *Folate antagonist:* Aminopterin, Methotrexate, Trimethoprim, Pyrimethamine
- *Metabolic disorders:* Diabetics, Phenylketonuria, hyperhomocystinuria
- *Viral infection:* Rubella, parvovirus, Epstein-Barr virus, etc.
- *Chromosomal causes:* Turners, Trisomy 13, 18, 21
- *Assisted reproductive techniques (ART):* Is associated with higher risk of CHD in the fetus, e.g. tetralogy of fallot (TOF) is associated with intracytoplasmic sperm injection (ICSI).

Syndromes associated with CHD
Marfan syndrome, Noonan's syndrome, Holt-Oram syndrome, Williams syndrome. Cri du chat syndrome Wolf-Hirschhorn syndrome

Q. 11. What should be done when a fetal cardiac anomaly is suspected?

History
- Detailed of family history to rule out familial syndromes
- Medical history of the mother to rule out chronic disease, viral infections
- History of teratogenic drug intake.

Scan
- NT scans at 11–14 weeks—increased NT is usually associated with cardiac anomalies.
- Detailed cardiac scan
- Extracardiac anomalies associated with CHD, Dandy-Walker syndrome, gastroschisis, holoprosencephaly, imperforate anus duodenal atresia, omphalocele, renal agenesis, hydrops fetalis, Meckel-Gruber syndrome, agenesis of corpus callosum, diaphragmatic hernia, microcephaly, skeletal dysplasia are associated with cardiac anomaly. If there are such anomaly then cardia should be carefully screened
- Fetal cardiac echo at 20–22 weeks to evaluate cardiac structure and function, arterial and venous flow, and rhythm.

Karyotype
Fetal karyotype (with screening for deletion in 22q11.2 when conotruncal anomalies are present).

Referral to a fetal medicine specialist, pediatric cardiologist, geneticist, and/or neonatologist to discuss prognosis of the baby.

Q. 12. What are the effects of maternal cardiac disease on the fetus?

Fetal death, fetal morbidity, intrauterine growth restriction (IUGR), fetal heart disease, fetal polycythemia, premature labor.

Q. 13. What are the Indications for LSCS?

- Cardiac disease itself is not an indication for lower segment cesarean section (LSCS). Usually indicated for obstetric reasons
- Marfan syndrome (root >4 cm)
- Coarctation of aorta with Berry's aneurysm
- Aortic dissection
- Ventricular arrhythmias when baby is near mature.

Q. 14. What are the contributory factors for CCF in pregnancy?

- *Infective causes:* Respiratory, endocarditis
- *Vascular operations:* Increased fluid intake or parental fluids
- *Fluid retention:* Excessive salt intake, PET
- *Over activity:* Physical, emotional
- *Associated conditions:* Hyperthyroidism, anemia, hypertension
- *Medications:* Steroids, beta mimetic.

Q. 15. What is the Rule of 5 in cardiac disease?

- *5 minutes:* Emptying of uterus—pulmonary edema
- *5 hours:* Congestive cardiac failure (CCF)
- *5 days:* Bacterial endocarditis
- *5 weeks:* Embolism.
- *5 months:* Cardiomyopathy.

Q. 16. What are the common complications that occur in heart diseases?

- Congestive cardiac failure
- Pulmonary edema
- Infective endocarditis
- Thromboembolism
- Auricular fibrillation.

New York Heart Association—Functional Classification of Cardiac Disease

New York Heart Association Cardiac Functional Classification

Class I: No functional limitation of physical activity. No symptoms of cardiac decompensating with activity.

Class II: Mild amount of functional limitation. Patients are asymptomatic at rest. Ordinary physical activity results in symptoms.

Class III: Limitation of most physical activity. Asymptomatic at rest. Minimal physical activity results in symptoms.

Class IV: Severe limitation of physical activity results in symptoms.

New York Classification has limitations as it is not able to judge the severity of the disease, not able to diagnose the lesion and it is not based on signs, but only symptoms.

Q. 17. What are the conditions where pregnancy is contraindicated or MTP is indicated?

- Pulmonary hypertension of any cause
- Severe systolic ventricular dysfunction left ventricle ejection fraction (LVEF)—<30%, New York Heart Association (NYHA) 3 and 4
- Previous peripartum cardiomyopathy with any residual impairment of left ventricle function
- Severe left heart obstructive lesions, mitral stenosis, aortic stenosis or coarctation.
- Marfan's syndrome with aortic root > 4 mm
- Eisenmenger's complex, and tetralogy of Fallots.

- Up to 7 weeks gestation, mifepristone is an alternative to surgery
- When prostaglandin E compounds are given, systemic arterial oxygen saturation should be monitored with pulse oximeter
- Prostaglandin F compounds should be avoided because they can significantly increase PAP and may decrease coronary perfusion.

WHO	Risk	Checkup	Conditions
1	Low risk	1–2 in pregnancy	Mild pulmonary stenosis and mitral valve prolapsed, PDA, repaired ASD, VSD, PDA, anomalous pulmonary venous drainage
2	Low to moderate	1/each trimester	WHO 2 and 3 Unoperated ASD/VSD, repaired tetralogy, arrhythmias, Mild left ventricular impairment, native tissue valvular heart disease
3	High risk	2–4 weeks	Or not considered WHO 1 and 2 are Marfan's syndrome with or without aortic dilatation, repaired coarctation, aorta <45 mm with bicuspid aortic valve
4	Very high risk		Pregnancy is contraindicated

Q. 18. What are the other classification of heart disease?

Since disease series specific risk is too small predictors are used. There are 3 different types classification. Carpreg, Zahara and WHO classification. Carpreg study includes acquire and congenital heart disease whereas study is based on population with congenital heart diseases. WHO classification includes all known maternal cardiovascular risk factors including the underlying present heart diseases and common abnormalities. Hence, it is recommended by task force. Carpreg score: 0-5%, 1-27% and >1-75%.

Q. 19. What are the maternal predictors of neonatal events in woman with cardiac disease?

There can be a neonatal event if the mother has a cardiac disease, who is she is on oral anticoagulants or who is fitted with mechanical prosthesis or with left heart obstruction or with NYHA class 2 with/without cyanosis.

Q. 20. What contraception advice is given to these patients?

Hormones: Minipill, cerazette, can be used in all patients except it is not recommended in WHO 3 and 4 category and pregnancy is high risk.

Injectable progesterone can lead hematoma at the site if patient is on anticoagulants.

Condom is safe. Cu-T is not advised in cyanotic heart disease where HCT>55% as there is more chances of menorrhagia.

Levonorgestrel an emergency contraception also can be used in all patients but with caution if the patient is on warfarin [risk category 3].

Long-acting progesterone like Mirena, implanon, depo provera produce amenorrhea which is advantageous to both cyanotic and anticoagulated patients.

Mirena is contraindicated in pulmonary hypertension, Fontan or other condition where vagal reaction would be poorly tolerated

Vasectomy—not very suitable because usually male partner outlives his cardiac female partner and may need some times new partner.

Sterilization

Abdominal tubectomy is better than laparoscopy as there is no increased intraabdominal pressure or head low position is required.

Risk of contraception in heart diseases

WHO 1—always stable
WHO 2—broadly stable
WHO 3—caution required
WHO 4—do not use.

WHO 1: Always stable—all cases congenital lesions repaired, mild mitral valve prolapse with trivial regurgitation, mild pulmonary stenosis, repaired coarctation with no hypertension or aneurysm.

WHO 2: Broadly stable—prosthetic valve lacking WHO 3 and 4 criteria, uncomplicated mild mitral aortic disease, most arrhythmias other than fibrillation, or flutter, and hypertrophic cardiomyopathy lacking WHO 3 or 4 criteria.

WHO 3: Caution use—thrombotic risk factor with warfarin, mechanical valves, arrhythmias, dilated left atrium >4 cm

WHO 4: Do not use—thrombotic episode risk even on warfarin, ischemic heart diseases, dilated cardiomyopathy and LV dysfunction of any cause, pulmonary hypertension of any cause and mechanical valve Starr Edward Bjork any tricuspid valve.

The risk of congenital heart disease in offspring (Lupton and coleagues—2002)

Lesion	Previous sibling affected	Father affected	Mother affected
Marfan's	–	50%	50%
Aortic stenosis	2	3	15–18
Pulmonary stenosis	2	2	6–7
VSD	3	2	10–16
ASD	2.5	1.5	5–11
PDA	3	2.5	4
Coarctation	–	–	14%
TOF	2.5	1.5	3

Hereditary transmission: Marfan syndrome, ASD, VSD, PDA, obstructive left sided, obstructive right sided, Fallots, Ebstein anomaly, etc. Transposition of great vessels, etc.

Q. 21. How do you do prepregnancy counseling in a cardiac patient?

In counseling, the following areas should be considered:

- The underlying cardiac lesion
- Maternal functional status
- The possibility of further palliative or corrective surgery and residual disease after surgery
- Review of drugs and to stop statins if she is taking, need for anticoagulant
- Additional risk factors
- Maternal life expectancy
- Ability to continue pregnancy and care for a child
- Abortion, preterm birth, stillbirth, neonatal deaths morbidity, mortality
- Importance of frequent visit to the hospital
- Economic factor and insurance coverage
- Hereditary transmission of the cardiac disease
- Investigations-specific
- Distance of the hospital from the home
- Transportation.

Q. 22. How often should be seen in antenatal period?

The follow-up plan should be individualized and needs to be flexible.

In general prenatal visits should be scheduled every month till 28 weeks from mild disease NYHA 1–2.

Moderate and severe disease once in fort night till 28 weeks an there after weekly once.

Q. 23. What will be chief aim of management of the patient in pregnancy in antepartum care?

The chief aim of management of the patient in pregnancy is to keep patient within her cardiac reserve. It is preferable to have detailed baseline information prior of pregnancy.

Nocturnal cough and basilar crepts may the first warning signs of failure.

Q. 24. What are the admission policy?

NYHA 1: To admit at or near term.

NYHA 2: Admit at 28 weeks in case of unfavorable social surroundings.

NYHA 3 and 4: At diagnosis
Limiting activity is helpful in severely affected women with ventricular dysfunction, left heart obstruction, or class III or IV symptoms.

Hospital admission by mid-second trimester may be advisable for some.

Q. 25. What are the drugs used in premature labor?

Drugs used in premature labor are Atosiban, $MgSO_4$.

Indomethacin can cause premature ductal closure and beta mimetics like terbutaline and ritodrine can cause tachycardia and hypotension, Hence, they are contraindicated in valvular heart disease, arrhythmias and ischemic heart disease. Calcium channel blockers are also not indicated where there is bradycardia, conduction defects.

Q. 26. What is the role of hematinics and heparin in cyanotic heart disease?

Hematinics are indicated in CHD even though Hb and Hct is high because the RBC's and platelets are dysfunctional to maintain the Hb in the optimum range routinely iron and folic acid are advised. Prophylactic heparin is not recommended unless there are high-risk factors like auricular fibrillations.

Q. 27. What is the role of anticoagulants?

- For pregnant women with mechanical valves mainly
- Valvular hear diseases Severe stenosis, pulmonary hypertension
- Arrhythmias
- History of thromboembolism, deep vein thrombosis
- Dilated cardiomyopathy.

Warfarin is more effective than heparin, but teratogenic. Warfarin from 13 weeks to 36th week can be given to avoid fetal effects. Should be stopped at least 2 weeks before labor to avoid fetal brain bleeding. It warfarin emryopathy. It is dose dependent. Warfarin embryopathy—causes facial anomalies, nasal bone hypoplasia and bridge depression, skeletal anomalies, stippled noncalcified epiphyses, shortened fingers, brachydactyly, nail hypoplasia, scoliosis. Should be stopped at least 2 weeks before labor to avoid fetal brain bleeding.

Q. 28. What is the recommended antibiotic prophylaxis?

American Heart Association recommends only in:
- Prosthetic cardiac valves
- Previous endocarditis
- Congenital heart disease
- Unrepaired cyanotic congenital heart disease, including palliative shunts and conduits
- Completely repaired congenital heart defects with prosthetic material or device whether placed by surgery or catheter intervention during the first 6 months after the procedure (prophylaxis is recommended because endothelialization of prosthetic material may be incomplete within 6 months of the procedure)
- Repaired congenital heart disease with residual defects at the site or adjacent to the site of a prosthetic patch or prosthetic device
- Cardiac transplantation recipients who develop cardiac valvulopathy.

If the patient is undergoing genitourinary or dental procedures, she should be given antibiotic prophylaxis.

High-risk patient

Ampicillin—2 g IM or IV, plus gentamicin sulfate 1.5 mg/kg IV 30 min before procedure and Ampicillin, 1 g. IV, or amoxicillin, 1 g PO 6 hours after procedure.

High-risk patient who have penicillin allergy

Vancomycin: HCl 1 g IV infusion within 1-2 hours plus, Gentamicin sulfate, 1.5 mg/kg IV 30 min before procedure.

Other antibiotics used are cephalosporins, like—ceftriaxone, cefixime and macrolides like azithromycin, clindamycin, etc.

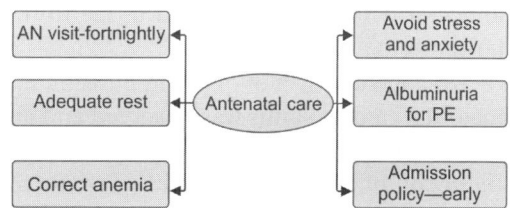

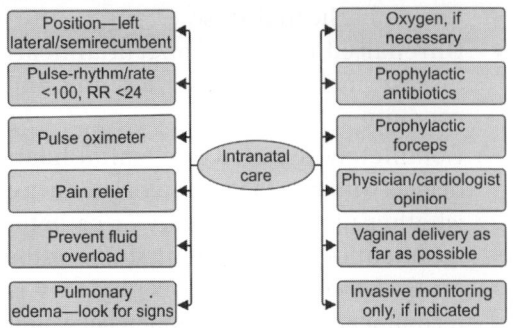

Q. 29. What is the role of induction of labor in cardiac disease?

Preterm induction is rarely indicated, but once fetal lung maturity is assured induction can be planned. When indicated. Most of the time, they end up in spontaneous labor. Oxytocin drip is safe during labor.

Oxytocin and artificial rupture of the membranes are indicated when the Bishop score is favorable. A long induction time should be avoided if the cervix is unfavorable. While there is no absolute contraindication to misoprostol or dinoprostone, there is a theoretical risk of coronary vasospasm and a low risk of arrhythmias. Dinoprostone also has more profound effects on BP than prostaglandin E1 and is therefore contraindicated in active CVD. Mechanical methods such as a Foley catheter would be preferable to pharmacological agents, particularly in the patient with cyanosis where a drop in systemic vascular resistance and/or BP would be detrimental.

Heparin anticoagulation is discontinued at least 12 hours before induction, or reversed with protamine if spontaneous labor develops, and can usually be resumed 6–12 hours postpartum.

No adverse effect of oxytocin infusion on maternal cardiac status was observed and all of the women went home in good condition. Induction of labor with a modified oxytocin infusion is a safe and effective alternative for selected gravidas with cardiac disease where elective delivery is warranted.

Vaginal delivery is not advised if the patient is already on warfarin within two weeks prior to delivery, or if there is history of recent myocardial infarction or she has symptomatic aortic stenosis.

Postpartum Care

Ergometrine is contraindicated as it causes vasoconstriction, oxytocin can be given slowly to control PPH. Prostaglandins are useful in selected cases of PPH when the pulmonary artery pressure is within normal limits.

Q. 30. How will you provide pain relief during labor?

Catecholamines can cause tachycardia.

Epidural anesthesia with adequate volume preloading is the technique of choice (but can increase CHF and pulmonary edema). IV analgesia also suitable for some.

GA also is suited for some (Nitrous oxide+ Succinylcholine+Pentothal+oxygen).

Q. 31. How will you manage the fluid intake?

- Keep AS patients on a wet side (125–150 mL/h)
- Most patients to be kept on the dry side (75 mL/h)
- Desaturation not responding to O_2 may suggest pulmonary edema.

Q. 32. What prophylactic measures will you take in cardiac patients?

- Antibiotics—in selected cases.
- Antiarrhythmic—Only if indicated (tight stenosis)
- Anticoagulation—to be continued— Heparin/low molecular weight heparin (LMWH)/warfarin.

Peripartum care

Extended monitoring is required for at least 72 hours post-delivery as the hemodynamics do not return to baseline rapidly. Breast feeding is advised if the mother is not in failure and also early ambulation and stockings will help in high risk patients to avoid embolism.

Congenital Cardiac Disease in Pregnancy

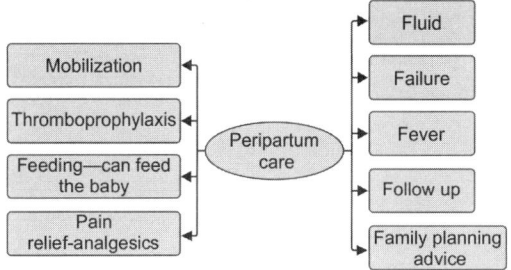

Q. 33. When you do cardiac surgery?

Cardiac surgery during pregnancy is advised only when oral medication or less invasive procedures like per cutaneous interventions have failed. Fetal morality (14–33%) and maternal morbidly (20%) is due to intraoperative hypotension, embolic complications, placenta hyperperfusion. Preterm labor is common. Outcome depends upon advanced maternal age, duration of operative procedure, emergency surgery, associated maternal illness, gestational age, etc.

Neonatal outcome is strongly correlated with maternal outcome. Similar to maternal risk factors, several predictors for neonatal outcome have been described such as baseline NYHA class >II or cyanosis, left heart obstruction, smoking during pregnancy, the use of oral anticoagulants during pregnancy, mechanical valve prosthesis, and multiple gestation. Cardiac surgery causes high fetal mortality during pregnancy (up to 30%).

Q. 34. What are the conditions where dissection of aorta is possible?

Conditions where dissection of aorta is possible:
- Ehler Danlos
- Marfans syndrome
- Coarctation of aorta

Q. 35. What are the indications for mitral valvotomy during pregnancy?

- Size <1—suare cm (mitral stenosis)
- CCF not responding to treatment
- Auricular fibrillation
- Symptomatic—palpitation, dyspnea, easy fatigability. Massive hemoptysis, etc.

Q. 36. What are the surgeries done in cardiac diseases?

Stenotic lesions	Balloon valvuloplasty, percutaneous trans mitral commissurotomy (PTMC), valve replacement
Regurgitation lesions	Valve replacement, repair
Coronary artery	Coronary artery bypass grafting (CABG)
Hypertrophic cardiomyopathy	Septal myectomy
Peripartum cardiomyopathy	Heart transplantation
ASD<VSD<PDA	Surgical closure, device closure
Coarctation of aorta	Balloon angioplasty, repair
Ascending aortic diameter >50 mm	Replacement
Transposition of great vessels, Ebstein's anomaly	Repair

Q. 37. What is Interventional treatment?

An intervention may arise when cardiac function deteriorate during pregnancy or when a cardiac condition is either unknown or underestimated before pregnancy. In emergency situations, interventional procedures are justified. Ultrasound-guidance and abdominal shielding can help to limit fetal radiation exposure to acceptable doses. The uterus receives radiation scattered from the irradiated area, which is more important than the direct exposure (only 2%). The actual risk depends on the dose and stage of development of the fetus. Radiation doses to the fetus higher than 50–100 mGy place the child at risk for growth retardation, malformation, or miscarriage. For low doses to the fetus, the principal risk is radiation-induced cancer.

Q. 38. What are the points to be remembered in treating cardiac disease with pregnancy?

- Prepregnancy risk assessment is required
- Genetic counseling if there is congenital cardiac disease
- LSCS on obstetric indication
- If X-ray is necessary then shield the abdomen
- Surgery preferably in the second trimester
- MTP can be done if there is contraindication for pregnancy
- Vaginal delivery is safe
- ASD prone for—supraventricular tachycardia, arrhythmia, embolism, pulmonary hypertension and Eisenmenger's syndrome
- Better to close the ASD before child goes to school, so that physical growth and health will be normal and in adult pregnancy
- Fetus may inherit the congenital heart disease in 4–10% of cases and it is more if mother is suffering from the disease
- If cardiac lesion is seen then other lesions should be looked for
- Avoid tachycardia in mitral stenosis, Marfan's syndrome, and hypertension in peripartum cardiomyopathy, Marfan's, ASD, VSD, PDA, and hypotension in Eisenmenger's syndrome, ASD and aortic stenosis
- Caution should be taken while prescribing drugs causing tachycardia
- Cardiovascular surgery can be followed after cesarean in necessity
- *ECHO:* It shows suitability for PTMC
- Pregenetic diagnosis of inherited cardiac diseases can be done by NGS
- Continuous telemetry is indicated till 48 hours after delivery if there is history of or ongoing arrhythmias with decreased ventricular function
- MRI can be of help to evaluate the extra-cardiac vascular structures and aorta and left ventricle.

		Drug class
1.	Penicillin group:	
	Ampicillin/Amoxicillin	A/B
2.	Cephalosporins: Cephalexin, ceftriaxone, cefazolin	A/B
3.	Macrolides:	
	Clindamycin/Azithromycin	B/C
4.	Glycopeptide-antibiotic: Vancomycin	B
5.	Anticoagulant:	
	Warfarin	X
	Heparin	C
6.	Antiarrhythmic drugs:	
	Lidocaine	B
	Procainamide	C
	Adenosine	C
	Amiodarone	D
7.	To control heart rate and BP:	
	Atenolol	D
	Labetalol	C
	ACE inhibitors	D
	Alpha methyldopa	B
	Hydralazine	C
8.	Diuretics:	
	Furosemide	C

Bibliography

1. Bagga R, Choudhary N, Suri V, et al. First and second trimester induced abortions in women with cardiac disorders: a 12-year analysis from a developing country. J Obstet Gynaecol. 2008;28(7):732-7.
2. Barth WH Jr. Cardiac surgery in pregnancy, Cardiac surgery: Cardiac surgery during pregnancy should only be done if all other treatment modalities (medication and percutaneous intervention) have failed. Clin Obstet Gynecol. Volume 5.
3. Belfort MA, Saade GR, Foley MR, et al. Critical Care Obstetrics, 5th Edition. Nov 2010. ISBN: 978-1-405-15273-0
4. Copel JA, Pilu G, Kleinman CS. Congenital heart disease and extracardiac anomalies: Associations

and indications for fetal echocardiography. Am J Obst Gynec. 1986;154(5):1121-32. doi:10.1016/0002-9378(86)90773-8.
5. Embil JM, Kwan-Leung C. The American Heart Association 2007 endocarditis prophylaxis guidelines: A compromise between science and common sense. Can J Cardiol. 2008 Sep;24(9):673-5. PMCID: PMC2643171.
6. Gandhii M, Amir A, Shamshirsaz. Cardiac lesions in the critical care setting. Critical care obstetrics for the obstetrician and gynecologist. 2016;43(4): 710-28.
7. Gopalakrishnan PP, Shukla SK, Tahir Tak. Clinical Medicine and Research .2009 sept: 7(3):63-68
8. Head CEG, Thorne SA. Congenital heart disease in pregnancy. Postgrad Med J 2005; 81:292-8. doi:10.1136/pgmj.2004.026625
9. James AH, Jamison MG, Biswas MS, et al. Acute myocardial infarction in pregnancy: a United States population-based study. Circulation. 2006 Mar 28;113(12):1564-71. Epub 2006 Mar 13.
10. Lupton M, Oteng-Ntim E, Ayida G, et al. Cardiac disease in pregnancy. Curr Opin Obstet Gynecol. 2002 Apr;14(2):137-43.
11. Oliver Ruiz JM. Congenital heart disease in adults: residua, sequelae, and complications of cardiac defects repaired at an early age. Rev Esp Cardiol. 2003 Jan;56(1):73-88.
12. Pieper PG, Hoendermis ES, Drijver YN. Cardiac surgery and percutaneous intervention in pregnant women with heart disease. Neth Heart J. 2012;20: 125-8.
13. Regitz-Zagrosek V, Blomstrom Lundqvist C, Borghi C, et al. The Task Force on the Management of Cardiovascular Diseases during Pregnancy of the European Society of Cardiology (ESC), Endorsed by the European Society of Gynecology (ESG), the Association for European Paediatric Cardiology (AEPC), and the German Society for Gender Medicine (DGesGM). ESC Guidelines on the management of cardiovascular diseases during pregnancy. Eur Ht Jr. 2011;32: 3147-97. doi:10.1093/eurheartj/ehr218.
14. Regitz-Zagrosek V, Lundqvist CB, Borghi C, et al. ESC Guidelines on the management of cardiovascular diseases during pregnancy: the task force on the management of cardiovascular diseases during pregnancy of the European society of cardiology (ESC). Eur Heart J. 2011;32: 3147-97.
15. Richards AA, Garg V. Genetics of Congenital Heart Disease. Curr Cardiol Rev. 2010 May; 6(2): 91-7. doi: 10.2174/157340310791162703 PMCID: PMC2892081.
16. Roberts DJ, Genest D. Cardiac histologic pathology characteristic of trisomies 13 and 21. Hum Pathol. 1992;23:1130-40.
17. Roberts DJ, Genest D. Cardiac histologic pathology characteristic of trisomies 13 and 21. Hum Pathol. 1992;23:1130-40.
18. Roos-Hesselink JW, Kerstjens-Frederikse WS, Meijboom FJ, et al. Inheritance of congenital heart disease. Neth Heart J. 2005 Mar; 13(3): 88-91. PMCID: PMC2497309.
19. Roos-Hesselink JW, Kerstjens-Frederikse WS, Meijboom FJ, et al. Inheritance of congenital heart disease. Neth Heart J. 2005;13: 88-91.
20. Sau AK, Vasishta K, Dhar KK, et al. Induction of labor in pregnancy complicated by cardiac disease. J Obstet Gynaecol. 1993 Feb;33(1):37-9.
21. Secher NJ, Thayssen P, Arnsbo P, et al. Effect of prostaglandin E2 and F2 alpha on the systemic and pulmonary circulation in pregnant anesthetized women. Acta Obstet Gynecol Scand. 1982;61:213-8.
22. Tanous D, Siu SC, Mason J, et al. Silversides, B-type natriuretic peptide in pregnant women with heart disease, J Am Coll Cardiol. 2010;56: 1247-53.
23. Tararbit K, Lelong N, Khoshnoo B. The risk for four specific congenital heart defects associated with assisted reproductive techniques: a population-based evaluation. Hum Reprod. 2013 Feb;28(2): 367-74.
24. Thorne S, MacGregor A, Nelson-Piercy C. Cardiovascular risk of progestogen only contraceptive methods Heart. 2006;92(10):1520-5.
25. Vitale N, De Feo M, De Santo LS, et al. Dose-dependent fetal complications of warfarin in pregnant women with mechanical heart valves. J Am Coll Cardiol. 1999;33(6):1637-41.
26. Wilson RD, Calgary AB. SOGC clinical practice guidelines; 2015.

CHAPTER 4B

Heart Diseases and Pregnancy: Cardiologist's Perspective

Nagesh CM

CASE 1

A 22-year-old female patient with 5 months of amenorrhea presented to us with history of exertional dyspnea and palpitations of 2 months duration. Also gives history of one episode of paroxysmal nocturnal dyspnea. No history of swelling of limbs, abdominal distension or facial puffiness. No previous history of rheumatic fever or penidure prophylaxis. On examination, pulse, blood pressure and jugular venous pulse (JVP) were normal cardiovascular examination revealed loud first heart sound with mid-diastolic murmur in mitral area and loud pulmonary component of second heart sound. Rest other systems were normal.

Q. 1. What is your diagnosis?

Rheumatic heart disease: Severe mitral stenosis, pulmonary hypertension in sinus rhythm, NYHA class II, with no signs of infective endocarditis.

Q. 2. How did you diagnose RHD in this patient without history of rheumatic fever?

In 50% of patients may not have history of rheumatic fever or penidure prophylaxis in the past. Most common valve lesion in pregnancy is mitral stenosis and etiology of MS is rheumatic in 99% of cases.

Q. 3. What are the normal hemodynamic changes during pregnancy?

Shown in the Table 1.

Table 1: Physiological changes during pregnancy and childbirth

Pregnancy	Childbirth
• Increase in cardiac output by 30–50% by the end of T1 and continues to rise thereafter • Augmentation of stroke volume resulting in a systolic murmur of grade 2/6 early pregnancy • Blood volume increase by a maximum of 40% by 24 weeks • Heart rate increase by 1–30 beats in late pregnancy • Reversible chamber dilatation in up to 30% of women • Vena caval compression–decreased venous return-reduction in preload	• Cardiac output increases by another 15% in early 1st stage, by 25% in late 1st stage and by up to 50% during expulsive part of 2nd stage • Heart rate and BP may increase due to anxiety and pain
	After childbirth
	• Acute increase in preload due to elimination of vena caval compression, edema resolution and backflow from involuting uterus—partially compensated by blood loss during delivery
• Systemic vascular resistance decreases secondary to placental circulation being low resistance and also vasoactive substance change in levels	

Heart Diseases and Pregnancy: Cardiologist's Perspective

Q. 4. What are the differentiating symptoms and cardiac findings during pregnancy between physiological and pathological changes?

Symptoms and signs of pregnancy may mimic cardiac disease due to the physiological changes (Tables 2 and 3).

Table 2: Signs and symptoms common for both pregnancy and cardiac disease

Symptoms	Signs
- Easy fatigability - Palpitations - Pedal edema - Syncope, urinary frequency - Breathlessness	- Tachycardia - Collapsing pulse - Precordial heave - S3 being heard - Systolic murmur up to grade 3 - Dilated neck veins

Table 3: Signs and symptoms that should rise the suspicion of cardiac disease

Symptoms	Signs	
- Dyspnea at rest - Orthopnea and PND - Progressive symptoms - Repeated syncope attacks - Above ankle and persistent edema	- Bradycardia <50 - Pulmonary rales - Severe tachycardia >150 - Raised JVP - Diastolic murmur - Grade 4 onwards systolic murmur	- Cyanosis - Clubbing - Pulmonary rales - Cyanosis - Clubbing - Cardiomegaly

Q. 5. What are etiologies of valvular heart diseases in women of child-bearing age?
Given in Table 4.

Table 4: Etiology of cardiac disease in women of reproductive age group

Valve	Congenital	Rheumatic	Cardiomyopathy	Others
Mitral	- Stenosis - MVP	- Stenosis - Regurgitation	- Tethered valve - Hypertrophic CMP anterior leaflet motion during systole	- Prior infective endocarditis - Prosthetic valve
Aortic	Bicuspid valve	- Stenosis - Regurgitation		- Marfan - Ehler danlos - Turner - Prior Infective endocarditis - Prosthetic Valve - Connective tissue disorder - Ross procedure
Pulmonary	Stenosis Noonan's syndrome Postoperative —TOF			- Postoperative residual regurgitation - Prosthetic valve
Factors altering the outcome			- Arrhythmias - IHD - Prior heart failure - Anticoagulation - Ejection fraction <40%	- Severe pulmonary hypertension - Aortic coarctation - Aortic root dilatation - History of stroke or TIA

Q. 6. How does the hemodynamic changes of pregnancy affect mitral stenosis?

The increase in heart rate limits the available time for left ventricle (LV) filling, resulting in increasing left atrial and pulmonary pressures leading to pulmonary edema.

Increased volume load and tachycardia cause patient to deteriorate and advance from one NYHA to higher.

The risk of maternal death is greater during labor and postpartum period due to increase in preload from autoperfusion of uterus which flood central circulation leading to pulmonary edema.

Q. 7. What are the causes for decompensation of stable valvular heart disease (MS) in pregnancy?

- Intercurrent infections
- Anemia
- Pulmonary embolism
- Atrial fibrillation
- Severe preeclampsia.

Q. 8. How do you investigate this patient?

- Routine investigations
  - Hb for anemia
  - Total and differential counts, ESR-infections
  - Renal function tests and electrolytes
  - Thyroid function tests
- ASLO (antistreptolysin antibodies), CRP (C-reactive protein)
- Electrocardiogram (ECG)
- Echocardiogram
  - To confirm rheumatic heart disease etiology
  - Assess valve lesions and their severity
  - Assess valve suitability for PTMC
  - Any clot in left atrium or appendage.
  - Other investigations routinely done in pregnancy along with an anomaly scan.

Q. 9. How do you monitor pregnancy with valvular heart disease?

Patient with known valvular heart disease must undergo proper prepregnancy counseling.

Patients decompensate usually during 20–22 weeks and around 30 weeks when cardiac output is high, so regular follow-up recommended before pregnancy, after pregnancy confirmation.

Regular penidure prophylaxis every 3 weeks to be continued.

Patient should be monitored for precipitating factors like anemia, thyrotoxicosis, infections, atrial fibrillation and recurrent rheumatic activity, preeclampsia and promptly treated.

Q. 10. How do you manage the case of mitral stenosis (MS) during pregnancy?

- *Mild-to-moderate MS:* Only medical management. Pregnancy is tolerated well unless decompensation occurs.
- *Symptomatic moderate-to-severe MS.*

Medical management (Valvular heart disease)

Table 5 summarizes the medical management of all valvular lesions.

Table 5: Summary of medical management of valvular lesions in pregnancy

Mitral stenosis	Mitral regurgitation
Beta-blockers—Metoprolol, atenolol (Class D) rarely propranlol Diuretics—Thiazide, and loop diuretics Anticoagulants Prophylaxis with antibiotics	Nitrates and hydralazine as vasodilators Diuretics rarely Anticoagulants Prophylaxis with antibiotics
Aortic stenosis	**Aortic regurgitation**
Beta-blockers—metoprolol, atenolol (Class D) rarely propranolol Diuretics—Thiazide, and loop diuretics (LVF) Anticoagulants Prophylaxis with antibiotics	Diuretics Vasodilators (ACE and ARBs not to be used)

Invasive Management

PTMC (Percutaneous trans mitral commissurotomy)

- Done in symptomatic MS refractory to medical therapy, forestall need for MVR (mitral valve replacement)
- Second trimester is the best time

- Most accepted, reported success up to 100%
- Done using shielding of abdomen to prevent radiation.

Advantages: Maternal mortality rates for percutaneous mitral valvuloplasty were 0.2%, and fetal mortality rates were 2%, which included elective terminations; overall, the procedural success rate was 98%.

Mitral Valve Replacement

Usually deferred until postpartum, unless hemodynamically compromised not responding to medical or PTMC.

Disadvantages
- Maternal mortality—3%
- Fetal loss—12-20%

Obstetric Management
- Cesarean section indicated only for obstetric reasons.
- Endocarditis prophylaxis guidelines do not recommend antibiotic prophylaxis for vaginal delivery in women with VHD.
- Invasive monitoring including pulmonary artery pressure (PAP) and systemic vascular resistance (SVR) should be considered.
- After delivery oxytocin 10-20 units in 1,000 units of crystalloid administered to lower SVR and PVR, resulting in lower cardiac output.

Q. 11. What is the role of digoxin nowadays?

Digoxin is recommended only to the patients with atrial fibrillation for rate control in RHD and heart failure patients due to its inotropic effect. No mortality benefit noted with digoxin.

Q. 12. How do you manage this case?

As described earlier since patient has severe MS and second trimester is ideal time for PTMC, I would ask her to undergo PTMC to prevent further complications.

Q. 13. When do you refer for surgery?

- Deferred until postpartum, unless hemodynamically compromised not responding to medical or PTMC.
- Patient developing acute severe mitral regurgitation after PTMC.

14. What are the potential risks of valvular heart disease in pregnancy?

Table 6: The answer is depicted

Valve lesion	Potential risks in pregnancy
Tricuspid regurgitation	Associated with other cardiac lesions but usually well tolerated
Pulmonic stenosis/ insufficiency	Usually well tolerated or asymptomatic prior to pregnancy. May be of greater concern after surgery for congenital heart disease
Mitral stenosis	Atrial fibrillation, cerebral or systemic thromboembolism, pulmonary edema
Mitral regurgitation	Well tolerated and may decrease with decreased afterload
Aortic stenosis	Arrhythmia, heart failure, or syncope
Aortic insufficiency	Well tolerated and may decrease with decreased afterload

Q. 15. How do you manage aortic stenosis (AS) during pregnancy?

The etiology of AS in pregnant mother is usually congenital, bicuspid aortic valve.

Many asymptomatic women with AS have symptom onset during pregnancy due to increased systemic metabolic demands and limited ability to increase stroke volume.

Congestive heart failure is the most common complication.

Patient education and frequent maternal monitoring are used in asymptomatic patients.

In symptomatic, treatment options include bedrest, oxygen supplementation and beta-blockers.

Balloon aortic valvuloplasty and aortic valve replacement in severe AS who failed medical therapy.

Q.16. How do you manage regurgitant lesions mitral and aortic regurgitation during pregnancy?

In theory the decrease in the SVR (systemic vascular resistance) and shortened diastole of pregnancy decreases the regurgitation severity and are well tolerated.

17. How do you manage right sided valve lesions?

- *Pulmonary stenosis:* Usually congenital. Mild to moderate lesion well tolerated. if severe and symptomatic pulmonary balloon valvuloplasty can be performed safely during second trimester.
- *Tricuspid stenosis:* Rare, but treatment with percutaneous balloon commissurotomy has been successful.
- *Right sided regurgitant lesions:* Well tolerated.

18. How do you advise prophylaxis in this rheumatic fever?

As shown in the underlying Table 7.

Table 7: Secondary prophylaxis for patients with rheumatic fever

Condition	Prophylaxis
Rheumatic fever with carditis and residual valvular lesions	For 10 years or till the age of 40 years (whichever is longer) or lifetime
Rheumatic fever with carditis and residual valvular lesions	For 10 years or till the age of 21 years (whichever is longer)
Rheumatic fever without carditis	For 5 years or till the age of 21 years (whichever is longer)

Table 8: Drugs used for secondary prophylaxis

Drug used	Dosage
Benzathine penicillin	Weight <27 kg—6L units IM 4 weekly Weight >27 kg—12L units IM 4 weekly
Penicillin V potassium	0.25 g orally twice daily
Sulfadiazine	Weight <27 kg—0.5g orally once a day Weight >27 kg—1g Orally once a day
Macrolide or azalide (For penicillin allergic patients)	Varies

Q. 19. How do you grade a pregnant patient with valvular heart disease?

NYHA classification of cardiac disease in pregnancy

NYHA class I—No limitation of routine activities.
NYHA class II—Slight limitation of routine activities.
NYHA classs III—Severe limitation of activities.
NYHA class IV—Symptomatic at rest.

20. What is the role of invasive monitoring in mitral stenosis and pregnancy?

Invasive cardiac monitoring like radial artery cannulation and pulmonary catheter are beneficial in assessing the cardiac output, pulmonary artery pressure and for guiding fluid and drug therapy, especially in NYHA III and IV patients.

CASE 2

Cardiomyopathies

Patient Mrs X wife of Mr Y, resident of Karnataka, belonging to lower socioeconomic class, is 29-year-old primigravida, para one with one living issues, with 33 weeks period of gestation with regular ANCs referred to cardiac OPD with complaints of:
- Amenorrhea since 8 months

- Swelling of lower limbs since 7 days
- Breathlessness since last 7 days.

Patient complains of swelling of both lower limbs since 7 days which has gradually increased to involve up to mid thigh region. Pedal edema increases during evening hours and reduces on lying down. Patient also complaints of breathlessness since last 15 days. Patient gets breathlessness on immediately on lying down. It is not associated with palpitations or any chest pain. There is no history of fever, cough or decreased urine output. There is no history of asthma or chronic cough or previous cardiac diseases. No history of penidure prophylaxis.

Obstetric History
She is gravida 1, uneventful.

Past History
There is no history of cardiac disease or no history of fever, joint pain or recurrent sore throat in the past.

Personal History
My patient is a housewife. She does not have any kind of addiction.

Family History
There is no history of similar complaints in any of the family member.

Socioeconomic History
She belongs to lower middle class according to modified Kuppuswamy scale.

On Examination
My patient is conscious and well oriented to time, place and person. She is thin built.

Her height is 5 feet and weight is 50 kg. Her gait is normal.

Vitals
- Her pulse rate is 100/min regular, good in volume, bilateral synchronous without any radiofemoral delay.
- Her BP is 90/60 mm Hg
- Her JVP is raised. She is afebrile
- Her respiratory rate is 30/min

General Physical Examination
- There is no pallor or icterus
- There is bilateral pitting pedal edema.

Systemic Examination
Cardiovascular: Apex beat is present in 5th intercostals space and is heaving S1S2 normal.

Pan systolic murmur grade III is heard best over mitral area radiating to left axilla.

Respiratory: Air entry equal on both the sides. No added sounds or crepts heard.

CNS: No abnormality detected.

Q. 21. What is the final diagnosis ?
This patient with no history of past cardiac disease has presented with symptoms suggestive of biventricular failure and hence peripartum cardiomyopathy diagnosis should be kept in mind.

Q. 22. Define peripartum cardiomyopathy (PPCMP)?
Pericardiac cardiomyopathy is cardiac failure occurring in the last few weeks of pregnancy to the first five months after delivery in a pregnant lady usually with no pre-existing cardiac disease.

Q. 23. What are the risk factors associated with PPCMP?
Several risk factors are associated with PPCM include the following:
- Elderly pregnant women
- Multiparous women
- Multiple pregnancy
- Race (Negroid)
- Hypertensive disorders of pregnancy
- Cocaine exposure
- Some of the tocolytics
- Family history.

Q. 24. How do you diagnose PPCMP?

National Heart, Lung and Blood Institute (NHLBI), with the National Institutes of Health (NIH), have given the following criteria for the diagnosis of PPCMP.

Cardiac failure occurring in a pregnant woman in the last few weeks of pregnancy or within the first five months after delivery who gives no history of previous cardiac disease and in whom no other cause for heart failure can be identified. Along with these, left ventricular malfunctioning has to be demonstrated with a fall in the ejection fraction to <45% or end diastolic dimensions of the left ventricle ≥ 2.7 cm/m^2

Cardiac Disease in Pregnancy Risk Score— One point for each 1. History of past cardiac event or arrhythmia 2. Cyanosis or NYHA >II 3. Mitral valve area <2 cm^2/aortic valve area <1.5 cm^2/ LV outflow gradient >30 mm Hg 4. LV ejection fraction <40% The cardiac disease in pregnancy (CARPREG score)	Chance of cardiac complication: 0 points = 5% 1 point = 27% ≥2 points = 75% Contraindication for pregnancy

Q. 25. What is the clinical presentation of PPCMP?

Early signs and symptoms of PPCM may often mimic normal physiological findings of pregnancy and include:
- Pedal edema, dyspnea on exertion, orthopnea, PND, and persistent cough.
- Abdominal discomfort secondary to hepatic congestion, dizziness, precordial pain, and palpitations, and, in the later stages, postural hypotension can occur. Arrhythmias and asymptomatic LV dysfunction may occur.

Signs of biventricular failure:
- Edema
- Raised JVP
- Resting tachycardia
- Hypertension
- Basal crepitations
- Signs of pulmonary/systemic embolism
- Cardiac signs: S3 gallop, loud P2, arrhythmias, murmur of mitral regurgitation.

In the majority of patients, symptoms develop in the first 4 months after delivery (78%). Only 9% of patients present in the last month of pregnancy. 13% present either prior to 1 month before delivery, or more than 4 months postpartum.

Q. 26. What is the etiopathology of PPCMP?

The etiopathogenesis of PPCMP is not understood and hence various factors have been thought to be responsible, some of them being:
- Inflammatory etiology—substantiated by increase in CRP, IL6, IFN, etc.
- Autoimmunity-association with hypertension, familial occurrence, etc.
- Increased apoptosis—elderly women, multiparous women showing more risk
- Endothelial dysfunction—association with hypertensive disorders of pregnancy
- Genetic—racial and familial occurrence
- Cerium
- Nutritional aspects
- Increased soluble forms like tyrosine kinase levels—Association with preeclampsia
- *Peripartum oxidative stress:* Proinflammatory and proapoptotic factor formation (16kDa prolactin). This hypothesis has led to potential therapeutic strategy with blockade of prolactin by bromocriptine.

Q. 27. What investigations will you order in a case ?

Ans: Following Investigations are done in this case
- CBC, urine routine, LFT, RFT, electrolytes along with magnesium and calcium levels
- ESR, CRP

- T3, T4, TSH
- Chest X ray
- Echocardiogram-clinches the diagnosis by demonstrating LV dysfunction.

Neither cardiac catheterization nor biopsy is required.

Q. 28. How do you manage this case?

PPCMP is a type of dilated cardiomyopathy and managed in the same lines as the other CMPs. The principles of management are:
- Improve hemodynamic status
- Minimize the patient discomfort
- Improve long-term outcome.

The following interventions are useful in the treatment:
- Sodium restriction
- Inotropes—digoxin
- Diuretics—furosemide, spironolactone
- Vasodilators—hydralazine, nitrates, beta-1 selective blockers
- Anti-coagulation especially with low EF or when bromocriptine is used
- Bromocriptine.

Newer Modalities
- Devices to assist left ventricle—as a bridge before transplantation
- Implantable cardioverters for resynchronization.

Transplantation: More of rejection anticipated

Experimental therapy: Immunosuppressive and immunomodulating therapy (pentoxifylline).

Q. 29. What are the complications of PPCMP?

Maternal Complications
- Low output state can lead to chronic hypoxia, slow circulation leading to thromboembolism, arrhythmias
- Delay in diagnosis as it may be misdiagnosed as preeclampsia
- It can be undertreated because of fetal concerns.

Fetal Complications
- Fetal distress due to maternal hypoxia or drug induced hypovolemia.

Q. 30. How do you manage during labor?

Route of Delivery

As cesarean delivery is more often associated with infections and embolic events, vaginal delivery is the most preferred.

Other interventions are:
- Adequate pain control
- Take care of infection
- Manage anemia, preeclampsia energetically
- Sodium restriction is helpful
- Confining to bed in pregnancy helps to maintain uteroplacental circulation.

Q. 31. What is the prognosis and follow-up data on PPCMP?

- Recovery—50%
- Maintained on drugs—25%
- Deterioration—25%.

ACE inhibitors and β-blockers are continued for at least 1 year after normalization of ejection fraction.

Q. 32. What is the risk of subsequent pregnancy?

It is known to recur in 30% and hence further pregnancies need to be discouraged.

Q. 33. What are the other types of cardiomyopathies seen in pregnancy?

Pregnancy may be associated with other varieties of CMPs like dilated cardiomyopathy (DCM) and hypertrophic cardiomyopathy (HCM).

Q. 34. How do you manage DCM during pregnancy?

Only women with EF >50% can attempt pregnancy, ones with EF between 40–50% if with poor exercise tolerance pregnancy is contraindicated. If <30% pregnancy should never be attempted.

Other pregnant women with DCM are symptomatically managed along the same principles as PPCMP is managed.

Q. 35. How do you manage HCM during pregnancy?

Prepregnancy symptomatic patients do not do well in pregnancy, otherwise HCM patients tolerate pregnancy better than others.

They are managed with beta-blockers of increased dose (keeping in mind the fetal side effects).

Labor is cut short in the second stage and CS done only for obstetric indications.

CASE 3

Coronary Artery Disease

A 35 years female of Indian origin in her twenty-fifth-week of pregnancy presented to the emergency department with acute onset progressive chest pain and diaphoresis. She did not have any documented cardiovascular risk factors and denied any complications during prior normal vaginal pregnancy 7 years ago. She was taking her multivitamin pills and no other prescribed medications. Her parents and sibling did not have CAD and DM.

Initial assessment revealed an afebrile pregnant lady with blood pressure 117/79 mm Hg, pulse 88 beats per minute, pulse oximetry 99% on room air. There were no signs of congestive heart failure with clear lungs and no jugular venous distension. The precordial auscultation revealed normal sounds with physiological splitting. Electrocardiography (EKG) showed ST-segment elevation in anterolateral leads V1–V4, I and aVL with reciprocal ST depressions in inferior leads II, III and AVF. Coronary catheterization was performed through right radial artery access after shielding the patient's back and abdomen with lead aprons to minimize fetal radiation exposure. Angiogram showed total occlusion of the proximal left anterior descending (LAD) artery with normal right and left circumflex coronary arteries. Patient received 325 mg aspirin and loading dose of (600 mg) clopidogrel. Mechanical thrombectomy was performed, and a bare metal stent was deployed in the LAD. Intra-arterial heparin was used to maintain anticoagulation during coronary intervention. Post-angioplasty EKG showed resolution of ST-segments. She had an uncomplicated hospital course. Pre-discharge transthoracic echocardiography revealed normal left ventricular function without any wall motion abnormality. She was discharged on 81 mg aspirin, 75 mg clopidogrel, 25 mg metoprolol tartrate twice a day regimen. She delivered on due date at 38 weeks period of gestation without any complication, and underwent cesarean section for labor arrest. Antiplatelet regimen was not interrupted during labor and delivery in our patient. She remained asymptomatic during follow-up with optimal medical management. Atorvastatin was added to her regimen 6 months after pregnancy.

Q. 36. What are the options to manage acute MI and pregnancy?

MI in any patient has two options of management:
1. Thrombolysis and
2. Coronary angiography.

Thrombolytics are better avoided in pregnancy without the correct information about coronary vascular anatomy. This may increase the risk of hemorrhage and further dissection of atherosclerotic plate in coronary vessels.

The main concern with coronary angiography is radiation exposure, but the following facts would clarify the concerns.

- The radiation exposure is to the tune of 0.02–0.1mGy which is far below the teratogenic threshold.
- Utilizing radial artery approach than femoral minimizes the risk of radiation.
- It helps to differentiate between organic obstruction or spasm of the vessel.
- It helps to place a stent and thus it is therapeutic too.

The main controversy is about continuing antiplatelet therapy, its duration, management during labor. Some recommend dual antiplatelet therapy combining clopidogrel and aspirin for at least 4 weeks.

Q. 37. What care to be taken during labor?

Post-MI a patient ideally should deliver at least 2–3 weeks later if feasible.

Vaginal delivery can be considered except for obstetric reasons, women on clopidogrel, or the ones in failure.

Ergots should be avoided in them. The ones who are planning pregnancy should do so after an year of MI, after evaluation for revascularization especially after weaning them from the teratogenic drugs.

Q. 38. What are the risk factors for CAD in pregnancy?

- Chronic hypertension/preeclampsia
- DM
- Dyslipidemia
- Smoking
- Family history of CAD
- Previous use of combined OC pills.

Q. 39. What are the causes for myocardial infarction in pregnancy?

- Atherosclerosis
- Coronary spasm/dissection
- Coronary vascular thrombosis
- General vasculitis
- Autoimmune factors associated with collagen vascular diseases
- Amniotic fluid embolism
- Tumor of adrenal medulla (pheochromocytoma)
- Cocaine abuse.

Q. 40. What time during pregnancy is MI common?

MI tends to occur mostly in women in labor or in the postpartum period.

It is more commonly found in the ones who are hypertensives and diabetics.

CASE 4

PPI

A 27-year-old G1P0 presented for prenatal care in the first trimester of pregnancy. She had a significant past medical history of bradycardia, hypotension and syncope that required permanent cardiac pacemaker placement 6 years earlier. In the early second trimester, the patient began experiencing light-headedness and breathlessness with exertion. Pacemaker interrogation done and reprogrammed, with resolution of the patient's symptoms. The remainder of the pregnancy progressed unremarkably. The patient underwent primary cesarean section at 39 weeks gestation with delivery of a healthy term infant. Preoperative anesthesia consultation was obtained. The postoperative course was uneventful. Pre-pregnancy pacemaker settings were re-established after the postpartum period.

Q. 41. How do you manage patient with PPI with pregnancy?

Management during Pregnancy

- Obtain detailed history regarding symptoms like palpitations, syncope, dizziness, seizures, exersional dyspnea.

- Interrogate the pacemaker preferably as a part of prepregnancy counseling or at least in the first trimester specially to know the patient dependency on the device.
- Detailed cardiac evaluation by ECG and ECHO preferably before or at least in the first trimester of pregnancy has to be done.
- Every visit ask for symptoms
- Though they tolerate pregnancy well, decompensation may occur in third trimester
- May present with RVF, AF, any of these may result inintrauterine fetal demise also.

Q. 42. Which mode of delivery is better in patients on PPI?

PPI perse does not indicate an option for route of delivery. Decision is based on obstetric indications. Otherwise PPI patients can have a vaginal delivery.

Q. 43. What are the anesthetic considerations in patients with PPI?

Epidural is preferred over subarachnoid block.

Anesthetist should be aware of the details of pacemaker including durability and battery life.

Close monitoring throughout surgery and in the immediate postoperative period is crucial to pickup any dysfunction of pacemaker and resulting reduction in cardiac output. The signs are not well appreciated in an anesthetized patient and ECG interpretation is very important.

Any other factor which can alter the heart rate like potassium level fluctuations on either side should be monitored. Associated hypertension, use of antihypertensive like beta-blockers, calcium-channel blockers which can have an effect on the heart rate needs to be considered throughout the monitoring.

Q. 44. What other surgical precautions need to be taken?

- Avoid monopolar cautery as this can cause asystole.
- Use small bursts of bipolar cautery. Keep the cautery grounding plate as away as possible from the pacemaker, but as close to the surgical area as possible
- If the pacemaker is still affected then the pacemaker may be converted to a continuous asynchronous pacing mode (VOO) by programming or by placement of a magnet over the device.

Post-surgery monitoring:

Post-surgery change the settings of pacemaker if the pacemaker was reprogrammed before.

CASE 5

Pregnancy and Hypertension

A 35-year-old lady at 32 weeks of gestation in her first pregnancy goes to your office for a minor upper respiratory tract infection. Incidentally, her blood pressure is found to be 155/90 mm Hg with a pulse rate of 85/min. The cardiovascular examination and chest examinations are otherwise unremarkable.

Q. 45. What is your first impression about this case?

This could be a case of a pregnancy with any form of hypertension. This needs to be considered as hypertensive disorder of pregnancy is defined as any systolic reading above 140 mm Hg and diastolic reading above 90 mm Hg on 2 occasions 6 hours apart.

But here only one reading has been taken, so repeat recording for confirmation is to be done.

But sometimes if the initial reading itself is >160/110 mmHg, strong consideration of the diagnosis has to be made as therapy becomes very essential at this level of blood pressure.

Q. 46. How do you classify hypertension in pregnancy?

Table 9: Classification of hypertension in pregnancy

Hypertensive type	Definition/description
1. Chronic hypertension	Hypertension BP 140/90 mmHg before pregnancy or that is diagnosed before the 20th week of pregnancy
2. Gestational hypertension	• New HTN with BP>140/90 mm Hg on two separate occasions without proteinuria after the 20th week of gestation or BP normalizes by 12 weeks postpartum • It is often a retrospective diagnosis
3. Preeclampsia superimposed on chronic hypertension	Increased BP above the patients baseline, a change in proteinuria or new onset proteinuria after 20 weeks, or evidence of end organ dysfunction
4. Preeclampsia-Eclampsia	Proteinuria >0.3g during 24 hours or grade ++ in two samples in addition to new hypertension after 20 weeks of gestation. In the absence of proteinuria, the disease should be suspected when increased BP is associated with headache, blurred vision, epigastric pain, nausea and or vomiting, low platelets, or abnormal liver enzymes

Q. 47. What are the antihypertensive drugs commonly used in pregnancy?

Antihypertensive used in hypertensive disorders of pregnancy belong to different categories:
- *Centrally acting*: Methyl dopa is the drug that has extensively been used from a long time, safe in pregnancy both for the mother and the baby. It may be associated with postpartum psychosis in some and hence it is not preferred by all after delivery.
- *Beta-blocker:* Though beta-blockers are the commonly used drugs in nonpregnant hypertensive, it is not the first line drug as it is associated with FGR, neonatal hypoglycemia, bradycardia, etc.
- *Calcium-channel blockers:* Nifedipine is the drug from this group that is used in HDP, but is the second line drug, used in addition to alpha-methyldopa or labetalol.
- *Labetalol:* Which is both alpha and beta blocker is nowadays the most commonly used drug in HDP. But, its long-term effects are not studied and safety not proved beyond doubt.
- *Diuretics:* Diuretics are not used in hypertension as they worsen the hemoconcentration associated with HDP and may compromise uteroplacental circulation. Their use is restricted to situations like massive edema especially postpartum and in the emergency management of pulmonary edema or initial stages of acute renal failure associated with hypertension.
- *Emergency use:* IV labetalol, oral nifedipine, can be used as emergency management option. If available hydralazine also may be used.

A detailed discussion of HDPs is available in Chapter 8.

Arrhythmias and Pregnancy

Q. 48. What are the mechanisms of arrhythmias in pregnancy?

Mechanisms implicated are:
- Increased heart rate and cardiac output
- Reduced SVR
- Increased plasma catecholamines and adrenergic receptor sensitivity
- Atrial stretch

- Increased intravascular volume and end diastolic volumes
- Hormonal and emotional changes.

Q. 49. What are the diagnostic modalities used in pregnancy to diagnose arrhythmias?

- Resting ECG
- Echocardiogram
- Pharmacological testing. For example adenosine in narrow QRS tachycardias.
- Electrophysiological testing-rarely done in pregnancy.

CASE 6

Congenital Heart Disease and Pregnancy

Congenital heart diseases could belong to any of the following group:
- Acyanotic heart diseases
- Cyanotic heart diseases
- Left to right shunts.

A 29-years-old lady with history of 30 weeks of amenorrhea incidentally detected to have ejection systolic murmur (ESM) in pulmonary area on regular antenatal check-up was referred for cardiac evaluation. Patient was asymptomatic. On examination, hemodynamically stable. Cardiac examination revealed wide, fixed split S2 with grade 2 ESM. Other systems were normal.

Q. 50. What is your diagnosis?

Probably atrial septal defect (ASD).

Q. 51. What are the types of ASDs?

ASD may be classified as:
- Ostium secundum ASD—common type
- Ostium primum ASD
- Sinus venous type
- Coronary sinus type—rare type.

Q. 52. How do you investigate this patient?

ECG is to be done and depending on the findings the ASD may be categorized:
- *Incomplete right bundle branch block:* Ostium secundum ASD.
- *Left axis deviation:* Ostium primum ASD.
- *Inverted P waves:* Sinus venosus ASD.

Q. 53. How do you manage a case of ASD and pregnancy?

- ASD is well tolerated usually
- Presence of pulmonary hypertension/atrial fibrillation worsens the prognosis
- Postpartum DVT and paradoxical embolism should be kept in mind and prevented.

Q. 54. What are the other shunt lesions seen and their effect on pregnancy?

a. *Ventricular septal defect (VSD):* VSD is well tolerated in pregnancy, but pregnancy is contraindicated in women with reversal of shunt and pulmonary hypertension.
b. *Patent ductus arteriosus (PDA):* The pregnancy outcome depends on pressure gradient across, and small communications with normal pressures are not detrimental to a pregnant mother, but again pulmonary hypertension contraindicates pregnancy.

Coarctation of Aorta (CoA)

Aortic coarctation reveals most often as secondary hypertension in pregnancy.

Lower extremity impairment in circulation is the cause of renal hypertension, can cause IUGR, occasional fetal death due to uteroplacental insufficiency.

Anti-hypertensives, surgery, stenting may have to be considered in these patients.

Cyanotic Congenital Heart Disease (CCHD)

Q. 55. What is the effect of pregnancy on cyanotic heart disease?

Normal physiological changes in pregnancy which decreases the peripheral resistance worsens the right to left shunt. Hypoxia, cyanosis will cause polycythemia, increases the risk of thrombosis in the mother and fetal growth restriction in the baby.

Q. 56. What are potential complications of common congenital heart diseases seen during pregnancy?

Cardiac lesion	Potential complications during pregnancy
Atrial septal defect	• Paradoxical embolus • Eisenmenger's physiology and cyanosis
Ventricular septal defect	• Endocarditis • Eisenmenger's physiology and cyanosis
Patent ductus arteriosus	• Eisenmenger's physiology and cyanosis
Eisenmenger's syndrome	• Cyanosis • Fetal growth retardation • Maternal mortality
Coarctation of the aorta	• Decreased uterine perfusion • Hypertension • Aortic dissection • Intracranial hemorrhage • Bicuspid aortic valve pathology
Ebstein's anomaly	• Increased tricuspid insufficiency • Right ventricular failure • Arrhythmias; heart block

Complex Cyanotic Congenital Heart Disease

With the advances in the management of congenital heart disease and successful childhood surgeries, many of the girls are reaching the age of childbearing and the outcome of pregnancy is uniformly good. Early interventions have resulted in these women with normal pulmonary artery pressures and absence of cyanosis which are the predictors of good prognosis.

Post repair patients may show tachyarrhythmias, bradyarrhythmias, heart blocks, which may necessitate antiarrhythmic therapy.

Complex cyanotic CHD
- Tricuspid stenosis atresia
- Double-outlet right ventricle
- Single ventricle
- Transposition of the great arteries
- A variation of these entities

Infective Endocarditis (IE)

This is one of the grave complications during pregnancy in a woman with pre-existing cardiac disease-maternal mortality 29% and fetal mortality 23%.

It is the infection of the endocardium, endothelium of thoracic great vessels, prosthetic valves or diseased valves.

Incidence is 0.006%, more common on the left side.

Hence women with high risk lesions are usually given prophylaxis for infective endocarditis.

Prophylaxis is recommended for those with a prosthetic valve, a history of infective endocarditis, cyanotic congenital heart disease and cardiac transplant recipients with valvulopathy.

Anticoagulation and Pregnancy

Q. 57. What are the indications for antithrombotic agents in pregnancy?

- Acute VTE
- Mechanical prosthetic valves
- Prevention of pregnancy-related complications in women with antithrombin deficiency, antiphospholipid antibody (APLA) syndrome, or other thrombophilia's who have had a prior VTE.

Q. 58. Why there is increased risk of thrombosis during pregnancy?

Normal pregnancy is associated with a hypercoagulable state, which arises from the following:

- *Increased serum levels of procoagulants:* Including fibrinogen and factors II, VII, VIII, X and XII.
- Decreased protein S levels.
- *Increased resistance to activated protein C:* Observed in the second and third trimesters of pregnancy.

- Increased serum plasminogen activator inhibitor-1 (PAI-1) and placental PAI-2 levels lead to a decreased fibrinolytic state.
- *Venous stasis:* Resulting from pressure of the gravid uterus on the inferior vena cava and decreased venous tone.
- Increased platelet adhesiveness.

Q. 59. What are the complications of anticoagulation during pregnancy?

- Use of anticoagulants in the breastfeeding mother: Heparin and LMWHs are not secreted into breast milk, and 2 reports have shown that maternal administration of warfarin does not induce an anticoagulant effect in the breastfed infant. Thus, women using these agents can safely breastfeed.
- Fetal complications of anticoagulants during pregnancy:
  - Warfarin crosses the placenta and can cause fetal bleeding and teratogenicity, later occurring mainly during the first trimester.
  - Neither UFH nor LMWH cross the placenta, therefore, these agents do not cause fetal bleeding or teratogenicity, although bleeding at the uteroplacental junction and fetal wastage are possible.
- Maternal complications of anticoagulants during pregnancy:
  - Major bleeding in 2%.
  - Immune thrombocytopenia (heparin-induced thrombocytopenia [HIT]) in 3%, which predisposes them to venous and arterial thrombosis.
  - Heparin-induced osteoporosis causes vertebral fracture in 2–3% of patients, and significant reduction in bone density is seen in about 30% of patients receiving long-term UFH. LMWH causes less osteoporosis and HIT than UFH.

Q. 60. How do you maintain anticoagulation in pregnant patient with mechanical prosthetic valves?

The main principle of management depends on:
- *Type of the valve:* Ball in cage highest risk followed by tilting disc then bi-leaflet valves.
- *Valve position:* Prosthetic valve at tricuspid region has highest risk of thrombosis followed by mitral and aortic valve.

Q. 61. What are the advantages and disadvantages of various anticoagulant drugs use in pregnancy?

- *Heparin:* Heparin is safe for fetus, does not cross placenta, and provides appropriate anticoagulant effect at appropriate doses. Disadvantage being osteoporosis and heparin induced thrombocytopenia.
- *Warfarin:* More efficacious than UFH for thromboembolic prophylaxis of pregnant women with mechanical valves. Unfortunately, warfarin therapy in the first trimester of pregnancy is associated with a substantial increase in fetal anomalies, fetal wastage (30%), prematurity (45%), and low birth weight (50%).
- Adverse effect of warfarin is dose dependent with dose >5 mg/day, fetal complications occurred in 88% and embryopathy in 8% compared with lower dose <5 mg/day which is 15% and embryopathy 0%.
- Low molecular weight heparin-attractive alternative to heparin because of ease of its use and superior bioavailability. It does not cross placenta, so no embryopathy. However, its use is associated with valve thrombosis and maternal deaths.

Q. 62. Which type of anticoagulation is better—heparin or warfarin?

In a systematic review of fetal and maternal outcome of pregnancy in patients with mechanical heart valves, the regimen associated with the lowest risk of valve thrombosis (3.9%) was warfarin throughout pregnancy. Using it through an entire pregnancy, however, was associated with warfarin embryopathy in 6.4% of live births. This risk was eliminated when heparin was substituted for warfarin at or prior to 6 weeks and continued until 12 weeks, although using heparin only from 6–12 weeks gestation was associated with an increased risk of valve thrombosis (9.2%).

Q. 63. What are the various regimens for anticoagulation during pregnancy?

Regimen 1: Stop warfarin from 6–12 weeks gestation and anticoagulate with unfractionated heparin. Continue warfarin up to 36 weeks with goal of PT/INR 2.5–3.0. Restart heparin 2 weeks prior to planned delivery.

Regimen 2: Recent concept is if dose of warfarin required is, 5 mg/day continue the same throughout pregnancy. Change over to heparin 2 weeks prior to planned delivery.

Bibliography

1. AHA Guidelines on Prevention of Rheumatic Fever and Diagnosis and Treatment of Acute Streptococcal Pharyngitis. Am Fam Physician. 2010;81(3):346-59.
2. Batra YK, Bali IM. Effect of coagulating and cutting current on a demand pacemaker during transurethral resection of the prostate: A case report. Canadian Anaesthetists' Society Journal. 1978;25:65-6.
3. Benrey J. Indications and Choices in Pacemaker Therapy. Texas Heart Institute Journal. 1991;18:170-8.
4. Bowater SE, Thorne SA. Management of pregnancy in women with acquired and congenital heart disease. Postgrad Med J. 2010;86(1012):100-5
5. Caramella JP, Mentre B, Jattiot F, et al. Reprogrammation d'un stimulateur cardiaque induite par le bistouriélectrique. Annales Françaisesd' Anesthésieet de Réanimation. 1987;6:214-6.
6. Cockburn J, et al. Final report of study on hypertension during pregnancy: the side effects of specific treatment on the growth and development of the children. Lancet. 1982;1:647-9.
7. Constantine G, et al. Nifidipine as a second line antihypertensive drug in pregnancy. Br J ObstetGynaecol. 1987;94:1136-42.
8. Duran N, Günes H, Duran I, et al. Predictors of prognosis in patients with peripartum cardiomyopathy. Int J Gynaecol Obstet. 2008;101:137-40.
9. Frontera JA, Gradon JD. Right-side endocarditis in injection drug users: review of proposed mechanisms of pathogenesis. Clin Infect Dis. 2000;30:374-9.
10. Gerber MA, Baltimore RS, Eaton CB, et al. Prevention of rheumatic fever and diagnosis and treatment of acute streptococcal pharyngitis circulation. 2009;119:1541-51
11. Hameed A, Mehra A, Rahimtoola S. The role of catheter balloon for severe mitral stenosis in pregnancy.Obstet Gynecol. 2009;114:1336-60.
12. Hermmings GT, Whalley DG, O'Connor PH. Invasive monitoring and anesthesia management of patients with mitral stenosis. Can J Anaesth. 1987;34:182-5.
13. Hilfiker-Kleiner D, Meyer GP, Schieffer E, et al. Recovery from postpartum cardiomyopathy in 2 patients by blocking prolactin release with bromocriptine. J Am Coll Cardiol. 2007;50:2354-5.
14. Iadanza A, Del Pasqua A, Barbati R, et al. Acute ST elevation myocardial infarction in pregnancy due to coronary vasospasm: A case report and review of the literature. Int J Card. 2007;115:81-5.
15. Jessurun CR, Adam K, Moise KJ, et al. Pheochromocytoma induced myocardial infarction in pregnancy. Tex Heart Inst J. 1993;20:120-2.
16. Kao DP, Hsich E, Lindenfeld J. Characteristics, adverse events, and racial differences among delivering mothers with peripartum cardiomyopathy. JACC Heart Fail. 2013;1:409-16.
17. Lampert MB, Lang RM. Peripartum cardiomyopathy. Am Heart J. 1995;130:860-70.

18. Montoya ME, Karnath BM, Ahmad M. Endocarditis during pregnancy. South Med J. 2003;96:1156-7.
19. Pearson GD, Veille JC, Rahimtoola S, et al. Peripartum cardiomyopathy: National Heart, Lung, and Blood Institute and Office of Rare Diseases (National Institutes of Health) workshop recommendations and review. JAMA. 2000;283:1183-8.
20. Plouin PF, et al. Comparison of antihypertensive efficacy and perinatal safety of labetalol and methyldopa in the treatment of hypertension in pregnancy: a randomized controlled trial. Br J Obstet Gynaecol. 1988;95:868-76.
21. Roth A, Elkayam U. Acute myocardial infarction associated with pregnancy. J Am Coll Cardiol. 2008;52:171-80.
22. Rubin PC, et al. Nifidipine and platelets in preeclampsia. Am J Hypertension. 1988;1: 175-7.
23. Schenker JG, Polishuk WZ. Mitral valvotomy during pregnancy. Surg Gynecol Obstet. 1968;127:593-7.
24. Sibai BM, et al. A comparison of labetalol plus hospitalization versus hospitalization alone in the management of preeclampsia remote from term. Obstet Gynecol. 1987;70:323.
25. Simpson J. Anesthesia and the Patient with Co-existing heart disease. Little Brown & Co, Boston. 1993;474.
26. Siu SC, Sermer M, Colman JM, et al. Prospective multicenter study of pregnancy outcomes in women with heart disease. Circulation. 2001;104:515-21.
27. Sliwa K, Hilfiker-Kleiner D, Pieske B, et al. Current state of knowledge on aetiology, diagnosis, management, and therapy of peripartum cardiomyopathy: a position statement from the Heart Failure Association of the European Society of Cardiology Working Group on Peripartum Cardiomyopathy. Eur J Heart Fail. 2010;12:767-78.
28. Stout KK, Otto CM. Pregnancy in women with valvular heart disease. Heart. 2007;93:552-8.
29. Sugrue D, Blake S, Troy P, et al. Antibiotic prophylaxis after normal delivery—is it necessary? Br Heart J. 1980;44:499-502.
30. Thaman R, Curtis S, Faganello G, et al. (2011). Cardiac outcome of pregnancy in women with a pacemaker and women with untreated atrioventricular conduction block. Europace, 13, 859-863. http://dx.doi.org/10.1093/europace/eur018.
31. Van Zweiten PA, et al. Differential pharmacological properties of beta-adrenoceptor blocking drugs. J Cardiovasc Pharmacol. 1983;5(suppl 1):S1-7.
32. Wilson W, Taubert KA, Gewitz M, et al. Prevention of infective endocarditis guidelines from the American Heart Association. Circulation. 2007;116:1736-54.
33. Witlin AG, Mabie WC, Sibai BM. Peripartum cardiomyopathy: an ominous diagnosis. Am J Obstet Gynecol. 1997;176:182-8.

CHAPTER 4C

Pregnancy with Mitral Stenosis and Mitral Regurgitation and Cardiac Failure

IB Vijayalakshmi

Introduction

Pregnancy with rheumatic heart disease (RHD) may increase the maternal and fetal risks. Depending on the type and severity of maternal RHD, patients respond differently to the hemodynamics of pregnancy resulting in abnormalities of functional capacity, left ventricular (LV) function and pulmonary pressure. Hence, in the management of the most common RHD like mitral stenosis (MS) and or mitral regurgitation (MR) in pregnant women, prompt bedside diagnosis, appropriate investigations and treatment are important, to reduce the morbidity and mortality in both mother and the child.

CASE 1

Pregnancy with Mitral Stenosis

History of Present Illness

A 26-year-old full term pregnant lady presented with the history of coughing out ½ liter of frank blood every day for the past three days. Cough not associated with any fever. One week back there was acute nocturnal respiratory distress. Patient had mild breathlessness on exertion since 6th month of amenorrhea which had gradually progressed to grade III in severity. No history of chest pain, pain or swelling of legs, syncope or neurological deficit.

Trimester History

First Trimester

- Spontaneous conception
- No history of exposure to X-ray or consumption of sedatives or antidepressants or antiepileptics
- No history of fever with rash, suggestive of rubella fever
- No history of hyperemesis.

Second Trimester

- She perceived quickening at 5th month
- Only single ANC visit
- She has received one dose of tetanus immunization from local dispensary
- No history of high blood pressure (BP) records, pedal edema, headache, epigastric pain, blurring of vision. But had mild exertional dyspnea which was not taken on a serious note by obstetrician
- No past history of sore throat, migratory polyarthritis or admission for heart disease.

Etiology of Mitral Stenosis

In our country the etiology of MS is almost always rheumatic. Congenital (parachute mitral valve with stenosis), systemic lupus erythematosis (SLE), carcinoid syndrome, endocarditis, mucopolysaccharidosis are the other very rare causes. In about 40% of MS is isolated. There is a female preponderance which is observed with nearly 2/3 of all MS patients being females. In developed countries, the time interval between onset of rheumatic fever to development of symptoms of RHD is nearly two decades. Whereas in India, like other developing countries, it is 5–15 years.

Obstetric History

She is a primigravida.

Past History

- There is a history of blood transfusion 2 days ago. There is no history of jaundice, any chronic illness or recurrent urinary tract infection.
  She experienced only mild exertional dyspnea during her nonpregnant state. She was a diagnosed case of MS since her early adulthood (15 years of age). She had definite history of rheumatic fever in her childhood (5 years of age). The patient was on tablet furosemide 40 mg twice a day and potassium chloride syrup 2 tsf thrice a day with prophylactic injection benzathine penicillin once in every 21 days.
- There is no past history of tuberculosis. She is not a known case of asthma.

Personal History

Patient is a housewife.

Socioeconomic History

She belongs to lower middle class according to modified Kuppuswamy scale.

Dietary History

Total calorie intake is 1500 kcal and protein intake is 17 g/day which is grossly inadequate.

Examination

Patient is conscious and well oriented to time, place and person. She is thin built. Her height is 5 feet and 2 inches weight is 48 kg. She is breathless and not able to lie down (orthopneic).

Vitals

- Her pulse rate is 108/min regular, low volume, bilateral, synchronous without any radiofemoral delay.
- Her BP is 94/74 mm Hg
- Her jugular venous pulse (JVP) is not raised. She is afebrile.
- Her respiratory rate is 32/min.

General Physical Examination

- Hair shows signs of malnutrition:
- Pallor is seen in the conjunctiva, nails and skin
- There is no icterus
- There is no angular stomatitis, glossitis or cheilosis
- Nails show platonychia
- There is no pedal edema, no puffiness of face.

Systemic Examination

Cardiovascular System

Inspection: No chest deformity, except mild precordial bulge. On palpation, the apex beat is in the left 5th intercostal space (ICS) ½ inch medial to the left mid clavicular line (MCL) and tapping in nature. Diastolic thrill is palpable in the mitral area which is best felt in left lateral position at the end of expiration. On auscultation, M1 is short, sharp and accentuated in the mitral area. A2 is audible and P2 is loud in pulmonary area. Opening snap is heard just after S2. A low-pitched mid-diastolic rumbling murmur of intensity 4/6 with presystolic accentuation is heard in the mitral area without any radiation. This murmur is best heard with the bell of the stethoscope, in left lateral position, at the height of expiration.

Respiratory System

Bilateral vesicular breath sounds with basal crepitation.

Central Nervous System

Examination of cranial nerves—normal. No tremors or muscle wasting is seen. The power and tone in both upper and lower limbs—normal. Deep tendon reflexes—normal.

Obstetrical Examination

Uterine size—36 weeks. Position is left occipito-anterior. The fetal heart sounds (FHS)—160/min, regular.

Investigation

Electrocardiogram (ECG) showed evidence of left atrial enlargement—wide and notched P wave (P mitrale) which is most prominent in lead II. There is right ventricular hypertrophy with right axis deviation.

Chest X-ray (Fig. 1) shows slight increase in the transverse diameter of heart with straightening of the left border of heart. There is double contour of the right border of heart. The evidence of pulmonary arterial hypertension (PAH) is seen as dilated pulmonary artery at hilum with peripheral pruning.

On transthoracic echocardiography (TTE) interrogation, she was diagnosed to have RHD with critical MS. The mitral valve orifice area (MVOA) was 0.4 cm² and the transmitral valve (MV) gradient was 38/22 mm Hg (Table 1 for echo grading). She was immediately taken for emergency balloon mitral valvuloplasty (BMV) as she had hypotension despite blood transfusion given by the obstetrician. Next day she had a normal vaginal delivery.

Provisional Diagnosis

A full-term primigravida, with chronic rheumatic heart disease with mitral stenosis, in sinus rhythm, with pulmonary apoplexy.

Pathology

There is diffuse thickening of the MV leaflets and the commissures and chordae tendinae are fused and shortened. Also the valve cusp becomes rigid with reduced mobility especially the posterior mital leaflet. Initially rheumatic valvulitis causes damage to the MV but later the damage is due to trauma to the initial valve deformity caused by altered flow pattern. At a later stage sometimes the valve may be calcified. There may be occurrence of thrombus formation and arterial embolization.

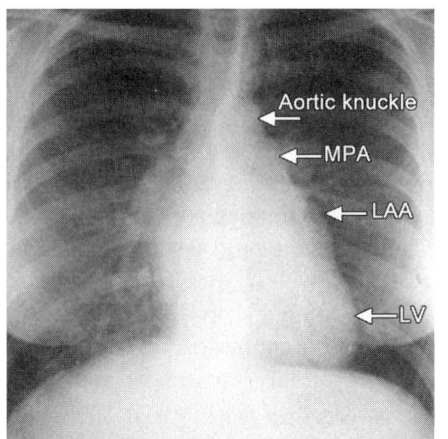

Fig. 1: Chest X-ray in PA view, in a case of mitral stenosis shows straightening of left border of the heart formed by aortic knuckle, dilated main pulmonary artery prominent left atrial appendage and under filled LV. Cephalic veins are prominent

Table 1: Echo grading of mitral stenosis

Severity	Mitral valve area (MVOA) (sq cm)	Diastolic trans-mitral pressure gradient (mm Hg)
Mild	1.4–2	<5
Moderate	1–1.4	5–12
Severe	<1	>12

Cardiovascular Physiology during Pregnancy

During pregnancy, the most important cardiovascular changes that occur are (i) increase in blood volume, (ii) decrease in systemic vascular resistance (SVR), and (iii) increase in the heart rate. In normal pregnancy there is an increase in the following hemodynamic parameters: cardiac output (CO) (30–50%), heart rate (10–20 beats per minute) and blood volume (40–50%).[1] These changes start during the first trimester and peak by 20–24 weeks of pregnancy and then are sustained until term.[2] During labor, the CO and BP increases with uterine contractions. During labor pain and uterine contractions, the stroke volume is augmented by auto-transfusion. Also there is an increase in heart rate due to the increase in sympathetic tone due to pain.[1] After delivery there is further increase in CO due to the decompression of the vena cava and the return of uterine blood into the systemic circulation.[3] After delivery, the stroke volume, heart rate and CO remain high for 24 hours with rapid intravascular volume shifts in the first 2 weeks postpartum.[1] The cardiovascular adaptations associated with pregnancy regress by about six weeks after delivery.

Anemia during pregnancy may result from an unbalanced increase in plasma volume over erythrocyte mass.[4] There is a higher risk of thromboembolism due to state of hypercoagulability contributed due to a series of changes in hemostasis.[5,6] There is doubling of the resting gradient across the stenotic valve due to combination of increase in heart rate, intravascular volume and CO.[4] Also in regurgitant lesions there is worsening of the symptoms of heart failure due to increase in volume overload on the heart.

Consequences of Valvular Heart Disease during Pregnancy

In women with left-sided obstructive lesions, pregnancy is poorly tolerated due to increase in the heart rate, blood volume and CO. But in pregnant women with regurgitant lesions, the decrease in SVR often is beneficial until delivery, when the abrupt increase in vascular resistance may precipitate pulmonary edema. An exceptionally high-risk group are women with pulmonary hypertension who are particularly intolerant to the hemodynamic changes of pregnancy.

Mitral Stenosis

The most common acquired valvular heart disease in pregnant women is rheumatic MS and moderate or severe stenosis may be associated with pulmonary congestion, edema and atrial arrhythmias during pregnancy or soon after delivery.[3] In pregnant women with moderate or severe MS (valve area <1.5 cm^2), particularly during the second and third trimesters, heart failure is progressive and eventually pulmonary edema can occur.[7-9] An increase in left atrial and pulmonary pressures contributes to atrial wall stress and the development of atrial arrhythmias. Also even in previously asymptomatic women hemodynamic decompensation can occur due to fever, anemia and any increase in heart rate (sinus tachycardia, AF). This occurs mainly because there is shortened diastolic filling period which causes decreased time for left arial emptying and increased pressure gradient across MV and increased left atrial pressure. There is a direct relationship between maternal and fetal outcomes and severity of MS and the prepregnancy New York Heart Association (NYHA) functional class.[10] There is additional risk of thromboembolic events with AF though it is <15%. Mortality is between 0 and 3%.[7-9]

The prematurity rates are 20–30%, stillbirth 1–3% and intrauterine growth retardation 5–20%.[8,9] In patients with severe MS, the fetal morbidity has been estimated at approximately 33% compared with 28% in patients with moderate MS and 14% in patients with mild MS.[7] Despite the reported morbidity, the absolute mortality appears to be low.[9,11]

Management

In these patients, the two main goals of medical therapy are to reduce the heart rate and reduce the left atrial pressure. Physical activity should be restricted and β1-selective blockers commenced in symptomatic patients or with pulmonary arterial hypertension (PAH) (echocardiographically estimated systolic pulmonary artery pressure [PAP]>50 mm Hg).[12,13] Diuretics may be used if symptoms persist, avoiding high doses. But diuretics should be used with caution to avoid associated uteroplacental hypoperfusion, as this is directly related to adverse fetal outcomes.[10] In patients with AF, digoxin can be used for control of ventricular rate and is generally considered safe, well tolerated and has few adverse fetal effects. During pregnancy, amiodarone is contraindicated and should not be used to control ventricular rate.[14] Anticoagulation is recommended therapeutically in case of paroxysmal or permanent AF, left atrial thrombosis or prior embolism.[12,13] It should also be considered in patients with moderate or severe MS and spontaneous echocardiographic contrast in the left atrium, large left atrium (≥40 mL/m^2), low CO or congestive heart failure, because these women are at very high thromboembolic risk.[15]

During pregnancy, clinical and echocardiographic follow-up to be done at 3 and 5 months and every months thereafter. In patients unresponsive to medical therapy PMC/BMV to be considered after 20th week of gestation. CMC during pregnancy still practiced in developing world CPB during pregnancy risk is same to mother as non-pregnant state but fetal mortality is high.

During labor and delivery, hemodynamic monitoring is indicated especially in patients with moderate to severe MS in order to optimize LA pressure and avoid the development of pulmonary edema. Vaginal delivery is the usual approach, with the use of epidural anesthesia to achieve effective pain control and with the use of assisted-delivery devices during the second stage of delivery (eliminating the need for pushing).[10] It is considered in patients with mild MS and in patients with moderate or severe MS in NYHA class I/II without pulmonary hypertension. Cesarean section should be performed in patients with moderate or severe MS who are in NYHA class III/IV or have pulmonary hypertension despite medical therapy, in whom percutaneous transvenous mitral commissurotomy (PTMC) cannot be performed or has failed.[15] Cesarean section is also considered when there are obstetrical indications for it.

Role of Interventions during Pregnancy

In patients where the hemodynamic compromise persists despite appropriate medical treatment, PTMC may be needed. It is preferably performed after 20 weeks gestation and is only considered in women with NYHA class III/IV and/or estimated systolic pulmonary pressure >50 mm Hg at echocardiography despite optimal medical treatment, in the absence of contraindications and with favorable valve anatomy.[12,13] It should be performed by an experienced operator and in experienced hands has a low complication rate. The benefit of restoring normal placental blood flow outweighs the procedural risk and the radiation risk to the fetus is minimized using an abdominal lead apron as shown in Figure 2. The radiation dose should be also be minimized by keeping screening time as short as possible[12,13] and the procedure should be assisted by echocardiography and Doppler instead. Complications, such as thromboemboli, stroke, pericardial effusion, atrial arrhythmias and new onset MR have been reported. Severe MR requiring MV repair or replacement is rare. Other

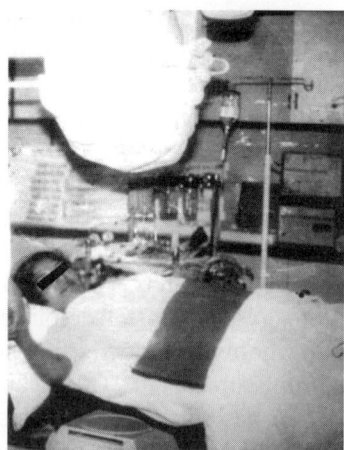

Fig. 2: Pregnant lady covered with abdominal lead apron during PTMC procedure

complications include excessive blood loss, uterine contractions and precipitous labor. The use of the Inoue balloon catheter (Toray, Houston, Texas) seems to be preferred, in view of its shorter procedure times and hence less radiation exposure for the fetus.[13] Due to the risk of complications, BMV should not be performed in asymptomatic patients. Open-heart surgery should be reserved for cases in which all other measures fail and the mother's life is threatened or there is concurrent mitral regurgitation or other contraindications to BMV.[12]

Mitral Regurgitation

In pregnancy as decreased SVR regurgitant volume, mitral regurgitation is usually well tolerated. But due to the increase in both venous return and vascular resistance, they can experience difficulty during labor, delivery and the early postpartum period. Depending on regurgitation severity, symptoms, and LV function the maternal risk is stratified.[7] There is poor tolerance in patients with acute severe regurgitation and severe regurgitation with LV dysfunction. Arrhythmias are the most frequent complications in asymptomatic women with preserved LV function.

Management

Prepregnancy surgery favoring valve repair should be recommended in all patients with severe regurgitation and symptoms or compromised LV function or LV dilatation.[12] Follow-up should be done every trimester in mild/moderate regurgitation, and more often in severe regurgitation in pregnant patients. The medical therapy is after load reduction and diuretics in symptomatic patients with valvar regurgitation and LV dysfunction. Drugs like angiotensin-converting-enzyme inhibitors as well as angiotensin receptor blockers are highly teratogenic and therefore contraindicated during pregnancy and other agents, such as hydralazine or nifedipine, should be substituted.[3,16] The vaginal delivery is preferable; shortened second stage is advisable and in symptomatic patients epidural anesthesia is preferred. In the first 24–48 hours postpartum, diuresis may be needed and after load reduction may be helpful.[17] Surgery is unavoidable during pregnancy in acute severe regurgitation with refractory heart failure. Delivery should be undertaken prior to cardiac surgery if the fetus is sufficiently mature.

Conclusion

In women with RHD pregnancy can be a difficult situation. For the best patient outcomes in pregnant women with RHD, precise, prompt diagnosis and appropriate therapeutic management guided by accurate quantification of valve dysfunction is necessary. Due to the sustained long-term benefits early intervention is recommended for rheumatic MS. At experienced centers, when valve anatomy is favorable for a successful repair early intervention may also be considered in selected patients with MR. To optimize the best patient outcomes pregnant women with RHD should be managed by a multidisciplinary team from preconception counseling until the postpartum visit. In women with significant valve lesions it is better to correct the valve disease before pregnancy is contemplated.

PATHOPHYSIOLOGY

Mitral Stenosis

Q. 1. Why does pregnancy aggravate the symptoms of mitral stenosis?

Increase in blood volume by 30–50% -increase in capillary hydrostatic pressure—pulmonary edema. Decrease in SVR, increase in HR 10-20 beats/min—reduced diastolic filling time of LV, increase in CO by 30–50%—increase in transvalvular gradient—rise in LA pressure.

During labor and delivery sympathetic stimulation—rise in HR and CO.

Sudden rise in venous return due to autotransfusion and IVC compression—decompensation. Atrial enlargement in pregnancy—atrial fibrillation.

Hypercoagulability—thromboembolic risk

During pregnancy patient symtomatic status increases by 1 or 2 NYHA class.

Symptoms

- **Shortness of breath (SOB)**—Most common (in mild MS, by sudden change in HR, volume, status or CO, e.g. severe exertion, excitement, fever, severe anemia, paroxysmal AF or other tachycardia, pregnancy, thyrotoxicosis. As MS progress, lesser stress ppt. dyspnea and also orthopnea, PND) (Flowchart 1).
- **Palpitations**
- **Cough**
- **Hemoptysis** (from rupture of pulmonary bronchial venous connections secondary to PVH/never fatal).
- **Attacks of acute respiratory distress** (pulmonary edema).
- Atypical angina—Chest pain in 10-15% of patients, even in the absence of atherosclerosis; etiology often remains unexplained but may be emboli in the coronary circulation or acute right ventricular pressure overload.
- Patients may develop hoarseness as a result of compression of the left recurrent

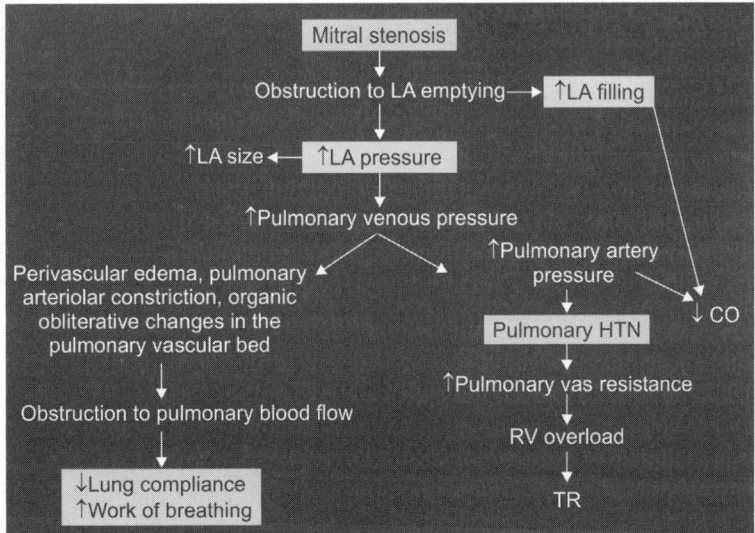

Flowchart 1: Pathophysiology of mitral stenosis

laryngeal nerve by the enlarged LA leading to hoarseness (Ortner's syndrome or cardiovocal syndrome).
- Fatigue due to the reduction in CO.LV function is normal in the majority with pure MS, but impaired LV function may be encountered in up to 25% of patients and presumably represents residual damage from rheumatic myocarditis or coexistent hypertensive or IHD.
- Malar flush in face.

Dyspnea or SOB

- Defined as an abnormally uncomfortable awareness of breathing
- Subjective feeling of difficulty in breathing
- Principal symptoms of cardiac and pulmonary disease and ranges from an increased awareness of breathing to intense respiratory distress
- At rest or on exertion
- Exertional dyspnea—cardiac failure, chronic pulmonary disease or poor physical condition.
- Left ventricular failure (LVF)or MS—pulmonary congestion. The interstitial and alveolar edema stiffens the lungs, make them less compliant and stimulates respiration by activating "J" receptors in the lung—tachypnea, retractions
    - ↑ Pulmonary blood flow (PBF) will have its vasculature engorged, resulting in interstitial edema → act as an barrier for proper gaseous exchange → ↓ oxygen diffusion → hypoxemia → compensate the respiratory rate and effort manifesting as respiratory distress.
    - Less frequently, cardiac dyspnea occurs secondary to a reduced CO, without pulmonary engorgement—TOF
    - Cardiac output limitation (i) valvular-decreased effective stroke volume – RVOT, LVOT), (ii) myocardial—decreased ejection fraction and stroke volume
    - Anemia - ↓ oxygen carrying capacity
- Orthopnea = shortness of breath on lying supine, within 1–2 minutes and relieved on sitting
- Recumbent position → ↓ pooling in LL and abdomen → blood displaced from extravascular to intravascular compartment → ↑ preload → failure of LV to pump → ↑ PV congestion and capillary pressure → interstitial edema → ↓ in lung compliance, ↑ airway pressure, ventilation perfusion mismatch
- Diaphragm is elevated decreasing lung volume
- Paroxysmal nocturnal dyspnea = sudden wakening from sleep with shortness of breath
    - Slow absorption of ECF from the dependent areas → extravascular to intravascular compartment → ↑ in preload
    - Elevation of diaphragm due to ↑ intra-abdominal pressure → ↓ vital capacity
    - ↓ LV adrenergic support during sleep → ↓ LV contraction
    - Depression of respiratory center during sleep
    - HR ↑ during sleep especially REM sleep. Violent dreams may play a role by ↑ sympathetic activity
    - Transient nocturnal arrhythmias.

Wood has differentiated between several kinds of hemoptysis complicating MS:
1. Sudden hemorrhage (previously called "pulmonary apoplexy"). Often profuse, rarely life-threatening. It results from the rupture of thin-walled, dilated bronchial veins, caused by acute rise in LA pressure. With persistence of pulmonary venous hypertension, the walls of these veins thicken appreciably. Hemoptysis tends to disappear as MS progresses.

2. Blood-stained sputum associated with attacks of paroxysmal nocturnal dyspnea.
3. Pink, frothy sputum characteristic of acute pulmonary edema with rupture of alveolar capillaries.
4. Pulmonary infarction due to pul embolism – necrosis and hemorrhage into alveoli
5. Blood-stained sputum complicating chronic bronchitis due to edematous bronchial mucosa.

On Examination

Decubitus: May be orthopneic.

Cyanosis: Present in severe MS with ac. Pulmonary edema

Edema: Bilateral pedal edema, accentuated in CCF

Neck vein: Engorged in CCF prominent 'a' wave in PAH

1. Pulse—low volume. Rhythm—usually regular, irregular in AF.
2. BP—usually low. Cold extremities.
3. *Respiration:* May be tachypneic

Engorged pulsatile neck veins, pedal edema, tender hepatomegaly (signs of RV failure). In patient with sinus rhythm and severe PAH or associated TR, JVP reveals prominent 'a' wave due to vigorous right atrial contraction and a gradual pressure decline after MV opening (Y-descent).

Systemic CVS: Inspection—no deformity of precordium, - no venous prominence seen, visible pulmonary arterial. Pulsation in left 2nd ICS in PAH.

Palpation: Apex beat- left 4th ICS, outside MCL, tapping in character. *Thrill—diastolic thrill over apical area, best palpable in left lateral position at the height of exp. *Left parasternal heave- in pulmonary HTN. *Left parasternal impulse (rt ventricular tap). *Palpable S2

- Auscultation—S1-short, sharp, accentuated
- Opening snap—audible just after S2 (just medial to apex)

Mitral area—low pitched mid-diastolic rumbling murmur with presystolic accentuation of varying intensity without any radiation and best heard in left lateral position at the height of expiration with the bell of the stethoscope.

Pulmonary area—pulmonary ejection click with ejection systolic murmur in pulmonary HTN (due to relative obstruction). P2 accentuated closely split S 2 systolic murmur - due to TR following RV dilatation

The arterial pulses are reduced in volume due to the decreased stroke volume, AF.

- When MS is severe, increase vasoconstriction, resulting in pinkish-purple patches on the cheeks (mitral facies).
- Pulmonary hypertension and right ventricular hypertrophy-prominent "a" wave (atrial contraction). The "a" wave is absent in patients with AF and only a prominent "v" wave (atrial filling during ventricular systole when the tricuspid valve is closed) is seen. If present, tricuspid regurgitation can lead to a prominent "c-v" wave (reflecting regurgitation of blood into the right atrium) and the neck veins are very pulsatile.
- Palpation and percussion of the chest wall reveals an apical impulse that is generally normal.
- However, if pulmonary hypertension is present, there may be a right ventricular heave (substernal lift) and a palpable S2.
- Advanced disease may be associated with the signs of right-sided heart failure.

Heart Sounds

As a result of the elevated left atrial pressure, the stenotic (but noncalcified) mitral leaflets are still widely separated at the onset of ventricular contraction. Thus, the first heart sound (S1) is loud, reflecting the increased excursion of the leaflets. As the leaflets become more rigid and calcified, their motion is limited and S1 becomes soft.

The second heart sound is initially normal but, with the development of pulmonary hypertension, P2 becomes increased in intensity and may be widely transmitted. As pressure increases further, splitting of S2 is reduced and ultimately S2 becomes a single sound.

A third heart sound of left ventricular origin is never heard in pure MS because of the obstruction to flow across the MV. However, it may be present if there is coexisting aortic or mitral regurgitation or may be generated from the right ventricle.

A fourth heart sound may be heard, most often originating from the right ventricle when it is hypertrophied and dilated and the patient is still in sinus rhythm.

Opening Snap

An opening snap (OS) of the MV is heard at the apex when the leaflets are still mobile.

The OS is due to the abrupt halt in leaflet motion in early diastole, after rapid initial rapid opening, due to fusion at the leaflet tips. It is best heard at the apex and lower left sternal border. The OS following S2 may be mistaken for a split S2.

As the MS progresses and left atrial pressure is higher, the OS occurs earlier after S2 or A2. Thus, the shorter the A2-OS interval, the more severe the mitral stenosis.

Diastolic Murmur

- Low-pitched diastolic rumble that is most prominent at the apex, patient lying on the left side in held expiration and by using the bell of the stethoscope, after exercise (very light pressure also may help (strong pressure will instead completely eliminate the low frequencies of MS)
- Although the intensity of the diastolic murmur does not correlate with the severity of the stenosis, the duration of the murmur is helpful since it reflects the transvalvular gradient
- This early diastolic murmur is decrescendo, becoming softer as the left atrial pressure falls and the transvalvular gradient decreases. If the patient is still in sinus rhythm, the increase in atrial pressure after atrial contraction, results in an increase in the loudness of the murmur, termed "presystolic accentuation"
- The diastolic murmur may be inaudible or absent when MS is very severe, due to the very slow flow across the mitral valve.
- The diastolic murmur and OS are diminished with inspiration, but augmented with expiration (in contrast to tricuspid stenosis). With inspiration, the A2-OS interval widens and a distinct P2 may be heard
- Increasing venous return, e.g. by lying the patient down and lifting the legs, augments the gradient; as a result, the diastolic murmur lengthens while the A2–OS interval shortens. Similar changes are seen in response to exercise. In contrast, reducing venous return with amyl nitrate, the Valsalva maneuver, or squatting shortens the murmur and lengthens the A2–OS interval.

Additional Sounds, Murmurs

- A pulmonary ejection sound, which diminishes with inspiration when the pulmonary arteries dilate
- With the development of tricuspid regurgitation, there is a holosystolic murmur best heard along the right sternal border which increases with inspiration
- A faint and brief murmur of pulmonic regurgitation (Graham Steell murmur) may be heard at the base

- Murmurs of mitral or aortic regurgitation may also be present if these valve lesions coexist with MS.

Pulmonary Changes

Pulmonary changes VC, TLC, max breathing capacity and O_2 uptake/unit of ventilation—may reduced. Also the elevated pulmonary venous pressure and PAWP: ↓ CL, contribute to exertional dyspnea.

Clinical Assessment of Severity

1. Assessing the A2–OS gap.
2. Assessing the severity of PAH.
3. Intensity or duration of the diastolic murmur.

Modified New York Association Functional Classification of Heart Disease

Class I: Asymptomatic except during severe exertion.
Class II: Symptomatic with moderate activity.
Class III: Symptomatic with minimal activity.
Class IV: Symptomatic at rest.

Q. 2. What is the current use of digoxin?

Digoxin is not used liberally like in the past for either MS or MR patients. Infact it is contraindicated in mitral regurgitation and aortic regurgitation as it worsens the regurgitation. Digoxin is used:
- To control the heart rate in case of atrial fibrillation with fast ventricular rate; in patients who are notresponding or who have contraindication for beta-blockers and calcium channel blockers.
- In heart failure with reduced LV function, digoxin can decrease number of hospitalizations, increase exercise tolerance, though there is no benefit of reduction in mortality (Class II a). The benefit is irrespective of cause of LV failure, concomitant heart failure medication or rhythm (sinus or AF).

Q. 3. How much fluid should be given in case of mitral stenosis?

Fluid restriction is not done in mild to moderate MS. Only in patients of severe MS with paroxysmal nocturnal dyspnea fluid restriction is done especially in the evening to avoid PND till emergency BMV is done.

Q. 4. When to refer the case for surgery?

All the symptomatic patients of severe mitral regurgitation with compromised LV function or LV dilatation should be referred for pre-pregnancy valve repair. The severe mitral regurgitation with refractory heart failure should be referred for valve replacement surgery during pregnancy. If the fetus is sufficiently mature, delivery should be undertaken prior to cardiac surgery. If heart failure is in term patient then cardiac surgery and cesarean sections can be done simultaneously.

Indication for surgery in MS
- MS with LA body thrombus is referred for open mitral commissurotomy, or valve replacement.
- Surgery is indicated in severely symptomatic patients (NYHA class III to IV) with severe MS (mitral valve area <0.5 cm^2, stage D) who are not candidates for balloon mitral valvotomy or who have failed previous BMV (Class I B)and are not high risk for surgery.
- Mitral valve surgery is reasonable for severely symptomatic patients (NYHA class III to IV) with severe MS (mitral valve area <0.5 cm^2, stage D), provided there are other operative indications (e.g. aortic valve disease, CAD, TR, aortic aneurysm). (Class IIaC)

- Concomitant mitral valve surgery may be considered for patients with moderate MS (mitral valve area 1.6 cm² to 2.0 cm²) undergoing cardiac surgery for other indications. (Class IIbC)
- Mitral valve surgery and excision of the left atrial appendage may be considered for patients with severe MS (mitral valve area <0.5 cm², stages C and D) who have had recurrent embolic events despite receiving adequate anticoagulation. (Class II b C). Anticoagulants are contraindicated during pregnancy.

Q. 5. How to monitor the patient during pregnancy?

In pregnant patients, follow-up should be done every trimester in mild/moderate regurgitation, and more often in severe regurgitation (Figs 3 and 4 for radiological appearance).

Before Pregnancy
All patients with suspected valve stenosis should undergo a clinical evaluation and transthoracic echocardiography before pregnancy and mitral valve gradient, valve area, and pulmonary pressures should be evaluated. (Level of Evidence: C)

During Pregnancy (see flowchart 2)
- Anticoagulation should be given to pregnant patients with MS and AF unless contraindicated. (Level of Evidence: C)
- Use of beta blockers as required for rate control is reasonable for pregnant patients

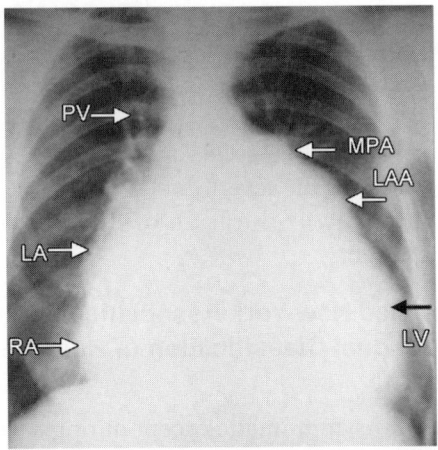

Fig. 3: Chest X-ray in PA view in a case of mitral regurgitation shows cardiomegaly. CT ratio >70% double shadow, left atrial border beyond right atrium indicating gross dilatation of LA. MPA is prominent, aneurysmally dilated left atrial appendage dilated left ventricle with prominent cephalic pulmonary viens

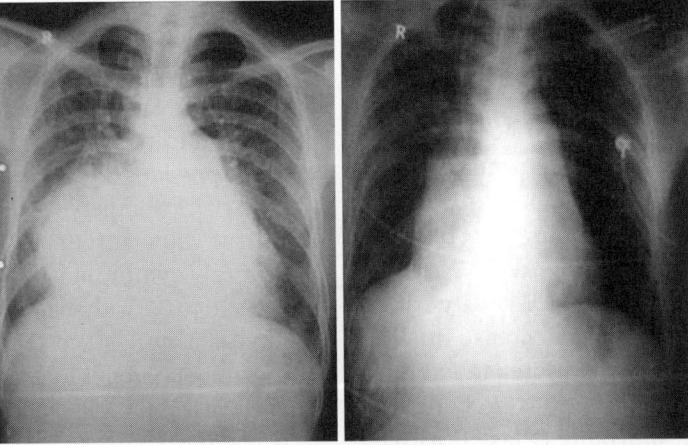

Fig. 4: Chest X-ray before and after LA plication is a case with severe mitral regurgitation

Flowchart 2: Rationale of treatment in mitral stenosis

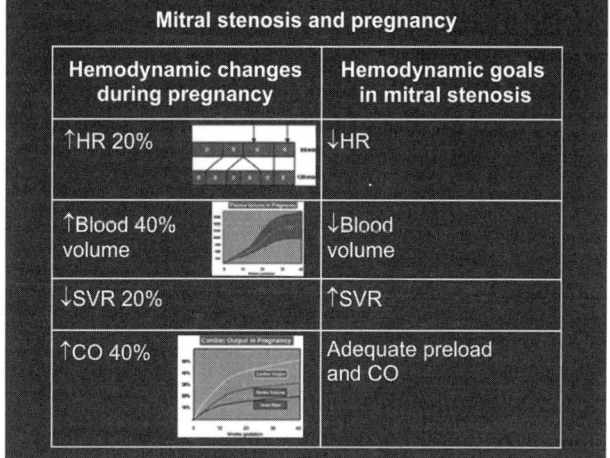

with MS in the absence of contraindication if tolerated. (Level of Evidence: C)
- Mitral stenosis, which tends to worsen during pregnancy because of the increase in cardiac output coupled with the increase in heart rate; this shortens the diastolic filling time and exaggerates the mitral valve gradient
- The cornerstone of therapy for the symptomatic patient is beta-blockade. This pharmacologic mode slows the heart rate, prolongs the diastolic filling time, and can result in marked clinical improvement with control of symptoms.
- Bed rest also may be helpful to slow the heart rate and to minimize cardiac demands.
- The judicious use of diuretics is appropriate if pulmonary edema is present.
- When the mother fails to respond adequately to medical management, balloon valvuloplasty may be performed if the valve anatomy is favorable and concomitant mitral regurgitation has been ruled out.
- Surgical valvotomy may be performed but should be reserved for patients with symptoms refractory to medical therapy in whom balloon valvotomy is contraindicated.
- Closer monitoring during pregnancy usually is warranted.
- Early delivery may be necessary in the setting of maternal hemodynamic compromise.

Q. 6. Primary and secondary prevention of rheumatic fever.

Primordial Prevention
- Nothing but prevention of occurrence of streptococcal infections in society.
- Improvement of social conditions and increasing access to primary health care.
- Primarily improvement of the socio-economic status of people at high-risk for the development of rheumatic fever.

Primary Prevention

Treatment of streptococcal infections to prevent rheumatic heart disease.

- Antibiotic treatment of proven or presumed GAS pharyngitis is effective in reducing the attack rate of rheumatic fever by 70%.
- Intramuscular penicillin is superior to all other regimens of oral penicillin and erythromycin.

Secondary Prevention

These are strategies to prevent recurrent rheumatic fever episodes once the patient has rheumatic heart disease:

- IM benzathine penicillin superior over all other strategies (oral sulfonamide (e.g. sulfadiazine, sulfadoxine, sulfisoxazole), erythromycin, penicillin V).
- Injections every 2 weeks, superior over every 4 weeks in endemic regions, though every 3 week regimen is optimal.
- The duration of prophylaxis should be individualized and take into account the socioeconomic conditions and risk for GAS exposure in that patient.
- Individuals who have suffered carditis, with or without valvular involvement are at higher risk for recurrent attacks and should receive prophylaxis well into adulthood and perhaps for life.
- If the valvular heart disease persists, prophylaxis should be life-long.
- Patients who have not suffered rheumatic carditis may receive prophylaxis until 21 years of age or 5 years after the last attack.

References

1. Maganti K, Rigolin VH, Bonow RO. Valvular heart disease in women. CurrCardiovas Risk Rep. 2008; 2:217-26.
2. Van Oppen ACA, Van Der Tweel I, Alsbach GPJ, et al. A longitudinal study of maternal hemodynamics during normal pregnancy. ObstetGynecol. 1996;88:40-6.
3. Reimold SC, Rutherford JD. Clinical practice. Valvular heart disease in pregnancy. N Engl J Med. 2003;349:52-9.
4. Carpenter AJ, Camacho M. Valvular heart disease in women: the surgical perspective. J ThoracCardiovasc Surg. 2004;127:4-6.
5. Thorne SA. Pregnancy in valve disease. Heart. 2004;90:450-6.
6. Oakley C, Child A, Iung B, et al. Expert consensus document on management of cardiovascular diseases during pregnancy. Eur Heart J. 2003;24:761-81.
7. Lesniak-Sobelga A, Tracz W, KostKiewicz M, et al. Clinical and echocardiographic assessment of pregnant women with valvular heart diseases—maternal and fetal outcome. Int J Cardiol. 2004; 94:15-23.
8. Hameed A, Karaalp IS, Tummala PP, et al. The effect of valvular heart disease on maternal and fetal outcome of pregnancy. J Am CollCardiol. 2001;37:893-9.
9. Silversides CK, Colman JM, Sermer M, Siu SC. Cardiac risk in pregnant women with rheumatic mitral stenosis. Am J Cardiol. 2003;91:1382-5.
10. Vasu S, Stergiopoulos K. Valvular heart disease in pregnancy. Hellenic J Cardiol. 2009;50:498-510.
11. Zelop C, Heffner LF. The downside of cesarean delivery: short- and long-term complications. ClinObstet Gynecol. 2004:47;386-93.
12. Vahanian A, Alfieri O, Andreotti F, et al. Guidelines on the management of valvular heart disease (version 2012). Joint Task Force on the Management of Valvular Heart Disease of the European Society of Cardiology (ESC); European Association for Cardio-Thoracic Surgery (EACTS). Eur Heart J. 2012;33:2451-96.
13. Elkayam U, Bitar F. Valvular heart disease and pregnancy part I: native valves. J Am CollCardiol. 2005;46:223-30.
14. Bonow RO, Carabello BA, Chatterjee K, et al. American College of Cardiology/American Heart Association Task Force on Practice Guidelines. 2008 focused update incorporated into the ACC/AHA 2006 guidelines for the management of patients with valvular heart disease: a report of the American College of Cardiology/American Heart Association Task Force on Practice Guidelines (Writing Committee to revise the 1998 guidelines

for the management of patients with valvular heart disease). Endorsed by the Society of Cardiovascular Anesthesiologists, Society for Cardiovascular Angiography and Interventions, and Society of Thoracic Surgeons. J Am Coll Cardiol. 2008;52:e1-142.
15. Regitz-Zagrosek V, Blomstrom L, Undqvist C, Borghi C, et al. ESC Guidelines on the management of cardiovascular diseases during pregnancy: the Task Force on the Management of Cardiovascular Diseases during Pregnancy of the European Society of Cardiology (ESC). Eur Heart J. 2011;32:3147-97.
16. Cardiovascular drugs in pregnancy. In: Elkayam U, editor. Cardiac Problems in Pregnancy. 3rd ed. New York: Wiley- Liss; 1998. p. 339-450.
17. Stout KK, Otto CM. Pregnancy in women with valvular heart disease. Heart. 2007;93:552-8.

CHAPTER 5

Diabetes in Pregnancy

Lalithambica Karunakaran

CASE

History

Date of examination: August 1, 2015.
23-year-old Mrs A, resident of Alappuzha, Kerala, homemaker, married since 2½ years, G3A1E1 with previous history of 1st spontaneous abortion and 2nd tubal ectopic managed conservatively.
LMP: 23/10/2014
EDC: 30/7/2015, with irregular cycles usually delayed by 2–3 weeks
Corrected EDC 18/08/2015, by first trimester scan
POG: 37 weeks 4 days of gestation (corrected dates) admitted on 28th July with abnormal GTT for further management.

Presenting Complaint

Abnormal glucose tolerance test (GTT), detected at 37 weeks of gestation. Admitted for control of diabetes and safe confinement.

History of Presenting Illness

Patient was apparently normal till 35 weeks of gestation. During routine antenatal checkup height of fundus was more than period of gestation (POG). USS was done, which showed hydramnios. A 75 g GTT was done which was normal. Repeat scan done after two weeks (GA 37 weeks) revealed hydramnios and macrosomia. 75 g GTT was repeated, reported as 160 mg/dL.

History of Present Pregnancy

Pregnancy was confirmed with UPT after 25 days of missing periods. Then she consulted a doctor who examined her and did a scan. She was told that her dates were wrong and her EDD would be 18/8/2015.

1st Trimester

- Patient had regular ANC
- Took folic acid, had 1st dose of tetanus toxoid
- USS done and her EDC was reassigned.
- No history of (h/o) radiation exposure/teratogenic drug intake.
- No h/o UTI /discharge per vaginum
- No h/o bleeding per vaginum.

2nd Trimester

- Quickening felt at around 20 weeks of gestation

- 2nd dose of tetanus toxoid taken, iron and calcium tablets taken
- Anomaly scan done around 20 weeks and was reported to be normal
- 75 g GTT done, at 24 weeks-was normal
- No h/o UTI or discharge p/v
- No h/o GDM/GHTN
- No h/o abdominal pain/bleeding p/v/leaking p/v.

3rd Trimester

- No h/o abdominal pain/bleeding/leaking p/v
- Appreciates fetal movements well
- Doctor told her that size of uterus on clinical exam at 35 weeks was more than POA. So, USG was done at 35 weeks of gestation and was said to have hydramnios
- 75 g screening test repeated and the value was said to be normal, repeat scan done after two weeks, was reported to have hydramnios and macrosomia, 75 g screening test repeated, reported as 160 mg/dL
- FBS and PPBS done-values were 105 mg% and 160 mg% respectively. She was advised medical nutrition therapy and simultaneously she was started on regular insulin 4-4-4 unit s/c half hour before food and NPH 4 units at 10 pm.

Past History

No history of diabetes mellitus (DM)/hypertension (HTN)/thyroid disease/bronchial asthma.

No surgical history.

Family History

No h/o DM/HTN in family members.

Menstrual History

Menarche attained at 13 years of age. Irregular cycles—delayed up to two weeks.

Marital History

Married 2½ years, nonconsanguineous marriage. No history of infertility treatment/contraception usage.

Obstetric History: $G_3 A_2$

1st pregnancy—conceived spontaneously 8 months after marriage, spontaneous abortion at 1½ months.

2nd pregnancy—conceived 8 month after 1st abortion, said to have tubal ectopic, expectant management, beta-hCG checked serially, resolved.

3rd present pregnancy.

Personal History

Takes a nonvegetarian diet
Sleep—normal, bowel and bladder habits-normal.

Socioeconomic Status

Socioeconomic Class III (Modified Kuppu-Swamy scale).

General Examination

Patient is moderately built and nourished. Patient is afebrile. No pallor/cyanosis/clubbing/icterus/pedal edema/lymphadenopathy.

Prepregnancy wt 69 kg, BMI 26.32. Present wt—82 kg. Weight gain in pregnancy 13 kg—162 cm.

PR—86/min regular, normal volume and character, no radiofemoral delay. BP 130/80 mm Hg in left upper limb in left lateral position.

Breasts—normal changes of pregnancy seen. Nipples not retracted.

A skin lesion suggestive of fungal infection seen in inframammary area.

CVS—S1S2 normal no murmur.

RS—bilateral air entry equal, no added sounds.

CNS—higher mental functions normal. No focal deficits.

Abdomen Examination

Inspection

Abdomen longitudinally distended, uterus appears overdistended. linea nigra (+), striae gravidarum (+), umbilicus flushed to surface, all quadrants moves equally with respiration. No visible dilated veins, pulsations or scars. Hernial orifices—normal.

Palpation

Symphysiofundal height—42 cm, abdominal girth 44 inches.

Height of fundus corresponds to term pregnancy. Fundal grip—soft, broad, non-ballotable mass suggestive of breech.

Umbilical grip-on the right side, irregular nodules felt corresponding to fetal limb buds.

On left side—uniform resistance felt corresponding to fetal spine.

1st pelvic grip—hard, round, ballotable mass suggestive of head.

2nd pelvic grip—findings of 1st pelvic grip confirmed. Sinciput is felt at same level as occiput corresponds to deflexed unengaged head.

Liquor appears excess, EFW—3.8 kg clinically.

Auscultation

Fetal heart sound heard on the left side below umbilicus—138/min.

Summary

A 23-year-old G3A2 37 weeks 4 days of gestation, admitted with abnormal GTT value of 160 mg/dL detected at 37 weeks with normal GTT value at 24 weeks now admitted for management of GDM and safe delivery. She is on medical nutrition therapy and insulin.

General Examination

Unremarkable except for fungal infection in inframammary area.

Obstetric Examination

Reveals overdistended uterus with singleton fetus, longitudinal lie, vertex presenting, LOA with excess liquor and good fetal heart sound, EFW—3.8 kg.

Diagnosis

A 23-year-old G3A2 P0, 1 abortion and 1 ectopic managed conservatively, now 37 weeks 4 days vertex presentation with unengaged head. GDM, macrosomia, hydramnios on medical nutrition therapy and insulin.

Discussion

Q.1. Define GDM.

Glucose intolerance that either commences or is first diagnosed in pregnancy. This includes two categories:
1. Undiagnosed diabetes mellitus that existed before pregnancy.
2. Diabetes mellitus developing during pregnancy.

Q. 2. Why do some women develop gestational diabetes although anti-insulin factors are present in all pregnancies?

Due to production of anti-insulin factors by placenta, insulin requirement during pregnancy almost doubles. Those women whose pancreatic reserves are poor, cannot increase the insulin production to the required amount. So, women with poor pancreatic reserves develop GDM.

So, GDM is a station in the road to the development of type II DM.

Q. 3. What are the anti-insulin factors present in pregnancy?

Placental products like human placental lactogen, placental insulinase, estrogen, progesterone, tumor necrosis factor alpha, leptin and fetoplacental product—cortisol are the anti-insulin factors. They antagonize the physiological effects of insulin (insulin reduce the plasma glucose by inhibiting, glycogenolysis and lipolysis promoting glucose uptake by cells and glycogen synthesis) and thereby try to increase blood glucose level.

Q. 4. Why GDM usually occurs in second half of pregnancy?

The anti-insulin factors are mainly produced by the placenta. Significant amount of these agents are produced from 24 to 28 weeks of gestation onwards when placental mass is increasing in size.

Q. 5. In the case of your patient, GTT was normal at 24 weeks. Still she developed macrosomia and hydramnios. And GTT detected to be abnormal at 37 weeks. What is the reason?

Anti-insulin factors are produced in increasing amounts as pregnancy advances. Insulin resistance also increases. So, GDM may be manifest any time during pregnancy. That depends on pancreatic reserve of the woman. So even if GTT is normal at 24–28 weeks it is better to repeat at 32 and 36 weeks.

Q. 6. How does the fetus act as a marker for diagnosis of GDM?

Hyperglycemia leads to hydramnios and macrosomia. So, if these are identified, repeat GTT, even if previous values were normal. So as in this case, a 3rd TM USS can pickup undiagnosed GDM.

Q. 7. Comment on the CHO metabolism in early normal pregnancy.

Insulin production increases and metabolism is anabolic, i.e. glycogen and fat synthesis increase, glycogenolysis decrease, FBS lowered, i.e. fasting hypoglycemia.

Placenta-hormones and insulinase increase blood glucose levels.
- Baby-alanine usage deprives mother of major gluconeogenic source
- Mother-Lipolysis as glucose is mobilized to baby.

These lead to fasting hypoglycemia and postprandial hyperglycemia.

Q. 8. What happens to CHO metabolism in late pregnancy?

- "Diabetogenic"—decreased glucose tolerance. Increased insulin resistance
- Decreased hepatic glycogen stores
- Increased hepatic glucose production
- Facilitated anabolism during feeding Accelerated starvation during fasting
- Ensures continuous supply of glucose and amino acids to fetus.

Q. 9. How is fuel metabolism altered in diabetic pregnancy?

Facilitated anabolism is reduced, i.e. underutilization of exogenous fuels in fed state.

Overproduction of endogenous sources in fasting state, i.e. hyperaccelerated starvation.

Q. 10. What are the causes of glycosuria in pregnancy?

There are many reasons for glycosuria in pregnancy. They give the urine sugar test positive. Decreased renal threshold, lactosuria, frank diabetes and some times impaired glucose tolerance can causes glycosuria.

Q. 11. If a known diabetic woman approaches you and seeks opinion regarding conception, how will you counsel her?

I will evaluate following points before allowing her to conceive:
- Find out the type of diabetes mellitus, whether type I or type II
- Duration of diabetes

- Convince her the need for strict glycemic control before conception
- Evaluate for vasculopathy, retinopathy, nephropathy if not evaluated recently
- Whether on OHA and if yes, what type, if needed change to insulin
- If on ACE inhibitors or ARB, then switch over to safer and least teratogenic antihypertensive drugs
- Previous obstetric history of pregnancy loss or congenital anomaly
- Folic acid supplementation—5 mg/d
- Convince the need for weight reduction BMI <27 before conception
- Check HbA1C, it should be <6 while pregnancy is attempted
- HbA1C should not be routinely used for assessing glycemic control in 2nd and 3rd trimester
- Table 1 shows other aspects that need to be discussed with the couple.

Table 1: Risks of pre-existing diabetes on pregnancy

8–16 weeks of pregnancy–51% recurrent episodes of hypoglycemia		
23% enter pregnancy with retinopathy, 9% are newly diagnosed		
Rapid optimization of glycemia may accelerate progress of retinopathy		
12% nephropathy have pre-existing nephropathy		
Incidence of preeclampsia in diabetes <10 years duration is 11%, >10 years without vasculopathy-22%, with vasculopathy 36%		
Anomalies		CEMACH study- 43/1000 for type 2 DM, 48/1000 for Type 1, i.e. >2 times for general population
HbA1C	Anomaly	
10	8%	
12	14%	
14	20%	
4.2-fold increased neural tube defects, 3.4 times is the risk of congenital heart diseases		

Q. 12. What are the specific points in ANC other than the routine?

- More frequent visits—every 2 weeks till 28 weeks, every week thereafter till delivery
- Strict glycemic control, teach self-monitoring of glucose
- Every visit
  - Screen for urine albumin, urine culture each trimster
  - Check BP
  - Look for monilial infections
- Each trimester—optic fundus examination by ophthalmologist with experience in diabetic retinopathy
- Frequent USS needed
- Screening for aneuploidy—beta-hCG and PAPP-A are unaffected by diabetes unlike alpha FP. NICE recommends T1 aneuploidy screening as T2 screening may not be reliable.

Q. 13. What are the indications for USS in a diabetic pregnancy?

- Accurate gestational age assessment at 7–10 weeks
- NT scan—as a screen for trisomy and cardiac anomaly. This can also detect certain other anomalies like anencephaly, holoprosencephaly, exomphalos.
- Anomaly scan at 18–20 weeks
- Fetal echo is optional
- Growth scans from 28 weeks: AC >/= 75th centile—more rigid glycemic control required
- 3rd trimester: Antepartum surveillance
- BPP- Falacies:
  - Liquor: May be excess
  - Fetal movements: May be exaggerated in hypoglycemia
  - Fetal breathing movements: More in hyperglycemia
- So, these parameters do not ensure fetal well-being in diabetes as in other high risk pregnancies
- Doppler study of umbilical artery and MCA: Doppler will be normal, unless there is vasculopathy.

Q. 14. What is role of non-stress test (NST)?

- Not indicated till 40 weeks if patient is GDM on diet, well controlled without any complications and no previous pregnancy loss.
- Twice weekly NST starting at 32 weeks with BPP as back-up test in:
  - Women with history of stillbirth
  - Those who develop hypertension or preeclampsia or growth restriction
  - Gestational diabetes requiring insulin
  - Pregestational diabetes
- Doppler evaluation if FGR.

Q. 15. How will you manage preterm labor in a pregnancy with GDM?

In case of preterm labor, tocolysis should be with nifedipine. Salbutamol can increase blood sugar.

Antenatal corticosteroids should be administered with intensified blood glucose monitoring for the next 5–7 days.

Q. 16. How corticosteroids administered for fetal lung maturity affects a diabetic pregnancy?

Two days after steroid administration insulin requirement may increase up to 40%, then it declines and reaches previous level after 5 days. Blood sugar should be monitored and insulin dose increased accordingly, or mother can even go for diabetic ketoacidosis (DKA).

Q. 17. How will you decide timing and mode of delivery in your patient?

My patient was detected to have diabetes 3 days ago. I have to control her diabetes as quickly as possible and terminate pregnancy at least by 8th August, i.e. 10 days prior to EDC. If termination is done before control of diabetes, neonatal complications are more like RDS, hypoglycemia. If termination is delayed, IUD is the risk, since there is macrosomia and hydramnios.

Q. 18. When will you terminate a case of GDM usually?

GDM well controlled on diet without any complications can be taken to till 40 weeks. GDM on insulin is usually induced after completed 38 weeks.

Q. 19. How will you decide route of delivery and plan termination?

- Cesarean sections are done only for obstetric indications. Indications for elective cesareans include previous CS, macrosomia estimated fetal wt >4 kg
- Elective section for diabetes are best planned as first case in the morning. The night dose of regular and NPH insulin is given while morning dose is omitted
- Labor induction depends on the Bishops score.
  - If the score is poor, mechanical methods like Foley's induction and then local prostaglandins used. Patient can take her regular meals and insulin till she goes into labor.
  - If the score is favorable, then induction started in the morning, morning insulin and meal is omitted. The dose of NPH the night before need not be omitted.

Q. 20. What are the indications to terminate <38 weeks?

- Fetal compromise
- Maternal hypertension
- Worsening retinopathy
- Worsening nephropathy.

Q. 21. How will you manage this case intrapartum?

- Intrapartum glycemic control is important and directly correlates with the incidence of neonatal hypoglycemia and fetal distress. Mean blood glucose level of 80–110 mg/dL should be maintained. If blood sugar is

high >140 mg%, NS and insulin should be given. If <100 mg % D5 is given
- Close fetal monitoring with continuous CTG, if not one-to-one intermittent auscultation
- Good analgesia as pain stimulates adrenergic pathways and disturbs blood sugar control
- Partogram to monitor progress and early diagnosis of dysfunctional labor.
- Avoid using regular dose of insulin if induction is done or elective LSCS is planned
- Monitor blood sugar hourly
- Use short acting insulin depending on blood sugar levels.

Q. 22. If there is delay in 2nd stage of labor, in this patient, what will you anticipate?

As there is macrosomia, shoulder dystocia should be anticipated

Q. 23. Why shoulder dystocia is more in macrosomic baby of a diabetic mother than macrosomic baby of a nondiabetic mother?

In uncontrolled DM, baby has hyperinsulinemia, Insulin is an anabolic hormone. It increases the synthesis of fat which is selectively deposited in the cheeks and shoulders of fetus. Also insulin stimulates growth of long bones. So clavicle is longer which along with extra fat over shoulders increase bisacromial diameter → shoulder dystocia.

Q. 24. What is the postpartum management in diabetes?

- There is a sharp fall in the patient's insulin requirements after delivery.
  - For pregestational diabetes, adjust to half the dose of insulin taken before delivery or the prepregnancy dose according to blood sugar level. Sometimes up to 48 hours even pregestational diabetic lady may not require insulin
  - If the patient had a cesarean section, rapid acting insulin is used to keep blood glucose levels between 120 and 150 mg/dL by multiple dose injections or continuous insulin infusion until she is orally allowed
  - GDM on diet can revert to their normal diet postpartum
  - GDM on insulin usually do not require insulin postpartum.
- Women with pre-existing diabetes can resume or continue with metformin and glibenclamide while breastfeeding but other ovarian hyperstimulation syndrome (OHSs) should be avoided
- Fasting and postprandial glucose levels should be checked in those who were on insulin, before discharge. All gestational diabetes should have a GTT tested at 6 weeks and annually thereafter
- Counsel regarding diet, exercise and weight reduction which can reduce the chance of developing type II diabetes later
- Breastfeeding encouraged as soon as possible in all diabetic women that helps to reduce risk of neonatal hypoglycemia.

Q. 25. What contraception you will advise?
- Copper IUDs, barrier methods and natural family planning methods can be used without restriction
- Hormonal methods like pills, patch, vaginal rings, injectables, implants LNG-IUS should be avoided in diabetics with vasculopathy.
- Tubal ligation can be offered if family is completed, with caution in those with vasculopathy and hypertension.

Q. 26. What are the adverse effects of DM on fetus in first trimester?
- Malformations
- Early growth restriction
- Fetal wastage.

Q. 27. What is the mechanism of congenital malformation in DM with pregnancy?

- Maternal metabolic abnormality exposes the embryo to abnormal fuel or nutrients during organogenesis
- Disruption of normal functioning of yolk sac
- Oxidative metabolism and generation of free oxygen radicals toxic to embryos
- Hyperglycemia induced mutations in embryonic DNA
- Ketoacidosis.

Q. 28. How can you prevent congenital malformations in a diabetic pregnancy?

- Fuel mediated teratogenesis can be avoided by excellent control of glycemic status before conception and should be maintained during 1st 8 weeks after conception.
- Periconceptional folic acid supplementation is also important.

Q. 29. What are the effects of uncontrolled DM on a 2nd trimester fetus?

- Hypertrophic cardiomyopathy
- Polyhydramnios
- Pleural effusion (PE)
- Fetal loss.

Q. 30. What are the effects of uncontrolled DM on 3rd trimester fetus?

- Macrosomia
- Intrauterine fetal death.

Q. 31. What are the factors contributing to sudden fetal death in diabetes?

- Vasculopathy and placental insufficiency
- Hyperglycemia
- Hypoglycemia
- Chronic intrauterine hypoxia
- Increased HbA1c → shift to left in oxygen dissociation curve → decreased oxygen release → fetal hypoxia
- Villous edema → impaired diffusion of oxygen across placental barrier
- Increased metabolic rate in macrosomia → increased oxygen demand by fetus
- Ketoacidosis
- Hypokalemia leading on to cardiac arrhythmia in the baby
- Placental dysfunction
- Congenital anomaly
- Preeclampsia and its complications.

Q. 32. What is the incidence of congenital malformations in diabetes? What are the anomalies?

2-6-fold increase in major malformations. The most common is cardiac anomalies, i.e. VSD and TGV. CNS malformations like anencephaly, holoprosencephaly and open spina bifida are also common. The most specific is sacral agenesis/caudal regression syndrome which is rare.

Q. 33. Can you predict risk of congenital anomaly in a pregestational diabetic mother?

It has a correlation with HbA1C in the periconceptional period (Table 2).

Table 2: Anomaly risk association with HbA1C levels

HbA1c	% of anomaly
< 6.1	3.7
6.1–9	5.2
9.1–12	8.2
12.1–15	32.2
>15	41.7

Q. 34. What is the mechanism of increased anomalies in diabetes?

- Metabolic abnormality during organogenesis—hyperglycemia, hypoglycemia, hyperketonemia
- Increased free oxygen radicals.

Q. 35. What are the effects of GDM on the neonate?

- Respiratory distress syndrome
- Hypoglycemia

- Hyperbilirubinemia
- Hypocalcemia
- Hypomagnesemia
- Birth injuries
- Increased operative delivery
- Polycythemia
- Macrosomia

Q. 36. Define neonatal hypoglycemia.

Blood glucose < 35 mg/dL.

Q. 37. Why baby develops hypoglycemia? Who explained the mechanism?

It is a complication of uncontrolled DM. In utero fetus is exposed to high levels of glucose, amino acids, and fatty acids. All these stimulate fetal islets to secrete more insulin. Islets undergo hyperplasia and hypertrophy. After birth, islets continue to produce excess insulin, but fuel supply has been cut off. So baby develops hypoglycemia. This is called Pederson's hypothesis.

Q. 38. How can one prevent this complication?

By maintaining euglycemia in the third trimester and intrapartum period.

> Explanations for neonatal complications. Page 1130 Williams Obstetrics 24th edition.

Q. 39. Why is RDS more common in babies of diabetic mothers?

Maternal hyperglycemia and consequent fetal hyperinsulinemia impairs pulmonary surfactant production by suppressing cortisol surge in mother.

Q. 40. Why is hypocalcemia more common in IDM?

Failure of neonatal parathyroid to increase parathormone secretion which in turn may be due to hypomagnesemia.

Q. 41. Why neonatal jaundice more in IDM?

Fetal hyperinsulinemia → increased fetal anabolism → increased oxyen requirement → polycythemia → excessive hemolysis after delivery.

Q. 42. What precaution taken at the time of delivery can decrease neonatal hyperinsulinemia?

Early cord clamping.

Q. 43. What are the long-term consequences of GDM on fetus?

Hyperglycemia leads to epigenetic changes in offspring by altered methylation and expression of genes associated with fat deposition and metabolic control, including leptin and adiponectin.

Hence, subsequent metabolic risk in adolescents develops, i.e. obesity and later on development of diabetes mellitus.

Other complications could be impaired cognitive development and impaired motor function.

Q. 44. What are the adverse effects of diabetes on the pregnant mother?

- More prone for ketoacidosis than non-pregnant state
- Increased incidence of preeclampsia due to placentomegaly
- Increased incidence of UTI, asymptomatic bacteriuria especially pyelonephritis
- Monilial vulvovaginitis
- Hydramnios
- Preterm labor
- Increased induction of labor
- More operative deliveries including instrumental deliveries
- Increased incidence of atonic and traumatic postpartum hemorrhage (PPH)
- Failure of lactation
- Increased febrile morbidity due to endometritis and wound infection

Diabetes in Pregnancy

- In pregestational diabetes, there will be worsening of diabetic nephropathy and proliferative retinopathy
- Type 2 DM (40–50%), and CVS diseases.

Q. 45. What is the policy for screening GDM in your institution?

We follow the DIPSI recommendation. It is a 'single step, diagnostic procedure for all patients (universal screening). In the antenatal clinic, after preliminary examination, the pregnant woman is given 75 g oral glucose load, irrespective of her fasting status or previous meal timing. GDM is diagnosed if the post two-hour blood glucose value is >/= 140 mg/dL. The rationale behind this test is that a normal glucose-tolerant woman would maintain euglycemia despite the glucose load, while in the GDM patient, the glycemic excursion exaggerates latent insulin deficiency. A summary of all the methods is given in Table 3.

GOI recommendations

Consume 75 g glucose in 300 mL water, drink in 5 minutes and also if vomits within 30 minutes, repeat the test on a different day.

Q. 46. What are the advantages of this single step diagnostic test?

- Pregnant woman need not be fasting
- The test can be performed in the first visit itself, can be repeated in the second and third trimester
- It hardly affects the daily routine of the woman
- It is both a screening as well as a diagnostic procedure.

Q. 47. What is the current IADPSG recommendation for screening and what is the basis for this recommendation?

IADPSG recommendation is 75 g OGTT, based on the HAPO study. The test is positive if any value is equal to or more than the cutoff.

Table 3: Diagnostic criteria for GDM

Criteria	FBS		2 Hr-PPBS	
WHO Plasma Glucose after 75 g glucose load	Either >126 mg		Or 140 mg	
	FBS	1 hour	2-hour	3-hour
ADA	95 mg	180	155	140 mg
HAPO consensus— Plasma glucose after 75 g glucose load	92 mg	180 mg	153 mg	
DIPSI– Plasma glucose after 75 g glucose load irrespective of fasting status- 2 hours	>140 mg			

Source: (High risk obstetrics-James)

Table 4: IADPSG recommendation for GDM diagnosis with 75 g glucose

Fasting plasma glucose	1 hour plasma glucose	2 hour plasma glucose
≥ 92 mg/dL	≥180 mg/dL	≥= 153 mg/dL

Q. 48. Who are the pioneers in developing screening for GDM?

O' Sullivian and Mahan.

Q. 49. What was the recommendation for diagnosis of GDM with 100 g GTT?

Refer Table 5.

Table 5: Cut off values

FBS	90
1 hour postprandial	165
2 hours postprandial	140
3 hours postprandial	120

If any 2 values were equal to or more than the cutoffs GDM was diagnosed

Later on, these values were modified to 105,190,160,140, respectively.

Q. 50. Why was this modification made?

The original values derived by O'Sullivan and Mahan was blood sugar estimation done from whole venous blood. Later on, the technique changed to that of estimating plasma glucose. Here, the values were 15% higher than that of whole venous blood.

Q. 51. What are the cutoff values recommended by Carpenter and Couston for 100 g glucose GTT? What was the basis of this change?

Table 6: Cutoff values for 100 g GTT

FBS	95
1 hour	180
2 hours	155
3 hours	135

Two or more of these values should be equal to or more for a diagnosis (Table 6)

There was a change in the technique of blood glucose estimation. Previously, Somogyi Nelson method was used where, in addition to glucose, other oxidizing agents in blood were also included. But in modern technique of glucose estimation, only glucose is detected and measured by glucose oxidase method. So, values were naturally less. Carpenter and Couston found that perinatal complications were less when these lower values which represented the true glucose values, were taken as cutoff.

Q. 52. What is the normal fasting blood glucose in a nondiabetic pregnant lady?

69 ± 9 mg%.

Q. 53. Name a few studies related to diabetes and pregnancy.

- DIPSI—Diabetes in Pregnancy Study Group India
- HAPO—Hyperglycemia and Adverse Pregnancy Outcomes
- ACHOIS—Australian Carbohydrate Intolerance Study
- DAPIT—Diabetes and Preeclampsia Intervention Trial
- MiG—Metformin in Gestational Diabetes
- M-FMUN—Maternal and Fetal Medicine Units Network study.

Q. 54. What is the key to successful management of diabetes in pregnancy?

Patient education and achieving and maintaining euglycemia in periconceptional period and throughout pregnancy and intrapartum.

Q. 55. Would you prefer universal or selective screening for GDM? Why?

Universal screening, i.e. all pregnant women will be screened because by ethnicity, all Indian women fall into medium risk category for GDM (see Table 7).

- If the prevalence is <3%, screening is done based on historic risk factors
- If >3% provocative testing with 50 g OGCT/ 75 g GCT is recommended.

Table 7: Historic risk factors and rationale for universal screening

Risk factors	Screening
• BMI >30 • Previous macrosomia • Past pregnancy with GDM • 1st degree relative with GDM • Ethnic origin—Asia, Arab, black Caribbean • Previous abnormal glucose tolerance • Poor obstetric outcome earlier • Previous LGA infant • PCOS • Age >25 years	• ADA-no routine screening for low risk • All criteria if applied only 10% of pregnant population form low risk • Selective screening will miss 30% cases • So in the interest of simplicity, many recommend universal screening

Q. 56. Once you make a diagnosis of GDM, how will you manage the case?

To achieve and maintain euglycemia is the aim.

Medical nutritional therapy, exercise and insulin/hypoglycemic agents like metformin, glyburide or a combination are the three modalities of treatment.

- *Exercise:* Half an hour of mild to moderate upper limb exercise or walking after each meal will help to control postprandial hyperglycemia
- *Medical nutrition therapy:* This is done in consultation with a nutritionist, taking into account the dietary habits and cultural preferences. The total calorific value according to the BMI of the woman is:
  - BMI<25 kg/sqm—3000 cal/day
  - Overweight (BMI 25-30 kg/sqm)—2500 cal/day
  - Morbid obesity (BMI >40 kg/sqm)—1250 cal/day.

The total calorie requirement should consist of <45% carbohydrate, 30% protein and 25% fat (mainly unsaturated fats). This is met through three major meals and three minor meals at equal intervals. Also, high fiber diet and one that has a low glycemic index is able to avoid insulin therapy to a large extent (Details given in Table 8).

A close watch on the weight gained during pregnancy at each antenatal visit is important as both obesity and diabetes are associated with macrosomia. Similarly, excessive weight gain and edema may be an early sign of developing preeclampsia.

- Insulin
- Metformin
- Glyburide

Table 8: Glycemic index of food and their importance

• It is the extent of rise in blood sugar in response to a food in comparison indicates with the response to an equivalent amount of glucose

Contd...

Contd...

• The CHO that produces only small fluctuation in blood glucose and insulin levels are called low GI foods and are recommended for use by GDM women

Low glycemic index foods will enhance in vivo sensitivity to endogenous insulin causing decrease in the requirement of drugs, and decreased complications.

Low GI	Legumes and lentils, dried beans, peas, green gram, Bengal gram (rich in fiber) (30–40%)
Medium GI	Fruits (45–55%)
High GI	Cereals like rice, white bread, root vegetables-potato, carrot, candy bars and syrupy foods (65–70%)

Q. 57. What are the indications for starting insulin along with MNT?

Usually we wait for 1–2 weeks to see whether MNT and exercise will achieve euglycemia. But insulin is started immediately if:

- Fasting hyperglycemia
- Macrosomia
- GDM diagnosed near EDC as in the case of my patient (no time to wait for MNT to control the blood sugar levels)
- Wait for 2 weeks with MNT and exercise, if 2 hours PPBS is <120 mg continue MNT and monitor FBS and PPBS once in 2 weeks till 28 weeks and once a week later
- If 2 hr PPBS >120 mg start insulin and monitor FBS and PPBS once in 3 days till levels are stabilized by adjusting insulin dosage and later weekly monitor.

Q. 58. What are the therapeutic targets recommended?

- FBS ≤95 mg/dL
- 1hr PPBS ≤140 mg/dL
- 2hr PPBS ≤120 mg/dL

- Before each meal: 60–105 mg/dL
- 2 AM to 6 AM: >60 mg/dL

Q. 59. Is there any difference in therapeutic targets based on the fetal biometric parameters?

- AC >75th centile, a more rigid glycemic control needed, i.e. maintain
- FBS < 80 mg/dL
- 2 hr PPBS <100 mg/dL
- Very stringent control of sugars to FBS < 86 mg may put >20% babies to the risk of SGA.

Q. 60. What is the mechanism of development of macrosomia?

Macrosomia is a complication of uncontrolled diabetes.

Maternal hyperglycemia → Fetal hyperglycemia → Fetal islet hyperplasia → Fetal hyperinsulinemia → Increased fetal anabolism → Macrosomia (Pederson's hypothesis).

Q. 61. All hyperglycemic mothers do not have macrosomic babies and some babies may even be growth restricted. Why?

This may be due to glucokinase gene mutation in the fetus which affects the birth weight. Glucokinase in the pancreas senses glucose levels in the blood and controls the insulin release. Mutant gene → defective insulin secretion. In case of fetal glucokinase mutation, maternal hyperglycemia will not induce fetal hyperinsulinemia. Hence, there will not be macrosomia and may even result in a growth retardation.

Q. 62. What is the effect if mother has a glucokinase mutation?

The maternal hyperglycemia transmitted to the fetus, will lead to fetal hyperinsulinemia and hence macrosomia. This usually is known as MODY 2 (maturity onset diabetes of the youth) which is being diagnosed more frequently and known to run in different generations of the family.

Q. 63. What is the effect if both the mother and fetus has glucokinase mutation?

There will not be any change in the baby weight.

Q. 64. What are the different types of insulins used in pregnancy?

Refer Table 9.

Table 9: Recombinant human insulins and insulin analogs can be used

Insulin preparation used in pregnancy	Onset of action	Peak action	Duration of action
Short-acting			
Human regular insulin	½–1 hr	2–4 hr	4–6 hr
Intermediate acting			
NPH	3–4 hr	10–16 hr	20–24 hr
Biphasic (premixed)			
NPH + regular (mixtard)	0.5 hr	2–10 hr	12–18 hr

Q. 65. What advise you will give the patient regarding insulin administration?

- Teach her about symptoms of hypoglycemia
- Encourage self glucose monitoring. In case symptoms s/o hypoglycemia occurs, GRBS should be done and if low she should take some sugar which should be always available nearby
- Ask her to take insulin 30 min before meal. never omit a meal after insulin
- Diet should have a consistent pattern, i.e. High fluctuation in CHO content day to day not advisable.

Q. 66. Why insulin is given 30 min before meal? Why not along with meal?

While in storage form insulin remain as hexamers. After s/c injection it will split into monomers and then only it can get absorbed. The process takes about 30 min.

Q. 67. How will you decide on type and dose of insulin to be started?

If blood glucose is not controlled with MNT and exercise or otherwise insulin is indicated, the glucose profile is evaluated. If FBS is normal and PPBS values are higher regular insulin is given ½ hour before each major meal. If FBS is also high, NPH is added at bed time. NPH should not be given earlier because peak action will occur after midnight when hypoglycemia may be missed.

Insulin resistance is maximum in the morning because of diurnal variation in secretion of anti-insulin hormones. So 2/3 of total dose of insulin is given in the morning and 1/3 in the evening

For pregestational DM already on insulin dose can be adjusted for the desired control. To start insulin, dose can be 0.5 units/kg for pregestational and 0.2 units/kg for GDM. Then according to blood glucose values before and after each meal dose can be adjusted. For example, if post-breakfast value is high, morning dose of regular insulin should be increased. If FBS is high, bedtime dose of NPH is increased.

Q. 68. For managing pregestational DM in pregnancy, would you prefer premixed insulin?

It has the advantage of twice daily administration. But proportion of intermediate acting and regular is fixed, so we cannot adjust each according to each patient's blood sugar profile. So, in pregnancy where rigid control is aimed, regimen of regular and intermediate insulins given separately is preferred.

Q. 69. What are insulin analogs?

- They are agents structurally similar to insulin produced by substituting or changing the position of one or more aminoacids from the native insulin. Confers altered pharmacokinetic properties
- Better qualities to mimick endogenous insulin
- They lower blood sugar in a pattern mimicking endogenous insulin
- They have different pharmacokinetics different preparations have different onset of action and duration of action
- In pregnancy short-acting analogs like aspart and lispro are used. Long-acting analogs like glargine are also now reported to be safe in pregnancy.

Q. 70. What are the advantages of analogs over recombinant human insulin?

- It can be given just before food
- No need to wait as it is absorbed fast
- The blood level mimicks that of natural insulin
- Risk of hypoglycaemia is less.

Q. 71. What is the importance of diagnosing and treating diabetes in pregnancy?

Refer Table 10.

Table 10: Treatment of diabetes in pregnancy

Risks of not treated	Treatment will significantly reduce some of the adverse maternal and neonatal outcomes
Preeclampsia—increased by 21% Shoulder dystocia—18% Primary C section rates—8–11% ACHOIS- Intervention vs nonintervention groups	PTL, NICU admissions, hyperbilirubinemia-depended not on FBS but 1 and 2 hours values
Serious perinatal outcomes—1% vs 4% Preeclampsia—12% vs 18% Postpartum depression—8% vs 17% LGA—13% vs 22% PNM—5 deaths vs none in intervention group (p value—0.07) Shoulder dystocia—not significant—1% vs 3%	ACHOIS study M-FMUN study Landon et al.

Bibliography

1. ADA Diagnosis and Classsification of Diabetes Mellitus. Diabetes Care. 2009;32:S62-7.
2. American College of Obstetricians and Gynecologists. Gestational Diabetes Mellitus. Practice Bulletin Number. 2013;137.
3. Bhide A, Arulkumaran S, Damania KR, et al. Arias' Practical Guide to High-risk Pregnancy and Delivery. 4th edition. Elsevier; 2015.
4. Bradley RJ, Nicolaides KH, Brudenell JM. Are all infants of diabetic mothers 'macrosomic'? BMJ. 1988;297:1583.
5. Buchanan TA, Kjos Sl, Montoro MN, et al. Use of fetal ultrasound to select metabolic therapy for pregnancies complicated by mild gestational diabetes. Diabetes Care. 1994;17:275-83.
6. Correa A, Gilboa SM, Besser LM, et al. Diabetes mellitus and birth defects. AMJ Obstet Gynecol. 2008;199:237.
7. Cunningham, Leveno, Bloom, et al. Williams Obstetrics. 24th edition. McGraw Hill Education; 2014.
8. De Marini S, Mimouni F, Tsang RC, et al. Impact of metabolic control of diabetes during pregnancy on neonatal hypoglycemia: a randomized study. Obstet Gynecol. 1994;83:918.
9. Getahun D, Fassett MJ, Jacobsen SG: Gestational diabetes: risk of recurrence in subsequent pregnancies. AMJ Obstet Gynecol. 2010; 203:467.
10. Hattersley AT, Beards F, Ballantyne E, et al. Mutation in the Glucokinase Gene of the fetus results in reduced birth weight. Nat Genet. 1998;19:268-70.
11. Hunt KJ, Logan SL, Conway DL, et al. Postpartum screening following GDM: How well are we doing? Curr Diab Rep. 2010;10:235.
12. International Association of Diabetes in Pregnancy Study Group Consensus Panel: Recommendations on diagnosis and classification of Hyperglycemia in pregnancy. Diabetes Care. 2010;33(3).
13. Jovanovic- Peterson L, Durak EP, Peterson CM. Randomized trial of diet Vs diet plus cardiovascular conditioning on glucose level in gestational diabetes. Am J Obstet Gynecol. 1989;161:415.
14. Kerlan V. Postpartum and contraception in women after gestational diabetes. Diabetes Metab. 2010;36:566.
15. Kitzmiller JL, Block JM, Brown FM et al. Managing pre-existing diabetes for pregnancy. Diabetes Care. 2008;31(5):1060.
16. Kjos SL, Schaefer-Graf UM. Modified therapy for Gestational Diabetes using high risk and low risk fetal abdominal circumference growth to select strict vs relaxed maternal glycemic target. Diab Care. 2007;30:S200-5.
17. Landon MB, Mele L, Spong CY, et al. The relationship between maternal glycemia and perinatal outcome. Obstetrics and Gynecol. 2011;117(2):218.
18. Langer O, Conway Dl, Berkus MD, et al. A comparison between glyburide and insulin in women with GDM. N Engl J Med. 2000;343:1134.
19. Langer O, Yogev Y, Zenakis EMJ, et al. Insulin and glyburide therapy: dosage, severity level of gestational diabetes and pregnancy outcome. AMJ Obstet Gynecol. 2005;192:134.
20. Metzger BE, Lowe LP, Dyer AR, et al. Hyperglycemia and Adverse Pregnancy Outciome. N Eng J Med. 2008;358:1991-2002.
21. Misra R. Ian Donald's Practical Obstetric Problems. 7th edition. Wolters Kluwer; 2014.
22. National Institute for Health and Clinical Excellence: Diabetes in pregnancy. Management of DM and its complications from preconception to postnatal period: Clinical Guideline No. 63; 2008.
23. O'Sullivan JB, Mahan CM. Criteria for the Oral Glucose Tolerance test in Pregnancy. Diabetes. 1964;13:278-85.
24. Raymond O Powrie, Michael F Greene, William Camann. De Swiet's Medical Disorders in Obstetric Practice. 5th edition. Wiley-Blackwell; 2010.
25. Reece EA. Diabetes induced birth defects: What do we know? What can we do? Curr Diab Rep. 2012;12:24.
26. Sheshiah V. Handbook on diabetes mellitus. 4th edition. All India Publishers and Distributers; 2009.
27. Studd J, Lin Tan S, Chervenak FA. Current progress in obstetrics and gynecology-1. Tree Life Media; 2012.

CHAPTER 6

Fever in Pregnancy

D Leela

CASE

Mrs R. aged 28 years, a primigravidae at 32 weeks of gestation, presented to the antenatal outpatient department with following complaints:
- High-grade fever with chills and rigors of 3 days duration
- Weakness, fatigue and occasional headache
- Abdominal discomfort with burning micturition
- Nausea and occasional vomiting.

Initially, her fever was low grade and intermittent. She had cold and throat pain for which she took an antipyretic. In a day, it became a high grade, continuous fever with chills and rigors, followed by sweating. Due to the fever, she had nausea and could not eat anything. As the weakness and fatigue increased along with fever, she was brought to the hospital.

Obstetric History

- Married for 2 years
- Nonconsanguineous marriage
- Regular menstrual cycles
- Spontaneous conception LMP:_____ EDD:_____
- Regular antenatal checkups from 8 weeks of gestation
- Underwent all required antenatal investigations
- Dating ultrasound scan confirmed expected date of delivery
- Combined screen with nuchal translucency and biochemistry ruled out trisomies
- Anomaly scan at 18 weeks ruled out structural anomalies. First growth scan at 28 weeks confirmed satisfactory fetal growth
- Immunised against tetanus
- On oral iron, folate and calcium supplementation
- Nutrition is adequate.

Medical and Surgical History

No comorbidities.

Family History

No medical disorders, no congenital anomalies.

Personal History

No addictions. Belonged to the middle income group, graduate, home maker; husband is a bank employee. Both hail from Visakhapatnam.

General Examination

Vitals

Temperature: 38.4°C, Pulse: 120/minute, BP: 100/70 mm Hg., Respiratory rate: 30/minute.

She was pale, dehydrated, anicteric, with no rash, petechiae or lymphadenopathy.

Systemic Examination

CVS and respiratory systems: No abnormality.
CNS: Conscious and coherent with no neck rigidity or motor weakness.
Breasts: Normal, with physiological changes of pregnancy.
Abdominal examination: No hepatosplenomegaly.

Obstetric Examination

- Uterine fundal height corresponded to 32 weeks gestation
- A singleton fetus with cephalic presentation was felt. Fetal heart sounds were well heard with pocket Doppler
- Liquor appeared adequate
- Clinically, the fetus was not growth restricted
- Mild generalized abdominal tenderness at examination
- However, no regular uterine activity was noted.

Pelvic Examination

Not done as there was no vaginal discharge or history suggestive of preterm labor.

Discussion

Q. 1. What are the possible causes of fever in this patient?

Common causes for fever with this type of clinical picture would be:
- Malarial fever
- Urinary tract infection
- Dengue fever
- Viral influenza including H1N1 fever
- Typhoid fever.

Q. 2. What investigations do you do to confirm your diagnosis of malaria?

The following investigations will help to arrive at diagnosis (Figs 1 and 2):
- Peripheral blood smear examination:
  - Stained with Giemsa or Wright stain
  - Thick smear helps identify the presence of malarial parasite
  - Thin smear is to identify the type of malarial parasite and degree of parasitemia
  - It is the gold standard test to confirm malarial infection
  - In a febrile patient, *three negative smears* over a 12–24-hour period can safely rule out the diagnosis of malaria
- Rapid diagnostic tests (RDT):
  - Help diagnose malarial antigens in the blood in 15–20 minutes
  - Dipstick method from the blood sample
  - Presence of specific bands in the test window confirm the type of malarial parasite infection
  - Useful in places where microscopy is not readily available.

Q. 3. What is severe and complicated malaria?

If parasitized red cells are more than 2% in the maternal blood it results in severe disease with complications.

Q. 4. What are the maternal complications of malarial fever?

The following complications are seen if the infection is severe (complicated malaria)
- Anemia
- Hypoglycemia
- Pulmonary edema
- Respiratory distress
- Renal failure
- Convulsions and altered sensorium due to cerebral malaria
- Jaundice
- Bleeding diathesis
- Septicemia
- Shock.

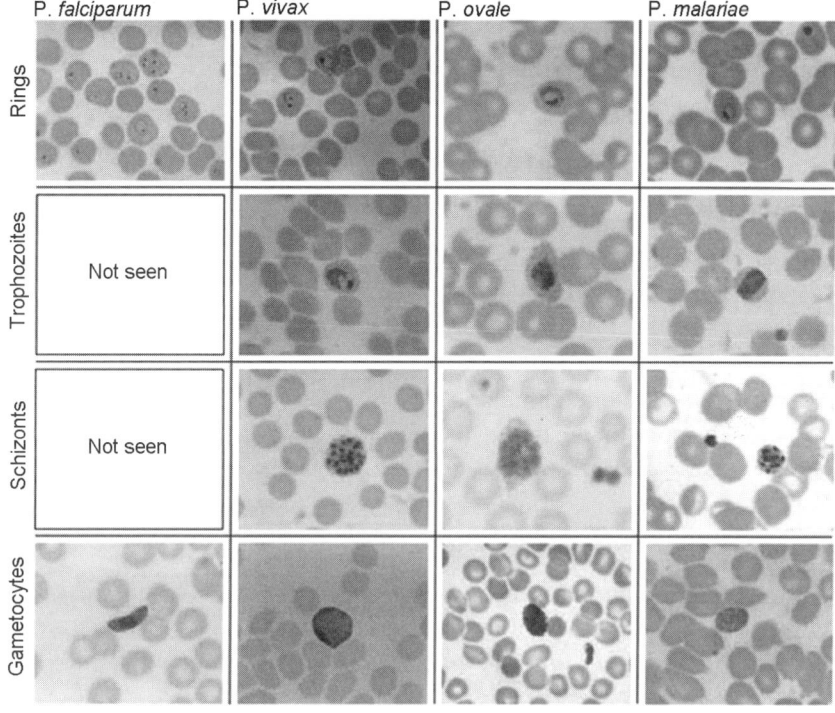

Fig. 1: Identification of species of malaria based on forms seen on blood smears
(*Source:* Taken from internet images—Protozoan Infections part I)

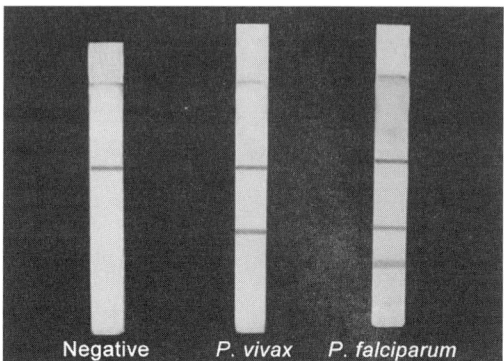

Fig. 2: Rapid diagnostic tests for malaria parasites
(*Source:* Taken from Clinical Microbiology Reviews. 2002;15(1):66-78)

Q. 5. How do you assess the severity of malarial fever?

There are some ominous signs of malaria:

- Pallor, jaundice, altered sensorium, tachycardia, hypotension, respiratory distress, point to a seriously ill patient
- The degree of parasitemia in peripheral smear: >2% of parasitized RBC indicates overwhelming infection
- Confirmatory tests: Hb <8 g/dL, thrombocytopenia. Blood sugar <40 mg/dL, oliguria, urine output <0.4 mL/kg body wt/hour, acidosis, gram-negative septicemia.

Q. 6. What are the principles of treatment of malaria in pregnancy?

- Assessing the severity of infection and hospitalization
- Supportive care, if necessary, intensive care
- Team approach—obstetrician, laboratory support, infectious disease specialist and intensivist
- Prompt treatment with antimalarial agents as per national guidelines
- Antenatal care for rest of the pregnancy with fetal surveillance.

Q. 7. What is the drug treatment for malaria?

The choice of drug depends on the type of the malarial parasite causing fever, severity and gestational age.

Primaquin should not be used in pregnancy, but can be given postdelivery.

If patient has vomiting intravenous route is preferred.

Uncomplicated *Plasmodium falciparum* infection (Table 1)

Table 1: Drugs used and their dosage in malaria and their safety in pregnancy

Drug	Dose	Indications
Chloroquine	Loading dose of 600 mg followed by 300 mg 6–8 hours later on 1st day 1, 300 mg OD on day 2 and day 3	Does not work if there is resistance. Safe in pregnancy
Quinine	10 mg/kg body weight × 8th hourly × 7 days. Can be combined with clindamycin 450 mg × 8th hourly	Safe in 1st trimester. Drug of choice in chloroquine resistant cases
Artesunate	4 mg/kg orally in divided doses on day 1 followed by 2 mg/kg orally for next 6 days	Useful in 2nd and 3rd trimester
Artesunate Pyrimethamine + Sulfadoxine	50 mg × 4 tablets on days 1, 2 and 3 25 mg + 500 mg × 3 tablets on day 1 only	Recommended in 2nd and 3rd trimester

Uncomplicated *P. vivax* and other types of infection:

Oral chloroquine 600 mg initially, followed by 300 mg after 6 hours on day 1 and 300 mg single dose on days 2 and 3.

Complicated falciparum malaria (Table 2)

Table 2: Treatment for complicated malaria

Drug	Dose
Quinine	Loading dose of 20 mg/kg in 5% dextrose IV infusion over 4 hours, followed by 10 mg/kg × 8th hourly till patient can be started on oral medication to finish 7 day course
Clindamycin	10 mg/kg IV × 8th hourly, followed by oral medication of same dose till 7 day course is completed
Artesunate	2.4 mg/kg IV at 0, 12 and 24 hours followed by OD dose till patient is able to take orally to complete 7 day course

Q. 8. What is cinchonism?

Side effects of quinine are described as cinchonism:

- Tinnitus
- Blurring of vision
- Headache
- Nausea
- Diarrhea
- Altered auditory acuity.

Q. 9. How do you manage the complications of malaria?

- Anemia: It is more commonly seen in women who are not immune to malaria, If Hb is <8 g/dL. Packed cell transfusion is indicated

- Hypoglycemia: Develops due to infection as well as from quinine. Treated with a bolus of 25–50 mL of 50% glucose followed by infusion of 5% glucose
- Pulmonary edema: Managed with close monitoring and fluid restriction
- Renal failure: May need dialysis
- Circulatory collapse and DIC: Blood and blood products are to be supplemented
- Septicemia: Full work up for infection along with parenteral broad spectrum antibiotics are indicated
- Cerebral malaria: Oxygenation to avoid hypoxia, correction of hypoglycemia, prevention or treatment of convulsions with benzodiazepines, dilantinize all patients with more than 2 seizures, maintain fluid balance and correct anemia. Be ready to ventilate.

Q. 10. Congenital malaria.

- Development of malaria in the newborn due to transmission of malarial parasites or infected red cells in utero or at the time of delivery, but not by mosquito bite
- Incidence is 0.3% and 1–4% in newborns of immune and nonimmune mothers respectively
- Feeding problems, fever, restlessness, anemia, jaundice and hepatosplenomegaly are some of the clinical problems.

Q. 11. What are the effects of pregnancy on malaria?

- Pregnant women are at greater risk due to low immunity
- Primi gravidae and adolescents are at greater risk
- Infection is more severe in 2nd trimester due to placental sequestration
- Associated HIV infection increases the severity
- Severity is related to splenic sequestration and placental sequestration of parasitized red cells
- Mortality in pregnancy can be as high as 50%.

Q. 12. What is the specific obstetric management in malaria?

Management of malaria in pregnancy is shown in Flowchart 1.

- 1st trimester:
  - Treat the infection as per the severity
  - No indication for termination of pregnancy
  - Miscarriages may happen due to severe infection/hyperpyrexia
  - Continue regular antenatal care
  - Advise about prevention of recurrence
- 2nd trimester and 3rd trimesters:
  - Treat the infection as per the severity
  - Antenatal care as recommended with monitoring of hemoglobin, platelets and blood glucose
  - Steps to prevent recurrence once the infection is cleared
  - Weekly 300 mg of chloroquine until delivery and breastfeeding completed in non-falciparum malaria to prevent recurrence
  - Monitor fetal growth and well-being as there is risk of fetal growth restriction and stillbirth
  - Risk of preeclampsia
  - Risk of preterm labor: Tocolysis and steroids can be considered if there is no contraindication
  - If fetal growth restriction or fetal heart abnormalities are detected, management is individualized as per the severity and gestational age with team approach involving obstetrician, neonatologist, fetal medicine specialist and infectious disease specialist.

Peripartum malaria
- Women should be informed of vertical transmission and risk of congenital malaria to the newborns and infants

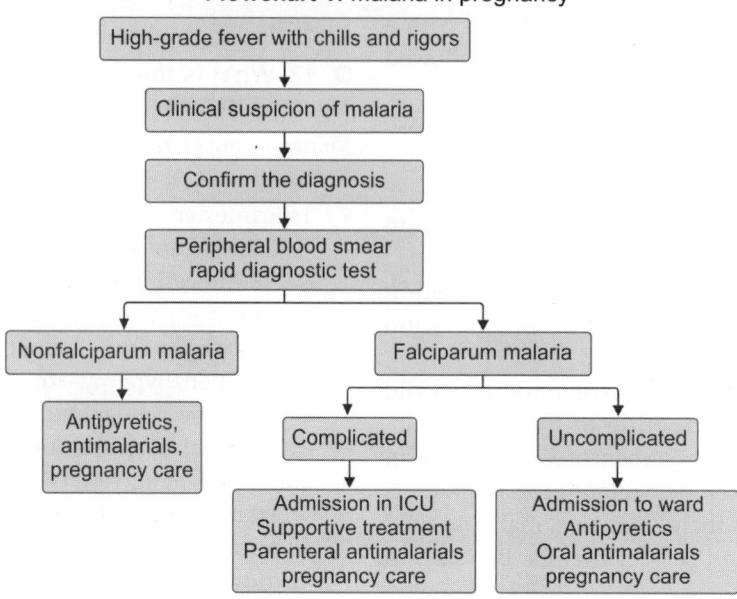

Flowchart 1: Malaria in pregnancy

- Histology of placenta, blood films from placenta, umbilical cord and newborn will help diagnose congenital infection.

Delivery
- No role for elective induction or elective LSCS
- No role for instrumental delivery in 2nd stage due to malaria
- Risk of postpartum hemorrhage if there is thrombocytopenia.

Postpartum:
- No contraindication for breastfeeding
- Primaquin can be given for eradication if there is no risk of G-6-PD deficiency in non-falciparum malaria. Dose is 15 mg base/day × 14 days.

Q. 13. Preventive measures recommended by WHO.

- Use of long-lasting insecticidal nets (LLIN)
- Indoor residual spraying of insecticides
- Intermittent preventive treatment in pregnancy using pyrimethamine and sulfadoxine from 2nd trimester onwards this practice is stopped in India from 2010.

Q. 14. Preventive measures recommended by Government of India.

Prevention of mosquito breeding in clean still and standing water:
- Do not allow stagnation of water around houses
- Properly cover all water storage containers
- Release mosquito eating Gambusia fish into wells, ponds and large pools of water
- Houses should be sprayed with insecticides
- To prevent mosquito bites, use bednets and mosquito repellents
- Full course of treatment for malaria be taken if there is a clinical attack.

Note

1. *Definition of fever in pregnancy and puerperium:*
   A rise in body temperature by 38°C once or 37.5°C on two occasions, 2 hours apart, during pregnancy or puerperium.
2. *Low-grade fever:*
   Fever that does not exceed 37.8°C and usually rises by evening, e.g. tuberculosis.

3. *Conditions of hyperpyrexia:*
   - Temperature >41.5°C is called hyperpyrexia
   - Malaria
   - Septicemia
   - Tetanus
   - Encephalitis
   - Pontine hemorrhage.
4. *Conditions of hyperthermia:*
   The body temperature is set high due to outside source without fever, e.g. heat stroke.
5. *Malignant hyperthermia or malignant hyperpyrexia:*
   An autosomal dominant condition in which affected person develops rapid rise in body temperature and muscle contractions when exposed to volatile anesthetic gases.
6. *Causes for fever during antenatal period:*
   These can be due to infections affecting specific organ in the body or can be due to noninfectious causes (Table 3).

Table 3: Causes of fever in pregnancy

Infections	Organ-specific infections	Non-Infectious causes
Viral: Influenza, rubella, CMV, herpes, dengue, chikungunya, etc. **Bacterial:** Streptococcus, E.coli, Pseudomonas, enteric fever **Protozoa:** Malaria, Toxoplasma, amebiasis **Fungal (Rare):** Candida	**UTI:** Cystisis, pyelonephritis **Respiratory:** Bronchitis, pneumonia, tuberculosis **Uterine:** Chorioamnionitis **GIT:** Hepatitis, enteritis, pancreatitis, appendicitis **Cardiac:** Subacute bacterial endocarditis **Neurological:** Meningitis, malaria	**Adnexal accidents** Ovary: Torsion, hemorrhage, rupture or infection Uterus: Red degeneration of fibroid **Endocrine/ metabolic** Diabetic ketoacidosis, pheochromocytoma, hyperthyroidism

Contd...

Infections	Organ-specific infections	Non-Infectious causes
		Thrombosis DVT, pulmonary embolism **Malignancy** Leukemia, lymphoma **Other causes** Hyperemesis, sickle cell crisis, malignant hyperthermia **Pyrexia of unknown origin**

The investigations need to be individualized and done based on the clinical suspicion of a diagnosis.

The following may give a clue to the diagnosis:
- Respiratory symptoms, direct towards RS
- Urinary frequency, fever with chills, dysuria point towards UTI
- Endemicity of a disease
- Local epidemics like chikungunya fever, dengue, etc.
- Family history of a diagnosed pyrexia
- Low platelet count toward dengue
- Typhoid epidemics/bradycardia.

7. *Causes of fever during intrapartum period:*
   - Chorioamnionitis
   - Dehydration
   - Epidural analgesia
   - All the causes of fever in the antenatal period
   - Drug induced-misoprostol.
8. *Common causes of fever during puerperium:*
   - Genital tract infection: Endomyometritis, pelvic abscess
   - UTI: Cystitis, pyelonephritis
   - Breast: Engorgement, acute mastitis, breast abscess

Contd...

- Wound infection: LSCS site, episiotomy and perineal tears
- Misoprostol in excess used to control PPH.

9. *Types of fever:*
   - Continuous: Temperature remains above normal and does not fluctuate >1°C in 24 hours, e.g. typhoid, meningitis, lobar pneumonia and urinary infection
   - Remittent: Temperature remains above normal but fluctuation is >1°C in 24 hours, e.g. infective endocarditis
   - Intermittent: Temperature remains elevated for certain period of time and later cycles back to normal
   - Quotidian fever: Periodicity of 24 hours, falciparum malaria
   - Tertian fever: Periodicity of 48 hours, vivax and ovale malaria
   - Quartan fever: Periodicity of 72 hours, malariae malaria
   - Pel-Ebstein fever: High fever for a few days followed by low-grade fever in cyclical form, Hodgkin's lymphoma.

10. *Fever with chills and rigors*
    - Malaria
    - Filariasis
    - Urinary tract infection
    - Cholangitis
    - Abscesses
    - Pneumonia
    - Infective endocarditis
    - Septicemia
    - Kala-azar.

11. *Fever with rash:*
    - Chickenpox
    - Zoster
    - Measles
    - Rubella
    - B19 parvovirus
    - Typhus
    - Allergy.

12. *Fever with petechiae:*
    - Dengue
    - Leptospirosis.

13. *Fever with membrane in the throat:*
    - Diphtheria
    - Infectious mononucleosis
    - Candidiasis
    - Agranulocytosis
    - Vincent's angina.

14. *Fever with delirium:*
    - Encephalitis
    - Typhoid
    - Meningitis
    - Pneumonia
    - Liver disease
    - Cerebral malaria.

15. *Important features in history taking:*
    - Onset and duration
    - Grade and pattern
    - Relief with antipyretics
    - Contact with people having fever
    - Travel to endemic areas
    - Associated symptoms: mostly relate to:
      - Cause of fever
      - Any drug consumed
      - Exposure to animals, insects
      - Infected fellow traveler while traveling
      - Immunization status
      - Marital history, history of partner, change of partner, etc.
      - Chills and rigors
      - Cough with/without sputum, cold, throat pain
      - Urinary frequency, burning
      - Nausea, vomiting, loose stools
      - Abdominal pain—site, severity and nature
      - Headache
      - Calf pain
      - Convulsions
      - Vaginal discharge
      - Fetal movements

16. *Important signs to check in clinical examination:*
    - Record the temperature, pulse rate, respiratory rate and BP
    - Look of the patient; flushed, toxic, ill looking
    - Rash: type and distribution
    - Tongue for pallor, hydration and icterus
    - Conjunctiva for pallor and icterus
    - Throat for congestion, tonsillar enlargement
    - Neck nodes
    - CVS and respiratory system examination
    - Tenderness in the renal angles, both loins, right and left hypochondria, epigastrium and suprapubic area
    - Calf tenderness, knee joint tenderness
    - Obstetric examination
    - Vaginal examination if needed.

Fever with lymphadenopathy (generalized or localized)
Generalized in—syphilis, toxoplasmosis and viral infections.
Localized in—
a. Inguinal STD like syphilis, chancorid, LGV, etc.
b. Cervical—*Streptococcus*, TB, EBV

17. *Recommended investigations for fever:*
    Infections are to tailored to the clinical picture

    Commonly done investigations are:
    - Full blood count with differential count
    - Peripheral smear
    - Mid-stream urine sample for microscopy and C/S
    - Swabs for C/S
    - Blood culture—both aerobic and anaerobic if fever is high-grade and persistent.

    Other Investigations
    - Liver function tests, serum electrolytes, renal function tests
    - Serological tests if viral or dengue fever are suspected
    - Swabs: Throat, wound site, vaginal, endocervical, endometrial or placental
    - Sputum for AFB and C/S
    - Chest X-ray (abdominal shielding during antenatal period)
    - 2D echo
    - USG of abdomen including fetal well being
    - Leg vein Doppler
    - Lumbar puncture
    - V/Q scan if pulmonary embolism is suspected.

Normally fetal core temperature is more than maternal core temperature and thus allowing transfer of heat only one way that is from fetus to mother. But when the maternal temperature becomes very high heat is transferred to fetus and causes all problems as the temperature regulation is not matured in the baby.

18. *Effects of fever on fetus:*
    The effects depend on:
    a. Gestational age
    b. Severity
    c. Cause of fever
        - 1st trimester:
            - Miscarriages
            - Fetal structural defects mostly CNS, cardiac and eye
        - 2nd and 3rd trimester:
            - Preterm labor
            - Preterm premature rupture of membranes
            - Intrauterine growth restriction
            - Stillbirth
            - Neonatal morbidity and rarely mortality due to congenital infections and sepsis.

19. *Modes of transmission to fetus/neonate:*
    - Transplacental transfer via umbilical blood flow or direct spread to amniotic fluid
    - Ascending infection from cervix and uterus to amniotic fluid
    - Intrapartum exposure to maternal vaginal secretions and blood

- Postpartum exposure to maternal respiratory infections and breast milk.
20. *USG findings of in utero fetal infections:*
    - IUGR
    - Echogenic bowel
    - Intracranial calcification
    - Hydrocephalus
    - Microcephaly
    - Isolated ascites
    - Pericardial or pleural effusion
    - Nonimmune hydrops.
21. *'Chorioamnionitis':*
    Infection of amniotic fluid, membranes, placenta and or decidua, also called as 'intra-amniotic infection'
    Causes
    - Premature rupture of membranes (PROM) resulting in ascent of infection from cervix and vagina
    - Bacteremia causing transplacental spread
    - Iatrogenic: due to invasive procedures like amniocentesis, CVS and fetal surgery.
22. *Clinical presentation of chorioamnionitis:*
    - Fever >37.8°C
    - Maternal tachycardia >100 beats/minute
    - Fetal tachycardia >160 beats/minute
    - Uterine tenderness
    - Foul smelling vaginal discharge
    - Leukocytosis of >15,000 cell/mm^3.
23. *Maternal effects of fever:*
    - Transient illness
    - Hospitalization in certain fevers
    - Prolonged usage of medication, e.g. TB, recurrent UTI
    - Anxiety about pregnancy
    Rare complications
    - Pulmonary edema
    - Renal failure
    - Disseminated intravascular coagulation (DIC)
    - Convulsions, delirium
    - Septicemia, adult respiratory distress syndrome
    - Maternal mortality.
24. *Steps of management of fever in antenatal period (Flowchart 2):*
    - Good history
    - Thorough clinical examination
    - Necessary investigations
    - Team approach—obstetrician, physician, microbiologist and neonatologist
    - Inpatient/outpatient management depending on the severity
    - Hydration, cold sponging, antipyretics and antibiotics based on the cause of fever
    - Prompt control of fever to minimize adverse fetal effects
    - Plan delivery as per the clinical situation.
25. *Steps of managing intrapartum fever:*
    - Control of temperature with oral or parenteral paracetamol
    - Intravenous hydration if necessary
    - Intravenous broad spectrum antibiotics administration if fever remains high or there is any suspicion of infection without delay
    - Blood cultures and other cultures are to be taken before starting antibiotics
    - Continuation of parenteral antibiotics during labor and immediate postpartum
    - Oral antibiotics to be given for a minimum of 5 days
    - Labor may need to be augmented to minimize maternal and fetal effects.
26. *Steps of managing postpartum fever:*
    - Good history and examination to find out the cause
    - Oral or parenteral paracetamol
    - Adequate hydration and nutrition
    - Broad spectrum antibiotics
    - Encourage breastfeeding, teach correct method if there is breast engorgement or crack nipples

Flowchart 2: Fever in pregnancy and management protocol

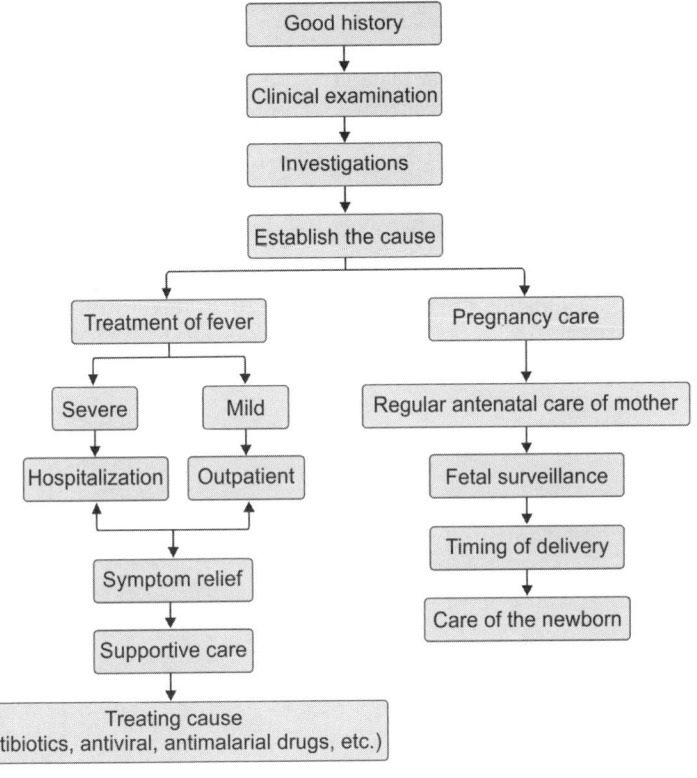

- Perineal hygiene if episiotomy site is infected
- Abdominal wound drainage in case of LSCS.

27. *Commonly used antibiotics in pregnancy and puerperium (Table 4):*

Table 4: Drugs and their dosage for puerperal sepsis

Drug	IV dose	Oral dose
Co-amoxiclav	1.2 g × 12th hourly or 8th hourly	375 mg or 625 mg TID
Cefuroxime	1.5 g × 8th hourly	Cephalexin 500 mg TID
Clindamycin	900 mg × 8th hourly	300 mg, 6–8 hourly

Contd...

Contd...

Drug	IV dose	Oral dose
Gentamicin	3–5 mg/kg body wt. in divided doses	
Metronidazole	500 mg × 8th hourly	400 mg, 8th hourly

Broad spectrum antibiotics are recommended
- Second or third generation cephalosporins, e.g. cefotaxime, ceftriaxone
- ß-lactam plus inhibitor combination, e.g. ampicillin plus sulbactam, piperacillin plus tazobactam, co-amoxiclav, ticarcillin plus clavulanate potassium
- Combination of aminoglycoside plus clindamycin.

Bibliography

1. Guidelines for the treatment of malaria. 3rd edition WHO 2015.
2. Julianna Schantz-Dunn, Nawal M Nar. Malaria and pregnancy: A global health prospective. Reviews in Obstetrics and Gynacology 2009; 2(3):186-92.
3. Maharaj D. Fever in Pregnancy Infectious Disease and Antimicrobial Therapy in antimicrobe.org
4. Management of pyrexia in the pregnancy and the intrapartum period. Developed using NICE and RCOG Clinical Guideline 12032 Middle Essex NHS Trust, UK
5. Newton E. Global Library Women's Medicine (ISSN: 1756-2228) 2008; DOI 10.3843/GLOWM. 10175
6. Sundarravindran TK. Factsheet malaria in pregnancy in India for Common Health in partnership with Rural Women's Social Education Centre (RUWUSEC) and Society for health alternatives (SAHAJ).
7. The diagnosis and treatment of malaria in pregnancy, green top guideline No. 54b April 2010. Royal College of Obstetricians and Gynaecologists, UK.

CHAPTER 7

Anemia in Pregnancy

Sunanda R Kulkarni

CASE

Patient by name X, wife of Y, from low socio-economic status aged 32 years, a G2P1L1 presented to the OPD for the first time with history of amenorrhea of 8 months duration with following complaints:
- Exertional dyspnea of 1 month
- Palpitations since 2 months
- History of bleeding per rectum since 2 months.

History of Present Pregnancy

First Trimester
- Spontaneous conception
- No history of fever with chills
- No history of drug intake/bleeding/hyperemesis/hematemesis.

Second Trimester
- Quickening in 4th month
- Had ANC only once in 5th month
- IFA prophylaxis taken regularly
- Two doses of injection tetanus toxoid (TT) taken
- History of bleeding per rectum since 3 months.

Menstrual History
- MC: 3–4/30days, normal flow, no history of menorrhagia
- Last menstrual period (LMP)
- Estimated date of delivery (EDD)

Obstetric History
- G2P1L1.

Previous Baby
- Full term normal delivery at home 4 years ago
- No PPH. No IUCD or OCP usage.

Past History
- Nothing significant.

Personal History
- She is a home maker
- Socioeconomic status
- Belongs to lower socioeconomic status according to Kuppuswamy classification.

Dietary History

Vegetarian
- Total caloric intake—1,500 kcal
- Protein intake deficient by 30% (requires 50 g but takes 35 g).

On Examination

Patient was conscious, well oriented to time, place and person and breathless. She was thin built and her height was 5 feet and weight 50 kg.

Vitals

- Pulse rate: 120 beats/minute
- Blood pressure: 110/70 mm Hg
- JVP increased
- Respiratory rate: 32 cycles/min, mostly thoracic.

General Physical Examination

- Pallor +++, no jaundice, no lymphadenopathy
- Pedal edema ++
- Angular stomatitis
- Platyonychia.

Inspection

- Apex beat in the 5th intercostal space.

Palpation

- Apex in the left 5th intercostal space at midclavicular line.

Auscultation

- First sound accentuated, S2 normal.
- Ejection—systolic murmur of grade 2 in pulmonary area, non-radiating
- Respiratory system (RS)
- Trachea—central, air entry equal on both sides, crepitation at the base of both lungs.

Abdominal Examination

Inspection

- Abdomen uniformly distended
- Striae gravidarum +, linea nigra +
- No scars, hernial orifices intact.

Palpation

- Mild hepatomegaly present—tender
- Fundal height: 30–32 weeks, SFH—30 cm
- Abdominal girth: 31"
- Fundal grip: Broad, soft, irregular mass s/o breech
- Lateral grip: Left—smooth curved structure—spine
- Right: Hard knob like structures—limb buds
- Pelvic grip: Hard globular mass—head
- Auscultation—FHS+

Local Examination

External hemorrhoids not seen.

Q. 1. Summarize your case.

A 32-year-old lady coming from low socio-economic status, G2P1L1 with 32 weeks of gestation in cephalic presentation with anemia in failure.

Q. 2. What are the reports of her investigation?

- Hb: 5.8 g%
- Indices: RBC—3.4 L/µL; MCH—14.3 aL pg, MCV—53.2 CL fl; MCHC—26.9 aL g/dL; RDW 22 aH %, HCT—19.3 aL %, Platelets—353000/µL.
- WBC—5800/µL, neutrophils—67.8, lymphocytes—19.3, monocytes—12.2; eosinophil—3 and basophil—0.0/103/µL.
- Peripheral blood smear: Microcytic hypochromic anemia with RBCs showing anisocytosis, and poikilocytosis
- Stool: Ova, cyst are absent
- ECG: Sinus tachycardia
- ECHO: Mildly dilated LV with trivial MR with good LV function.

Q. 3. What other investigations would you like to do?

- Blood group and Rh factor
- HIV1 and 2
- VDRL
- HBsAg
- RBS
- Thyroid profile
- Ultrasound scan of abdomen and obstetric
- Urine routine.

Q. 4. Would you like to take opinion of any other speciality in your case?

Physician's reference and surgical opinion for hemorrhoids.

Q. 5. What is your management plan for this patient?

- HDU care
- Failure management
- Anemia correction
- Fetal surveillance
- Hemorrhoids management
- Team approach
- Obstetric management.

Cardiac Failure Management

Propped-up Position

Pulse oxymeter and O_2 administration if saturation is <95%, at the rate of 4–6 L/m.

If saturation is low, central venous pressure monitoring for fluid policy and intensivist consultation for intubation.

Injection
- Furosemide 40 mg IV and repeat SOS
- IV line is maintained
- Fluid restriction
- Prophylactic antibiotics
- Get arterial blood gas analysis.

Q. 6. How will you correct anemia in this patient?

Blood transfusion is the mainstay as:
- It is severe anemia
- Patient has cardiovascular signs and symptoms of heart failure (packed cell transfusion with correction of heart failure)
- Rapid correction is required to prevent the severe consequences of anemia on pregnancy outcome
- In addition she has on going blood loss (bleeding hemorrhoids).

Q. 7. What are the effects of folic acid deficiency on pregnancy?

- Effects on the fetus—abortion, malformation of the fetus, especially neural tube defects, IUGR, prematurity
- Effects on mother—abruptio placentae.

Q. 8. What are the effects of iron deficiency anemia on pregnancy?

- On fetus: IUGR, prematurity, low fetal iron stores, prone for infection
- Effects on mother: Sepsis, shock, PPH, subinvolution of the uterus, CCF, PE, embolism, DVT, poor lactation, precipitate labor. Effects of deficiency of both iron and folic acid are not very specific and may overlap each other.

Q. 9. How do you manage labor?

Induction

Most often they go for spontaneous and preterm labor, occasionally precipitate labor. Induction is rarely required. If required PGs can be used. Augmentation to be done carefully to avoid fluid overload.

- 1st stage
  - Propped up position
  - Keep blood ready
  - Prophylactic antibiotics
  - No over loading of fluids
  - Analgesics
  - If there is failure—diuretics, oxygen, packed cells.
- 2nd stage
  - Prophylactic forceps
  - Avoid episiotomy, if possible
  - Delayed cord clamping conserves 80–100 mL of blood.
- 3rd stage
  - Active management with oxytocin or misoprostol to be done
  - Severe anemia—platelet concentrates transfusion.

Q. 10. How do you manage puerperium?
- Antibiotics for prevention of infection
- Repeat Hb after 48 hours
- I will look for DVT
- I will look for subinvolution and lactation failure
- Protein rich diet
- Non-compliant patients TDI of iron may be considered
- Ferric carboxymaltose injection.

Q. 11. What are the causes of anemia in postpartum period?
- LSCS
- Forceps delivery
- Perineal tear
- APH—abruptio placentae, placenta previa]
- Postpartum hemorrhage
- Already anemic
- Big baby, twins, induced labor.

Some studies have shown that postpartum hemorrhage is more when the Hb level is <10 g.

Hemoglobin should be checked after 48 hour. If it is <10 g then it should be treated. If it is severe <7 g—packed cell transfusion.

Mild and moderate anemias can be treated by oral iron or FCM if the patient is not compliant and it also reduces the duration of hospital stay.

Q. 12. Define and classify anemia.
Definition of anemia
- Is defined as pathological deficiency of O_2 carrying component of blood measured in unit volume of hemoglobin
- Is defined as a condition of low circulating volume of Hb in which Hb is below a threshold of 2 standard deviation below the median health population of the age, sex and state of pregnancy
- Is defined as a reduction in the concentration of circulating oxygen carrying capacity of blood below the level that is expected for a healthy person of the same age, sex in the same environment.

Classification of anemia

WHO Classification
- Mild: 10–10.9 g/dL
- Moderate: 7–9.9 g/dL
- Severe: <7 g/dL

ICMR Classification
- Mild: 10–10.9 g/dL
- Moderate: 7–9.9 g/dL
- Severe: 4–6.9 g/dL
- Very severe: <4 g/dL

Q. 13. What are the desired hemoglobin levels in each timester?
- First trimester Hb—11 g
- Second trimester Hb—10.5 g%
- Third triemster—11 g%.

Q. 14. What do you mean by physiological anemia of pregnancy?
Physiological anemia
- Hemodilution of plasma volume: 40–50%
- Increase in RBCs: 20–30% (300–400 mL)
- Total blood volume: 1,500 mL (30–40%)

Erythrocyte dilution occurs by 15%, because of hemodilution hemoglobin concentration decrease and results in physiological anemia. This is a protective mechanism of the body to deal with shunting of blood to the fetus and the blood loss during labor except in case of cardiac disease in pregnancy.

Q. 15. What are the hematological findings before the clinical manifestation of anemia?
Before signs and symptoms of anemia develops:
- RDW >15%
- Heterogeneous population of red cells
- Ferritin level <12 mg/L
  (1 µg of ferritin = 10 mg of storage Fe)

Q. 16. What are the food sources of iron?

Sources of iron	Sources of B_{12}	Sources of folic acid
Veg sources: Green leafy vegetables, drumstick leaves, spinach jaggery, dates Non-veg: Beef, pork, chicken, sea-food, turkey and lamb	Stored in muscle, serum and red cell. Veg sources: B_{12} is present in water, cows milk, nodular roots, legumes Non-veg: Beef liver, salmon	Spinach, beans, lettuce, broccoli, asparagus, cooked lentils

Q. 17. What is the mechanism of iron absorption and iron metabolism?

Iron is absorbed by the following mechanism:
- Iron regulatory proteins
- Hypoxic inducible factor (HIF)
- FPN protein—this is negatively regulated.

Hepcidin is a hormone secreted by hepatocytes which regulates the absorption of iron.

Iron is absorbed by both active and passive mechanism: Active transport is by mucosal block theory. Here absorption is controlled by apoferritin. When ferritin is fully saturated no more iron is absorbed. In passive absorption iron in combination with serine and glycerine diffuses across the border. Apart from this it is also regulated by placental progesterone oxygen levels in the tissue amount of anemia, high altitude, placental lactogen, etc.

Iron absorption
- Heme absorption > non-heme
- Ferrous > ferric
- Acidic media > alkaline
- Severe deficiency > mild deficiency.

Hemoglobin contains heme and globin. Life span of normal RBC is 90–120 days. When the life span of RBC is over it is engulfed by reticuloendothelial cells. It is destroyed in the spleen. The globin part goes to amino acid pool and iron from the heme goes to the labile pool of the iron where it is recycled. Iron excretion is 1–2 mg/day. Excreted in the form of sweat, and shedding epidermal of skin cell and mucosal lining of GI tract.

Iron Metabolism
Body iron component
- Total iron: 50 mg/kg body weight in male and 40 mg in female
- Storage iron: 30% (ferritin, hemosiderin) stored in liver, hepatocytes, reticuloendothelial cells, and skeletal muscles, when iron stores are in excess it is converted and stored as hemosiderin.
- This leads to iron deposition as amorphous called hemosiderin.
- Transport iron: 1%
- Hb iron: 65%
- Tissue iron (myoglobin, enzyme). 4%
- Iron stores: Ferritin, myoglobin, liver—4 g
- Transport iron: Transferritin is a protein where it binds to metals. It delivers iron to cells by binding to specific cell membrane receptors.
- Basal Fe requirement: 3 mg/kg/day.
- Menstruating women: 0.7–0.9 mg/day (lost)
- Pregnant women:
  - 1 mg/day in the first trimester
  - 5–7 mg/day in 2nd and 3rd trimester
- Facilitators of iron absorption: Vitamin C, HCl
- Inhibitors of iron absorption: Milk and its products, legumes, cereals, nuts, seeds.
- Increased requirements in pregnancy: Increased demand, shunting to the fetus, loss during labor, diminished intake and absorption, decreased prestores, demand, etc.
- Other heme proteins certain enzymes also: Contain heme as part of their prosthetic group (catalase, peroxidase, tryptophan, mitochondrial cytochromes).
- Trace elements needed for the production are cobalt, copper, chromium. Hormone responsible for hemoglobin production is:

Erythropoietin. Thyroxine is also linked in the production. Proteins are also necessary.

Iron economy
- Uterus and its contents: 500–600 mg
- Blood loss during labor: 150–200 mg
- Lactation: 150–200 mg
- Total demand: 700–1400 mg
- Saved iron: 25 × 9 = 225 mg
- Iron deficiency: 600–700 mg.

Q. 18. How do you diagnose anemia?
- Clinical diagnosis and laboratory diagnosis
- Laboratory methods
- Visual method
  - Tallquist paper method
  - Sahli's method
- Photoelectrical calorimetry
  - Cyanmethemoglobin
  - Oxyhemoglobin
  - Alkali hematin method
  - Clinically—pallor, pale conjunctiva, platonychia, koilonychias, angular cheilitis, glossitis, etc. Symptoms like weakness, tiredness, etc.

Tallquist method
- Advantages: Inexpensive, rapid, simple, no reagents or electricity required
- Disadvantages: Results influenced by lighting, size and thickness of blood spot, temperature and humidity.

Sahli's method
- Advantage: Cheap and simple
- Disadvantages: Less accurate. Color developed is unstable. Interobserver variability. Use of manual pipetting prone to error. No international standard.

Cyanmethemoglobin method
- Advantage: Measurement of cyanmethemoglobin—a stable compound. More accurate. Standard reference available. This is commonly used method in auto analyzer.

Hemoglobin color scale:
- Advantages: Simple and economical. Portable electricity not required.
- Disadvantage: Interobserver variability.

Copper sulphate method:
- Advantage: Inexpensive, simple, rapid interpretation, electricity not required.
- Disadvantages: Inaccurate, provides only ranges of hemoglobin levels. Difficult to conduct in rural areas. Requires fresh solutions. Proper disposal of standard solution.

Sodium lauryl sulfate method:
Cyanide free sodium lauryl sulfate method is safe method and it is also an accurate method.

Q. 19. What is the importance of peripheral blood smear in anemia?
- Blood smear: Malarial parasite—malaria sickle cells: Sickle cell disorders
- Howell-jolly bodies: Megaloblastic anemia, thalassemia, sickle cell anemia
- Heinz bodies: Thalassemia
- Spherocytes: Spherocytosis
- Schistocytes: Microangiopathic hemolytic anemia
- Hypersegmented neutrophils: Megaloblastic anemia
- Microcytic hypochromic: Iron deficiency, thalassemia.
- Bite cells: G6PD deficiency
- Nucleated red cells: Hemolytic anemia
- Basophilic stippling: Thalassemia, megaloblastic anemia, lead poisoning
- Burr cells: Uremia
- Target cells: Liver pathology
- Clumping of RBCs: Hemolytic anemia.

Q. 20. Which type of anemias need special investigation?
Hemolytic anemias require some special tests:
- Sickle cell anaemia: Sickling demonstration
- Thalassemia: Hb electrophoresis
- Spherocytosis: Osmotic fragility tests, etc.

Anemia in Pregnancy

Q. 21. Name the parasites and worm infestations causing anemia?

- Ancylostoma duodenale 0.2 mL/worm/day
- *Necator americanus* 0.03 mL/worm/day
- Malarial parasite
- Leishmania
  - *Entamoeba histolytica*
  - *Diphyllobothrium latum*
- Some of the parasites like giardia can cause malabsorption and bloody diarrhea
- Schistosomiasis, trichuriasis and ascariasis can cause anemia indirectly.

Q. 22. What are the causes for microcytic, hypochromic anemia?

- Fe deficiency
- Thalassemia
- Sideroblastic anemia
- Chronic diseases (Rheumatoid arthritis and renal disease)
- Drug induced—alcohol, anti-TB drugs, chloramphenicol, etc.

Q. 23. What are the causes of megaloblastic anemia?

Folic acid and B_{12} deficiency.

Q. 24. What are the laboratory findings in Fe deficiency anemia?

- Microcytic hypochromic anemia
- Hb: <10 g
- Serum iron: <30 µg/100 mL
- MCHC: <30%
- MCV: <75 fl
- Serum ferritin: <30 µg
- % of iron saturation < 10%
- TIBC: >400 µg/mL
- Serum bilirubin: Not raised
- MCH: <25 pg
- Microcytic hypochromic smear
- Increased TIBC, low serum iron and transferrin saturation
- Increased soluble transferritin receptors
- Bone marrow: Micronormoblast, absence of stainable iron.

Q. 25. How will you diagnose folic acid deficiency?

- Peripheral smear: Macrocytosis and normochromic, anisopoikilocytosis, basophilic stippling, Howell-Jolly bodies, Cabot rings, decreased platelets.
  - Red cells folate level is more important as it is not fluctuated by dietary intake like serum—150–700 µg/L
  - Serum folate level—3.1–17.5 ng/mL.

Q. 26. How will you diagnose B_{12} deficiency?

- Serum B_{12} estimation
- Peripheral smear hypersegmented neutrophils >5
- Reticulocyte count
- Folic acid—liver 10 mg
- B_{12}—3,000 µg in adult and 50 µg in newborn—liver.

Pernicious anemia

Pernicious anemia is due to intrinsic factor deficiency.

Q. 27. What are the causes of megaloblastic anemia?

- Decreased intake—diet, alcohol, prolonged parenteral therapy
- Decreased absorption—tropical sprue, coeliac diseases, malabsorption
- Increased demand—multiple pregnancy
- Multigravida, hemolytic anemia
- Medication—antiepileptic drugs, oral pills, pyrimethamine, primidone, zidovudine.
- Cooking—prolonged cooking.

Q. 28. How do you diagnose megaloblastic anemia?

- Hypersegmented neutrophils (<5 lobes)
- Macrocytosis, anisocytosis

- Giant polymorphism, Howell-Jolly bodies
- MCV: >100 microns to the power of 3
- MCHC: Normal
- MCH: >33 pg
- Serum folate: <3 ng/mL
- Serum bilirubin may be raised
- Serum iron: Normal or high
- Serum B_{12}: <90 pg/mL
- Leukopenia and thrombocytopenia.

Q. 29. How do you treat a case of megaloblastic anemia?

Folate prophylaxis is 400 µg/day for 6 months in pregnancy and 3 months post-partum and therapeutic dose is 1 mg/day and in neural tube defects 4 mg/day.

Cyanocobalamin or hydroxycobalamin

1 mg IM injection given 3 times a week for 2 weeks followed by every 3 months. In patients with neurologic involvement: dose is higher. 1 mg on alternate days until no further improvement is noted followed by 1 mg every 2 months.

Q. 30. How do you diagnose dimorphic anemia?

- In pregnancy dimorphic anemia is seen. Serum folate: <3 ng/mL
- Serum B_{12} <90 pg/mL
- Hypersegmented neutrophils, Howell-Jolly bodies
- Smear: Macrocytic or normocytic and hypochromic or normochromic.

Q. 31. How do you classify anemias and describe each?

- Based on production of RBCs: Impaired production and increase destruction
- Based on cell size: Normocytic normochromic, macrocytic hypochromic and microcytic hypochromic
- Clinical classification: Cause of anemia, blood loss, destruction
- Quantitative classification:
  - Hematocrit
  - Hemoglobin
  - Blood cell indices (MCV, MCH, MCHC)
  - Reticulocyte count
- Etiological classification: Fe, folic acid, B_{12}, deficiency, etc.

Normochromic, normocytic anemia (normal MCHC, normal MCV)

- Anemias of chronic disease
- Hemolytic anemias (those characterized by accelerated destruction of RBCs)
- Anemia of acute hemorrhage
- Aplastic anemia (those characterized by disappearance of RBC precursors from the marrow).

Hypochromic, microcytic anemia (low MCHC, low MCV)

- Iron deficiency anemia
- Thalassemia
- Anemia of chronic disease (rare cases).

Normochromic, macrocytic anemia (also see Flowchart 1) (normal MCHC, high MCV)

- Vitamin B_{12} deficiency
- Folate deficiency.

Classification

Category	Serum Ferritin µg/L	Hb %	Diagnosis
1	>12	>11	No anemia
2	<12	>11	Fe stores decreased
3	<12	<11	Fe deficiency anemia
4	>12	<11	Other causes

	Iron deficiency	Megaloblastic anemia	Dimorphic anemia
MCV:	<75	>100	>100
MCHC:	<30%	30–36%	<30%
S B_{12}:	Normal	Decreased	Decreased

Contd...

Anemia in Pregnancy

Contd...

S folic acid: Normal	Low	Low
S ferritin: Low	Normal	Decreased
S iron: Low	Normal	Low
Smear: Microcytic	Macrocytic	Normal or macrocytic
Hypochromic	Normochromic, ovalocytes	Hypo or normochromic
High RDW	In vitamin B_{12} deficiency	High RDW: Mainly applies to normocytic normochromic situations
Microcytic hypochromic anemia		

Q. 32. What is the role of stool examination?

Stool shows—ova and cyst of ankylostomiasis, giardia, *Entamoeba histolytica*.

Ankylostomiase egg appears as oval or elliptical shaped, not bile stained, size 60 × 40 microns.

Flowchart 1: Classification of anemia based on serum ferritin

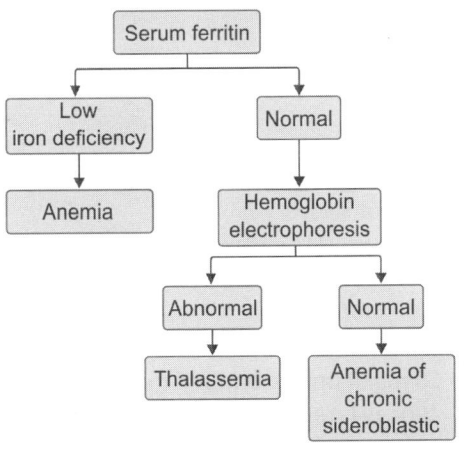

Q. 33. What are the government programs for control of anemia?

- 100 mg element Fe^+ 500 folic acid for 100 days in pregnancy followed by postpartum 100 days.
- De-worming in pregnancy
  - Albendazole can be given
  - Mebendazole can be given
  - Piperazine citrate
  - Levamisole 2.5 mg/kg single dose.
- Pyrantel pamoate can be given but it is controversial.

Q. 34. What are the WHO recommendations?

Daily oral iron and folic acid supplementation is recommended as part of the antenatal care to reduce the risk of low birth weight, maternal iron deficiency anemia and iron deficiency.

Suggested scheme for daily iron and folic acid supplementation in pregnant women.

- Dose: Iron—60 mg of elemental iron folic acid—400 µg (0.4 mg)
- Frequency: One supplement daily
- Duration: For 6 months in pregnancy. If 6 months cannot be achieved in pregnancy the continue postpartum or increase the dosage to 120 mg in pregnancy. If prevalence is more than 40% then continue postpartum.
- *National anemia prophylaxis program:* Distribution of pediatric dose for—1–5 years (6–60 months)
- From 5 years to 18 years—30 mg of iron and 250 µg of folic acid/day for 100 days in a year. Priority is given to adolescent girls.

Q. 35. What are the NRHM guidelines?

NRHM guidelines 2014: Treatment of anemia in different periods of gestation for different levels of Hb.

NRHM guidelines for management of anemia in pregnancy

Hb level (g)	14–16 weeks	20–24 weeks	20–30 weeks	30–34 weeks
<7	Blood transfusion (BT)/refer to higher center	BT/refer to higher center	BT/refer to higher center	BT/refer to higher center
>11	Prophylactic iron	Prophylactic iron	Prophylactic iron	Prophylactic iron
9–11	Therapeutic iron	Therapeutic iron	Therapeutic iron	Therapeutic iron
7.1–8.9	Therapeutic iron	Iron sucrose injection	Iron sucrose injection	Blood transfusion

Other recommendations
- All pregnant patients should be dewormed at first visit. Albendazole 400 mg single dose
- In all 4 visits hemoglobin tests should be performed by cyanmethemoglobin method
- Iron sucrose injection 100 mg in 100 mL of normal saline. Totally 400 mg to be given in 4 divided doses with an interval of 2–4 days.
- If the patient has received iron sucrose already but still hemoglobin is not improved then top up with 2 doses of iron sucrose injection each 100 mg.
- Prophylactic dose—100 mg of elemental iron and 0.5 mg of folic acid. Single dose daily for 100 days.
- Therapeutic dose—100 mg of iron BD.

BT (blood transfusion): Blood transfusion when the hemoglobin is less than <7 g in any trimester.

All pregnant patient should also receive vitamin B_{12}, 15 μg and vitamin C 100 mg.

Fe-deficiency anemia—prevention
- Primary prevention
  - Supplementation
  - Diet
  - Preschool children
  - Adolescence—heavy bleeding
- Secondary
  - Prevention by screening.

Cord clamping at birth
- Providing additional placental blood to the preterm baby by either delaying cord clamping for 30–120 seconds, rather than early clamping, seems to be associated with less need for transfusion, better circulatory stability, less intraventricular hemorrhage (all grades) and lower risk for necrotizing enterocolitis.
- Umbilical cord milking is a safe procedure and it improves Hb and iron status at 6 weeks of life among term and near term neonates.
- In term babies 1–3 minutes dealy in cord clamping is beneficial is beneficial as per WHO.

Q. 36. How do you calculate parenteral iron dosage

A.
- 0.3 × weight in pounds × [100 – Hb %] + 50% for stores
- 250 mgs × [14 – Hb of patient]
- Body weight × [targeted Hb – actual Hb × 2.4 + stores

B.
- 25 mg of iron is required to raise 1% of Hb.
- 100 mg is required to raise 0.55 g%/100 mL

Hb estimation by	1st visit	2nd visit	3rd visit	4th visit
Cyanmethemoglobin method	14–16 weeks	20–24 weeks	26–30 weeks	30–34 weeks

Anemia in Pregnancy

Parenteral Iron Therapy
- *1st generation*—iron dextron, iron sorbitol citric acid complex
- *2nd generation*—iron sucrose, ferric gluconate
- *3rd generation*—ferric carboxymaltose, carbonyl Fe-highly purified elemental iron, in stomach converted to HCL salt, less toxic, slow absorption but continued release.

Ferrous gluconate, fumarate—are tasteless, (ferrous aspartoglycinate) which is a chelated iron.

Parenteral Iron Therapy

Type of iron	Test dose	Route	Dose	Reactions	Advantage
Imferon Iron dextran	Yes	IM/IV	1.5 mg/kg weight	Anaphylaxis, arthralgia	–
Jector Iron sorbitol Citric acid complex	Yes	IM, Z track	50 mg	Skin discoloration Arthralgia, fever	–
Iron sucrose	No	IV	200 mg in 200 mL saline/15–20 minutes	Anaphylaxis is rare, vomiting, hypotension	–
Iron carboxy polymaltose	No	IV	1000 mg in 100 mL NS in 15 minutes		1,000 mg at a time

Q. 37. What are the contraindications for IV iron?

- Allergic reactions to the test dose/previous hypersensitivity to IV iron
- Acute renal failure
- Chronic liver failure, asthma
- Signs and symptoms of inflammation
- First trimester of pregnancy
- Anemia not attributable to iron deficiency
- Iron overload
- Acute infection/inflammation.

Preparation	Iron compound (mg/tab)	Elemental iron mg/tab (%)
Fe-sulfate (hydrous)	300	60 (20%)
Fe-sulfate (dried)	200	65 (32.5%)
Fe-fumarate	200	66 (33%)
Fe-gluconate	300	36 (12%)

Contd...

Preparation	Iron compound (mg/tab)	Elemental iron mg/tab (%)
Fe-succinate	100	35 (35%)
Fe-bisglycinate	300	60 (20%)
Carbonyl iron	100	98 (98%)
Na-feredetate	231	33 (14%)

Q.38. What instructions have to be given about taking iron?

- Iron supplementation either on empty stomach or 2 hours after a meal
- Cook in iron pot
- Diet leafy vegetables, jaggery, etc.
- Milk and milk products between meals
- Take tablet along with citrus fruit
- Vitamin C tablets
- Increase the dose slowly
- Avoid tea or coffee 2 hours before taking tablets.

Q. 39. How do you assess the response to treatment?

- Rise of Hb 1 g/dL—3-4 weeks
- Hct rise by 3%-4 weeks
- 0.1 g rise/day
- Reticulocyte appear—8-10 days increased appetite feeling of well being to note the color of the stools for compliance.

Q. 40. What causes poor response to oral iron therapy?

- Iatrogenic—inappropriate choice and time of administration of iron preparation
- Patient—noncompliance, skipping the dose, half dose, decreased duration
- Concurrent inhibitors of iron absorption like antacids, H_2 blockers, calcium salts, phytates in food
- Coexistent chronic inflammatory conditions
- Ongoing blood loss
- Coexistence of vitamin B_{12} and folic acid deficiency
- Hypoproliferative anemia in pregnancy with low erythropoietin levels and no renal disease can be treated with recombinant human erythropoietin.

Comparison of different methods of iron therapy

Route of iron	Efficacy	Cost	Side effects	Problems	Medical supervision required
Oral iron (tablets/syrup)	Excellent	Cheap	Constipation, discomfort		
Discoloration of teeth (syrup)	Inhibitors	Not required			
Parenteral iron	Good	Inexpensive	Joint pain, fever	Skin discoloration	Day care procedure
Blood transfusion	Very good	Expensive	Transfusion reactions	Hepatitis, HIV, shock and death	Day care procedure
Dietary iron	Inhibitors	Expensive	Large amount	Increase time	Not required

Q. 41. Indications for blood transfusion?

- Excessive bleeding
- Anticipating surgery
- Refractory anemia
- Advanced pregnancy
- Hemolytic anaemia
- After delivery if there is PPH
- Severe anemia in any duration of pregnancy.

Exchange transfusion

Required only in sideroblastic and sickle cell anemias.

Rule of 3

Hb (g/dL) = 3 × RBC (million)/cmm—Hb in gms/dL × 3 = PCV in %

Mainly apples to normocytic normochromic situations.

Q. 42. When will you suspect thalassemia?

- If the patient is not responding to treatment
- No other cause for anemia
- Patient is coming from a particular area where there is prevalence (North western part of India) or from a particular community (Sindhis, Gujaratis, Bengalis, etc.)

Q. 43. How do you diagnose a case of thalassemia?

- Blood—microcytic hypochromic, anisocytosis, poikilocytosis, target cells, Howell-

Jolly bodies, basophilic stippling, red cells, Heinz bodies.
- Tests for inclusion bodies by supravital staining will show unpaired alfa chains aggregates in RBCs
- Hemoglobin electrophoresis—increased fetal Hb—10-98%
- Acid elution test—reveals heterogeneous distribution of Hb F in red cells
- Unconjugated serum bilirubin increased
- Serum Fe also increased (multiple transfusion), TIBC ferritin Fe binding capacity, transferrin saturation normal or increased
  - Iron overload test—serum ferritin,
  - MRI- noninvasive and shows liver and cardiac iron
- Osmotic fragility test—to rule out spherocytosis, sickle cell
- HPLC—detection, identification, and quantification of hemoglobin variants.

Q. 44. How do you differentiate between iron deficiency anemia and beta thalassemia?

- Mentzer index, MCV/RBC <13, in thalassemia >13, iron deficiency anemia
- RDW normal in thalassemia increased in iron deficiency anemia (11.5–14.5) carrier screening
  - Red cell indices—low MCH, and MCV in ethnic group—then exclude iron deficiency anemia and chronic anemias, DNA testing
  - Electrophoresis or HPLC for quantification of Hb A2
    - ◊ If >3.5%—beta thalassemia minor
    - ◊ If <3.5%—alfa thalassemia trait—confirm by genetic analysis
- Hb electrophoresis at alkaline pH.

Q. 45. What is the pathology of thalassemia?

Pathogenesis of iron overload in thalassemia: Ineffective erythropoiesis increased absorption—iron binding capacity of transferritin is exceeded uptake by liver, heart and endocrine cells generation to reactive species with oxidant cells damage. Organ dysfunction.

Differential diagnosis of anemia

	Iron deficiency	Beta thalassemia
MCV	Decreased	Increased
RDW	Increased	Normal
Red cell morphology: Microcytic hypochromic with basophilic stippling, polychromasia		
RBC count	Decreased	Normal
Serum iron	Decreased	Normal
TIBC	Increased	Normal
Transferritin saturation—decreased: Normal or increased		
Serum ferritin	Decreased	Normal
Hb electrophoresis	Normal	Hb A2 >3.5%
Bone moat row	Lower or absent	Normal
Oral iron can be given. Oral not advised usually		
Reticulocyte count	Normal RDW	Increased RDW
>2%	Thalassemia	Hemolytic anemia
<2%	Chronic disease	Iron deficiency anemia

Q. 46. How do you counsel the patient?

Screening—screening of the partner:
- Thalassemia trait and silent carrier, fetus 25%, Hb Barts, 25% normal and 50% trait
- Thalassemia trait couples—25% normal and 50% trait and 25% Hb Barts.
- PGD should be discussed in case of IVF and ICSI. NIPT in first trimester. Evaluate the maternal prepregnancy status for thyroid status diabetes, liver dysfunction
- Counseling about osteoporosis and vitamin D intake
- Councel about cardiac status by ECHO.

Q. 47. How do you manage a case of thalassemia in pregnancy?

Beta thalassemia—major and minor.

Beta thalassemia major: After birth fetal hemoglobin is not replaced by adult hemoglobin. Repeated blood transfusion is required, can be recognized clinically by typical thalassemia facies, short height, frontal bossing etc. Life span is short. Repeated blood transfusion is required. Iron chelating therapy with desferioxmine may be necessary. Pregnancy is rare but MTP may be required to save the mother.

Beta thalassemia minor: This may not be symptomatic and go without notice in few cases, suffers from mild anemia, parenteral iron should not be given, even if husband is heterozygous, fetus has 25% chance of getting the disease.

β-thalassemia intermediate varity is usually late in onset, rarely transfusion dependent. During pregnancy they should be counseled about FGR and they should be given oral iron and folic acid supplementation.

Q. 48. How do you treat a pregnant woman with thalassemia?

- Folic acid 5 mg/day.
- During early pregnancy, screen the partner for carrier status. If negative no further testing required.

  If partner is positive there is risk of thalassemia to the baby, hence do DNA analysis, if mutation is identified then MTP is advised. If DNA analysis is normal then can continue the pregnancy.
- Iron replacement depending on the hematinic indices.
- TSH done to rule out thyroid dysfunction since 75% thalassemia major suffer from thyroid problems. Blood sugar for diabetic status.
- Aggressive chelation in pre pregnancy can reduce iron burden and end organ damage. Desferoxmine 20 mg/kg/day 4–5 days in a week.
- Regular antenatal check-ups—2-3 weeks.
- Routine USG to rule out IUGR.

[In future, hemopoietic stem cell transplantation in utero, when HSCT is given as the fetus is in immune compromised status graft versus host reaction is not there and the cell is well accepted. After birth HLA matched transplantation of the bone marrow of the sibling within the first year of life. Instead peripheral blood stem cell is preferred now a days. HLA matched geno identical cord blood equally effective stem cell sources.]

Labor—close monitoring

Breastfeeding—no contraindication.

Different hemoglobin in adults

Hemoglobin type	Globin chain	%
HbA adult type	Alfa 2 beta 2	95%
HbA2	Alfa 2 delta 2	<3%
HbF	Alfa 2 gamma 2	<2%

Typical clinical and laboratory features in alfa thalassemia

Type	Genotype	Anemia	Red cell changes	Hb electrophoresis		Clinical features
				Newborn	Adult	
Silent carrier	α α/α–	Absent	None	1–2% Hb Bart's	Normal	Asymptomatic
α thalassemia	α –/α – – α α /– –	Absent or mild	Microcytic hypochromic	5–15% Hb Bart's	Normal	Usually asymptomatic

Contd...

Anemia in Pregnancy

Contd...

Type	Genotype	Anemia	Red cell changes	Hb electrophoresis		Clinical features
				Newborn	Adult	
Hb H disease	α−/−−	Moderate	Microcytosis, target cells	20–40% Hb Bart's	HB H	Moderate anemia, hepatosplenomegaly
Hydrops fetalis	−−/−−	Severe	Numerous erythroblasts	8–100% Hb Bart's	–	Fetus has hydrops, mother develops severe PET. Fetal-death in utero or after birth

Q. 49. Describe genesis of thalassemia?

Silent carrier: Loss of one gene, clinically may not be noticed.

Alfa thalassemia minor: Deletion of 2 genes. Mild anemia, oral iron can be given, laboratory diagnosis shows iron deficiency picture. No parenteral iron. Electrophoresis shows—HbA2.

Sometimes blood transfusion may be required. Fetus carries the genes.

Hb H—deletion of 3 genes, suffers from chronic hemolytic anemia, stress should be avoided, blood transfusion may be required. Homozygous alfa thalassemia—deletion of all 4 genes, Hb Barts has increased affinity for oxygen. Can develop PET in pregnancy. Fetal hydropic is possible.

Diagnosis of types of thalassemia

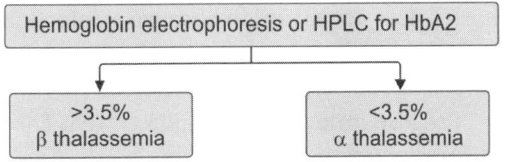

Q. 50. What are the investigation for sickle cell anemia?

- Peripheral blood smear—sickle cells
- Peripheral smear—increased reticulocytes
- Unconjugated bilirubin increased
- ESR decreased
- Identification of HbS—slide test by using sodium meta bisulfate 2% or electrophoresis
- HPLC—high performance liquid chromatography Hb electrophoresis
- Slide test will not differentiate between trait and sickle cell disorder
- Fetal Hb test—alkali denaturation test—for knowing severity of sickle cell anemia
- Prenatal diagnosis:
  - Fetal blood analyses,
  - Fetal DNA
    ◊ Amniotic fluid
    ◊ CVS.

Q. 51. How do you manage a case of sickle cell anemia in pregnancy?

Sickle cell trait does not require any specific treatment.

Q. 52. How do you do prepregnancy counseling in a case of sickle cell anemia?

Prepregnancy:
- Check sickle cell status of the partner.
- Hyrdoxyurea, ACE should be stopped 3 months prior to pregnancy.
- Counselling regarding the maternal condition, fetal outcome, importance of regular check-ups.
- If both parents are heterozygous, 1 in 4 chance for the fetus to be affected.

- Antibiotic prophylaxis. If the patient is sensitive to penicillin the erythromycin should be given.
- Vaccination—*Haemophilus influenzae*, meningococcal vaccine should be given.
- Avoid air traveling

Q. 53. How do you manage during pregnancy?

- Ante natal visits every 2–3 weeks.
- Avoid stress factors like stress, exercise, cold, dehydration.
- Investigations: Complete blood count, ferritin level, reticulocyte level, folate level,
- Transfusion of blood in pregnancy is controversial.
- To screen for most common minor red cell antigens so that phenotypically matched blood will be available for transfer.
- Check for urine culture and sensitivity to rule out asymptomatic bacteriuria.
- Low dose aspirin
- Exchange transfusion only in case of acute sickle cell disease. Blood should be matched for an extended phenotype including full Rh typing C, D, E, as well Kell typing and CMV negative.

During pregnancy they may suffer either from:
- Chronic hemolytic anemia
- Vaso occlusive crisis
- Fetal effects like FGR, placental abruption, preeclampsia, stillbirth, prematurity, etc.

Q. 54. What are the complications of sickle cell disease and their management?

- *Vaso-occlusive or painful crisis:* Obstruction of blood vessels leads to hypoxia, infarction, and pain. This is the most common crisis and most common reason for hospitalization. Fetal effects like FGR, placental abruption, preeclampsia, still birth, prematurity, etc. Good hydration, careful fluid balance, adequate analgesia, oxygen supplementation, IV antibiotics covering encapsulated organisms, 5 mg FA daily. Patient should be kept warm.
- *Acute chest syndrome:* Should be differentiated from pneumonia.

Monitor saturation and blood gas volumes
Management during labor:
- Keep the pregnant woman warm. Maintain good hydration, oxygenation. Pain relief to be given.
- Monitoring of her vitals—pulse, blood pressure, oxygen saturation.
- Transfusion of blood if Hb <8g/dL, prophylactic blood transfusion is controversial. Avoid prolonged labor.
- Avoid acidemia
- Anesthesia: Epidural than GA for LSCS. Continuous fetal monitoring.
- Acute anemia and neurological events due to thrombotic cerebrovascular accidents are also complication of sickle cell disease
- Breastfeeding is allowed. No hydroxylurea if the patient is breastfeeding
- Early ambulation and hydration advised.
- Low molecular weight heparin for 7 days in case of normal delivery and for 6 weeks incase of LSCS.

Contraception
- No oral pills because of crisis. Progesterone only pill can be given.
- ICUDs—with caution because of infection and bleeding.
- Barrier contraception is advised.
- Progesterone containing pills DMPA. They are known to prevent crisis.

Q. 55. What preventive measures can be taken?

Health Education
- Avoiding consanguineous marriages in the affected caste
- Carrier screening in specific caste group located in particular geographical area

- Prenatal diagnosis
- Gene therapy in future.

Q. 56. What is the role of erythropoietin?

Hypoproliferative anemia in pregnancy with low erythropoietin levels and no renal disease can be treated successfully with recombinant human erythropoietin.

Q. 57. What is refractory anemia?

Refractory anemia refers to those anemias which are unresponsive to all known therapy except transfusion. There is no known cause of like liver disease, kidney disease, etc. Refractory anemias with cellular or hypocelluar bone marrow is used to exclude aplastic anemia. In practice refractory anemia with hypercelluar or bone marrow also pancytopenia and with or without splenomegaly.

Q. 58. What is the role of erythropoietin in pregnancy?

It can be used in pregnancy safely as it does not not cross the placenta, including renal disease in pregnancy.

Points to Remember
1. Early regular antenatal check-up is associated with early detection of anemia and possibility of treatment.
2. Anemia is associated with warning symptoms like hemorrhoids, menorrhagia. These problems should be treated before pregnancy. For this awareness should be created.
3. Anemia is usually seen in multipara and with decreased interval between the consecutive pregnancies
4. In endemic areas, better to advise deworming.
5. In severe microcytic hypochromic anemia or those who do not respond to the treatment, suspect rare type of anemias.
6. Patient who are not compliant should be given FCM therapy before discharging.
7. Along with IV infusion other nutrients like folic acid, B_{12}, should be prescribed as most of our patients will be having deficiencies.

Bibliography

1. ACOG women's healthcare physicians, Committee opinion Number 543, December 2012 (Reaffirmed 2014).
2. Adamkiewicz TV, Silk BJ, Howgate J, et al. Effectiveness of the 7-valent pneumococcal conjugate vaccine in children with sickle cell disease in the first decade of life. Pediatrics. 2008;121(3):562-9. doi:10.1542/peds.2007-0018.
3. Anemia: When is it not iron deficiency? Annette Carley Pediatr Nurs. Jannetti Publications, Inc. 2003;29(3):205-11. Posted 07/16/2003.
4. Cochrane Database of Systematic Reviews: Early cord clamping versus delayed cord clamping or cord milking for preterm babies.
5. Dacie and Lewis Practical Hematology. In: Lewis SM, Bain BJ, Bates I (eds). Churchil Livigstone; 2002.
6. Fina Lubaki JP, Musiti Ngolo JR, Zikudieka Maniati L. Active management of third stage of labour, postpartum haemorrhage and maternal death rate in the Vanga Health Zone, Province of Bandundu, Democratic Republic of the Congo. Afr J Prm Health Care Fam Med. 2010;2(1), Art. #76, 3 pages. DOI: 10.4102/phcfm.v2i1.76
7. Green top guidelines No 61, 2011. ROOG Nice accreditation.
8. Green top guidelines No 66, March 2014. Nice accreditation.
9. Harris SA, Payne G Jr, Putman JM. Erythropoietin treatment of erythropoietin-deficient anemia without renal disease during pregnancy. Obstetrics & Gynecology. 1996; 87(5):812-4.
10. Iron therapy. Am J Hematol. 2004:76(1).
11. Kaima A. Frass postpartum hemorrhage is related to the hemoglobin levels at labor: Observational study. Alex J Med. 2015:51(4); 333-7.
12. Kawthalkar S. Essentials of haematology. Jaypee. 2013
13. Makrydimas G, Lolis D, Lialios G, et al. Recombinant human erythropoietin treatment of postpartum anemia Preliminary report. rHuEpo administration is useful for a more rapid amelioration of hematological indices in women with postpartum anemia.

Further, the dos International Journal of Obstetric Anesthesia. July 1996;5(3):202–205, doi:10.1016/S0959- 289X(96)80033-1

14. Milman N. Postpartum anemia I: definition, prevalence, causes, and consequences. Ann Hematol. 2011;90(11):1247-53. doi: 10.1007/s00277-011-1279-z. Epub 2011 Jun 28
15. National Nutritional Anemia Prophylaxis Program in India; 1990.
16. Patil SS, Khanwelkar CC, Patil SK. Conventional and newer oral iron preparations. JMPS. 2012;2(3):2012.
17. Pavord S, Myers B, Robinson S, et al. UK guidelines on the management of iron deficiency in pregnancy. British Committee for Standards in Haematology. BCHS; 2011.
18. Petrea M, Stepheni CJ. Penicillin prophylaxis in children with sickle cell diases. J Paedtr Pharmcol. Ther. 2010;3:152-9.
19. Prata N, Hamza S, Gypson R, et al. Pott Misoprostol and active management of the third stage. Int J Gynec & Obst. 2006;94(2):149-55. doi:10.1016/j.ijgo.2006.05.027
20. Rees DC, Williams TN, Gladwin MT. Sickle-cell disease. Lancet. 2010;376(9757):2018-31. doi: 10.1016/S0140-6736(10)61029-X. Epub 2010 Dec 3.
21. Rodgers GP, Young NS. Bethesda's Handbook of Hematology. Lippincott williams and wilkins; 2013.
22. Serjeant GR, et al. Fecundity and pregnancy outcome in a cohort with sickle cell-haemoglobin C disease followed from birth. BJOB. 2005;112:1308-14.
23. Sienas L, Wong T, Collins R, et al. Contemporary uses of erythropoietin in pregnancy: a literature review. Obstet Gynecol Surv. 2013;68(8):594-602. doi: 10.1097/OGX.0b013e3182a2d51c.
24. Srivastava T, Negandhi H, Neogi SB, et al. Methods for Hemoglobin Estimation: A Review of "What Works". J Hematol Transfus. 2014;2(3):1028.
25. Upadhyay A, Gothwal S, Parihar R, et al. Effect of umbilical cord milking in term and near term infants: randomized control trial. Am J Obstet Gynecol. 2013;208(2):120.e1-6.
26. Walters MC. Hematology. Stem cell therapy for sickle cell disease: transplantation. Am Soc Hematol Educ Program. 2005:66-73.

8

Hypertensive Disorders of Pregnancy

Muralidhar V Pai

Definitions

Gestational Hypertension

Gestational hypertension is defined as blood pressure more than 140/90 mm Hg (Korotkoff phase V is used to define diastolic pressure) observed on at least two occasions 6 hours apart, after 20 weeks of gestation in a woman with previously normal blood pressure.

Preeclampsia

Preeclampsia is diagnosed when gestational hypertension is associated with either proteinuria of ≥300 mg/24 hours (Dipstick 1+) or Protein: Creatinine ratio ≥ 0.3.

As per 2013 ACOG's Task Force on hypertension in Pregnancy,[1] preeclampsia may also be diagnosed if gestational hypertension is associated with any one of the following:
- Thrombocytopenia—platelets <100,000/μL
- Renal insufficiency—creatinine >1.1 mg/dL or doubling of baseline
- Abnormal liver function—AST and ALT twice the normal
- Cerebral symptoms—headache visual disturbances
- Pulmonary edema.

Eclampsia

When preeclampsia is complicated by convulsions, it is called eclampsia.

Chronic Hypertension

Presence of hypertension prior to pregnancy or before 20 weeks of pregnancy. This may be further classified as:
- Primary hypertension (essential)
- Secondary hypertension due to:
  - Chronic renal disease
  - Thyrotoxicosis
  - Connective tissue disease (systemic lupus erythematosus)
  - Pheochromocytoma
  - Coarctation of aorta.

Preeclampsia Superimposed on Chronic Hypertension

In this variety, a pregnant woman with chronic hypertension develops preeclampsia, which may be further classified as
- Chronic hypertension with preeclampsia
- Chronic hypertension with eclampsia.

Etiology of Preeclampsia

Predisposing Factors

- Preeclampsia in an earlier pregnancy
- Family history (mother or sister) of preeclampsia, hypertension
- Primigravida (immunological)
- Vascular diseases, such as essential hypertension, renal disease, diabetes mellitus

and connective tissue disease (systemic lupus erythematosus)
- Antiphospholipid syndrome
- Multiple pregnancies
- Diabetes mellitus/gestational diabetes
- Molar pregnancy and hydrops fetalis
- Others—obesity, maternal age (young or elderly), hyperhomocysteinemia, and metabolic syndrome.

Signs of Imminent Eclampsia

- Symptoms—headache, blurring of vision, epigastric pain, oliguria, etc.
- Signs—persistently elevated blood pressure, papilledema, exaggerated reflexes, pulmonary edema
- Laboratory values—S. creatinine >1.1 mg/dL, S. uric acid >7.4 mg/dL, AST/ALT doubled
- Platelets <100,000/mL.

Pathophysiology of Preeclampsia (Flowchart 1)

Obstetric Case History

A 22-year-old primigravida at 30 weeks gestation with history of high blood pressure (150/100 mm Hg) referred to further management.

No history of headache, giddiness or blurring of vision.

Past History

- There is no history of hypertension prior to pregnancy and no other medical disorder.
- Table 1 gives the differenciating points for chronic past existing hypertension and preeclampsia.

Personal History

Nonsmoker/nonalcoholic.

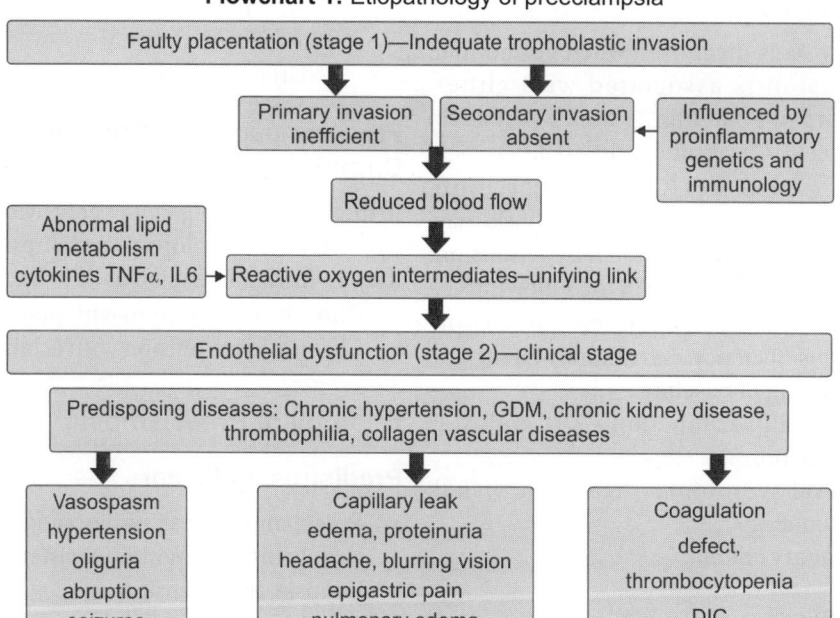

Flowchart 1: Etiopathology of preeclampsia

Hypertensive Disorders of Pregnancy

Table 1: Differences between chronic hypertension and preeclampsia

Chronic hypertension	Preeclampsia/gestational hypertension
Long history	Only in pregnancy
Elderly women	Young and elderly
Onset before 20 weeks of pregnancy	Onset usually after 28 weeks and sometimes after 20 weeks
Renal abnormalities may be marked Casts may be seen in urine microscopy	In severe cases renal dysfunction may be seen
Retinopathy may be present	Normal fundus usually
Cardiac changes like LVH may be present ECG changes may be seen	Not usual
Continues in postpartum period	Disappears in 10 days but not beyond 12 weeks
Needs to change the treatment in pregnancy	Initiation may be necessary

Family History

Mother is hypertensive, father is diabetic.

Socioeconomic History

Software engineer.

On Examination

- Moderately built and nourished
- Height is 5 feet 6 inches, and weight is 60 kg
- Pulse rate is 80/min regular, good in volume, bilateral synchronous. No radiofemoral delay
- BP is 150/100 mm Hg
- JVP is not raised. Afebrile
- Respiratory rate is 24/min
- No pallor or icterus
- Bilateral pedal edema + (No where else)
- Breasts show normal changes of pregnancy
- Heart sounds normal
- Air entry equal on both the sides. No added sounds or crepts
- No CNS abnormality.

Abdominal Examination

Inspection

- Abdomen uniformly distended
- Linea nigra and striagravidarum present
- No scar mark
- All hernia sites are free
- No hepatosplenomegaly.

Palpation

- Fundal height is around 28 weeks
- Symphysiofundal height is 28 cm
- Fundal grip—broad irregular mass suggestive of breech
- Lateral grip—back felt on right side and limbs felt on left side
- Pelvic grip—smooth hard ballotable mass suggestive of head felt
- Liquor appears to be adequate.

Auscultation

Fetal heart rate is 140/min regular.

Provisional Diagnosis

A 22-year-old primigravida at 30 weeks gestation with single live fetus in cephalic presentation having gestational hypertension/preeclampsia for evaluation.

Preeclampsia has to be confirmed by performing either 24 hours urine protein estimation or dip stick test.

Q. 1. What additional investigations need to be done once preeclampsia is confirmed?

Investigations to be done in a case of preeclampsia are:

Apart from routine investigations, such as blood group and type, hemoglobin, HIV, VDRL, HbsAg, GCT (if not done at 24 weeks), urine routine and microscopy, following specific investigations should be done at the time of diagnosis and repeated every week to look for deterioration of them.

> **Proteinuria testing**
> - *Quantitative:*
>   – Esbach's albuminometer
>   – Microalbuminuria determination method by immunoturbidimetry to detect very small amount of albumin
> - *Semiquantitative:*
>   – The Micral II test strip
>   – CLINITEK microalbumin
> - *Qualitative tests:*
>   – Heller's test
>   – Heat coagulation test
>   – Sulfosalicylic acid test
>
> Some of these could be semiquantitative too

- Hemoglobin and hematocrit (increased)
- Platelet count (decreased)
- Proteinuria quantification (increased)
- Renal function tests (serum creatinine, urea uric acid estimations)—elevated
- Liver function tests [elevated liver enzymes (transaminases)]—elevated
- Serum albumin estimation—decreased
- Coagulation profile—altered
- Serum electrolytes—imbalance
- Ultrasound to rule out FGR
- Fundoscopy.

Q. 2. What is the aim of the management of preeclampsia?

The aim is to prevent maternal complications, such as eclampsia, pulmonary edema, hepatorenal failure, HELLP syndrome and fetal death. Abruption is a complication which is difficult to prevent; however, one should be aware of that and once abruption occurs early intervention will prevent fetal death and maternal complications like DIC.

Q. 3. What should be the approach to management?

Once the diagnosis is confirmed, ideally the patient should be hospitalized especially if she hails from faraway place. In the hospital strict fetomaternal monitoring should be performed as follows:

Daily: Blood pressure (4th hourly), urine albumin, output, FHS (twice a day), fetal kick count.

Twice a week: Maternal weight gain (in severe cases, towards term), NST, AFI.

Weekly: Repeat all investigations, funduscopy, fetal biophysical profile scoring, Doppler studies (up to 36 weeks).

Once in 2 weeks: Fetal weight estimation to rule out FGR.

Q. 4. Outline management of preeclampsia.

Management essentially involves (a) control of hypertension (b) prevention of convulsion and (c) timely delivery.

a. Control of hypertension: Antihypertensive are started only when the diastolic BP (DBP) crosses 100 mm Hg. The target DBP is 90 mm Hg.

In current practice alpha-methyldopa, calcium channel blockers and labetalol are the mainstay of treatment in preeclampsia disorders. Diuretics are contraindicated during pregnancy as they may also cause neonatal thrombocytopenia, maternal hyperuricemia and may actually decrease the placental perfusion. However, diuretics may be used once the patient delivers and if the BP remains high.[2]

ACE inhibitors and ARBs are also contraindicated during pregnancy as they are associated with fetal anomalies and FGR (Table 2).

Table 2: Antihypertensives commonly used

Drug	Dosage	Remarks
Alpha-methyldopa	500–2000 mg in 4 equally divided doses	Time tested. Effect after 48 hours hence not the choice in emergency. Side effect—postural hypertension
Labetalol	200–2000 mg per day in divided doses	Choice for immediate action. Can be used as 20 mg IV stat if BP does not come under control follow up 40 mg after 20 min then 80 mg every 20 min (max 300 mg in 24 hours) in emergency. Caution in asthma
Nifedipine	10–20 mg per day in divided doses	Not to give sublingually can be used in emergency in the dose of 5–10 mg orally every hour until the DBP is lower than 100 mm Hg

b. Prevention of convulsions: Anticonvulsive therapy with magnesium sulfate (MgSO$_4$) should be started in all cases of severe preeclampsia/imminent eclampsia irrespective of the gestational age and mode of the delivery and to be continued through the labor/cesarean section and up to 24 hours after the delivery.

Magnesium sulfate (MgSO$_4$) regimen (Pritchard's regimen)[3]

- *At 0 hour:* Give 4 g of magnesium sulfate as a 20% solution intravenously at a rate not to exceed 1 g/min.
- Follow promptly with 10 g of 50% magnesium sulfate solution, one-half (5 g) injected deeply in the upper outer quadrant of both buttocks through a 3-inch-long 20-gauge needle. If convulsions persist after 15 min, give up to 2 g more intravenously as a 20% solution at a rate not to exceed 1 g/min. If the woman is large, up to 4 g may be given slowly.
- Every 4 hr thereafter give 5 g of a 50% solution of magnesium sulfate injected deeply in the upper outer quadrant of alternate buttocks, but only after ensuring that:
  - The patellar reflex is present (Loss of reflex begins with plasma Mg levels of 8–10 mg%).
  - Respirations are not depressed (not <14 breaths/minute). Respiratory arrest occurs at plasma Mg levels of 12 mg% or more.
  - Urine output the previous 4 hours exceeded 100 mL.
- The maintenance dose should be continued till 24 hours postpartum.
- The therapeutic magnesium blood levels should be 4–7 mg%.

Intravenous MgSO$_4$ regimen[4]
A loading dose of 6 g of 20% MgSO$_4$ in 100 mL 5% dextrose over 10–15 minutes is given. Maintenance dose of 2 g MgSO$_4$/h by infusion pump to obtain a serum magnesium level of 4 mg% in 6 hours and adjust the rate of infusion to keep serum magnesium between 4.0 and 7.0 mg% or clinically according to patellar reflex, urinary output and respiratory rate.

Zuspan regimen[5]
4 g IV loading followed by 1 g/hour infusion for maintenance × 24 hours.

Consultation to a neurologist is a prudent thing to do. They may start on short- to long-term anticonvulsive agents like levetiracetam or phenytoin sodium.

c. Delivery

Indications for delivery
- After completion of 37 weeks gestation (if there are no complications)
- Signs of severe/imminent eclampsia (as mentioned earlier)

- Eclampsia
- Placental abruption
- HELLP syndrome
- Hepatorenal failure
- Absent end-diastolic flow or reversal of flow in umbilical artery (one should not wait till the disappearance or reversal of 'a' wave in ductus venosus).

Indication for delivery at 37 weeks
PROM
- Development of severe features
- Placental abruption
- Oligohydramnios
- Estimated fetal weight <5th pct nonreassuring fetal testing
- Persistent BPP < or = 6/10
- Patient not willing to continue expectant management

Indication for hospitalization
- Development of severe features
- FGR
- Abnormal fetal heart tracing

Indication for delivery at 34 weeks
- *Worsening maternal condition:* Like increased hypertension or lab findings
- Nonreassuring testing like BPP < = 4/10, at least on 2 occasions 6 hours apart or recurrent late or variable decelerations
- Oligoamnios
- FGR
- Pulmonary edema
- Eclampsia
- Labor or rupture of membranes
- Placental abruption

Source: Jaitely M, Pauli. Prefer JT Best practice in high-risk pregnancy. Preeclampsia short- and long-term implications. Obstetrics and Gynaecology Clinics of North Am. 2015;42(2)299-313.

Mode of delivery
Depends on urgency to deliver. If fetomaternal condition is fair then labor may be induced using PGE2 gel or Misoprostol, provided extreme prematurity, severe FGR/oligohydramnios, CPD has been ruled out and Bishop score is favorable, else cesarean delivery is preferred.

Q. 5. What is the role of steroid prophylaxis?

Steroid prophylaxis should be considered all mothers less than 34 weeks of gestation. At an interval of 24 hours or 6 mg dexamthasone is given IM 12th hourly for 4 doses.

Q. 6. Outline the control of severe hypertension.

In emergency one or more of the following may be used in order to bring down the blood pressure immediately, as the situation demands.

Labetalol is the 1st line drug. Injection labetalol 10–20 mg IV stat and repeat 20–80 mg IV every 30 min to a maximum of 300 mg in 24 hours or constant labetalol IV Infusion with 1–2 mg/min.

Hydralazine may also be used. Inj hydralazine 5 mg IV/IM and repeat 5–10 mg IV every 20–40 min or constant infusion with 0.5–10 mg/hour. Higher or frequent dosage is associated with maternal hypotension, head ache and fetal distress hence, it is not used widely.

Nifedipine is the only oral antihypertensive that can be used in severe preeclampsia. It should never be given sublingually. Tab 10–20 mg orally stat and repeat in 30 min if needed then 10–20 mg orally every 2–6 hours.

Q. 7. Outline management of eclampsia.

The principles are the same as in the section on severe preeclampsia dealt with above. Certain special aspects relating to the management of an eclamptic seizure are as follows summarized in Flowchart 2.

General measures
The patient is ideally managed in a darkened, isolated room where there is minimum stimulation. Injury may be prevented by propping up the guard rails and keeping a padded tongue depressor at hand. A large bore intravenous line is established. Emergency investigations, such as complete blood count with peripheral smear and platelet count, liver

Hypertensive Disorders of Pregnancy

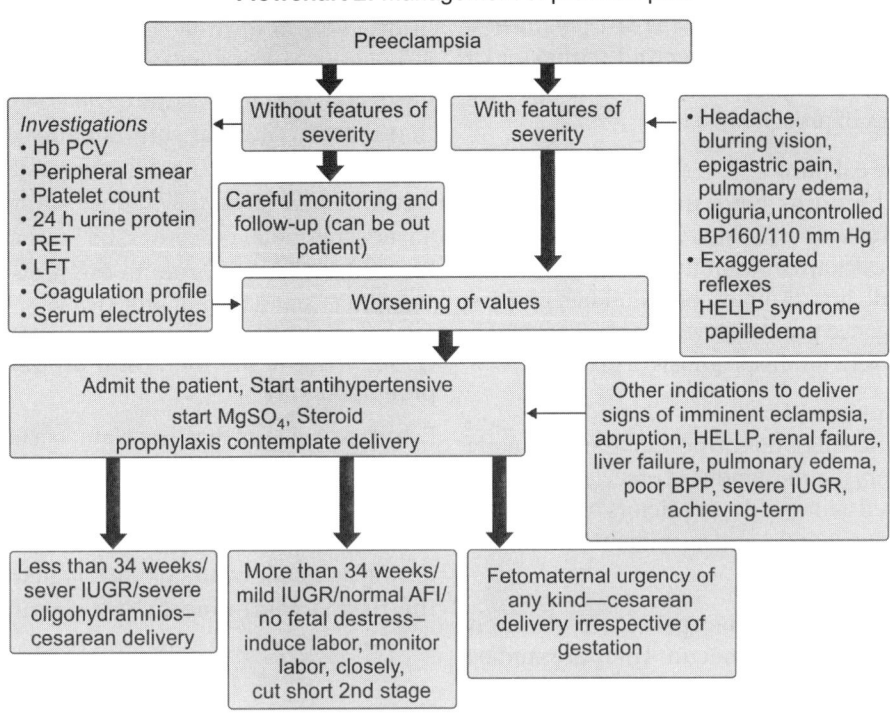

Flowchart 2: Management of preeclampsia

and renal function tests, arterial blood gases, serum electrolytes, bleeding time, clotting time, PT and PTT are ordered. Blood is crossmatched. Oxygen must be readily available and used as dictated by the patient's condition and arterial blood gas values. Maternal acidosis should be corrected when present.

Prevention of aspiration

The patient is nursed in a lateral position to facilitate drainage of secretions. Frequent oral suction is done. The chest must be auscultated after each convulsive episode and SOS chest radiography ordered if there is a doubt of aspiration.

Anticonvulsants

$MgSO_4$ is the drug of choice and the dose is same as given in imminent eclampsia.

Delivery should be accomplished speedily and with as little trauma as possible. In current practice tendency is to perform immediate caesarean section, especially if there is evidence of fetomaternal compromise and induction is deemed to take longer or fail.

Q. 8. Can preeclampsia be predicted/ what are the tests of prediction?

Since the etiology is not clearly understood its difficult to predict preeclampsia. Despite advancements in Doppler studies and biochemical markers like PAAP-A, etc. history, high-risk factors and clinical examination are still the best predictors. However, following tests have been in practice to predict preeclampsia.

Angiotensin sensitivity test

The abnormal vascular reactivity of patients may be detected using the degree of sensitivity to angiotensin II.

Roll-over test

A positive test is an elevation of 20 mm Hg or more in blood pressure when the patient rolls over from the lateral decubitus to the supine position. The test has poor sensitivity and poor specificity and of limited clinical value.

Mean blood pressure in the second trimester

Mean arterial pressure (MAP) [systolic + 2 (diastolic)/3] in the second trimester of pregnancy was proposed long time ago as a predictor of preeclampsia.

Urinary calcium

Several studies have demonstrated that preeclampsia is associated with hypocalciuria. A urinary calcium concentration equal or less than 12 mg/dL in a 24-hour collection has positive and negative predictive values of 85 and 91%, respectively, for the diagnosis of preeclampsia.

Serum uric acid

Hyperuricemia is one of the important and early laboratory manifestations of preeclampsia. It is suggested as one of the predictors but has poor sensitivity (0–55%) and specificity (77–95%).

Fibronectin

Patients with preeclampsia have elevated levels of plasma fibronectin. There are studies indicating that increased plasma levels of endothelium-originated fibronectin precede the clinical signs of preeclampsia and may be useful for prediction of the disease.

Uterine artery Doppler

Several investigations have suggested that transvaginal uterine artery color-Doppler velocimetry at 22–24 weeks is useful to identify women destined to develop preeclampsia. Early diastolic notches were present in both uterine arteries in 9.3% of the cases.

Q. 9. What is the role of bed rest, salt restriction aspirin, calcium, vitamin C and E in the prevention of preeclampsia?

Several large studies, the collaborative low-dose aspirin study in pregnancy (CLASP) has shown that aspirin does not have a role in prevention of preeclampsia in low-risk population but in high-risk group it reduces the overall risk. A few authors have suggested that dietary calcium supplements may be effective in preventing preeclampsia. Both calcium and aspirin may reduce severity and adverse perinatal outcomes. Bed rest and salt restrictions have no role in the prevention. Vitamin C and E are not effective

Q. 10. What is the long-term prognosis of preeclampsia?

Evidence suggests that preeclampsia like FGR and preterm birth, is a marker for subsequent cardiovascular morbidity and mortality; hence, women with hypertension identified during pregnancy should be evaluated during the first several months postpartum and counseled regarding long-term risks.

References

1. Hypertension in pregnancy, Task force on hypertension in pregnancy, ACOG. 2013.
2. Sibai BM. Etiology and management of postpartum hypertension-preeclampsia. Am J Obstet Gynecol. 2012;206(6):470.
3. Pritchard JA. The use of magnesium ion in the management of eclamptogenictoxemias. Surg Gynecol Obstet. 1955;100:131.
4. Sibai BM, Graham JM, McCubbin JH: A comparison of intravenous and intramuscular magnesium sulfate regimens in preeclampsia. Am J Obstet Gynecol. 1984;150:728.
5. Zuspan FP, problems encountered in the treatment of pregnancy induced hypertension a point of view. Am J Obstet Gynecol. 1978;131:591-7.

CHAPTER 9

ICU Rounds for Obstetricians

Sunil Karanth

Q. 1. What is the association of critical care medicine as a specialty in obstetrics?
Critical care medicine is a new specialty with its origins as recent as within the last three to four decades. Obstetric patients form a small but important part of this specialty. It is thus essential for both critical care physicians and obstetricians to be well-versed in the key management aspects of these patients.

The obstetric patients have unique demands, such as altered maternal physiology, demands of maternal care, demands of fetal care, etc.

Obstetric patients in ICU include patients during their pregnancy up to 6 weeks of termination of pregnancy.

These unique set of patients have brought the concepts of critical care into obstetrics. This concept of compartmentalizing of a specific subset of acutely ill patients in a geographic area with relevant infrastructure and personnel resulting in parcelation of medicine is now in obstetrics. Estimates across the world put the incidence of obstetric patients in a medical or multi-disciplinary ICU at 1-2%.

On the other hand, utilization of ICU services by obstetric patients is equal to around 1% across the world. Indian data correlate with the above numbers as well.

Q. 2. What are the different models of ICU care in relevance to management of an obstetric patient?
Critically ill obstetric patients would generally follow principles of critical care medicine, just like any other acutely ill patient. On the basis of the case mix, incidence of critically ill obstetric patients and the availability of trained personnel the following patterns of ICU can be adopted:

- Obstetric patients in a general intensive care unit
  - *Closed ICU model:* This is a structured intensivist-led model, wherein the intensivist or his team manages the critically ill patients in the intensive care unit.
  - *Open ICU model:* This is a more widely practised model of intensive care, where in the obstetric patient is admitted to a general intensive care under the obstetrician with other specialists, including intensivist playing supporting roles. The main advantage of this model is the continuity of care and most importantly the maintenance of the long standing physician–patient relationship.
- Obstetric ICU or high dependency unit (HDU)
- Virtual obstetric intensive care unit.

Considering the pros and cons of the above 2 systems of ICU a hybrid model of care could provide the advantages of both, and minimizing the disadvantages of each of the system. Furthermore, considering the fiscal viability and the need for such beds another

Flowchart 1: Multidisciplinary team approach in the care of a critically ill patient

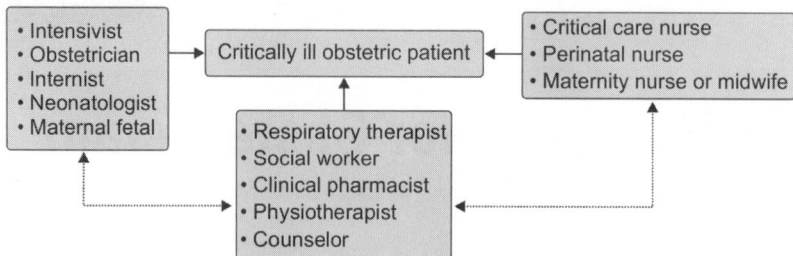

Modified from: Zeeman G, Wendel GD, Cunningham FG. A blueprint for obstetric critical care. Am J Obstet Gynecol 2003;188:532-6 and Marini JJ. Streamlining critical care: responsibilities and cost effectiveness in intensive care unit organization. Mayo Clin Proc. 1997;72:483-5.

model called "Virtual obstetric Intensive care unit" had been proposed.

Virtual Obstetric Intensive Care Unit

This is a novel concept proposed by certain authors in such institutions catering to high risk obstetric patients, but having a low prevalence of this subset of patients. As described, it would not be a viable proposition to have a separate specialized acute care area. In this concept, the multidisciplinary team (Flowchart 1) is brought to the acutely ill obstetric unit admitted in the general obstetric unit or birthing suite. This implies that if a parturient gets very ill the required specialists and the required organ specific support modalities (like mechanical ventilation, renal replacement therapy, vasopressors, etc.) are brought to the bedside of the patient.

Q. 3. Define admission criteria into the ICU for a critically ill obstetric patient.

According to a document by the Department of Health, London, critical care of an obstetric patient will encompass the concept of outreach services, paraphrased as "Critical care without walls." The level of critical care will depend on the acuity of illness, as defined by various Intensive care societies. The entire spectrum of care is defined as "comprehensive critical care."

Levels of care are categorized as below based on precise definitions:

- Level 0: Patients whose care can be met by normal ward care
- Level 1: Patients at risk of their condition deteriorating and needing a higher level of observation or those recently relocated from higher levels of care.
- Level 2: Patients requiring invasive monitoring/intervention that require support for a single failing organ system (excluding advanced respiratory support).
- Level 3: Patients requiring advanced respiratory support (mechanical ventilation) alone or basic respiratory support with support of at least one additional organ.

Q. 4. Which are the conditions requiring ICU admission during pregnancy and peripartum period?

The conditions requiring ICU admission during pregnancy and peripartum period could be arbitrarily classified into the following and in Table 1:

1. Conditions unique to pregnancy
2. Conditions causing increased susceptibility during pregnancy
3. Conditions unrelated to pregnancy
4. Preexisting that may worsen during pregnancy

Q. 5. Describe the ICU discharge criteria.

The two broad criteria for identifying patients suitable for discharge include:

Table 1: Conditions requiring ICU admission during pregnancy and peripartum period

Unique to pregnancy	Increased susceptibility during pregnancy	Unrelated to pregnancy	Preexisting disease that may worsen during pregnancy
Obstetric hemorrhage	Renal	Diabetic ketoacidosis	Cardiovascular
Placental abruption/placenta previa	Acute renal failure	CMV	Valvular disease
Retained placenta (accreta)	Infections	HIV infection	Eisenmenger syndrome
Pregnancy-induced hypertension	Urinary tract infections	Toxoplasmosis	Coarctation of aorta
HELLP syndrome	Listeriosis	Community acquired pneumonia	Cyanotic congenital heart disease
Acute fatty liver of pregnancy	Viral hepatitis E	Drug abuse	Primary pulmonary hypertension
Chorioamnionitis	*Plasmodium falciparum* malaria	Trauma	Respiratory
Amniotic fluid embolism	Coccidioidomycosis		Cystic fibrosis
Puerperal sepsis	Varicella pneumonia		Lung transplant
Pelvic septic thrombophlebitis	H1N1 pneumonia		Bronchial asthma
Peripartum cardiomyopathy	Hematologic		Obstructive sleep apnea
Ovarian hyperstimulation syndrome	Disseminated intravascular coagulation		Renal
Fetal mirror syndrome	Venous thrombosis		Glomerulonephritis
Tocolytic-induced pulmonary edema	Postpartum HUS/TTP		Chronic renal insufficiency
Gestational diabetes	Endocrine		Endocrine
Gestational hyperthyroidism	Sheehan syndrome		Prolactinoma
	Neurologic		Diabetes mellitus
	Intracranial hemorrhage		Hepatic
	Pulmonary		Cirrhosis
	Pulmonary thromboembolism		Hematologic
	Aspiration		Sickle cell disease
	ARDS		Anemia
			Rheumatologic
			Scleroderma
			Polymyositis
			SLE
			Neurologic
			Epilepsy
			Intracranial tumors
			Myasthenia gravis
			Multiple sclerosis

Modified from: Guntupalli KK, Hall N, Karnad DR, Bandi V, Belfort M. Critical illness in pregnancy. Part I: Approach to a pregnant patient in the ICU and common obstetric disorders. Chest. 2015;148(4):1093-1104.

a. When a patient's physiological state has been stabilized and the need for ICU monitoring and care is no longer needed.
b. When a patients physiological status has deteriorated and active intervention is no longer planned, discharge to a lower level of care is appropriate.

Q. 6. A 28-year-old primi, with 34 weeks gestation, normal antenatal period developed blurring of vision, increasing headache for 3 days. She was initially managed in a local hospital, where she was noted to have an elevated blood pressure (160/100 mm Hg). She was thus referred to a higher center. En route, she developed increasing drowsiness and noted to have a GCS of e3m4v1 at admission in the ER with pupils pinpoint and Doll's eye movement present. How do you approach a pregnant woman presenting with unconsciousness?

This patient with features of preeclampsia should be diagnosed with eclamptic seizures with postictal phenomenon. CVA should be considered in view of pinpoint pupils and Doll's eye movements. Though initial management is with Pritchard's regime, a neurologist's consultation and imaging of the brain is important

Generally, definition of consciousness has two elements—awareness and arousal.

Nearly half of obstetric patients admitted into the ICU in the developing world have neurological involvement. However, the causes for unconsciousness could be pregnancy specific or unrelated to the pregnant state.

On evaluating the various causes, the mechanisms of decreased consciousness group under the following categories:
- Failure or airway or breathing—hypoxia/hypercarbia
- Failure of circulation—hypotension/cardiac arrest
- Failure of central nervous system.

Q. 7. What are the frequent causes of unconsciousness?

Table 2 depicts various causes of uncosciousness in pregnancy and they are detailed below:

Trauma occurs in 6–7% of all pregnancies and is the leading cause of nonobstetric or co-incidental maternal death. The most common causes of trauma include motor vehicle accidents (55%), assault (22%), falls (22%), burns (1%) and suicides. Trauma puts both the mother and fetus at risk. It is estimated that fetal loss occurs in at least 40% of critically injured pregnant women. Fetal injuries are more likely with penetrating abdominal trauma in advanced pregnancy. The injuries could be classified as general and obstetric.

Preeclampsia and eclampsia are important causes of cerebral complications and consequent unconsciousness in pregnant women. It is the most common reason for referral of an obstetric patient to the ICU. The causes of unconsciousness in eclamptic patients could be excessive sedation, postictal state or raised intracranial pressure. The latter could result due to cerebral edema, cerebral hyperemia or intracranial hemorrhage.

Epilepsy affects only 0.5% of all pregnancies. Approximately one-third of patients experience worsening of seizures during pregnancy.

Other relevant causes of unconsciousness in a pregnant woman include **Amniotic fluid embolism, sepsis** (pregnancy-related, non-pregnancy related and nosocomial), HIV infection and its associated complications, intracranial hemorrhage, diabetic complications cerebral malaria, ischemic stroke, intracranial tumors, multiple sclerosis and electrolyte disturbances. Psychiatric issues also should be kept in mind.

Assessment and Initial Management of Unconscious Patient (Flowchart 2)

Management of unconscious eclamptic patients: Cerebral edema is seen in a significant number of patients with eclampsia. Further continued or frequent seizures, might further worsen the neurologic functioning. It may be sometimes important to differentiate eclampsia from other neurologic hypertensive emergencies.

Table 2: Causes of unconsciousness in pregnancy

Respiratory causes	Cardiovascular causes	Central nervous system causes	Metabolic disturbance	Others
Trauma	Trauma	Trauma	Hypo/Hyperglycemia	Autoimmune conditions
Airway obstruction	Cardiac disease	Epilepsy/eclampsia	Hypo/hypercalcemia	Iatrongenic
Respiratory failure	Myocardial infarction	Intracerebral hemorrhage	Hyponatremia	Anesthetic complications
	Septic shock	Drug overdose, including narcotics, barbiturates	Hypermagnesemia	Drug reactions
	Obstructive shock such as embolism—pulmonary or amniotic	Intoxications—alcohol	Hyperammonemia	Tocolytics
	Cardiac arrest—cardiac or non-cardiac origin	Cerebral infections including abscess		Magnesium sulfate
		Cerebral infarction,		Poisoning
		Cerebral edema		Psychiatric conditions
		Hypertensive encephalopathy		
		Vascular malformations		
		Space-occupying lesions		
		Sheehan's syndrome		
		Cerebral venous sinus thrombosis		

Modified from: Guntupalli KK, Hall N, Karnad DR, Bandi V, Belfort M. Critical illness in pregnancy. Part I: Approach to a pregnant patient in the ICU and common obstetric disorders. Chest. 2015;148(4):1093-1104 and Platteau P, Engelhardt T, Moodley J, et al. Obstetric and gynaecological patients in an intensive care unit: a one year review. Trop Doct. 1997;27:202-6.

Control of hypertension is very important in control of seizures.

Q. 8. A 28-year-old lady, with 38 weeks gestation underwent a normal vaginal delivery. Postoperatively, she developed PPH requiring emergency intervention and hysterectomy. Prior to the procedure, the family was unavailable to offer consent. What would be the most apt thing to do for the treating physician regarding the procedure and explain the legal position regarding cosenting in emergencies?

Prior to any procedure, counseling a patient and obtaining valid consent is mandatory. It is imperative that a patient scheduled for a procedure, comprehends all aspects of their health care and get involved in the medical decision-making.

Flowchart 2: General principles in the management of unconscious pregnant patient

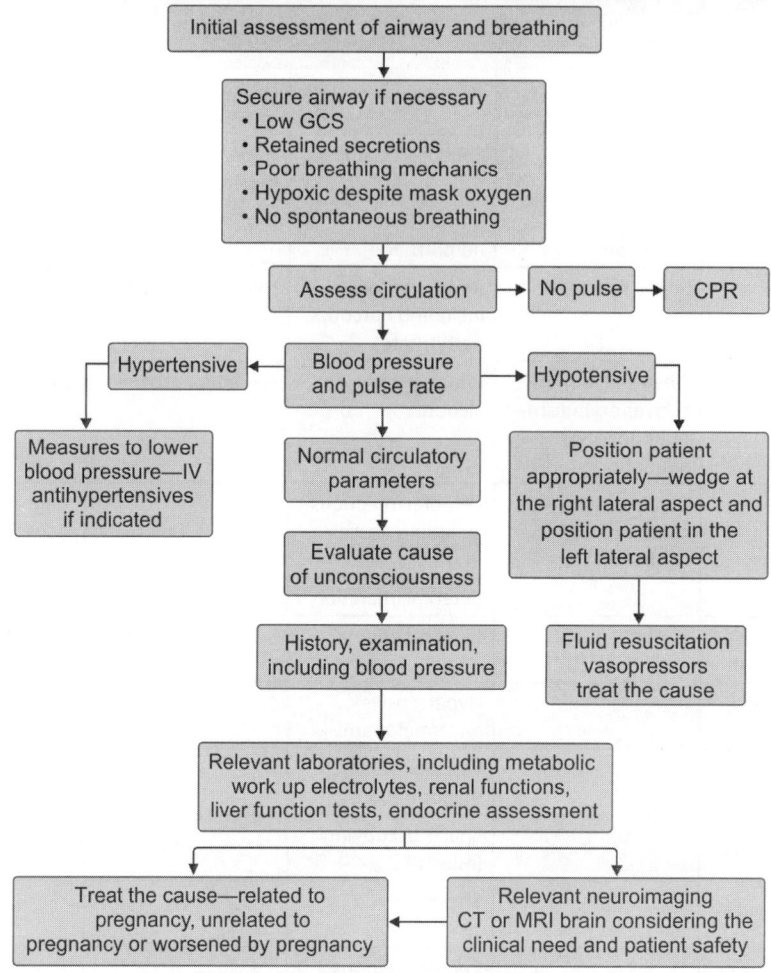

Modified from: Bobrowski R. Trauma in pregnancy. In James DK, Steer PJ, Weiner CP, Gonik B (Eds). High-risk pregnancy—management options. 2nd edition and Richards AM, Moodley J, Graham DI, et al. Active management of the unconscious eclamptic patient. Br J Obstet Gynaecol. 1986;93:554-62.

Failure to obtain a prior consent before physically handling or interfering with patient's body constitutes assault. Different types of consents exist. The one applicable in emergency situations is "presumed consent". It is a consent which is presumed and applicable only for emergency situations. Thus in the setting of a life threatening condition an emergency procedure or surgery that is needed has to be done. A "second opinion" may be sought, before performing any additional procedure not discussed, not lifesaving but mandatory. For the most part, an unconsented procedure may be performed at a later date after obtaining a fully informed consent. "The principle of beneficence may require healthcare professionals to act for the patient's benefit on her behalf, only when her life is at stake". In fact, delaying the procedure in these circumstances to obtain consent can be construed as negligence.

It may be appropriate to take the second opinion of a fellow colleague in writing if the latter has concurred with your decision for the procedure or surgery.

Q. 9. What are the principles of managing a major obstetric hemorrhage?

Nearly 50% of the maternal deaths occur due to major obstetric hemorrhage (MOH), most often due to hemorrhage in the postpartum period.

Definition of MOH

Antepartum hemorrhage is defined as hemorrhage occurring from 24 weeks of pregnancy and prior to delivery. This type of hemorrhage complicates 3–5% of all pregnancies.

Postpartum hemorrhage is defined as blood loss of 500 mL or more within 24 hours after birth. RCOG classifies postpartum hemorrhage as:
a. Minor 500–1000 mL
b. Major >1000 mL
c. Severe >2000 mL

The incidence of PPH is estimated to be 18% of all births with at least 4% categorizing as major variety of PPH (>1000 mL).

Management of MOH

The multidisciplinary team should include obstetricians, critical care physicians, anesthetists, neonatologists and obstetric physicians.

General preparations

Alert the team, when a high-risk patient is admitted. Following the trigger, a meeting of the team members (called perinatal huddle) to strategize and formulate a plan of management is essential. The preparation would also include appropriate arrangement of blood and blood products.

Blood blank protocols

Design appropriate blood bank protocols. It is also important that all members of the team are familiar with the protocol. The local transfusion guidelines should include the following:

a. Emergency blood release, including emergency release of blood if need be with O-negative group is appropriate.
b. Massive transfusion protocol: Standardized pathways are needed when massive transfusion is indicated. A protocol to this effect is called massive transfusion protocol. The protocol has a predetermined number of blood and blood products transfused in a prespecified ratio. Most data for this emerges from trauma literature. The current recommendation is to transfuse FFP:RBC in the ratio of 1 : 1 to 1 : 2 (Table 3).
c. A hemorrhage cart or medical kit allows easy access to medications and equipments needed to control obstetric hemorrhage.
d. Hemorrhage team: For fast, prompt and organized action, creation of a hemorrhage team or any such similar rapid response teams are important. Patients requiring activation of the hemorrhage team include:
   - Before delivery for patients refusing blood transfusion
   - Before delivery for patients expected to have placenta accreta
   - Before delivery for patients with full anticoagulation requiring surgery
   - Any PPH diagnosed as stage III
   - Any PPH in patients refusing blood transfusion.

Monitoring

Monitoring hemodynamic status refers to the standard monitoring of heart rate, blood pressure, peripheral perfusion, urine output and oxygen saturation. The physiological pregnancy state already mimics certain changes that occur consequent to blood loss. These changes mask the early signs of hemorrhage or blood loss. In order to identify shock at an early stage, a parameter called **shock index** was described. This is a ratio of heart rate to systolic blood pressure. A shock

Table 3: Massive transfusion protocol

Indications	Protocol					Drawbacks
Massive hemorrhage—anticipated need to replace 50% or more blood volume in 2 hours						Economic repercussions
Systolic blood pressure <90 mm Hg with a heart rate of >120/min	Round	PRBC	FFP	Platelets	Cryo PPT	Risk of wastage of products, especially plasma
Requirement for transfusion of 4 units of packed red cells within 1–2 hours	1	6	6	6	10	Risk of transfusion related acute lung injury (TRALI) and transfusion related immunomodulation (TRIM)
	2	6	6	6	10	
	3	Administer tranexamic acid				
Protocol will continue till deactivated by the surgical team	4	6	6	6		Risk of transfusion-related infections, transfusion related acute kidney injury (AKI), transfusion related circulatory overload
						Metabolic complications like hyperkalemia, hypocalcemia, iron overload and citrate toxicity

Modified from: Society of Obstetricians and Gynaecologists of Canada. Active Management of the Third Stage of Labour: Prevention and Treatment of Postpartum Hemorrhage. No. 235 October 2009 (Replaces No. 88, April 2000) and Pacheco Ld, Saade Gr, Gei AF, Hankins Gd. Cutting-edge advances in the medical management of obstetrical hemorrhage. Am J Obstet Gynecol. 2011;205:526-32.

index >1.1 predicts 3-fold increase in mortality, despite a systolic blood pressure which is >100 mm Hg. Thus emanating from trauma patients there is sufficient data to suggest the use of shock index as one of the guides to identify patients with hemorrhagic shock and consider early intervention despite the presence of normal blood pressure.

Laboratory changes

1. Hemoglobin and hematocrit: During acute hemorrhage, the hemoglobin and hematocrit always lag in response to the blood loss. A drop in hemoglobin/hematocrit by greater than 5 points or a low Hb (<25%), identified only 25% of the patients who eventually required a major intervention. On the other hand, a low value was suggestive of possible hemorrhage. Thus, a low value had good positive predictive value, though a normal hemoglobin does not suggest absence of hemorrhage.

2. Coagulation studies: The earliest and most consistent abnormality in hemorrhage-induced coagulopathy is abnormal fibrinogen level. Thus fibrinogen levels need to be an important part of the coagulation profile in bleeding patients. In the initial evaluation of women diagnosed to have postpartum hemorrhage fibrinogen level was found to be the best predictor of severe hemorrhage defined as decrease in hemoglobin >4 g/dL, transfusion of more than 4 units of RBCs or hysterectomy within the first 24 hours.

3. Acid–base changes: Significant anaerobic metabolism results in elevated lactates, lactate-induced metabolic acidosis and increased base-deficit. Thus lactate and metabolic acidosis can be measured as indirect markers of assessing the severity of shock and response to resuscitation. Elevated lactates with metabolic acidosis are strong predictors of morbidity and mortality.

Staging hemorrhage

Classification of hemorrhage has an important clinical significance, especially in the context of resuscitation and management. The classification proposed by the American College of Surgeons was modified for use in obstetric patients (Table 4).

Any hemorrhage needs following in summary:

Get help, arrange for blood and blood products, monitor the patient, evaluate the stage and deterioration.

Management

Management of peripartum hemorrhage is aimed at controlling the source of bleeding, adequate replacement of blood volume and supportive care.

a. Hemostasis: Choice of intervention for achieving hemostasis will depend on:
   - Etiology of the hemorrhage
   - Timing
   - Extent of interventions required
   - Rate of ongoing bleeding
   - Patient's acceptance of blood products
   - Availability of resources
   - Desire for future childbearing.

A management algorithm for 3 commonly encountered situations is proposed in the Flowchart 3.

b. Replacement therapy
c. Fluid management: Most data for hemorrhagic shock and fluid resuscitation emerges from trauma literature. However, the recent data show that in the long-term excessive administration of crystalloids results in poor outcomes, higher mortality, with exacerbation of the lethal triad of hypothermia, acidosis and coagulopathy. Thus, in a new paradigm in managing resuscitation called damage control resuscitation, the following principles are have been adopted:
   - Limitation of crystalloid therapy: Fluid therapy to a ratio of 1:1 or 2: to the EBL or <1.5 liters of fluids for every unit of PRBC is associated with a lower mortality.
   - Transfusion of blood products in ratios of whole blood
   - Permissive hypotension—when practiced is followed by less risk in comparison to massive transfusion.
d. Oxygen administration.

Table 4: Stages of peripartum hemorrhage

Stages	Blood loss	Clinical picture	Laboratory abnormalities
Stage 1	Vaginal delivery >500 mL LSCS >1000 mo	Normal	Normal
Stage 2	Estimated blood loss 1000–1500 mL	Normal	Normal
Stage 3*	Estimated blood loss >1500 mL or brisk bleeding of >500 mL in 10 minutes	Abnormal BP, pulse, shock index, urine output	Abnormal pH, base deficit, elevated lactate, >4 g% drop in hemoglobin
Stage 4	Cardiovascular collapse in the setting of severe hemorrhage	Profound hypovolemic shock (Blood loss not replaced) Amniotic fluid embolism with cardiovascular collapse	

*Stage 1 and 2 have normal clinical and lab parameters. Once the patient shows changes in clinical parameters the stage of hemorrhage is raised to stage 3 irrespective of the amount of blood loss

Modified from: Charbit B, Mandelbrot L, Samarin E, et al. The decrease of fibrinogen is a nearly predictor of the severity of postpartum hemorrhage. J Thromb Haemost. 2007;5(2):266-73 and Davis JW, Parks SN, Kaups KL, Gladen HE, O'Donnell-Nicol S. Admission base deficit predicts transfusion requirements and risk of complications. J Trauma. 1996;41(5):769-74.

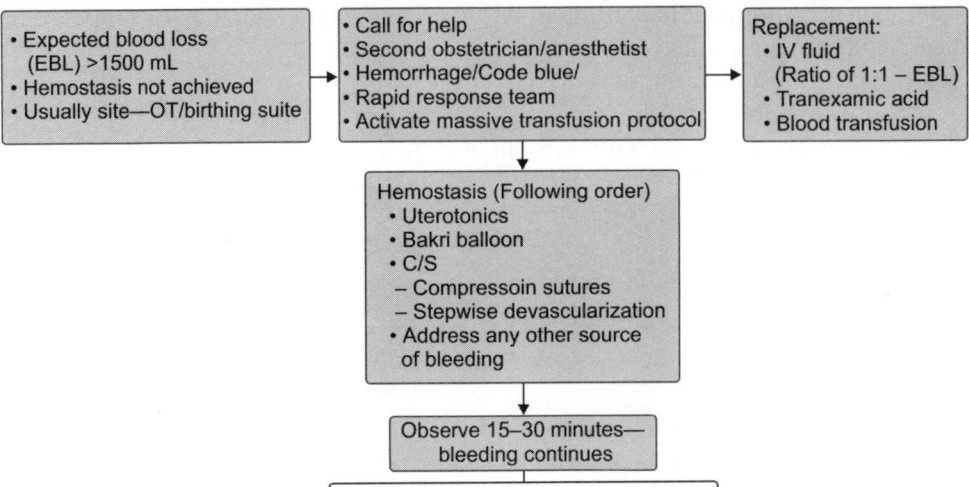

Flowchart 3: Management of severe PPH at the time of delivery

Modified from: RCOG. Postpartum hemorrhage, prevention and management. Green-top Guideline No. 52; 2009.

HAEMOSTASIS
H—**H**elp from seniors, fellow obstetricians, junior and supporting staff
A—**A**ssess the general condition—Shock index, Urine output, severity of bleeding
E—**E**valuate for other causes—4Ts—Tone, Tissue (Placenta, membranes), Trauma, Thrombin as cause for PPH, start **E**cbolics—Oxytocin, PGF2 alpha, methyl ergometrine, syntometrine, misoprostol
M—**M**assage the uterus, continue medical line of management
O—**O**xytocics to be continued
S—**S**urgical interventions
T—**T**amponade (Bakri balloon, condom tamponade, Sengstaken Blackmurray tube, Foley's balloon), bimanual compression
A—**A**pplication of compression sutures
S—**S**tepwise devascularization
I—**I**nterventional radiology use with uterine artery embilization
S—**S**ub-total/total hysterectomy

e. RBC transfusion: General recommendations and evidence in critically ill patients provide little justification for transfusion beyond Hb 7–8 g/L in the absence of active bleeding. However, this does not apply to patients who are constantly bleeding.

f. Coagulopathy: Again emanating from trauma literature, there is a suggestion that the most effective intervention to decrease risk of coagulopathy is early administration of FFPs. The evidence is to administer FFP:RBC in the ratio of 1:1 or 1:2 to decrease the risk of bleeding.

g. Antifibrinolysis: Hyperfibrinolysis is another important determinant of coagulation process resulting in increased risk of bleeding. Some data from surgical literature indicate a possible role for prophylactic administration of tranexamic acid, which reduces the risk of bleeding in high-risk patients and also decrease the amount of bleeding when administered in patients with hemorrhage.

Q. 10. What are the principles of blood transfusion in an obstetric patient? (Modified from the RCOG guidelines)

General principles of blood transfusion need to be followed prior any transfusion. These include:

a. Seeking a consent (retrospectively if the transfusion is very urgent).
b. Available group and screen, etc.
c. A high-risk patient with a significant likelihood of requiring emergency transfusion is evaluated every week for the group and cross match, development of new antibodies and ensuring adequate blood is available.
d. There is no role for preoperative autologous blood donation.
e. If the patient is at high risk of significant hemorrhage, intraoperative autologous transfusion may be an option. This is suggested only in centers with experience in this modality of transfusion.
f. Specifically in relation to major obstetric hemorrhage, it is recommended to have clear local protocols.
g. Firm criteria for initiation of RBC transfusion do not exist. This decision should be firmly based on clinical and hematological grounds. There is no requirement for transfusion if hemoglobin (Hb) >10 g/L. But if there is active bleeding with signs of shock or Hb <6 g/L, transfusion is indicated.
h. Fresh frozen plasma (FFP) and cryoprecipitate: FFPs should ideally be administered at a dose of 12–15 mL/kg for every 6 units RBC transfusion. Subsequent transfusion needs to be guided by results of clotting tests—PT/APTT. There is no role for anti-D prophylaxis if a patient with Rh-negative group receives a Rh-positive FFP or cryoprecipitate.

Platelet transfusions

In a patient who is actively bleeding platelet transfusions are indicated to maintain a count of >50,000/mm^3. However, transfusions are indicated when the counts dip below 75,000/mm^3 to maintain a margin of safety. It is ideal to transfuse group specific platelet. However, there seems to be no difference in the hemostatic effectiveness even if a non-identical group platelet is administered. If Rh-positive platelets are administered in Rh-negative women, anti-D immunoglobulin should be administered.

Q. 11. Discuss the role of rFVIIa and other agents in massive hemorrhage.

Many adjuvants have been trialled and tested over the years. Recombinant factor VIIa (rFVIIa) may be considered as one of the adjuvants to control life-threatening hemorrhage. However, it is extremely important to understand that rFVIIa, is not a replacement for a lifesaving procedure (surgery or embolization) nor transfer to an appropriate facility. rFVIIa was initially developed for management of inherited bleeding disorders. But over the course of years a number of off-label indications including its use in life-threatening hemorrhage has been proposed. Most of these data are limited to case series or registries. Accordingly rFVIIa can be used in PPH. The literature for this indication is largely based on case series. A scrutiny of this literature suggests possible benefit in the use of rFVIIa in terms of reducing bleeding or transfusion requirements. However, this benefit has to be outweighed against the risk of thrombotic complications with the use of rFVIIa, reported in around 2.5% of patients. However, it should also be emphasized that there is no role for prophylactic rFVIIa. In addition, for rFVIIa to be effective, attempts should be made to correct thrombocytopenia, acidosis and hypofibrinogenemia. Thus, use of rFVIIa should be very judicious, preferably under guidance by a hematologist with strong local protocols.

Fibrinogen concentrate is an adjuvant which could be considered as a replacement for cryoprecipitate with the advantages of faster reconstitution, ease of use and no requirement for thawing and ABO compatibility.

Fibrinolytic agents like tranexemic acid have been found to be effective in reducing blood loss in patients with trauma and after Ceserean section. However, at present there is no data available on mortality in PPH with the use of tranexemic acid.

Q. 12. A 35-year-old lady, delivered a male fetus of 4 kg. Postpartum she developed massive PPH, due to atonic PPH requiring an emergency hysterectomy and multiple transfusions. Despite the initial stability, she developed mucosal bleeding and oozing from the surgical site, 24 hours later. What is the likely diagnosis? How would you considering managing this patient?

The most likely diagnosis is *disseminated intravascular coagulation (DIC) in pregnancy*. The rate of DIC in obstetric patients ranges from 0.03 to 0.35%.

> **Causes for DIC in obstetrics**
> - Peripartum hemorrhage
> - Placental abruption
> - Spectrum of preeclampsia/eclampsia/HELLP syndrome
> - Retained stillbirth
> - Septic abortion and intrauterine infection
> - Amniotic fluid embolism
> - Acute fatty liver of pregnancy

In 2 different large cohort of patients the top 3 common obstetric causes of DIC included—placental abruption, postpartum hemorrhage and severe eclampsia.

Diagnosis of DIC

The diagnosis of DIC is largely based on clinical and set of abnormal laboratory investigations. Scoring systems based on the commonly available abnormal tests have been developed to aid in the diagnosis of DIC. These parameters include thrombocytopenia, prolonged prothrombin time (PT) and activated partial thromboplastin time (APTT), decreased fibrinogen and increased fibrin degradation product (FDP).

Point of care testing devices like thromboelastography (TEG) or thromboelastometry (TEM) may be useful for rapid diagnosis and management in obstetric coagulopathy disorders.

Multiple scoring systems have been proposed over the years for the diagnosis of DIC. The different scoring systems and their components are summarized in Table 5.

Treatment of DIC

a. The basic principles of managing DIC circles around:
   - Management of underlying condition which predisposes to DIC
   - Supportive care with blood products and related measures
   - Coagulation factors: Replacement guided by hemostatic indices. If PT/APTT are prolonged consider transfusion of FFPs at 15–30 mL/kg, or even higher if there is no sign of volume overload. If there is no suggestion of bleeding, correction of PT/APTT may not be warranted
   - Platelets: Aim for a platelet count of >50,000/mm^3 in the presence of DIC. But if there is ongoing active bleeding a higher threshold of 75,000/mm^3 may be considered.

Table 5: Scoring systems in DIC with their respective components

Parameters	ISTH score	JAAM score	Modified ISTH score
Platelet count (mm)^3	>100,000 = 0 <100,000 = 1 <50,000 = 2	<80,000 or >50% decrease within 24 hours = 3 < 80,000 but >120,000 or >30% decrease within 24 hours = 1 >120,000 = 0	< 50,000 = 1 50,000–100,000 = 2 100,000–185,000 = 3 >185,000 = 0
Fibrin related markers (FDP)	No increase = 0 Moderate increase = 2 Strong increase = 3	>/=25 = 3 >/=10 = 1 <10 = 1	-
Prothrombin time (value of patient/normal value)	<3 sec = 0 >3 sec but < 6 secs = 1 >6 sec = 2	>1.2 = 1 <1.2 = 0	<0.5 = 0 0.5–1 = 5 1.0–1.5 = 12 >1.5 = 25
Fibrinogen level	>1.0 = 0 <1.0 = 1		3.0 = 25 3.0–4.0 = 6 4.0–4.5 = 1 > 4.5 = 0
SIRS criteria	-	≥3 = 1 0-2 = 0	-
Calculated score	>5 = compatible with overt DIC; repeat scoring daily <5 = suggestive (not affirmative) for nonovert DIC; repeat next 1–2 days	≥4 = suggestive of disseminated intravascular coagulation	>26 high probability for DIC

Modified from: Erez O, Novack L, Beer-Weisel R, et al. DIC score in pregnant women--a population based modification of the International Society on Thrombosis and Hemostasis score. PLoS One 2014;9:e93240 and Thachil J, Toh CH. Disseminated intravascular coagulation in obstetric disorders and its acute haematological management. Blood Rev. 2009;23:167-76.

- Fibrinogen: Transfusion of Cryoprecipitate is advised if the serum fibrinogen level is <1.5 g/L
- Hemoglobin: The exact cutoff level of Hemoglobin to commence transfusion is unclear. Based on data from other critically ill patients, transfusions could be considered when the hemoglobin is <7 g/L if there is no active bleeding
- Crystalloid resuscitation: In a patient with multiple hemostatic abnormalities, resuscitation with IV fluids are likely to further worsen the process of DIC, by causing dilution of clotting factors and hemoglobin. Thus, in a patient with bleeding and shock secondary to DIC, transfusion of blood and blood products is more optimal than, crystalloids or colloids.
- Tranexemic acid: This antifibrinolytic agent may be useful in reducing bleeding. But, more evidence is still needed to recommend for routine use. Most guidelines suggest consideration if all other measures fail to control bleeding.
- Factor concentrates:
    ◊ Consideration can be given for fibrinogen concentrates if all measures fail and intractable PPH continues.

◊ rFVIIa has been considered in uncontrolled PPH across the world. It is considered as a global hemostatic agent. Use of this agent in PPH is associated with a lower mortality. Timing of administration is important for maximum efficacy of the drug. It is recommended that rFVIIa would act best when the coagulation parameters are corrected and there is no acidosis. However, administration of rFVIIa is associated with significant cost and increased risk of arterial thrombosis. Thus, guidelines suggest the use of rFVIIa before hysterectomy in the presence of massive PPH.

b. Regular clinical and laboratory surveillance: DIC is a dynamic process and constant assessment is essential to monitor the disease. There are no specific guidelines regarding the frequency of monitoring, but the principles include monitoring of hemostatic lab indices, clinical monitoring with reference to bleeding and worsening multiorgan failure. The frequency of the lab monitoring would depend on the rapidity of disease progression, stage of the illness and severity of the illness. The minimum laboratory investigations which would need monitoring include hemoglobin, PT/APTT, fibrinogen and FDP.

Q. 13. A 24-year-old lady, 36 weeks gestation, primi, progressed to labor. The intrapartum period was complicated and prolonged requiring assistance with ventouse device. She delivered a healthy female baby, but immediate postdelivery developed sudden onset of dyspnea and hypotension. A diagnosis of amniotic fluid embolism was considered and she was transferred to the ICU for further management. How do you confirm the diagnosis and manage the same?

Amniotic fluid embolism is a rare, but extremely lethal condition associated with pregnancy. Due to its rarity, literature on this clinical condition is sparse and despite optimal management the maternal and perinatal mortality and morbidity is high.

The basic pathophysiology is severe, extreme, abnormal activation of the pro-inflammatory cascade (similar to systemic inflammatory response syndrome) due to the entrance of materials from the fetal compartment into the maternal circulation. This intense activation of the inflammatory cascade results in the signs and symptoms associated with the disease.

Clinical Features

The typical triad is **sudden onset of hypoxia and hypotension followed by coagulopathy** occurring in relation to labor and delivery. In fact, most patients with AFE are likely to get admitted to ICU following this sudden collapse. Labor and delivery in the ICU is not common, and even if it does occur, AFE could be extremely rare. Hence, as in the non-ICU setting diagnosis of AFE in ICU is based on the clinical presentation and by exclusion of other causes. It is important to suspect AFE in any pregnant or postpartum woman developing sudden cardiovascular collapse, shock, seizures, cardiac arrest followed by coagulopathy. Rarely, AFE could also occur during first or second trimester, following termination of pregnancy or other procedures, such as amniocentesis.

Risk factors for AFE
- Operative delivery
- Placenta previa
- Placenta accreta
- Abruption of placenta
- Cervical lacerations
- Uterine rupture
- Polyhydramnios
- Multiple gestations
- Maternal age

This dramatic clinical presentation, may be preceded by a short history of anxiety, agitation, feeling of "imminent death or doom" followed by sudden cardiac arrest—asystole, VF or pulseless electrical activity (PEA). **In cases occurring prior to delivery fetal monitoring may show decelerations in fetal heart rate with loss of variability and terminal bradycardia**, usually secondary to decreased perfusion to the fetus consequent to shunting of oxygenated blood away from the uterus and catecholamine-induced hypertonicity causing further decrease in uterine blood flow.

DIC is present in over 83% of patients. Generally, the DIC develops after the episode of shock or collapse. Rarely, this could be the first sign of the disease. But, it is very important to identify the temporal sequence of events, and differentiate DIC occurring secondary to other obstetric problems like atonic uterus. DIC may benefit as generalized bleeding to catastrophic external or internal hemorrhage.

Management of patients with AFE (Flowchart 4)

Differential diagnosis:
- Myocardial infarction
- Pulmonary embolism
- Air embolism
- Anesthetic complications
- Anaphylaxis
- Eclampsia

Prognosis
AFE is associated with an extremely high mortality despite the best of care. Recurrence of disease in subsequent pregnancies have not been reported. However, this condition being extremely rare, the sample size is inadequate to ascertain this fact.

Q. 14. A 35-year-old diabetic, g2,p2, l1 with 26 weeks gestation presented to the emergency department with high-grade fever, chills and rigors. On further probing, she had a history of burning micturition

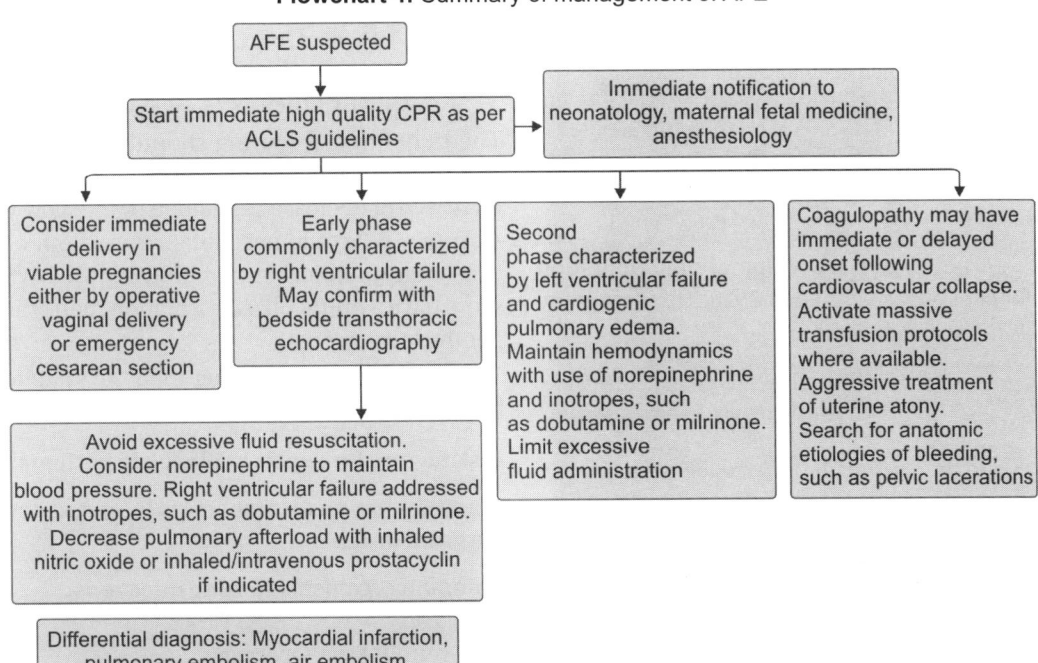

Flowchart 4: Summary of management of AFE

for 2 days. Initial evaluation revealed a systolic of <80 mm Hg with a heart rate of 130/min and temperature of 103°F. A diagnosis of urosepsis with septic shock was considered. How do you manage this patient?

Sepsis is one of the major reasons for admission of a pregnant woman to the ICU. The physiology in a pregnant woman is already in a state of compensation and a superadded insult like sepsis would have two potential problems—**firstly, the difficulty of diagnosis, and secondly, risk of rapid worsening and decompensation**. According to the WHO systematic analysis of causes for maternal death, sepsis accounted for 10.7% of maternal deaths. Despite the decrease in maternal mortality, deaths from sepsis seem to be on the increase. Definition of sepsis:

SCCM -2012

- Sepsis: Presence (suspected or documented) of infection together with systemic manifestations of infection
- Severe sepsis: Sepsis plus sepsis-induced tissue hypoperfusion or organ dysfunction
- Sepsis-induced hypotension: Systolic BP <90 mm Hg or Mean arterial pressure <70 mm Hg or decrease in Systolic BP >40 mm Hg or less than 2 SD below normal for age
- Septic shock: Sepsis-induced hypotension.

A newer and more operational definition for sepsis was defined in 2016. The details are as in the box below:

- Sepsis is defined as a life-threatening organ dysfunction caused by a dysregulated host response to infection
- Organ dysfunction can be identified as an acute changes in total sequential organ failure assessment (SOFA) score of ≥ 2 consequent to the infection
- The baseline score can assumed to be 0 if patients have no known preexisting organ dysfunction
- Patients with suspected infection who are likely to have a prolonged ICU stay or to die in the hospital can be promptly identified at the bed side with qSOFA, i.e. alteration in mental status, systolic blood pressure ≤ 100 mm Hg, or respiratory rate ≥ 22/min
- Septic shock is a subset of sepsis in which underlying circulatory and cellular/metabolic abnormalities are profound enough to substantially increase mortality
- Patients with septic shock can be identified with a clinical construct of sepsis with persisting hypotension requiring vasopressors to maintain MAP ≥ 65 mm Hg and having a serum lactate level >2 mmol/L (18 mg/dL) despite adequate volume resuscitation.

Sepsis and Pregnancy

Monitoring a obstetric patient suspected to have sepsis

Several scoring systems have been proposed for early detection of sepsis in an obstetric patient. scoring systems specifically for obstetric patients with sepsis have been evaluated and found to have a sensitivity of 89% and specificity of 78%. These include Modified Early Obstetric Warning score (MEOWS) and Sepsis in Obstetric Score (SOS). An example of MEOWS is given in Table 6. The frequency of scoring should be at least 12 hours. However, the frequency can be increased or decreased as guided by the scores. A score of > 3 could necessitate every hour or two-hourly monitoring. Centers using MEOWS score have a protocolized escalation matrix as per the local needs.

If the pulse rate is higher than the systolic blood pressure then score 2 for 'pulse'.

Risk factors for sepsis in obstetric patients

Common risk factors for sepsis in pregnancy are given in Table 7.

Common organisms causing infections:
- *E. coli*
- Group *B Streptococcus*
- Anaerobes

Table 6: Parameters in the MOEWS score

Score	3	2	1	0	1	2	3
Temperature		<35 °C		35–37 °C		37.5–39 °C	>39 °C
Systolic BP (mm Hg)	≤70	71–79	81–89	90–139	140–149	150–159	≥160
Diastolic BP (mm Hg)			≤45	46–89	90–99	100–109	≥110
Pulse		≤40	40–50	51–100	101–110	111–129	≥130
Respiratory Rate		≤8		9–14	15–20	21–29	≤30
AVPU				Alert	Responds to voice	Responds to pain	Unconscious
Urine output mLs/hr	≤10	≤30		Not measured			

Modified from: Singh S, McGlennan A, England A, et al. A validation study of the CEMACH recommended modified early obstetric warning system (MEOWS). Anaesthesia. 2012;67(1):12-8.

Table 7: Risk factors for sepsis in pregnancy

Antepartum factors	Intrapartum	Postpartum factors
Non white ethnicity	Protracted active labor	Retained products
Obesity	Premature rupture of membranes	Operative delivery
Lack of prenatal care	Multiple vaginal examinations	
Malnourishment	Perineal manipulation	
Impaired glucose tolerance	Instrumental delivery	
Diabetes mellitus	Unscheduled ceserean section	
Anemia		
Impaired immunity		
Patient's with sickle cell disease		
Group B colonization or infection		
Invasive procedures during pregnancy		
Primipara		
Preexisting medical problems		
Febrile illness		
Use of antibiotics in the two weeks prior to presentation		

- *Staphylococcus*
- *Enterococcus*
- *Klebsiella*
- *H. influenzae*

Specific infections and treatment
- Group A *Streptococcus*:
  – Common in the preantibiotic era
  – Reduced incidence after introduction of penicillin, but resurgence noted in 1980

- Produces exotoxin which results in extensive tissue and muscle necrosis.
- Treatment:
    ◊ Penicillin with clindamycin
    ◊ Vancomycin can be an alternative
- Bacterial pneumonia:
    - Preferred choice is macrolide ± β-lactam antibiotic. Depending on the setting and possibility of exposure to prior antibiotic, beta-lactam + beta-lactam inhibitor (BL-BLI) combination may be preferred, e.g. In the setting of an uncomplicated community acquired pneumonia, a combination of ceftriaxone and azithromycin may be preferred. Doxycycline is contraindicated.
    - Addition of an antiviral like oseltamivir may be considered if appropriate. It is important to note the higher predilection for viral pneumonias in pregnant woman due to a suppressed cell-mediated immunity.
    - Consider vancomycin if MRSA is suspected to be the source.
- Pyelonephritis:
    - Pregnancy is an important risk factor for urinary tract infections.
    - Common organisms causing pyelonephritis:
        ◊ *E. coli*—most common and a major pathogen
        ◊ *Klebsiella* and *Proteus*
        ◊ Less commonly more virulent organisms like *Pseudomonas*.
    - Antibiotic preferred
        ◊ Third generation cephalosporin
        ◊ If previous history of antibiotic exposure or instrumentation or hospitalization—BL + BLI combination may be preferred. Depending on the bacterial profile and the resistance patterns in the institution where the patient is admitted
        ◊ Aminoglycosides can be used as an additional antibiotic with care in view of the risk to the fetus
    ◊ Any structural abnormalities may have to be addressed surgically or through suitable instrumentation
- Chorioamnionitis:
    - The infection is typically polymicrobial.
    - Common organisms identified—genital *Mycoplasma*, group B *Streptococcus* and *E. coli*
    - Antibiotic cover should include both aerobic and anaerobic ones.
    - Suggested regimen:
        ◊ Ampicillin + gentamicin
        ◊ Clindamycin
        ◊ BL-BLI combination
- Endometriotis:
    - Typically polymicrobial infection
    - Anaerobes in 40% of patients with gram-positive and gram-negative facultative anaerobes.
    - Serious infections that are likely to progress to sepsis include—group A *Streptococcus*, staphylococci and *Clostridium* species.
    - Suggested combinations:
        ◊ Aminoglycoside with clindamycin
        ◊ Third generation cephalosporin with metronidazole
        ◊ Bl-BLI combination.

Management of Sepsis:
- Management principles and guidelines are predominantly guided by the surviving sepsis guidelines:
    - Protocolized, quantitative resuscitation of patients with sepsis-induced tissue hypoperfusion
    - Goals during the first 6 hours:
        ◊ CVP 8–12 mm Hg
        ◊ MAP ≥ 65 mm Hg
        ◊ Urine output ≥ 0.5 mL/kg/hour
        ◊ Central venous (superior venacava) saturation or mixed venous saturation 70% or 65%, respectively.
    - In patients with elevated lactate target resuscitation to normalize lactate levels at the earliest.

Recommended *surviving sepsis campaign care bundles to be completed within 3 hours:*
- Measure lactate level
- Obtain blood cultures prior to administration of antibiotics
- Administer broad spectrum antibiotics
- Administer 30 mL/kg crystalloid for hypotension or lactate ≥4 mmol/L

To be completed within 6 hours:
- Apply vasopressors (for hypotension that does not respond to initial fluid resuscitation) to maintain a mean arterial pressure (MAP) ≥ 65 mm Hg
- In the event of persistent arterial hypotension despite volume resuscitation (septic shock) or initial lactate ≥4 mmol/L (36 mg/dL):
  - Measure central venous pressure (CVP)*
  - Measure central venous oxygen saturation (ScVO$_2$)*
- Remeasure lactate if initial lactate was elevated*

*Targets for quantitative resuscitation included in the guidelines are CVP of ≥8 mm Hg, ScVO$_2$ of ≥70%, and normalization of lactate

- Screening for sepsis
- Diagnosis: Cultures if clinically appropriate prior to initiation of antibiotic.
- Antimicrobial therapy:
  ◊ Source control.
  ◊ Infection control
  ◊ Fluid therapy in Sepsis:
  ◊ Crystalloids are the preferred fluids in the early resuscitation of sepsis.
  ◊ Synthetic colloids are found to be harmful with an increased risk of Acute kidney injury.
  ◊ Albumin may be considered during resuscitation in patients with sepsis and septic shock if large volume of crystalloids are required.
  ◊ Initial fluid resuscitation is commenced with crystalloids at 30 mL/kg and further resuscitation guided by hemodynamic indices.
- Vasopressor therapy:
  ◊ Vasopressor therapy is initiated to target a MAP ≥ 65 mm Hg
  ◊ Norepinephrine is the first choice in the setting of septic shock.
  ◊ Epinephrine can be added or used as a substitute for nor-epinephrine.
  ◊ Vasopressin at a dose of 0.03 units/minute can be considered as a catecholamine sparing agent or increasing MAP.
  ◊ Dopamine is an alternative agent, though less preferred these days for septic shock, due to the risk of tachycardia, immunomodulation, etc.
  ◊ There is no role for low, renal dose of dopamine
- Inotropic agent:
  ◊ Dobutamine may be considered in patients with myocardial dysfunction, where in achieving a MAP>65 mm Hg is not possible despite optimal fluid resuscitation.
  ◊ Corticosteroid therapy: Low dose corticosteroids (hydrocortisone 200-300 mg/day) can be considered for early shock reversal in patients with septic shock, where in achieving target MAP is not possible despite vasopressors and fluid resuscitation. However, there is no evidence of better outcomes or harm with this practice.
- Glucose control: If 2 consecutive readings of capillary blood sugar (using a glucometer) are >180 mg%, commence insulin infusion. Infusion is administered in a protocolized manner to maintain an upper limit of GRBS of 180 mg%.
- Other ICU supportive measures.

Q. 15. What are the principles of managing acute respiratory distress syndrome (ARDS) in pregnancy?

ARDS is a form of acute respiratory failure due to ongoing pulmonary inflammation resulting in increased alveolocapillary permeability and consequent accumulation of inflammatory edema in the alveolar and interstitial spaces causing acute hypoxemia. The definitions of AROS are given in Table 8.

Table 8: Definition of terms in ARDS

Timing	Within 1 week of a known clinical insult or new or worsening respiratory symptoms
Chest imaging	Bilateral opacities—not fully explained by effusions, lobar/lung collapse, or nodules
Origin of edema	Respiratory failure not fully explained by cardiac failure or fluid overload. Need objective assessment (e.g. echocardiography) to exclude hydrostatic edema if no risk factor present
Oxygenation Mild	200 mm Hg < PaO_2/FiO_2 ≤ 300 mm Hg with PEEP or CPAP ≥ 5 cm H_2O
Moderate	100 mm Hg < PaO_2/FiO_2 ≤ 200 mm Hg with PEEP ≥ 5 cm H_2O
Severe	PaO_2/FiO_2 < 100 mm Hg with PEEP ≥ 5 cm H_2O

Obstetric-related ARDS is defined ARDS occurring during pregnancy or within 1 week postpartum. Some authors extend the period upto 1 month. Some authors describe obstetric ARDS as those occurring due to an obstetric cause or worsened by pregnancy. Prevalence of the disease has been estimated to be 15–70 cases per 10,000 pregnancies.

Some of the important differential diagnoses include—cardiac failure due to variety of causes including peripartum cardiomyopathy, different forms of non-infective pneumonitis (eosinophilic pneumonia, hypersensitivity pneumonitis), viral pneumonia, etc.

Etiopathogenesis of ARDS is classified as in Table 9.

Management of patients:

General principles of management of ARDS in pregnancy are similar to those in the general population. Important principles are:
- Treat the underlying cause, if a specific etiology has been identified.
- Management of ARDS:
  - Establish the diagnosis—as per the definition.
  - Fluid restriction

Recent studies have indicated that fluid restriction in the first few days of ICU stay, is associated with shorter ventilator and ICU stay.

Table 9: Classification of etiopathogenesis of ARDS

Unaffected by pregnancy	Modified by pregnancy	Unique to pregnancy
Direct/pulmonary • Pneumonia • Ventilator-associated lung injury • Chemical pneumonitis • Pulmonary contusion • Fat embolism	**Direct/pulmonary** • Aspiration of gastric contents • Viral pneumonia • Blastomycosis • Listeriosis • Venous air embolism	**Direct or pulmonary** • Amniotic fluid embolism • Tocolytic-induced pulmonary edema • Trophoblastic embolism
Indirect/extrapulmonary • Sepsis • Trauma • Burns • Acute pancreatitis • Transfusion-related acute lung injury (TRALI)	**Indirect/extrapulmonary** • Pyelonephritis • Malaria	**Indirect/extrapulmonary** • Preeclampsia • Eclampsia • HELLP syndrome • Chorioamnionitis • Endometriosis • Acute fatty liver of pregnancy

Adapted from: Cole DE, Taylor TL, McCllough DM, Shoff TC, Derdak S. Acute respiratory distress syndrome in pregnancy. Crit Care Med. 2005;33[Suppl]:S269-78.

- Termination of pregnancy: It may be appropriate to consider termination of pregnancy if the gestational age is consistent with fetal viability. If termination of pregnancy is feasible, it would facilitate easier management of ARDS and possibly better chance of fetal salvage. This decision, however, has to be taken on a case to case basis taking into consideration maternal or fetal factors.

Outcomes

The mortality and morbidity of ARDS in the general population ranges from 35 to 60%. In obstetric patients, the data is limited, but review of the existing literature predicts a mortality ranging from 25 to 50%. Among the survivors, less than 10% of patients are left with mild long-term disabilities (after 1 year), which is comparable to the similar patients in the general population.

Q. 16. Deccribe cardiac arrest associated with pregnancy.

The most common causes for cardiac arrest during pregnancy include hemorrhage, cardiovascular diseases (myocardial infarction, aortic dissection and myocarditis), amniotic fluid embolism, sepsis, aspiration pneumonia, pulmonary embolism and eclampsia. Iatrogenic causes could include hypermagnesemia and anesthetic complications.

Summary of guidelines in resuscitating a pregnant woman in cardiac arrest as derived from the American Heart Association (AHA) guidelines include:

- Patient position during CPR: Aortocaval compression is an important cause of decreased venous return in the supine position during singleton pregnancies after 20 weeks of gestation. Thus, in addition to all the regular protocols for resuscitating a patient with cardiac arrest one important addition in the AHA guidelines for BLS is optimal patient positioning. A left lateral tilt position can be provided and CPR delivered during the process of resuscitation. This could compromise the appropriateness of chest compression which is a very important step for the CPR process. Thus, it is recommended to use manual left lateral uterine displacement to patients with hypotension. The advantage of this maneuver over the left lateral tilt is facilitating appropriate chest compression during CPR.
- Chest compressions to be commenced at earliest without delay
- Lower half of the sternum to be the area of chest compression
- Chest compression should be "hard and fast" achieving a depth of at least 2 cm with adequate time for chest recoil.
- Drugs during CPR to be used in doses as in any other adults. Dose of DC current during CPR is also as in adults. However, care should be taken when the fetal monitor is connected regarding a theoretical risk of electrical arcing.
- If the patient is undelivered at the time of cardiac arrest consider expeditious delivery if fetal viability (>23 weeks) is reached. Operative vaginal delivery can be considered, if the process of labor has commenced. If not, emergency LSCS can be considered. Perimortem LSCS can be considered if return of spontaneous circulation (ROSC), is not achieved within 4 minutes of commencement of CPR. This timeframe is difficult to achieve. Hence, it is advisable to commence arrangement for a perimortem LSCS, as the CPR process is commenced.

Q. 17. Management of diabetic emergencies in pregnancy.

Two common complications are hyperglycemic states and less commonly hypoglycemia. Among the hyperglycemic states, Diabetic ketoacidosis seem to be the most commonly occurring complication.

Diabetic ketoacidosis (DKA)

Clinical features of DKA
- Initially: Nausea, vomiting, abdominal pain, hyperventilation, fruity breath, polydipsia, dry mucous membranes, tachycardia, weakness and polyuria and in later stages with more severe disease, hypotension, weight loss, mental status changes and organ dysfunction
- Characteristic laboratory findings include: Hyperglycemia (generally a blood sugar >300 mg%), elevated total count, metabolic acidosis with increased anion gap, positive serum and urine ketones, elevated serum osmolality and in severe cases evidence of prerenal acute kidney injury.

Management of DKA
- Identify and treat the precipitating cause
  - Search and treat for any underlying infection
  - Evaluate dietary and behavioral habits
  - Rule out any psychological stressors as precipitant cause
- Fluid resuscitation
  - Fluid resuscitation with crystalloids form the mainstay of immediate therapy
  - Important to identify the extent of fluid loss. This could be difficult in advanced pregnancy.
  - Static and dynamic indices can be used for assessment:
    ◊ Central venous pressure—important to be aware that low CVP has good sensitivity and specificity to indicate hypovolemia, but a normal and elevated CVP is a poor predictor of volume status
    ◊ Hourly urine output
    ◊ Clinical features, such as skin turgor
    ◊ Decreasing hematocrit
    ◊ Decreasing BUN-creatinine ratio (>20:1) indicates prerenal state
    ◊ Assessment of LV filling and inferior vena cava diameter and the response of these indices to a fluid challenge is a very sensitive indicator of fluid responsiveness
  - It is important to assess the extent of fluid loss and replace 75% of this volume in the first 24 hours.
  - Generally, the estimated fluid depletion can vary from 5–10 liters.
  - Start fluid resuscitation with 0.9% saline. Crystalloids in the form of 0.9% saline or 0.45% saline is to be continued until the blood sugar decreases to <250 mg%. Later on, change over to 5% dextrose with 0.45% saline.
  - The choice between 0.9% saline vs 0.45% saline is decided based on the corrected sodium. If the latter high, 0.45% saline may be preferred.
- Insulin infusion
  - Insulin infusion is critical to the treatment due to the insulin deficiency state.
  - Insulin is started at a dose of 0.1 U/kg/hour. The role for a bolus dose of IV insulin is controversial. Even if administered the dose should not exceed 0.1 u/kg.
  Following the initial bolus, the insulin is titrated to achieve a decrease in the blood sugar at the rate of 50–75 mg%. If the expected decrease does not occur or an increase is seen in the blood sugar the insulin dose is increased by 0.05 U/kg/hour. If the drop in blood sugar is >100 mg% decrease the dose of insulin by 0.05U/kg/hour.
- Potassium: It is important to keep a close watch on the potassium levels as DKA is a potassium depletion state. Despite a normal serum potassium, a deficit of 200–300 mmol may be present. As the treatment is continued, it is important to monitor the potassium closely every 2–4 hourly. If required potassium replacement at the rate of up to 20 mmol/hour (intravenously)

may be considered. In order to prevent large swings in the serum levels, potassium could also be added to the maintenance fluid and monitored cautiously.
- Correction of acidosis: The present day protocol do not advise the use of soda-bicarbonate even if the pH drops to the range of 6.8–7.1. In fact, a few studies have found this practice to be detrimental causing intracellular paradoxical acidosis and sudden hypokalemia.
- Oxygenation: It is important to perform all measures to maintain the uteroplacental circulation. But until the DKA has resolved there is no role for termination of pregnancy, even if fetal distress is present as this could be detrimental to the mother. In most instances, the fetal distress may be reversible if prompt and quick management is instituted.
- Preterm labor: If the patient is in labor at the time of presentation, further treatment will be based on the maternal condition. If the mother is very acidotic, tocolytics need to be used in an attempt to stall the process of labor, as the clinical condition of the mother puts her at risk if the labor continues. Magnesium sulfate is the preferred tocolytic under this clinical condition. Generally, the process of labor is stalled spontaneously with resolution of acidosis.

Q. 18. How to suspect cerebrovascular accident in hypertensive disorders of pregnancy?

Generally, it is not necessary to form imaging of the brain for diagnosis of eclampsia. The indications for performing a CT and suspect other pathologies like CVA include:
- Atypical presentation of eclampsia
  - Occurring before 20 weeks of gestation or
  - 48 hours postpartum
- Presence of focal neurological deficits.
- Pupillary abnormalities
- Status epilepticus or seizures refractory to magnesium sulfate
- Prolonged coma.

Q. 19. How do you manage status epilepticus in pregnancy?

Rarely, a patient has intractable seizures upon labor and delivery. In a patient who is a known patient of epilepsy, the diagnosis may be made with certainty. Otherwise, if there are features of preeclampsia, a diagnosis of eclampsia is made and treatment initiated with magnesium sulfate regime. Even otherwise, any convulsion in a previously normal patient after 20 weeks of gestation up to 48 hours of delivery too is treated as eclampsia.

When these last longer than 30 minutes with either (1) a continuous seizure or (2) a lack of full recovery between seizures, the patient is considered to be in status epilepticus/eclampticus.

Assuming that preeclampsia and eclampsia have been excluded, the protocol for managing status epilepticus is similar to the management of any seizure. The steps include:
- Assess airway, breathing and circulation
- If seizures difficult to control or GCS low with inability to protect airway, will need intubation and mechanical ventilation.
  - Simultaneously secure peripheral IV access.
- Aim to achieve rapid control of seizures
  - First line use of benzodiazepines:
    ◊ Lorazepam 0.1 mg/kg IV up to a maximum of 8–10 mg
    ◊ Midazolam 0.1 mg/kg IV up to a maximum of 10 mg
  - Second line
    ◊ Phenytoin 15–20 mg/kg slow IV
    ◊ Phenobarbital 15–20 mg/kg slow IV
    ◊ Levetiracetam 1–3 g slow IV
    ◊ Valproate 20–40 mg/kg
    Any of the above agent can be used.

There is no superiority of one over the other. Some evidence to support the superiority of valproate over other drugs.
- Third line:
    ◊ Propofol infusion
      1–2 mg/kg loading followed by 20 µg/kg/min
    ◊ Thiopental
      2 mg/kg loading followed by 0.5–5 mg/kg/hour infusion
    ◊ Midazolam
      0.05–2 mg/kg/hour infusion
- Identify the cause or precipitating factor, if present.

During this situation, the fetus must be monitored. In the setting of nonreassuring fetal testing results, establish an airway and attempt intrauterine resuscitation. If the seizure is not treated easily and the fetal testing results continue to be nonreassuring for longer than 10 minutes, a neuromuscular blocking agent can be administered and emergent cesarean delivery can be performed.

Q. 20. How do you manage cardiac failure in pregnancy?

- Anticoagulation is recommended in patients with intracardiac thrombus detected by imaging or with evidence of systemic embolism.
- Women with heart failure during pregnancy should be treated according to current guidelines for nonpregnant patients, respecting contraindications for some drugs in pregnancy
    - Fluid restriction
    - Diuretics
    - Beta-blockers
        ◊ ACEI are contraindicated
- Women with DCM should be informed about the risk of deterioration of the condition during gestation and peripartum
- In patients with a past history or family history of sudden death close surveillance with prompt investigation is recommended if symptoms of palpitations or presyncope are reported
- Therapeutic anticoagulation with LMWH or vitamin K antagonists according to stage of pregnancy is recommended for patients with atrial fibrillation
- Delivery should be performed with β-blocker protection in women with hypertrophic obstructive cardiomyopathy (HOCM)
- β-blockers should be considered in all patients with HOCM and more than mild Left ventricular outflow tract obstruction or maximal wall thickness >15 mm to prevent sudden pulmonary congestion. In HCM, cardioversion should be considered for persistent atrial fibrillation
- Due to high metabolic demands of lactation and breastfeeding, preventing lactation may be considered in peripartum cardiomyopathy
- Subsequent pregnancy is not recommended if LVEF does not normalize in women with Peripartum cardiomyopathy.

Bibliography

1. American College of Obstetricians and Gynecologists, Committee Opinion no. 560: Medically indicated late-pretermand early-term deliveries. 2013;560:1-3.
2. American College of Obstetricians and Gynecologists. Clinical management guidelines for obstetrician-gynecologists: postpartum hemorrhage. ACOG Practice bulletin no. 76. Obstet Gynecol. 2006;108:1039-47.
3. Aurangzeb I, George L and Raoof S. Amniotic fluid embolism. Crit Care Clin. 2004;20:643-50.
4. Barton JR, Sibai BM. Severe sepsis and septic shock in pregnancy. Obstet Gynecol 2012;120(3):689-706.
5. Baskett TF, Sternadel J. Maternal intensive care and near miss mortality in obstetrics. Br J Obstet Gynaecol. 1998;105:981-4.

6. Bhat PBR, Navada MH, Rao SV, et al. Evaluation of obstetric admissions to the intensive care unit of a tertiary referral center in coastal India. Indian J Crit Care Med. 2013;17(1):34-7.
7. Bobrowski R. Trauma in pregnancy. In: James DK, Steer PJ, Weiner CP, Gonik B (Eds). High risk pregnancy—management options. 2nd edition.
8. Bogert JN, Harvin JA, Cotton BA. Damage control resuscitation. J Intensive Care Med. 2014:1-10.
9. Bollinger D, Szlam F, Molinaro RJ, et al. Finding the optimal concentration range for fibrinogen replacement after severe haemodilution:an in vitro model. Br J Anaesth. 2009;102(6):793-9.
10. Brace V, Penney G and Hall M. Quantifying severe maternal morbidity: A Scottish population study. BJOG. 2004;111:481-4.
11. Brilli RJ, Spevetz A, Branson RD, et al. Critical care delivery in the intensive care unit: defining clinical roles and the best practice model. Crit Care Med. 2001;29:2007-19.
12. Brown J, Cohen M, Minei J, et al. J Trauma Acute Care Surg. 2012;73(2):358-64.
13. Brown L, Aro S, Cohen M. Trauma outcomes group. J Trauma. 2011;71(2):S358-63.
14. Callaway CW, Donnino MW, Fink EL, et al. Post cardiac arrest care: 2015 American Heart Association Guidelines update for cardiopulmonary resuscitation and emergency cardiovascular care. Circulation. 2015;132(suppl 2):S465-82.
15. Cantwell R, Clutton-Brock T, Cooper G, et al. Saving mothers' lives: reviewing maternal deaths to make motherhood safer: 2006-2008. the eighth report of the confidential enquiries into maternal deaths in the United Kingdom. BJOG. 2011;118(Suppl 1):1-203.
16. Charbit B, Mandelbrot L, Samarin E, et al. The decrease of fibrinogen is a nearly predictor of the severity of postpartum hemorrhage. J Thromb Haemost. 2007;5(2):266-73.
17. Chauhan A, Musunuru H, Donnino M, et al. The use of therapeutic hypothermia after cardiAC Arrest in a pregnant patient. Ann Emerg Med. 2012;60:786-9.
18. Clark SL, Hankins GD, Dudley DA, et al. Amniotic fluid embolism: analysis of the national registry. Am J Obstet Gynecol. 1995;172:1158-67; discussion 1167-9. (Level 388 II-2).
19. Clark SL. Amniotic fluid embolism. Obstet Gynecol. 2014;123:337-48. (Level III)
20. Cole DE, Taylor TL, McCllough DM, et al. Acute respiratory distress syndrome in pregnancy. Crit Care Med 2005;33[Suppl.]:S269 -S278.
21. Collins Pw, Lilley G, Bruynseels D, et al. Fibrin-based clot formation as an early and rapid biomarker for progression of postpartum hemorrhage: a prospective study. Blood 2014;124:1727-36.
22. Connolly AM, Katz VL, Bash KL, et al. Trauma and pregnancy. Am J Perinatol. 1997;14:331-6.
23. Cotton BA, Gunter OL, Isbell J, et al. Damage control hematology: The impact of a trauma exsanguination protocol on survival and blood product utilization. J Trauma 2008;64(5):1177-82.
24. Cotton BA, Harvin JA, Kostousouv V, et al. Hyperfibrinolysis at admission is an uncommon but highly lethal event associated with shock and prehospital fluid administration. J Trauma Acute Care Surg. 2012;73(2):365-73.
25. Cotton BA, Reddy N, Hatch QM, et al. Damage control resuscitation is associated with a reduction in resuscitation volumes and improvement in survival in 390 damage control laparotomy patients. Ann Surg. 2011;254(4):598-605.
26. CRASH-2. The importance of early treatment with tranexamic acid in bleeding trauma patients:an exploratory analysis of the CRASH-2 randomised controlled trial. Lancet. 2011;377:1096-101.
27. Cromey MG, Taylor PJ, Cumming DC. Probable amniotic fluid embolism after first trimester pregnancy termination. A case report. J Reprod Med. 1983;28:209-11. (Level III)
28. Davis JW, Parks SN, Kaups KL, et al. Admission base deficit predicts transfusion requirements and risk of complications. J Trauma. 1996;41(5):769-74.
29. Dellinger RP, Levy MM, Rhodes A, et al. Surviving Sepsis Campaign: international guidelines for management of severe sepsis and septic shock, 2012. Intensive Care Med. 2013;39(2):165-228.

30. Department of Health, London. Comprehensive Critical Care: A review of critical care services; 2000.
31. De Vaciana M. Diabetic ketoacidosis in pregnancy. 2013;37(4):267-73.
32. Elbourne DR, Prendiville WJ, Carroli G, et al. Prophylactic use of oxytocin in the third stage of labour. The Cochrane Database of Systematic Reviews. 2001;4:CD001808.
33. Erez O, Novack L, Beer-Weisel R, et al. DIC score in pregnant women—a population based modification of the International Society on Thrombosis and Hemostasis score. PLoS One 2014;9:e93240.
34. Fildes J, Reed L, Jones N, et al. Trauma: the leading cause of maternal death. J Trauma. 1992;32:643-5.
35. Fries D, Haas T, Klingler A, et al. Efficacy of fibrinogen and prothrombin complex concentrate used to reverse dilutional coagulopathy—a porcine model. Br J Anaesth. 2006;97(4):460-7.
36. Gando S, Iba T, Eguchi Y, et al. A multicenter, prospective validation of disseminated intravascular coagulation diagnostic criteria for critically ill patients: comparing current criteria. Crit Care Med. 2006;34:625-31
37. Glassford NJ, Bellomo R. Acute kidney injury: how can we facilitate recovery? Curr Opin Crit Care. 2011;17(6):562-8.
38. Guidelines for ICU Admission, Discharge and Triage. Society of Critical Care Medicine; 1999.
39. Guntupalli KK, Hall N, Karnad DR, et al. Critical illness in pregnancy. Part I: Approach to a pregnant patient in the ICU and common obstetric disorders. Chest. 2015;148(4):1093-104.
40. Hagiwara A, Kimura A, Kato H, et al. Hemodynamic reactions in patients with hemorrhagic shock from blunt trauma after initial fluid therapy. J Trauma. 2010;69(5):1161-8.
41. Hart LA, Sibai BM. Seizures in pregnancy: Epilepsy, Eclampsia, and stroke. Seminars in perinatology. 2013;37:207-24.
42. Hass BD. Critical care unit organization and patient outcomes. Crit Care Nurs Quart. 2005;28(4):336-40.
43. Hayashi K, Oshiro M, Takara I, et al. Coma caused by hypermagnesaemia in a pregnant woman complicated with HELLP syndrome [abstract]. Masui. 2003;52(7):783-5.
44. Health Service Executive. Early Warning Score Guidelines; 2012. http://www.hse.ie/eng/about/Who/ONMSD/practicedevelopment/MEWS/
45. Herrler T, Tischer A, Meyer A, et al. The intrinsic renal compartment syndrome: new perspectives in kidney transplantation. Transplantation 2010; 89(1):40-6.
46. Holcomb JB, Tilley BC, Baraniuk S, et al. Transfusion of plasma, platelets, 335 and red blood cells in a 1:1:1 vs a 1:1:2 ratio and mortality in patients with severe trauma: The PROPPR randomized clinical trial. JAMA. 2015;313(5):471-82.
47. Hossain N, Shansi T, Haider S, et al. Use of recombinant activated factor VII for massive postpartum hemorrhage. Acta Obstet Gynecol Scand. 2007;86:1200-6.
48. Iapichino G, Radrizzani D, Ferla L, et al. Description of trends in the course of illness of critically ill patients. Markers of intensive care organization and performance. Intens Care Med. 2002;28:985-9.
49. Ickx BE. Fluid and blood transfusion management in obstetrics. Eur J Anaesthesiol. 2010;27(12):1031-5.
50. Jeejeebhoy FM, Zelop CM, Lipman S, et al. Cardiac arrest in pregnancy: A scientific statement from the American Heart Association. Circulation. 2015;132:1747-73.
51. Jha UP, Swasthi. Quality in health. The law, science and art of consent—A gynaecologist's approach. Apollo Medicine. 2008;5(1):48-60.
52. Kanayama N, Tamura N. Amniotic fluid embolism: pathophysiology and new strategies for management. J Obstet Gynaecol Res. 2014;40:1507-17. (Level III)
53. Ker K, Prieto-Merino D, Roberts I. Systematic review, meta analysis and meta-regression of the effect of tranexamic acid on surgical blood loss. Br J Surg. 2013;100(10):1271-9.
54. Kittner SJ, Stern BJ, Feeser BR, et al. Pregnancy and the risk of stroke. N Eng J Med. 1996;335:768-74.

55. Knowles SJ, O'Sullivan NP, Meenan AM, et al. Maternal sepsis incidence, aetiology and outcome for mother and fetus: a prospective study. BJOG. 2015;122(5):663-71.
56. Knowles SJ, O'Sullivan NP, Meenan AM. Maternal sepsis incidence, etiology and outcome for mother and fetus: a prospective study. BJOG. 2015;122(5):663-71.
57. Koenig MA. Brain resuscitation and prognosis after cardiac arrest. Crit Care Clin. 2014;30:765-83.
58. Lapinsky SE, Kruzynski K, Seaward GR, et al. Critical care management of the obstetric patient. Can J Anaesth. 1997;44(3):325-9. ICM
59. Lapinsky SE. Obstetric infections. Crit Care Clin. 2013;29(3):509-20.
60. Lappen JR, Keene M, Lore M, et al. Existing models fail to predict sepsis in an obstetric population with intrauterine infection. Am J Obstet Gynecol. 2010;203(6):573.e1-5.
61. Lavigne-Lissalde G, Aya Ag, Mercier Fj, et al. Recombinant human FVIIa for reducing the need of invasive second-line therapies in severe refractory postpartum hemorrhage: A multicenter, randomized, open controlled trial. J Thromb Haemost; 2015.
62. Lavonas EJ, Chair Drennan IR, Gabrielli A, et al. Part 10: Special Circumstances of Resuscitation 2015 American Heart Association Guidelines Update for Cardiopulmonary Resuscitation and Emergency Cardiovascular Care Circulation. 2015;132 [suppl 2]:S501-18.
63. Levi M, Ten Ca'e H. Disseminated intravascular coagulation. N Engl J Med. 1999;341:586-92.
64. Levi M, Van Der Poll T. DisSEminated intraVascular coaGulation: a review for the internist. Intern Emerg Med. 2013;8:23-32.
65. Lewis G (Ed). The Confidential Enquiry into Maternal and Child Health (CEMACH). Saving Mothers' Lives: reviewing maternal deaths to make motherhood safer—2003-2005. The Seventh Report on Confidential Enquiries into Maternal Deaths in the United Kingdom. CEMACH, London; 2007.
66. Ley EF, ClonD MA, Srour MK, et al. Emergency department crystalloid resuscitation of 1.5 l or more is associated with increased mortality in elderly and non elderly trauma patients. J Trauma. 2011;70(2):398-400.
67. Li T, Zhu Y, Hu Y, et al. Ideal permissive hypotension to resuscitate uncontrolled hemorrhagic shock and the tolerance time in rats. Anesthesiology. 2011;114(1):111-9.
68. Mabie WC, Baha MS. Treatment in an obstetric intensive care unit. Am J Obstet Gynecol. 1990;162(1):1-4.
69. Mabie WC, Sibai BM. Treatment in an obstetric intensive care unit. Am J Obstet Gynecol. 1990; 162:1-4.
70. Mahutte NG, Murphy-Kaulbeck L, Le Q, et al. Obstetric admissions to the intensive care unit. Obstet Gynecol. 1999;94:263-6.
71. Mallampalli A, Guy E. Cardiac arrest in pregnancy and somatic support after brain death. Crit Care Med. 2005;33(10):S325-31.
72. Marini JJ. Streamlining critical care: responsibilities and cost effectiveness in intensive care unit organization. Mayo Clin Proc. 1997;72:483-5.
73. McLintock C and James AH. Obstetric hemorrhage. J Thrombosis and Haemostasis. 2011;9:1441-51.
74. Meier J, Kemming GI, Kisch-Wede IH, et al. Hyperoxic ventilation reduces 6-hour mortality at the critical haemoglobin concentration. Anesthesiology. 2004;100(1):70-6.
75. Miller RD. Transfusion therapy. Miller's Anesthesia. 6th edition. 1799;827.
76. Multz AS, Chalfin DB, Samson IM, et al. A "closed" medical intensive care unit (MICU) improves resource utilization when compared with an "open" MICU. Am J Respir Crit Care Med. 1998;157:1468-73.
77. Munnur U, Karnad DR, Bandi VDP, et al. Critically ill obstetric patients in an American and an Indian public hospital: comparison of case-mix, organ dysfunction, intensive care requirements, and outcomes. Intensive Care Med. 2005;31(8):1087-94.
78. Neal MD, Hoffman MK, Cuschieri J, et al. Crystalloid to packed red blood cell transfusion ratio in the massively transfused patient: when a little goes along way. J Trauma. 2012;72(4):892-8.
79. Nielsen N, Wetterslev J, Cronberg T, et al. TTM Trial Investigators. Targeted temperature management at 33°C versus 36°C after cardiac arrest. N Engl J Med. 2013;369:2197-206.

80. Pacheco Ld, Saade Gr, Gei Af, Hankins GD. Cutting-edge advances in the medical management of obstetrical hemorrhage. Am J Obstet Gynecol. 2011;205:526-32
81. Paradis N, Balter S, Davidson C, et al. Hematocrit as a predictor of significant injury after penetrating trauma. Am J Emerg Med. 1997;15(3):224-8.
82. PECkham CH, King RW. A study of intercurrent conditions observed during pregnancy. Am J Obstet Gynecol. 1963;87:609-24.
83. Platteau P, Engelhardt T, Moodley J, et al. Obstetric and gynaecological patients in an intensive care unit: a one year review. Trop Doct. 1997;27:202-6.
84. Poeran J, Rasul R, Suzuki S, et al. TranexaMIc acid use and postoperative outcomes in patients undergoing total hip or knee arthroplasty in the United States: retrospective analysis of effectiveness and safety. Br Med J. 2014;349:g4829.
85. Pollack MM, Katz RW, Ruttimann UE, et al. Improving the outcome and efficiency of intensive care: the impact of an intensivist. Crit Care Med. 1988;16:11-7.
86. Pronovost PJ, Angus DC, Dorman T, et al. Physician staffing patterns and clinical outcomes in critically ill patients a systematic review. JAMA. 2002;288:2151-62.
87. Rattray DD, O'connell CM, Baskett TF. Acute disseminated intravascular coagulation in obstetrics: a tertiary centre population review (1980 to 2009). J Obstet Gynecol Can 2012;34:341-7.
88. RCOG. Antepartum Haemorrhage, Green-top Guideline No. 63. 1st edn; 2011a. Available at: http://www.rcog.org.uk/files/rcog-corp/
89. RCOG. Blood transfusion in obstetrics, Green-top guideline. No. 47. 2nd edition. 2014. Available at: https://www.rcog.org.uk/globalassets/documents/guidelines/gtg-47.pdf
90. RCOG. Postpartum haemorrhage, prevention and management. Green-top Guideline No. 52; 2009. http://www.rcog.org.uk/files/rcog-corp/GT52Post partumHaemorrhage0411
91. Regitz-Zagrosek V, Lundqvist CB, Borghi C, et al. ESC Guidelines on the management of cardiovascular diseases during pregnancy. European Heart Journal. 2011;32:3147-97.
92. Revell M, Greaves I, Porter K. End points for fluid resuscitation in hemorrhagic shock. J Trauma. 2003;54(5):S63-7.
93. Richards AM, Moodley J, Bullock MRR, et al. Maternal deaths from neurological complications of hypertensive crises in pregnancy. S Afr Med J. 1987;71:487-90.
94. Richards AM, Moodley J, Graham DI, et al. Active management of the unconscious eclamptic patient. Br J Obstet Gynaecol. 1986;93:554-62.
95. Roberts CI, Algert CS, Knight M, et al. Amniotic fluid embolism in an Australian population-based cohort. BJOG. 2010;117:1417-21. (Level II-2)
96. Royal Australian and New Zealand College of Obstetricians and Gynaecologists. Management of postpartum hemorrhage. March 2011. Available at: http://www.ranzcog.edu.au/collegestatements-guidelines.html. Accessed Nov. 1, 2013.
97. Royal College of Obstetrician and Gynaecologists. Postpartum hemorrhage: prevention and management. April 2011. Available at: http://www.rcog.org.uk/womens-health/clinicalguidance/ prevention-and-management-postpartum-haemorrhage-green-top-52. Accessed Nov. 1, 2013.
98. Saving Mothers. The third Report on confidential enquiries into maternal deaths in South Africa. Pretoria: DOH;2004-4.
99. Say L, Chou D, Gemmill A, et al. Global causes of maternal death: a WHO systematic analysis. Lancet Glob Health 2014;2(6):e323-33.
100. Scott J, Foley MR. Organizing an obstetric critical care unit. In: Belfort MA, Saade G, Foley MR, Phelan GP, Dildy GA, editors. Critical care obstetrics. Fifth Edition: Blackwell Publishing Ltd; 2010.
101. Sharma P, Saxena R. A novel thromboelastographic score to identify overt disseminated intravascular coagulation resulting in a hypocoagulable state. Am J Clin Pathol. 2010;134:97-102.
102. Singer M, Deutschman CS, Seymour WC, et al. The third International concensus definition for sepsis and septic shock. JAMA.2016;315(8):801-810.doi:10.1001/jama. 2016.0287
103. Singh S, McGlennan A, England A, et al. A validation study of the CEMACH recommended

modified early obstetric warning system (MEOWS). Anaesthesia 2012;67(1):12-8.
104. Smith IF, Skelton V. An unusual intracranial tumour presenting in pregnancy. Int J Obstet Anesth. 2007;16(1):82-5.
105. Society of Obstetricians and Gynaecologists of Canada. Active Management of the Third Stage of Labour: Prevention and Treatment of Postpartum Hemorrhage. No. 235 October 2009. (Replaces No. 88, April 2000). Available at: http://sogc.org/guidelines/active-management-of-the-thirdstage-of-labour-prevention-and-treatment-of-postpartum-hemorrhage.
106. Spoerke N, Michalek J, Schreiber M, et al. Crystalloid resuscitation improves survival in trauma patients receiving low ratios of fresh frozen plasma to packed redblood cells. J Trauma. 2011;71(2):S380-3.
107. Tacconelli E, Cataldo MA, Dancer SJ, et al. ESCMID guidelines for the management of the infection control measures to reduce transmission of multidrug-resistant Gram-negative bacteria in hospitalized patients. Microbiol Infect. 2014;20 (Suppl. 1): 1-55.
108. Taylor Fb, Toh Ch, Hoots Wk, et al. Scientific Subcommittee on Disseminated Intravascular Coagulation (DIC) of the International Society on Thrombosis and Haemostasis (ISTH). Towards definition, clinical and laboratory criteria, and a scoring system for disseminated intravascular coagulation. Thromb Haemost 2001;86:1327-30.
109. Thachil J, Toh CH. Disseminated intravascular coagulation in obstetric disorders and its acute haematological management. Blood Rev. 2009;23:167-76.
110. The Advanced Life Support Group. Managing obstetric emergencies and trauma. In: Grady K, Howell C, Cox CS (Eds). The moet course manual. 2nd edition.
111. To WK, Cheung RTF. Neurological disorders in pregnancy. Hong Kong Med J. 1997;3:400-8.
112. Vandromme M, Griffin R, Kerby J, et al. Identifying risk for massive transfusion in the relatively normotensive patient: Utility of the Prehospital shock index. J Trauma. 2011;70(2):384-90.
113. Vandromme M, Griffin R, Weinberg J, et al. Lactate is a better predictor than systolic blood pressure for determining blood requirement and mortality: Could prehospital measures improve trauma triage? Jam Coll Surg. 2010;210(1):861-9.
114. Wafaisade A, Maegele M, Lefering R, et al. High plasma to red cell ratios are associated with lower mortality rates in patients receiving multiple transfusion (4 ≤ red blood cell 329 units <10) during acute trauma resuscitation. J Trauma. 2011;70(1):81-8.
115. World Health Organization. Recommendations for the prevention and treatment of postpartum haemorrhage. WHO, 2012. http://www.who.int/reproductivehealth/publications/maternal_perinatal_health/9789241548502/en/.
116. Yerby MS. Pregnancy and epilepsy. Epilepsia. 1991;32:S51-9.
117. Zeeman G, Wendel GD, Cunningham FG. A blueprint for obstetric critical care. Am J Obstet Gynecol. 2003;188:532-6.
118. Zielinski MD, Johnson PM, Jenkins D, et al. Emergency use of prethawed group A plasma in trauma patients. J Trauma Acute Care Surg. 2013;74(1):69-75.

Fetal Growth Restriction

Sunanda R Kulkarni

CASE

A patient, aged 30 years, a coolie, ANC card showed, belongs to a low socioeconomic class, Gravida 3, Para 2, living 2 with 8 months of pregnancy presented for the 1st time to OPD for antenatal checkup.

Gynecologic History

Menarche—14 years of age
MC = 3-4/28-30 days, cycles are regular with normal flow no dysmenorrhea.
LMP—8 months back.

Obstetric History

ML—6 years, nonconsanguineous marriage.
G3 P2 L2.

History of Present Pregnancy

1st Trimester

- Spontaneous conception
- No history of taking any medicine
- No history of fever
- No history of hyperemesis.

2nd Trimester

- Feeling of fetal movements since 5th month.
- Only single visit to the hospital at nearby PHC during 4th month
- Prophylactic iron and folic acid taken irregularly
- Record of BP, serological examination done
- Scan done at 4th month, showed no congenital anomalies, growth corresponds to gestational age
- No history of pain abdomen, bleeding.

3rd Trimester

Has come to our hospital for check up.

Past Obstetric History

Her babies delivered at home and according to her they were full term, normal delivery, No history of postpartum hemorrhage.

Past Medical and Surgical History

No history of jaundice, UTI, TB, or any other chronic illness.
No history of any operation.

Socioeconomic History

Patient is a coolie, husband also works as a coolie in mines. She is educated till 5th standard and husband up to 3rd standard.

Family History

There is no history of twins, congenitally malformed fetuses up to 2 generation on both sides.

Personal History

Her bowel habits are regular. She chews tobacco, and husband smokes beedies. She is hard working does not get good sleep at home.

Dietary History

Total calorie intake is about 1500 kcal and protein intake 20 g day. She often skips the meals. Large portion of her meal is carbohydrate.

Q. 1. What are the examination findings?

Patient is conscious, cooperative and well oriented to time, place and person. She is very thin built, her height is 5 feet and weight is 45 kg. Patient looks emaciated, no pedal edema and appears anemic.

Vitals

Pulse—80/minute regular, good volume BP—110/70 mm Hg, respiratory rate—20/minute.

Breast Examination

Breasts show normal changes of pregnancy.

Systemic Examination

Cardiovascular Examination
Apex beat in 5th intercostal space. 1st and 2nd heart sounds are heard well. No thrill/murmurs.

Respiratory System
Trachea is central, air entry on both sides normal. No sounds like crepitations or rhonchi.

Abdominal Examination

Inspection
Abdomen uniformly distended.
- Linea nigra and striaegravidarum are seen
- No scar
- Hernial orifices are normal.

Palpation
- Fundal height corresponds to 28 weeks of pregnancy
- Symphysio-fundal height 28 cm
- Abdominal girth—29 inches
- Fundal grip—broad irregular mass suggestive of breech
- Lateral grip—back felt on left side and limbs on right side
- Pelvic grip—Round, hard ballotable mass felt, in lower pole, suggestive of head
- Liquor—appears to be less.
- Auscultation—Fetal heart 148/minute regular.

Q. 2. Please tell the summary of the case?

Mrs X w/o Y aged 30 years, G3 P2 L2 with 32 weeks but clinically 28 weeks of gestation with a single live fetus in cephalic presentation in LOA position with suspected Fetal growth restriction (FGR).

Q. 3. What are the investigations findings of this patient?

- Hb—8g%
- Urine—albumin and sugar—Nil
- Blood group A positive
- Serology—HbsAg negative VDRLnegative HIV negative
- Scan:
A single live intrauterine gestation is seen in cephalic presentation.
- BPD 7.6 cm = 8th percentile;
- HC 27.0 cm = 2nd percentile;
- AC 25.0 cm = 2nd percentile;
- FL 5.4 cm = 2nd percentile;
- EFW 1.34 kg = 5th percentile;
- HC/AC 1.08 (normal) AFI = 10 cm
  50th percentile size of 29 weeks 2 days (3 weeks lag)

  Fetal movements are good. Umbilical artery doppler was normal.

Q. 4. What is the plan of action?

- Steroids 2 doses given in anticipation. Monitoring continued every 3rd day.
- Continue pregnancy until Doppler findings are stable. If there is deterioration

especially in the aortic isthmus or ductus venosus delivery has to considered. In this case, one should not wait till there is reversal of a wave which leads to severe acidemia. Follow up should be done with umbilical artery and Ductus venosus PI. If there is increased PI decision should be taken to terminate pregnancy.

Q. 5. How will you manage this case of FGR?

- Patient should be advised admission
- Advised high protein diet
- Stop Tobacco chewing
- Betamethasone—12 mg two doses, 24 hours apart or dexamethasone 6 mg, 4 doses 8th hourly for the maturation of the lungs
- Correction of anemia.

Q. 6. What is meant by SGA?

FGR and SGA are not synonyms. There are different reasons for small for gestation. They are: 1] wrong dates babies, 2] constitutionally small babies, 3] abnormally small babies [chromosomal defects] and 4] starved babies [placental insufficiency]. Wrong date should be ruled out first. Distinction between fetuses who are growth restricted, from those who are constitutionally small is important. The term SGA is descriptive term which includes constitutionally small and pathologically small fetuses whose weight at birth are less than expected (3-10% using standard curves for gestational age) regardless of the cause.

FGR is said to be present in those babies whose birth weight is below 10th percentile of average for the gestational age.

If AC less than 10th percentile or 2 SD deviations below the mean for the gestational age then all the other parameters like HC/AC, FL/AC should be seen.

Q. 7. What are the major and minor risk factors for FGR?

According to the RCOG guidelines one major or >3 minor factors should be subjected to monitoring for FGR.

Major factors are—smoking >11/cigarettes day, >40 years, cocaine, vigorous exercises daily, previous SGA, previous still birth, chronic hypertension, APA, heavy bleeding similar to menses, diabetes with vascular disease, paternal SGA, renal impairment, PAPP A <0.4, echogenic bowel.

Minor factors are—BMI <20, or 25-34.9, age >35, and pregnancy <6 months or >60 months, low fruit intake, nulliparity, IVF singleton pregnancy, smoking <10/cigarettes/day, etc.

For minor factors, uterine artery Doppler at 20-24 weeks and serial assessment of biometry and umbilical artery Doppler in 3rd trimester and for one major factor-serial assessment of fetal size and umbilical artery Doppler from 26-28 weeks should be seen from 26-28 weeks onwards and umbilical artery Doppler should be seen.

Q. 8. What are the causes of FGR?

Maternal Causes

- Low calorie diet—malnutrion
- Medications—Antimetabolites, anticonvulsants, warfarin
- Habits—Alcohol, Cocaine, Smoking, Illicit drugs
- Maternal diseases—Hemoglobinopathies, malaria, anemia, cardiac disease, collagen diseases, SLE, APA, TORCH, CHRONS disease, diabetes, hypertension etc.
- Uterine anomalies—unicornuate uterus
- Extremes of reproductive age.

Fetal Causes

TORCH, malaria, multiple gestation, in-born errors of metabolism.

Placenta and Cord Causes

Separation, hemorrhagic endovasculitis, small size, hemangioma, infarcts, Battlen door, circumvallate, Placental mosaicism, partial stricture, hypercoiling, thrombosis.

Investigations

- Scan—ecogenic bowel
- Biochemical—PAPPA—0.4 mom

Chromosomal Causes
13, 18, 21, X0, microdeletions, syndromes.

Miscellaneous Causes
High altitude.

Q. 9. How do you diagnose a case of FGR?
- Diagnosis—confirmation of date
- Clinically—SF height has less accuracy. It is not valid in the following conditions like fibroid with pregnancy, hydramnios, maternal BMI >35, uncorrected dextrorotation, individual bias, multiple pregnancy, etc. In these conditions, patient should be monitored by scan
- Clinical examination—Symphysio fundal height—less than 4 weeks, mild and >6 weeks is severe
  Usually it grows 1 cm/week from 24th week onwards till 36th week. Growth can be charted on gravidogram. Low sensitivity high positive rates and significant intra- and interobserver variation make the test unsuitable.
- Scan—for dating—1st trimester—usually CRL corresponds to the gestational age + or minus 5 days. CRL is measured from 7–13th week. PI—>2.5 and 1.45 unilateral and bilateral notches in uterine artery in 1st and 2nd trimester respectively, then it should be followed up for the evidence of uteroplacental ischemia. 2nd trimester- BPD—is measured from 13th week. BPD corresponds to the age of pregnancy ±7–12 days.

Anomalies also should be excluded. Oligohydramnios should be monitored.

If the date is not known review scan is done after 3 weeks and gestational age is assigned. If the abdominal girth or EFW is<10th PCT, then rescan should be every fortnightly or 3rd weekly.

The diameter of cerebellum almost equals the gestational age up to the age from 18th week to 24th weeks. The transverse cerebellar diameter (TCD) can better predict gestational age in cases in which there are variations of the fetal head shape such as dolichocephalic and brachycephalic or even when the fetus is in a direct occiput posterior position. Transverse cerebellar diameter measurement can be used for significant improvement in the accuracy of gestational age estimation in growth restricted fetuses.

3rd trimester—Dating should not be done in 3rd trimester

Fetal biometry and Doppler are to be done.

EFW and AC are important in diagnosing SGA. AC is sensitive but EFW is more specific.

FL/AC ratio—>23.5 indicates asymmetrical FGR and FL is measured from 14th week.

FL/AC ratio is 22 at all gestational ages from 21 weeks to term.

HC/AC ratio—normally >1 at <32 weeks, and <1 after 34 weeks.

Q. 10. How is fetal surveillance done?

Follow up is done by fetal biometry and Doppler. Serial umbilical artery Doppler—to monitor for SGA fetuses. In umbilical artery S/D ratio, reduced, absent, reversed flow should be monitored. If there is abnormality then MCA should be monitored to see the fetal adaptation.

Reversal of S/D ratio (UA>MCA) in FGR is called head sparing pattern.

CPR is cerebroplacental ratio. Normally it is 1.1. If it is <1—hypoxia. It is the PI ratio of MCA and umbilical artery.

Q. 11. How will you do follow up this patient?

If there is an abnormality in umbilical artery Doppler then middle cerebral artery and ductus venosus should be monitored. In DV PI should be monitored. If there is deterioration it leads to 'a' wave reversal.

Single deepest pocket of amniotic fluid is more valid than AFI. If the AFI <5 and single deepest pocket <2 cm predicts increased perinatal mortality. The decrease in amniotic volume is independent of biophysical profile and more closely relates to cardiovascular deterioration.

Growth charts—monitoring the growth on chart. If there is no growth then monitoring should done after a fortnight provided Doppler is normal. After rescan decision can be taken depending upon Doppler and period of pregnancy.

See Table 1.

Table 1: Long medium and short-term tests of fetal wellbeing

	Long	Medium	Short
Validity of tests	Valid for long time	Valid for 1–2 week	Valid for 1–3 days
Parameter used	Uterine artery Doppler	Umbilical artery Doppler	NST
Parameters altered		Amniotic fluid reduced	fetal arterial and venous Doppler
USG findings	Fetal biometry	Biophysical profile	—

Q. 12. What are the investigations for FGR?

- Noninvasive tests are, 1] Scan, 2] Doppler, 3] Echo. ECHO is done when scan shows structural abnormality.
- Invasive tests—Chorionic villous biopsy, amniocentesis and cordocentesis— these are indicated when chromosomal abnormalities are suspected.

Q. 13. What are the markers that show placental insufficiency?

They are PL13, PLGF SFLT1. All of them show placental insufficiency.

PL 13—is decreased in preeclampsia and FGR.

The sFlt-1/PlGF ratio is increased in preeclampsia and FGR.

If the cause for intrauterine growth restriction (IUGR) is preeclampsia then these markers are valid.

Low PAPP-A is associated with PE and is a marker of aneuploidy.

Q. 14. How do you monitor the FGR baby?

- Serial ultrasound biometry
- Umbilical artery, MCA
- DV
- AFI
- BPP
- CTG.

Q. 15. How do you manage a case of FGR?

General—Maternal nutrition—increasing calories:

- Bed rest—no role but if the woman is doing strenuous work then 8–10 hours rest
- Medications—Calcium channel blockers— no role
- Uterine relaxants—no role
- Progesterone supplementation—Maternal supplementation of progesterone for FGR—no role
- Aspirin—If associated with preeclampsia, if predicted in first trimester
- Oral hydration—No role.

Q. 16. What are the congenital anomalies associated with IUGR?

Cardiovascular, skeletal anomalies, renal, abdominal wall and chromosomal anomalies.

Q. 17. What are the sequences of Doppler Changes?

- Increased umbilical S/D ratio—Increased PI
- Middle cerebral artery PI <5th perfusion computed tomography (PCT) brain sparing effect
- Umbilical artery absent diastolic effect
- Umbilical artery reverse end diastolic flow
- Ductus venosus—increased PI
- Ductus venosus—reversed a wave
- Ductus venosus—decreased IVR and reversed a wave
- Umbilical vein—pulsations.

Fetal Growth Restriction

Main goals of prolonging the life

- Avoiding mortality in very small babies- 24-26 weeks
- Gaining survival – nearer to 28 weeks
- Avoiding morbidity 28-30 weeks
- Gaining maturity nearer to 32 weeks.

Q. 18. What are the differentiating points between constitutionally small and pathologically small FGR?

Refer Table 2 for answer.

Table 2: Difference between SGA and FGR

Small for gestation [constitutional]	Pathologically small
Ethnic and racial factors	Cause may be found
Ponderal index—normal	Normal
Subcutaneous fat—usually looks normal	Looks thin
RBC count—normal	May be increased with nucleated cells
Platelet count—normal	Thrombocytopenia
Doppler—usually normal	UA and UA analysis-Reduced or reversed End-diastolic flow

Q. 19. What are the Differentiating points between early and late FGR?

Refer Table 3 for answer.

Table 3: Difference between early and late FGR

Early FGR	Late FGR
Affects early	Late
Proportionally small	Asymmetry
Congenital infections	Hypertension, CVS, anemia
After birth—catch up less	More
Prognosis—poor	Good
Ponderal index—Normal	Increased
Less common	More common
Head—Normal to body	Appears big to abdomen
HC/ AC = Normal	HC/AC = increased

Contd...

Contd...

Early FGR	Late FGR
FL/AC—Normal	FL/AC increased
Catch up growth -poor	Good
Incidence 20%	80%
Cell hyperplasia affected	Cell hypertrophy affected
Increased placental disease	Less placental disease
Systemic CV adaptation	Central CVS adaptation
UA to DV normal	UA normal, abnormal CPR
tolerance to hypoxia	Placental disease low
Natural history	Tolerance no natural
Management is difficult	History diagnosis is
Mortality is more	Difficult less mortality.

Q. 20. Can you explain the mechanism of venous Doppler changes in FGR?

Normal fetus should have forward venous flow even at the end of diastole. Venous vessels exhibit a pulsatile triphasic wave form representing flow during systole [s wave], diastole [D wave], and atrial systole [a wave]. DV has highest forward flow velocity allowing the most oxygenated blood to by pass liver and directly enters the heart. It is directed through foramina of ovule towards the cerebral circulation.

In response to hypoxia dilatation of DV allows large propulsion of umbilical venous flow to pass into the right atrium through foramina and into the cerebral circulation in order to maintain oxygen to brain. This is manifested by pulsatile index for veins (PIV). As hypoxia increases, there will be increased academia and reversal of 'a' wave. Back flow in venous system leads to pulsation in intra-abdominal part of umbilical veins and reversal flow in the inferior vena cava. Reversal 'a' wave leads to decreased flow to coronary arteries, leading to death of the fetus.

Venous Doppler evaluation is beneficial when FGR occurs in earlier age. As the gestation increases cardia becomes more efficient.

Q. 21. What are the arterial changes and what is the brain sparing effect?

Abdominal circumference is affected first. Middle cerebral artery normally has high systolic and minimal diastolic velocities. In FGR, there is increased blood flow to the brain as there is decreased cerebral resistance. In which there is preferential perfusion of the brain, heart and adrenals at the expense of viscera and kidneys. This leads to decreased systolic/diastolic ratio as well as PI and resistance index in the MCA.

Arterial changes show brain damage and venous changes shows heart damage.

Q 22. What is the dilemma in delivering FGR babies?

Management is more complicated for pregnancies between 25 and 32 weeks' gestation, where each day gained in utero may improve survival by 1–2%. Early delivery of growth-restricted fetuses with abnormal umbilical artery waveform (after completion of antenatal steroid course) offers the benefit of a higher livebirth rate and disadvantage of a high neonatal mortality. Hence, one should balance between the risk of premature delivery and IUD. The current therapeutic goal is optimize the timing of delivery to minimize hypoxia and maximizing the gestational age and maternal outcome. Early term induction for SGA fetuses results in an increased risk of cesarean deliveries as well as neonatal metabolic and respiratory complications, with no apparent neonatal benefit. Less than 34 weeks, complications are more. Delayed delivery increases still births whereas early delivery increases complications of prematurity. Since, there is no effective interventions to improve the suboptimal fetal growth the goal is to manage FGR to deliver the most mature fetus while minimizing the hypoxic encephalopathy. Gestational age is more important to decrease the long-term effects of hypoxia. Less than 33 weeks, there is a dilemma of iatrogenic prematurity or hypoxia.

Stage-based management of FGR

Stage 1: EFW <3rd centile or CPR <5th centile or MCA—PI <5th centile

(Both persisting 12 hour apart) or mean UtA—PI >95th centile

If ≥37 weeks—Induction of labor

If ≤37 weeks repeat in 1 week.

Stage 2: UA absent EDF or AoI reversed diastolic velocities

(Both persisting 12 hours apart)

If ≥34 weeks then do elective lower segment cesarian section (LSCS)

If ≤34 weeks then repeat in 2–3 days.

Stage 3: DV pulsatility index >95th centile or UA reversed EDF

(Both persisting 12 hours apart)

If ≥30 weeks do elective LSCS

If ≤30 weeks repeat in 24–48 hours.

Stage 4: DV absent/reversed EDV (persisting 12 hours apart)

Or pathological CTG (reduced STV or deceleration pattern)

If ≥26 weeks, elective LSCS

If ≤26 weeks, repeat in 12–24 hours.

Refer Tables 4 and 5.

Table 4: Stage-based classification and monitoring of FGR

Stage	Pathophysiological correlate	Monitoring*
I	Severe smallness or mild placental insufficiency	Weekly
II	Severe placental insufficiency	Biweekly
III	Low-suspicion fetal acidosis	1–2 days
IV	High-suspicion fetal acidosis	12 hours

Table 5: Fetal growth rate according to gestation-

Growth rate	Weeks of gestation
5 g/day	15
15–20 g/day	24
30–35 g/day	34

Doppler becomes abnormal first. It is followed by abnormal CTG
computerized NST is more valid
Variability <3.5 ms is significant

Q. 23. What is the impact of IUGR on the fetus?

Intrapartum— Hypoxia

Neonatal—RDS, IVH, hypoglycemia, hypocalcemia, hyperviscosity syndrome [Hct—>65%], hypoinsulinemia, hypertriglyceridemia.

Encephalopathy, meconium aspiration syndrome, necrotizing enterocolitis, anemia, hypothermia, hyponatremia, hyperphosphatemia, cerebral palsy.

Long-term Effect

Fetal origin of adult disease. (Barker's hypothesis)—Cerebral palsy, ischemic heart disease, chronic renal disease, atherosclerosis, premature adrenarche, PCOD, non-insulin dependent diabetes, dyslipidemia, decreased growth, low IQ, cognitive behavioral defect.

If IUGR sets at <34 weeks may not catch up growth but if >34 weeks then after birth they may catch up the growth.

Q. 24. In which cases recurrence of FGR is seen?

Women with first pregnancy early-onset FGR, without concomitant maternal hypertensive disease, frequently develop FGR. Advanced maternal age is an independent risk factor for FGR. It also seen in smokers, drug addicts and maternal diseases like chronic hypertension, diabetes with vascular diseases, autoimmune kidney disease, maternal medication for epilepsy, etc.

Q. 25. What is BPP?

The BPP consists of 5 components:
1. Fetal breathing movements
2. Fetal tone
3. Gross body movements of fetus
4. AFI
5. NST.

Each component is given a score of 2 or zero and the maximum score is 10 (Manning score)
It should not be used for fetal surveillance in SGA, it also not recommended for pre-term babies
BPP has high false positive rate and is a poor predictor of intrauterine fetal death (IUFD)

Q. 26. What are the clinical application of Doppler and BPP?

When the BPP is >8 AFI normal with abnormal UA but normal MCA asphyxia is extremely rare but increased risk for intrapartum distress.

If there is low MCA, it shows brain sparing effect which may lead to hypoxia.

If the BPP is >6 and associated with oligohydramnios with umbilical artery showing absent or reversed flow it shows significant blood redistribution. This may lead to hypoxia, acidemia and fetal comprise. When DV shows increased pulsatility hypoxia is common and acidemia is more likely. When there is reversed 'a' wave or pulsatile UV shows cardiovascular instability, imminent still birth and high perinatal mortality irrespective of intervention.

Q. 27. What are the indications for termination of pregnancy?

- Maternal indication
- Doppler indication—Reversed a wave in DV, UA A/REDV
- BPP, 6
- Variability <5 in CTG
- Gestational age >37 weeks.

Q. 28. What are the indication for cesarean section?

Babies with DV abnormality, umbilical artery reversal, absent, an premature babies may not with stand the stress of labor and may need cesarean section.

Recent Advances

Aorto ischemic Doppler wave forms precedes the ductus venosus.

> **Points to remember**
> - Routine abdominal checkup may not detect FGR
> - Suspicion is required in low-risk patients
> - In high-risk patients, Doppler studies are required from second trimester
> - Follow up the case if there is uterine artery notch and look for PE
> - Aspirin in high-risk patients <16th
> - Add AFI along with biometry
> - Symmetrical and asymmetrical terms are not used. Instead early and late onset FGR are used FGR are used
> - When end diastolic flow is present delivery can be delayed
> - Absent and reverse diastolic flow is associated with increased perinatal mortality and morbidity.

Bibliography

1. Afshan A, Nadeem S, Asim SS. Fetal transverse cerebellar diameter measurement, a useful predictor of gestational age in growth restricted fetuses. Professional Med J. 2014;21(5):888-91.
2. Ananth CV, Kaminsky L, Getahun D, et al. Recurrence of fetal growth restriction in singleton and twin gestations. J Matern Fetal Neonatal Med. 2009;22(8):654-61. doi: 10.1080/14767050902740207.
3. Arora D, Desai SK, Sheth PN, et al. Significance of umbilical artery velocimetry in perinatal outcome of growth restricted fetuses. J Obstet Gynecol India. 2005;55(2):138-43.
4. Bamfo JEAK, Odibo AO. Diagnosis and Management of Fetal Growth Restriction. J Pregnancy. 2011;15. Article ID 640715. http://dx.doi.org/10.1155/2011/640715
5. Barbara Hoffman B, Horsager R, Roberts S. Williams Obstetrics Study Guide. New York : McGraw-Hill Education. 2014;24: 872.
6. Baschat AA, Weiner CP. Umbilical artery Doppler screening for detection of the small fetus in need of antepartum surveillance. Am J Obset Gynecol. 2000;182:154-8.
7. Carrera JM, Figueras F, Meler E. Ultrasound and Doppler Management of Intrauterine Growth Restriction. Donald School Journal of Ultrasound in Obstetrics and Gynecology. In: Kurjak A, Chervenak FA (Eds). July-September 2010;4(3):259-74.
8. Chafetz I, Kuhnreich I, Sammar M, et al. The importance of repeated measurements of the sFlt-1/PlGF ratio for the prediction of preeclampsia and intrauterine growth restriction. J Perinat Med. 2014;42(1):61-8. doi: 10.1515/jpm-2013-0074.
9. Del Río M, Martínez JM, Figueras F, et al. Severe intrauterine growth restriction. Ultrasound Obstet Gynecol. 2008;31(1):41-7.
10. Evers AC, van Rijn BB, van Rossum MM, et al. Subsequent pregnancy outcome after first pregnancy with normotensive early-onset intrauterine growth restriction at <34 weeks of gestation. Hypertens pregnancy. 2011;30(1):37-44. doi: 10.3109/10641955.2010.484080. Epub 2010 Sep 6.
11. Figueras F, Gardosi J. Intrauterine growth restriction: new concepts in antenatal surveillance, diagnosis, and management. Am J Obstet Gynecol. 2011;204(4):288-300. doi: 10.1016/j.ajog.2010.08.055. Epub 2011 Jan 7.
12. Figueras F, Gratacós E. Update on the diagnosis and classification of fetal growth restriction and proposal of a stage-based management protocol. Fetal Diagn Ther. 2014;36(2):86-98. doi: 10.1159/000357592. Epub 2014 Jan 23.
13. Goetzinger KR, Cahill AG, Macones GA, et al. Echogenic bowel on second-trimester ultrasonography: evaluating the risk of adverse pregnancy outcome. Obstet Gynecol. 2011;117(6):1341-8. doi: 10.1097/AOG.0b013e31821aa739.
14. Lausman A, McCarthy FP, Walker M, et al. Screening, diagnosis, and management of intrauterine growth restriction. Obstet Gynaecol Can. 2012;34(1):17-28. doi: 10.1016/S1701-2163(16)35129-5.
15. Mylonas I, Schiessl B, Jeschke U, et al. Expression of inhibin/activin subunits alpha (-alpha), beta A (-beta (A)) and beta B (-beta (B)) in placental

tissue of normal and intrauterine growth restricted (IUGR) pregnancies. J Molec Histol. 2006;37:43-52. PMID 16670820 DOI: 10.1007/s10735-006-9029-6.
16. Nicholas SS, Orzechowski KM, Weiner S. Making sense of Doppler ultrasound in obstetrics. Current progress in Obstetrics & Gynaecology. Studd J, Tan SL, Chervenak FA (Eds). 2012;1.
17. Odibo AO, Nelson D, Stamilio DM, et al. Advanced maternal age is an independent risk factor for intrauterine growth restriction. Am J Perinatol. 2006;23(5):325-8. Epub 2006 Jun 23.
18. Radu Vladareanu, Anea Burnei, Simona Containesu. Timing and mode of delivery of the Infant with IUGR. Current progress in Obstetrics & Gynecology. In: Studd J, Tan SL, Chervenak FA (Eds). 2012;2.
19. Rizzo G, Capponi A, Vendola M, et al. First-trimester placental protein 13 screening for preeclampsia and intrauterine growth restriction. Am J Obstet Gynecol. 2007;197(1):35.e1-7.
20. Schoofs K, Grittner U, Engels T, et al. The importance of repeated measurements of the sFlt-1/PlGF ratio for the prediction of preeclampsia and intrauterine growth restriction. J Perinat Med. 2014;42(1):61-8. doi: 10.1515/jpm-2013-0074.
21. Simchen MJ, Ofir K, Moran O, et al. Department of Obstetrics and Gynecology, Sheba Medical Center, Tel Hashomer, Israel. Eur J Obst, Gynec, and reproductive biology (Impact Factor: 1.7). 09/2013; 171(2). DOI: 10.1016/j.ejogrb.2013.09.016.
22. Stephen A, Walkinshaw, Cochrane L. Recent advances in Obstetrics and gynaecoogy 22nd edition Edited by john Bonner. Investgation & management of small fetus.
23. Tannirandorn Y, Phaosavasdi S. Significance of an absent or reversed end-diastolic flow velocity in Doppler umbilical artery waveforms. J Med Assoc Thai. 1994;77(2):81-6.
24. The investigation and management of the small-for-gestational-age fetus. Green-top Guideline No. 31 2nd Edition | February 2013 | Minor revisions – January 2014. The Journal of Obstetrics and Gynecology of India,
25. Tongsong T, Wanapirak C, Thongpadungroj T. Sonographic diagnosis of intrauterine growth restriction (IUGR) by fetal transverse cerebellar diameter (TCD)/abdominal circumference (AC) ratio. Int J Gynaecol Obstet. 1999;66(1):1-5.
26. Turan OM, Turan S, Gungor S, et al. Progression of Doppler abnormalities in intrauterine growth restriction. Update on the Diagnosis and Classification of Fetal Growth Restriction and Proposal of a Stage-Based Management Protocol. Ultrasound Obstet Gynecol. 2008; 32(2):160-7. doi: 10.1002/uog.5386.
27. Walkinsha SA. Lindsay Cochrane. Investigations and management of the small fetus. Recent advances in obstetrics and gynecology. In: Bonner J, Dunlop W (Eds). Page no. 17.

11

Liver Diseases in Pregnancy

Hemant Deshpande

Liver disease is rare but dramatic and tragic complication for both mother and infant. Because of physiology of pregnancy, certain disorders take more ominous course in pregnancy than in non-pregnant state (e.g. Hep E) while some are very unique to pregnancy (e.g. Acute fatty liver of pregnancy or cholestasis of pregnancy).

Here are some special case scenarios related with liver diseases in pregnancy.

CASE 1

A pregnant lady of 32 weeks of gestation came with complaints of pedal edema, jaundice, right upper quadrant pain, polyuria and polydipsia. On examination, there was e/o pedal edema, icterus, ascites, hypertension. Conjugated serum bilirubin was 6.4 mg/dL, serum transaminase 550 IU/L, platelets 1,00,000/mm³.

Q. 1. What is your diagnosis?

The most probable diagnosis in this case would be acute fatty liver of pregnancy or "acute yellow atrophy of pregnancy" or "acute obstetric fatty metamorphosis of liver". It most frequently complicates the third trimester and is commonly associated (or complicated) with preeclampsia (50–100%). It has high incidence of maternal (18%) and perinatal mortality (47%).

Q. 2. What are the diagnostic criteria for acute fatty liver in pregnancy (AFLP)?

The presence of more than 5 of 14 Swansea criteria support the clinical diagnosis of AFLP:

- Vomiting
- Abdominal pain
- Polydipsia and polyuria
- Encephalopathy
- Elevated transaminase (42 IU/L)
- Elevated bilirubin
- Hypoglycemia
- Elevated urate
- Renal impairment
- Elevated ammonia
- Leukocytosis
- Coagulopathy
- Ascites or bright liver on ultrasound.

Q. 3. Discuss the prognosis of AFLP.

Encephalopathy can occur in as high as 87% of cases. Polydipsia with or without polyuria, frequently is an early feature. After hours or a few days, some patients become lethargic and may decline into hepatic coma, or milder degrees of mental impairment. Ascites is usually transient and rarely prominent. After delivery, most patients improve slowly, and a full clinical and laboratory recovery may take from 1 to 4 weeks.

One of the keys to the diagnosis of AFLP is the rapidity with which LFT can deteriorate in the aggressive phase of the disease. Other pregnancy specific liver conditions do not impair liver function in this way.

Q. 4. What is the pathogenesis of AFLP?

Exact etiology is not known precisely. Recent research suggests that AFLP is associated with a Glu474Gln mutation in the long-chain 3-hydroxy acyl-coenzyme A dehydrogenase (LCHAD), a fatty acid β oxidation enzyme.

AFLP may occur because of an autosomal recessive abnormality in fetal long chain fatty acid beta oxidation.

Q. 5. Describe the relevant investigations in this case.

LFT abnormalities are:
- Conjugated hyperbilirubinemia (usually between 5 and 15 mg/dL)
- Increased alkaline phosphates (normal <170)
- Modest increases in serum aminotransferases (usually <1000 IU/L).

CBC and coagulation profile may show leukocytosis, thrombocytopenia and decreased clotting factors.

Blood sugar and RFT may show hypoglycemia and renal dysfunction also.

Confirmation of diagnosis is done by liver biopsy characterized by fatty metamorphosis. The hepatic architecture is intact and the lobules are swollen with compressed sinusoids. Centrilobular microvesicular fatty infiltration of hepatocytes and ballooning of hepatocytes seen.

Q. 6. What are the complications?

Course of disease is aggressive and patient deteriorates with rapidity. The complications that can occur are:
- Cerebral edema, renal failure (60%), hypoglycemia (53%), infections (45%), gastrointestinal hemorrhage (33%), coagulopathy (30%), fetal demise and postpartum hemorrhage.

Q. 7. What are the management principles?

The emergency therapeutic decisions usually are made without waiting for a histological proven diagnosis.

Ultrasound is most important in the exclusion of biliary tract disorders.

The mild jaundice and modest increase in serum aminotransferases are important signs against the diagnosis of fulminant hepatitis (viral or toxic).

The mild increase in blood pressure, hyperuricemia, and the intense thirst are uncommon in fulminant hepatitis and they favor the diagnosis of acute fatty liver of pregnancy. Liver biopsy is not indicated.

No specific treatment is available for AFLP. All patients should be hospitalized as soon as the diagnosis of AFLP is suspected.

Patients with any extrahepatic complications, should be attended in intensive care units.

It seems convenient to maintain glucose infusions because of the risk of a sudden hypoglycemia until a full metabolic recovery is obtained.

Prothrombin time and blood glucose should be repeated at least daily. Prothrombin time helps to assess the prognosis of liver failure and blood glucose detects a severe hypoglycemia.

Importance of interrupting pregnancy may seem questionable but a prompt delivery is preferable.

CASE 2

A pregnant lady with 36 weeks of gestation came to OPD with complaints of pruritus for 2 weeks, jaundice, malaise, vomiting. On examination, there was excoriation of skin over limbs, mild icterus. Serum bilirubin was 4.3 mg/dL, transaminase was 126 IU/L and serum bile acid was markedly increased.

Q. 8. What is the most likely diagnosis?

Pruritus and mild jaundice usually occurring in the last trimester of pregnancy points towards intrahepatic cholestasis. It can, however, occur in earlier gestational period also. It's incidence is 1 in 1,000 to 1 in 10,000 deliveries. It tends to recur in subsequent pregnancies, individuals with hepatitis C infection are more prone to it.

Q. 9. Describe pathology of cholestasis of pregnancy?

There is centrilobular cholestasis, canlicular bile plugs, retained biliary pigments in hepatocytes, lack of inflammation and necrosis. These changes tend to regress after pregnancy.

Q. 10. What are the clinical manifestations?

Patients usually begin having pruritus at night. Approximately 2 weeks later clinical jaundice develops in 50% of cases. The jaundice is usually mild, soon plateaus, and remains constant until delivery. The pruritus worsens with the onset of jaundice, and the patient's skin can become excoriated. The symptoms usually abate within 2 days after delivery.

Q. 11. What is the differential diagnosis?

1. Viral hepatitis
2. Gallbladder disease.

   There is usually no fever or abdominal discomfort, as in hepatitis and no nausea or vomiting as seen in hepatitis and gallbladder disease.

Q. 12. How do you investigate this case?

- LFT- Serum alkaline phosphatase is raised 5 to 10 folds.
- Bilirubin is elevated, but usually not above 5 mg/dL.
- Serum transaminase increased more than 10 times.
- Serum cholesterol and triglyceride levels and serum bile acids (chenodeoxycholic acid, deoxycholic acid and cholic acid) are increased more than 10 times the normal concentration.
- Prothrombin time is prolonged
- Screen for GDM
- Rationale: There is a primary change in the reductase metabolism of progesterone in cholestasis of pregnancy. Serum and urinary excretion of total sulfated progesterone metabolites are increased, whereas glucuronide metabolites are unchanged or low. Bile acids are deposited in the skin causing extreme pruritus. The degree of pruritus, however, is not always related to the serum level of bile acids. For diagnosing the fasting levels of serum bile acids should be at least three times the upper limit of normal

Carbohydrate metabolism is disturbed in patients with intrahepatic cholestasis of pregnancy. These patients should therefore be screened for **Gestational diabetes** when the diagnosis of cholestasis is made.

Q. 13. How do you treat this case?

Diphenhydramine, hydroxyzine, and other antihistamines can be used to relieve pruritus. Cholestyramine is an anion binding resin that interrupts the enterohepatic circulation, reducing the reabsorption of bile acids. A total of 8 to 16 g/day in three to four divided doses may be given.

Because cholestyramine also interferes with vitamin K absorption, the prothrombin time should be checked at least weekly. If prolonged, parenteral vitamin K should be administered. When the prothrombin time returns to normal, the frequency of injections can be decreased. Cholestyramine causes a sensation of bloating and often results in constipation. It can interfere with the absorption of other ingested medications. If the patient cannot tolerate cholestyramine, antacids containing aluminum may be used to bind bile acids. These medications are usually not as effective as cholestyramine.

Phenobarbital, in a dose of up to 90 mg daily given at bedtime, can be helpful. Phenobarbital induces hepatic microsomal enzymes, increasing bile salt secretion and bile flow. This medication usually takes more than 1 week to be effective. It has not been shown to change the serum concentration of bile acids. It is important to remember that phenobarbital must not be given within 2 hours of cholestyramine or the phenobarbital will be bound and excreted without being absorbed. The key to treating pregnancy-induced cholestasis is to begin therapy as soon as the diagnosis is made.

Dexamethasone has also been used with some success in treating pregnancy-induced cholestasis. Dexamethasone suppresses fetal—placental estrogen production, which is out of balance in the patient with cholestasis of pregnancy.

S-adenyl-methionine (SAM-e) works by reversing estrogen-induced impairment of bile secretion. Ursodeoxycholic acid (UDCA) is a naturally occurring hydrophilic bile acid that replaces other more cytotoxic bile acids. The dosage of UDCA is 14 to 16 mg/kg/day.

Intrauterine deaths are known to occur in this condition and thus antepartum fetal monitoring and timing of delivery are very important.

Delivery may be undertaken at term or as soon as fetal lung maturity has been documented. Jaundice usually disappears within 2 days after delivery.

CASE 3

A 38 weeks pregnant lady referred to tertiary care institute with H/O gross pedal edema, abdominal wall edema, with BP 160/110 mm of Hg, epigastric pain, vomiting, petechie over body. Serum bilirubin 2 mg/dL, LDH >600 IU/L, serum transaminases 78 IU/L, platelets 50,000 /mm^3. Peripheral smear shows presence of anisocytosis, burr cells, and spherocytes.

Q. 14. What is the diagnosis?

HELLP syndrome. This is considered to be a variant of preeclampsia, in some cases, HELLP symptoms are the first warning of preeclampsia and is characterized by hemolysis, elevated liver enzymes and thrombocytopenia. It can complicate 0.2–0.6% of all pregnancies. Superimposed HELLP syndrome develops in 4–12% of women with preeclampsia or eclampsia. Maternal mortality has been estimated to be as high as 2–24%. Perinatal mortality is equally high.

Most of the patients present with non-specific symptoms: generalized malaise, epigastric pain, nausea vomiting, and headache.

Right upper quadrant tenderness, hypertension and proteinuria may be absent or mild.

Q. 15. What are the differential diagnosis to be considered?

Hepatitis, idiopathic thrombocytopenic purpura, gallbladder disease, or thrombotic thrombocytopenic purpura.

Q. 16. What are the laboratory diagnostic criteria for HELLP syndrome?

Abnormal peripheral smear: spherocytes, schistocytes, triangular cells and burr cells.
- Total bilirubin level >1.2 mg/dL
- Lactate dehydrogenase level >600 U/L
- Serum aspartate amino transferase level >70 U/L
- Lactate dehydrogenase level >600 U/L
- Platelet count < 150,000/mm^3/ <1,00,000/mm^3
- Platelet count appears to be the most reliable indicator of the presence of HELLP syndrome.

Q. 17. What is the etiopathogenesis of this condition?

The hemolysis in HELLP syndrome is a microangiopathic hemolytic anemia. Red blood cells become fragmented as they pass through small blood vessels with endothelial damage and fibrin deposits. There is increase in bilirubin and lactic dehydrogenase levels. The elevated liver enzyme levels in the syndrome are thought to be secondary to obstruction of hepatic blood flow by fibrin deposits in the sinusoids. This obstruction leads to periportal necrosis and, in severe cases, intrahepatic hemorrhage, subcapsular hematoma formation or hepatic rupture. The thrombocytopenia has been attributed to increased consumption and/or destruction of platelets. With platelet activation, thromboxane A and serotonin are released, causing vasospasm, platelet agglutination and aggregation, and further endothelial damage.

Q. 18. Discuss the classification systems of HELLP syndrome.

Tennessee classification: Complete and partial.

Complete HELLP syndrome:
- All three criteria should be fulfilled
- Consider for delivery within 48 hours.

Partial HELLP syndrome:
- Any two of three criteria should be fulfilled

Mississippi system of classification
- Class I - platelet count <50000/mm^3
- Class II- platelet count 50000-100000/mm^3
- Class III- platelet count 100000-150000/mm^3.

Q. 19. Discuss the management of HELLP syndrome.

The treatment is based on the estimated gestational age and the condition of the mother and fetus.

Patients with HELLP syndrome should be treated prophylactically with magnesium sulfate to prevent seizures, whether hypertension is present or not.

Antihypertensive therapy should be initiated if blood pressure is consistently greater than 160/110 mm Hg despite the use of magnesium sulfate. The goal is to maintain diastolic blood pressure between 90 and 100 mm Hg. Prophylactic transfusion of platelets at delivery does not reduce the incidence of postpartum hemorrhage or hasten normalization of the platelet count.

Patients with DIC should be given fresh frozen plasma and packed red blood cells.

Termination of pregnancy has to be considered with worsening of the condition, fetal compromise or other complications.

CASE 4

A primigravidae with 10 weeks gestation came to emergency room with history of severe nausea and vomiting since one week, generalized weakness, oliguria. On examination patient was emaciated with sunken eyes, acidic smell from mouth, mild icterus was there with tachycardia and hypotension. She was little confused and disoriented. Laboratory findings suggestive of hyponatremia, hypokalemia, ketonuria and mild increased in blood urea levels.

Q. 20. What is the diagnosis in this patient?

This is an easily diagnosable condition of hyperemesis gravidarum (HG) which is defined as persistent vomiting that leads to weight loss greater than 5% of prepregnancy weight, with associated electrolyte imbalance and ketonuria. It occurs in about 1% of pregnancies. Seropositivity for *H. pylori* infection is more common in patients with hyperemesis.

Q. 21. How do you work up the case?

- Complete blood count
- Blood sugar
- Serum electrolytes

- Renal function test (RFT)
- Liver function test (LFT).

Abdominopelvic ultrasound

It is important to rule out other serious causes of vomiting. Ultrasound examination should be done to confirm pregnancy, to establish number of fetuses and to rule out vesicular mole. Laboratory investigations may reveal hyponatremia, hypokalemia and increased hematocrit. Liver function tests may be deranged in severe cases. There may be mild increase in total bilirubin (<4 mg/dL) and mild increase in ALT (2–3 times normal).

Q. 22. What are the complications of this condition?

They may be maternal and fetal complications.

Maternal complications

If left untreated, patient may present with Wernicke's encephalopathy as a result of thiamine deficiency. If it is untreated may lead to Korsakoff's psychosis or death.

Rapid correction of hyponatremia may cause central pontine myelinolysis.

Deep venous thrombosis may result from severe dehydration. Other risks include: Mallory-Weiss tear and hematemesis due to protracted vomiting.

Fetal risks include small for gestational age babies, prematurity. Fetal outcome is worse if mother develops Wernicke's encephalopathy.

Q. 23. Discuss the treatment.

1. *Correction of dehydration:* Rapid correction should be avoided to prevent central pontine myelinolysis. Dextrose fluids should be avoided because sodium content is less in them and Wernicke's encephalopathy may be precipitated because of high dextrose content.
2. *Correcting electrolyte imbalance:* Potassium supplementation should be given as required.
3. *Antiemetics:* Antiemetics like antihistaminics (doxylamine, promethazine) or dopamine antagonist (metaclopromide, domperidone) can be safely used as a first line drugs.
4. *Vitamin supplementation:* Pyridoxine-vitamin B6, has been proven to be non-teratogenic in combination with doxylamine. Thiamine should be replaced as either 50–150 mg orally or 100 mg diluted in 100 mL.

If patient is not responding to above treatment then 5-HT3 receptor antagonist (ondansetron) can be used. Corticosteroids have been reported to be an effective treatment in refractory cases. Corticosteroids should be avoided during the first trimester because of possible increased risk of oral clefting and should be restricted to refractory cases.

Alternative therapies, such as ginger supplementation, acupuncture, and acupressure, may be beneficial.

Eating small, frequent meals consisting of bland foods; avoiding fatty foods such as potato chips; and avoiding drinking cold, tart, or sweet beverages.

In refractory cases, worsening LFT, RFT, termination of pregnancy may have to be considered.

CASE 5

35-years-old multiparous referral patient with 34 weeks of pregnancy came to emergency room in shock with history of preeclampsia on treatment since 3–4 weeks, sudden onset pain in abdomen and tenderness. On examination, there was tenderness in right upper quadrant, guarding and rigidity. USG suggestive of moderate hemoperitoneum. FHS was absent.

Q. 24. What is the diagnosis?

The following differential diagnosis may have to be considered in this case:
- Ruptured uterus

- Abruptio placentae
- Spontaneous hepatic rupture

Silent uterine rupture is rare in unscarred uterus. Good uterine contour and absence of easy palpation of fetal parts rules out rutpured uterus.

Abruptio placentae may be seen in patients of preeclampsia, but absence of history of vaginal bleeding and no evidence of retroplacental clot, moderate hemoperitoneum disfavors diagnosis of abruption.

So diagnosis of spontaneous hepatic rupture should be kept in mind. It is a rare disorder seen in pregnancy. 94% associated with eclampsia/pre-eclampsia. Very high proportion is in multiparous women >30 years of age. In 85% of cases, right lobe of liver is affected. It may present with right upper quadrant pain, tenderness, diffuse abdominal pain and peritoneal signs.

Hepatic rupture is dangerous for mother and baby. Maternal mortality is 16–60% and perinatal mortality is between 40–60%.

Q. 25. How to manage this case?

Treatment of hepatic rupture is based on resuscitation and arresting the hemorrhage. If diagnosis is suspected, midline laparotomy should be considered along with delivery of baby. Various therapeutic maneuvers for hepatic rupture have been described. Currently the most successful one is Pringle's maneuver (digital compression of hepatic artery and portal vein to temporary arrest the hemorrhage), evacuation of residual hematoma, temporary packing with large dry gauze.

Unruptured small hematomas can be managed conservatively, following delivery of baby, with serial imaging.

CASE 6

35 weeks pregnant lady came to labor room with history of jaundice since 2–3 days, absent fetal movements since one day. She had history of outside food one week before. On examination, there was deep icterus, fetal heart sounds were absent. Serum bilirubin was 12 mg/dL, Serum transaminases were >1000 IU/L, platelets 68,000/mm^3. She was in active labor delivered a near term IUD within 2 hours, went into atonic PPH and died.

Q. 26. What is your likely diagnosis?

Hepatitis E infection is most likely cause in this case with rapid deterioration and high mortality in pregnancy. It is caused by the hepatitis E virus (HEV) via fecal-oral route. The infection is mild and self-limited without chronicity.

Q. 27. Explain the pathophysiology.

HEV is a nonenveloped, spherical, positive-sense, and single-stranded RNA virus. It is composed of viral protein and RNA. HEV is transmitted feco-orally, is a water-borne disease, and it has been associated with outbreaks through contaminated food or water supplies. HEV is excreted from the liver via the common bile duct into the duodenum of the small intestine, where it is relatively resistant to the acid, viral shedding in feces occurs during the incubation and early acute phase. The period of infectivity extends for up to 14 days after the onset of jaundice.

Q. 28. How will you diagnose and manage the case?

Laboratory evaluation of liver function test as urine bilirubin and urobilinogen, total and direct serum bilirubin, alanine aminotransferase (ALT) and/or aspartate aminotransferase (AST), alkaline phosphatase (ALP), prothrombin time (PT), total protein, albumin, complete blood cell (CBC) count, and in severe cases, serum ammonia.

Diagnosis is made by detection of IgM antibodies to HEV and presence of IgM anti-

HEV. Western blot assays detect IgM or IgG antibodies, IgG titers may remain elevated for years after infection.
- Pregnant women, have increased mortality secondary to hypertensive and renal complications. Severity of illness is due to attenuated cellular immunity which causes fulminant hepatitis with mortality up to 20% and perinatal mortality up to 33%.
- Good hygiene, clean water system, avoidance of food contamination can prevent hepatitis E infection. Management is done in conjunction with a gastroenterologist is mandatory to follow up patients in cases of acute disease. Hospitalization is done for fever, malaise, vomiting, weakness and abdominal pain. Supportive therapy for maintaining adequate fluid with high carbohydrate diet is given.

Patient should be monitored with serum bilirubin, SGOT, SGPT, platelet count, coagulation profile, BT/CT, blood sugar level. Active infection in labor should be managed at tertiary care level with multidisciplinary approach. PCV, FFP, platelets should be reserved and transfused whenever necessary. Strict monitoring of fetal well-being is necessary. Third stage of labor should be managed vigorously.

CASE 7

A 22-year-old primigravida came to follow up in ANC OPD with 38 weeks of gestation. She was HbsAg positive. All other investigations were normal. She was curious about this report.

Q. 29. What is the pathophysiology of HBsAg?

Hepatitis B disease is caused by hepatitis B virus, an enveloped partially double-stranded, circular DNA genome and from the family hepadnavirus. The core is surrounded by a lipoprotein coat or envelope, which is the HbsAg. The envelope lipoprotein is produced in excessive amounts and released into the circulation as HBsAg.

The concentration of HBV is high in blood, wound exudates, semen, vaginal discharge and saliva. The virus minimally detected in urine, feces, sweat, tears, and breast milk. Approximately 25% of the regular sexual contacts of infected individuals will themselves become seropositive. The average incubation period is 90 days from time of exposure to onset of symptoms, but may vary from 6 weeks to 6 months. HBV interferes with the functions of the liver during the replication in liver cells. HBV does not cross the placenta because of its size, and it cannot infect the fetus unless there have been breaks in the maternal-fetal barrier. Infected women can transmit HBV to the infant during labor. Perinatal transmission from the mother to baby is important mode of transmission. If a pregnant woman is an HBV carrier and is also positive for hepatitis B "e" antigen (HBeAg), her newborn baby has a 90% likelihood of becoming infected. Most HbsAg carriers are asymptomatic, potentially infectious, and a constant source of new infections.

Q. 30. What are the symptoms of acute infection?

Acutely infected individuals develop clinically apparent hepatitis with loss of appetite, nausea, vomiting, fever, abdominal pain and jaundice. Some may have dark urine and gray stool. About one-half of acute HBV infections in adults are symptomatic. About 1% of cases result in acute liver failure and death. Approximately 25% of infected infants will become chronic carriers.

Q. 31. Discuss the modes of transmission of hepatitis B and what are the sequelae of the infection?

Important modes of HBV transmission is due to contact with infected blood, body fluids, and by sexual intercourse, use of infected needles or blood transfusion. A break in the skin or mucosal barrier is required for transmission.

HBV infection is transient in about 90% of adults, approximately 5–10% of adults progress to become asymptomatic carriers and develop chronic hepatitis, cirrhosis and risk of hepatocellular carcinoma.

Q. 32. Discuss the different antigens and antibodies that are of diagnostic importance in hepatitis B infection.

- Surface antigen and antibodies (HBsAg and anti-HBs, respectively). The presence of HBsAg indicates that the woman is potentially infectious
- Core antigen and antibodies (HBcAg and anti-HBc, respectively)
- Precore antigen and antibodies (HBeAg and anti-HBe, respectively). HBeAg is indicative of infectivity and disease severity.

The risk of maternal-fetal transmission can be as high as 90% among women positive for HBsAg who are also positive for HBeAg. Anti-HBc is first antibody to appear and indicates acute HBV infection. Patients of hepatitis B should be tested for hepatitis D virus (HDV), HCV and HIV infections.

By definition, chronic HBV infection lasts for more than 6 months, with persistently positive HbsAg and anti-HBc IgG with absence of an anti-HBs response. HBeAg is often present and correlates with elevated levels of HBV DNA. The inflammatory response is milder and continuous process progressing to cirrhosis with risk of hepatocellular carcinoma.

Progression of disease depends upon viral replicative activity, which can be assessed by rising serum ALT concentrations.

After liver becomes cirrhotic, ALT concentrations decreases but there is rise in serum transaminases, bilirubin, antinuclear antibody (ANA), antimitochondrial antibody (AMA).

Q. 33. Discuss the management of hepatitis B.

Treatment with antivirals is recommended for patients with HBV DNA levels persistently greater than 10,000 copies/mL. Antivirals are not teratogens but information is limited during pregnancy. Lamivudine has been used in the latter half of pregnancy in attempt to prevent perinatal transmission of hepatitis B virus infection with mixed success.

- Avoid hepatotoxic drugs such as acetaminophen (Tylenol) that may worsen liver damage
- Abstain from alcohol use
- Do not donate blood, body organs, or other tissue
- Do not share any personal items that may have blood on them (e.g. toothbrushes and razors)
- Inform the infant's pediatrician, obstetrician and gynecologist, and labor staff that they are a hepatitis B carrier
- Make sure their baby receives hepatitis B vaccine at birth, one month, and six months of age as well as HBIG at birth
- Be seen at least annually by their regular medical doctor
- Discuss the risk for transmission with their partner and discuss the need for counseling and testing
- Liver function testing is recommended for women who test positive for HBsAg.

Q. 34. Discuss the labor management.

Standard precautions with blood and body secretions should be implemented as for care of all. Avoid the use of fetal scalp electrodes during fetal monitoring. Avoid fetal blood sampling.

Mode of delivery

Evidence is not conclusive to indicate that preferred mode of delivery is influenced by the likelihood of HBV transmission regardless of viremia. However, it may be prudent to follow the same recommendation as for delivery of Hepatitis C positive patients, i.e. if assisted delivery is required the use of soft cup for vacuum extraction or forceps is preferred over a metal cup which poses increased risk for scalp injury. Early cord clamping should be done. Standard precautions should be utilized when handling the baby.

Postpartum management

Instruct the patient on management of standard precautions for blood and body secretions.

Breastfeeding advice

Advise women who are Hepatitis B surface antigen positive there is no evidence that breastfeeding increases the risk of HBV transmission provided the neonate receives hepatitis vaccination and hepatitis B immunoglobulin (HBIG) at birth. Center for Disease Control and Prevention (CDC) and the World Health Organization (WHO) recommends that it is safe for an infected woman to breastfeed her child. All women with hepatitis B are encouraged to breastfeed their babies since the benefits of breastfeeding outweigh the potential risk of transmitting the virus through breast milk. In addition, since all newborns should receive the hepatitis B vaccine at birth, the risk of transmission is reduced even further. Advise HBV carrier women not to participate in breast milk donation. Breastfeeding is not recommended with some medications used in HBV treatments, e.g. lamivudine.

Bibliography

1. American Academy of Pediatrics. Work Group on Breastfeeding. Breastfeeding and the use of human milk. Pediatrics. 1997;100(6):1035-9. [Medline].
2. O'Brien JM, Shumate SA, Satchwell SL, et al. Maternal benefit of corticosteroid therapy in patients with HELLP (hemolysis, elevated liver enzymes, and low platelet count) syndrome: Impact on the rate of regional anesthesia. AJOG. 2002;186(Issue 3):475-9.
3. Isler CM, Barrilleaux PS, Magann EF, et al. A prospective, randomized trial comparing the efficacy of dexamethasone and betamethasone for the treatment of antepartum HELLP (hemolysis, elevated liver enzymes, and low platelet count) syndrome. American Journal of Obstetrics and Gynecology. 2001;184(Issue 7):1332-9.
4. Antiretroviral Pregnancy Registry Steering Committee. Antiretroviral Pregnancy Registry International Interim Report for 1 January 1989 through 31 January 2011 (issued June 2011). Wilmington, NC: Registry Coordinating Center; 2009. Available at http://www.apregistry.com/who.htm. Accessed August 16, 2011.
5. Audibert F, Friedman SA, Frangieh AY, et al. Am J Obstet Gynecol. 1996;175:460-4.
6. Barusruk S, Urwijitaroon Y. High prevalence of HGV coinfection with HBV or HCV among northeastern Thai blood donors. Southeast Asian J Trop Med Public Health. 2006;37(2):289-93. [Medline].
7. Bourliere M, Berman J, Ducrotte S, et al. Polyuro-polydipsie et steatose hepatique aigue gravidique. Discussion a propos d'un cas. J Gynecol Obstet Biol Reprod. 1989;18:79.
8. Brackett JC, Sims HF, Rinaldo P, et al. Two alpha subunit donor splice site mutations cause human trifunctional protein deficiency. J Clin Invest. 1995;95:2076-82.
9. Cammu H, Velkeniers B, Charels K, et al. Idiopathic acute fatty liver of pregnancy associated with transient diabetes insipidus. Br J Obstet Gynecol. 1987;94(2):173-8.
10. Carrat F, Bani-Sadr F, Pol S, et al. Pegylated interferon alfa-2b vs standard interferon alfa-2b, plus ribavirin, for chronic hepatitis C in HIV-infected patients: a randomized controlled trial. JAMA. 2004;292(23):2839-48. [Medline].
11. Castro MA, Ouzounian JG, Colletti PM, et al. Radiologic studies in acute fatty liver of pregnancy. A review of the literature and 19 new cases. J Reprod Med. 1996;41:839.
12. Effects of mode of delivery and infant feeding on the risk of mother-to-child transmission of hepatitis C virus. European Paediatric Hepatitis C Virus Network. BJOG. 2001;108(4):371-7. [Medline].
13. Erkan T, Kutlu T, Cullu F, et al. A case of vertical transmission of hepatitis A virus infection. Acta Paediatr. 1998;87(9):1008-9. [Medline].

14. Cottrell EB, Chou R, Wasson N, et al. Ann reducing risk for mother-to-infant transmission of hepatitis C virus: a systematic review for the U.S. Preventive Services Task Force Intern Med. 2013;158:109-13.
15. Fiore AE, Wasley A, Bell BP, et al. Advisory committee on immunization practices (ACIP), Prevention of hepatitis A through active or passive immunization: recommendations of the Advisory Committee on Immunization Practices (ACIP). MMWR Recomm Rep. 2006;55(RR-7):1-23.
16. Ganem D, Schneider RJ. Hepadnaviridae: the viruses and their Replication. In: Knipe DM, Howley PM, (Eds). 4th edition. Philadelphia, Pa: Lippincott Williams and Wilkins; 2001:2923-69.
17. Guilera M, Saiz JC, Lopez-Labrador FX, et al. Hepatitis G virus infection in chronic liver disease. Gut. 1998;42(1):107-11. [Medline].
18. Hamid SS, Jafri SM, Khan H, et al. Fulminant hepatic failure in pregnant women: acute fatty liver or acute viral hepatitis?. J Hepatol. 1996;25(1):20-7. [Medline].
19. Handa A, Brown KE. GB virus C/hepatitis G virus replicates in human haematopoietic cells and vascular endothelial cells. J Gen Virol. 2000;81(Pt 10):2461-9. [Medline].
20. Hollinger FB, Liang TJ. Hepatitis B virus. In: Knipe DM, et al. (Eds). Fields Virology, 4th edition. Philadelphia, Pa: Lippincott Williams and Wilkins; 2001:2971-3036.
21. Hou SH, Levin S, Ahola S, et al. Acute fatty liver of pregnancy. Survival with early cesarean section. Dig Dis Sci. 1984;29:449.
22. Kao JH, Chen W, Chen PJ, et al. Liver and peripheral blood mononuclear cells are not major sites for GB virus-C/hepatitis G virus replication. Arch Virol. 1999; 144(11):2173-83. [Medline].
23. Kim JP, Fry KE. Molecular characterization of the hepatitis G virus. J Viral Hepat. 1997;4(2):77-9.[Medline].
24. Koff RS. Hepatitis A. Lancet. 1998;351(9116):1643-9. [Medline].
25. Leikin E, Lysikiewicz A, Garry D, et al. Intrauterine transmission of hepatitis A virus. Obstet Gynecol. 1996;88(4 Pt 2):690-1. [Medline]
26. Lemon SM. Hepatitis A virus. In: Webster RG, Granoff A, (Eds). Encyclopedia of Virology. London, UK: Academic Press Ltd; 1994:546-54.
27. Lemon SM. Type A viral hepatitis: epidemiology, diagnosis, and prevention. Clin Chem. 1997;43(8 Pt 2):1494-9. [Medline].
28. Magann EF, Bass D, Chauhan SP, et al. Jr. Am J Obstet Gynecol. 1994;171:1148-53.
29. Magann EF, Perry KG, Meydrech EF, et al. Jr. Am J Obstet Gynecol. 1994;171:1154-8.
30. Martin JN, Blake PG, Perry KG, et al. The natural history of HELLP syndrome: patterns of disease progression and regression. Am J Obstet Gynecol. 1991;164(6 pt 1):1500-9.
31. Matern D, Hart P, Murtha AP, et al. Acute fatty liver of pregnancy associated with short-chain acyl- coenzyme A dehydrogenase deficiency. J Pediatr. 2001;138:585-8.
32. Naik SR, Aggarwal R, Salunke PN, et al. A large waterborne viral hepatitis E epidemic in Kanpur, India. Bull World Health Organ. 1992;70(5):597-604. [Medline]. [Full Text].
33. Ohto H, Ujiie N, Sato A, et al. Mother-to-infant transmission of GB virus type C/HGV. Transfusion. 2000;40(6):725-30. [Medline].
34. Reshetnyak VI, Karlovich TI, Ilchenko LU. Hepatitis G virus. World J Gastroenterol. 2008;14(30):4725-34. [Medline]. [Full Text].
35. Reyes H, Sandoval L, Wainstein A, et al. Acute fatty liver of pregnancy: A clinical study of 12 episodes in 11 patients. Gut. 1994;35:101.
36. Riely CA. Hepatic disease in pregnancy. Am J Med. 1994;96(1A):18S-22S.
37. Roberts EA, Yeung L. Maternal-infant transmission of hepatitis C virus infection. Hepatology. 2002;36(5 suppl 1):S106-13. [Medline].
38. Robinson WS. Hepatitis B virus and hepatitis D virus. In: Mandell GL, Bennett JE, Dolin R, (Eds). Principles and Practice of Infectious Diseases 4th edition. New York, NY: Churchill Livingstone; 1995:1406-39.
39. Rubio A, Rey C, Sanchez-Quijano A, et al. Is hepatitis G virus transmitted sexually? JAMA. 1997;277(7):532-3. [Medline].
40. Samuel D, Feray C. Recurrence of hepatitis C virus infection after liver transplantation. J Hepatol. 1999;31 Suppl 1:217-21. [Medline].

41. Samuels P, Cohen AW. Pregnancies complicated by liver disease and liver dysfunction. Obstet Gynecol Clin North Am. 1992;19:745-63.
42. Sherlock S. Acute fatty liver of pregnancy and the microvesicular fat diseases. Gut. 1983;24:265-9.
43. Stapleton JT, Lemon SM. Hepatitis A and hepatitis E. In: Hoeprich PD, Jordan MC, Ronald AR (Eds). Infectious diseases. 5th edition. Philadelphia: Lippincott Co; 1994:790-7.
44. Tan J, Lok AS. Update on viral hepatitis: 2006. Curr Opin Gastroenterol. 2007;23(3):263-7. [Medline].
45. Vanjak D, Moreau R, Roche-Sicot J, et al. Intrahepatic cholestasis of pregnancy and acute fatty liver of pregnancy. An unusual but favorable association? Gastroenterology. 1991;100:1123.
46. Vigil-De Gracia P, Lavergne JA. Acute fatty liver of pregnancy. Int J Gynaecol Obstet. 2001;72:193-5.
47. Visser W, Wallenburg HC. Temporising management of severe pre-eclampsia with and without the HELLP syndrome. Br J Obstet Gynaecol. 1995;102:111-7.
48. Wedemeyer H, Manns MP. Epidemiology, pathogenesis and management of hepatitis D: update and challenges ahead. Nat Rev Gastroenterol Hepatol. 2010;7(1):31-40. [Medline].
49. Wejstal R, Manson AS, Widell A, et al. Perinatal transmission of hepatitis G virus (GB virus type C) and hepatitis C virus infections—a comparison. Clin Infect Dis. 1999;28(4):816-21. [Medline].
50. Wolf JL. Liver disease in pregnancy. Med Clin North Am. 1996.
51. World Health Organization. Hepatitis A: fact sheet no. 328 (rev May 2008). Available at http://www.who.int/mediacentre/factsheets/fs328/en/index.html. Accessed August 16, 2011.
52. World Health Organization. Hepatitis C: fact sheet no. 164 (rev June 2011). Available at http://www.who.int/mediacentre/factsheets/fs164/en/index.html. Accessed August 16, 2011.
53. World Health Organization. Hepatitis E: fact sheet no. 280 (rev January 2005). Available at http://www.who.int/mediacentre/factsheets/fs280/en/. Accessed August 16, 2011.

12
CHAPTER

Multiple Pregnancy

S Habeebullah

CASE 1

Mrs X, 30 years, W/o Mr Y hailing from ZZ, primigravida belonging to lower middle class at 12 weeks of gestation presented to ANC with:

Excessive vomiting—2 weeks.

She had primary infertility for 5 years for which she was investigated and treated with clomiphene citrate. She confirmed her pregnancy with urine pregnancy test at 6 weeks. She had excessive vomiting at 10 weeks of gestation for which she was hospitalized and given IV fluids and antiemetics and discharged after 2 days.

She denied any history of bleeding per vaginum (PV), pain abdomen, fever, urinary symptoms, and exposure to teratogenic drugs or radiation. General examination revealed dehydration, mild pallor, pulse 110/min, BP 90/60. Abdominal examination revealed ≈16 weeks uterus. Speculum examination was unremarkable.

She was admitted with a diagnosis of hyperemesis gravidarum. Investigations were carried out and simultaneously she was treated with IV fluids and antiemetics. Hb, urine routine, microscopy and culture, ketone bodies and USG were carried out.

Multiple Pregnancy

Q. 1. What are the common causes of excessive vomiting in early pregnancy?

Multiple pregnancy, vesicular mole, pregnancy with urinary tract infection and gastritis. In view of uterine size more than period of amenorrhea, the first two conditions are more likely.

Q. 2. What USG findings should be looked for in early gestation in multiple pregnancy?

Number of gestational sacs (Fig. 1A), cardiac activity, dating (by measuring CRL, BPD, etc.) and gross abnormalities are to be verified. The chorionicity should also be established at this time. While dating twins CRL of larger twin is taken in first trimester as growth discrepancy starts early.

Twins being the most common type of multiple pregnancy, further discussions will be focused on twins.

Q. 3. What is superfecundation and superfetation?

Fertilization of two different ova in the same menstrual cycle by two acts of coitus is known as superfecundation, and two separate fertilizations by two different acts of coitus in

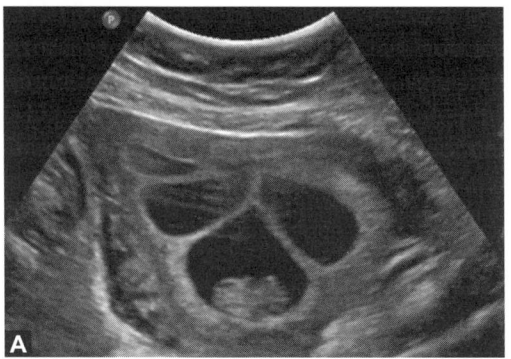 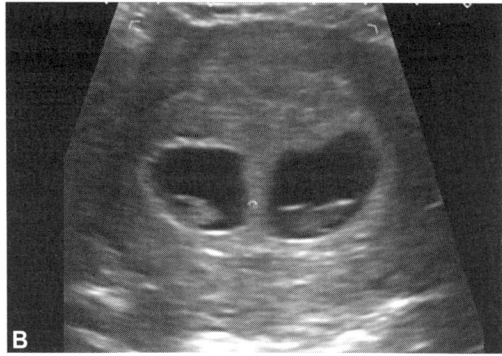

Figs 1A and B: (A) Multiple gestational sacs; (B) Dichorionic twins 8W 2D

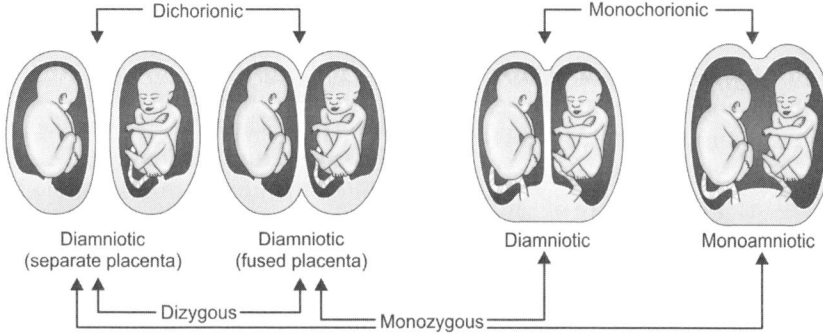

Fig. 2: Zygosity and chorionicity

two different menstrual cycles is superfetation. Here, the gestational ages of fetuses are different and may be of medicolegal importance.

Q. 4. What is zygosity and chorionicity?

Zygosity (Fig. 2) refers to the number of ova (zygotes) from which fetuses develop and so the genetic constitution. Twins can be monozygotic (30%) or dizygotic (70%). All over the world the frequency of monozygosity is constant, whereas dizygosity varies with race and other factors. In natural conceptions twin pregnancy occurs 1 in 80 whereas triplets 1 in 80^2, quadruplets 1 in 80^3 and so on (Hellin's rule). Due to wide availability of ART, the incidence of dizygotic twins and higher order births has increased and currently the incidence of twins is over 3%.

Chorionicity means the type of placentation of the fetuses (Fig. 2).

Dizygotic twins have two separate placentae which sometimes may be fused. They are dichorionic and diamniotic (DCDA) twins. In monozygotic twins depending on the timing of division of the embryo, various types of placentations develop. If the division of embryo occurs within 72 hours after fertilization (25–30%) two different blastocysts implant at two sites and DC DA twins develop. In the rest 75% the division occurs after day 3. If the division occurs between 4 days and 7 days when the blastocyst is already formed a single placenta develops which is shared by the twins and MC DA twins develop. If division is between 8 and 13 days (in 2% of monozygotic) MC MA twins are formed and after day 13 conjoint twins develop. About 75% of monozygotic twins are monochorionic, i.e. they share the same placenta, and this may result in complications (Fig. 2).

Q. 5. How is chorionicity determined?

Chorionicity is best determined by first trimester USG. If two separate gestational sacs are present each with its own fetus and a thick, echogenic chorion surrounding each embryo and a thick dividing membrane, they are DC DA twins (Fig. 1B). Twin peak sign, also known as lambda (λ) sign is an insinuation of triangular chorionic tissue between the layers of intertwin membrane (Fig. 3A). It is seen only in DC twins and best seen between 10-14 weeks. It may be less conspicuous or not present after 20 weeks.[1]

One gestational sac with 2 fetuses and a thin dividing membrane joining the placenta at right angle giving the 'T' sign is seen in MC DA twins (Fig. 3B). A single sac with 2 fetuses and no dividing membrane indicates MC MA twins.

Subsequently, discordant sex indicates dichorionic twins but if they are of same sex they may be DC or MC.

Q. 6. What is the significance of zygosity?

Mono and dizygotic twins have differences in complications and outcome which may influence the perinatal care they receive. Zygosity is important to a twin pair where questions of tissue compatibility in organ transplantation come. It has implication in research in twins. Postnatal zygosity testing is useful to distinguish genetic components from environmental factors in disease association studies on twins. Twins are always faced with the question whether they are identical. It may have effect on their bonding too.

Q. 7. What is the risk of chromosomal abnormalities in twins?

In monozygotic the risk is same as in singleton due to genetic sharing by the twins. In dizygotic for each of the twins the risk is same as for singleton; hence the risk is doubled.

Q. 8. How is screening for aneuploidy done?

In first trimester screening by NT scan between 11 and 13 + 6 weeks along with age is taken. In combined tests age and NT along with serum β hCG and PAPP-A are taken. In second trimester serum marker if done is taken with a different cutoff (almost double the value). Integrated screening improves the detection rate. If amniocentesis is needed in dichorionic twins both sacs should be separately sampled. After sampling the first sac indigocarmine (1-2 mL) is instilled into the sac to identify inadvertent sampling again from the same sac. In monochorionic single sample is taken (MZ twins need not be concordant for chromosomal abnormalities. Postzygotic nondisjunction can result in heterokaryotypic fetuses. So, it is always better to sample both sacs).

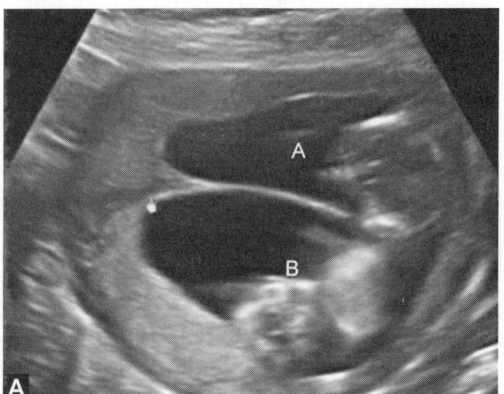 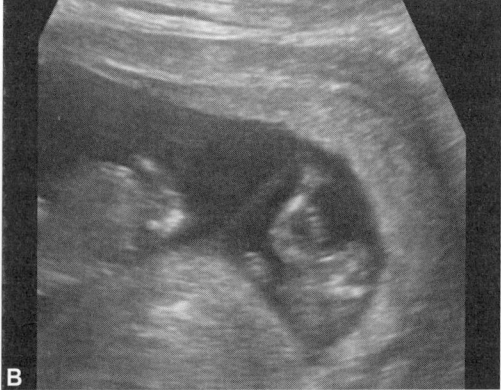

Figs 3A and B: USG zygosity and chorionicity

If there is karyotype abnormality in one, selective termination will be difficult unless the baby has structural malformation or subtle markers.

Q. 9. How is the screening for NTD done in twins?

MSAFP estimation in 2nd trimester is done for screening of NTD. However, the cutoff is 4.5 MOM instead of 2.5 for singleton. USG is always used to confirm the same.

Q. 10. How is twin pregnancy diagnosed clinically?

If risk factors in history are present or exaggerated pregnancy symptoms are present, one should rule out twins. Abdominal examination may show uterus more than the period of amenorrhea, increased abdominal girth >100 cm and polyhydramnios. Clinically, if at least 3 fetal poles are felt and 2 FHRs heard separately by two examiners with a difference of 10 beats/minute, the diagnosis is made.

Sometimes pelvic examination is helpful in detecting a presenting part which is not felt *per abdomen* in the pelvis.

Etiology of DZ twins
- Race
- Age (30–35 years)
- Family H/o twins (maternal)
- Previous H/o twins
- Multiparity (> para 4)
- OC pill usage immediately preceding the pregnancy
- Ovulation induction: clomiphene, gonadotropins
- Assisted-reproductive techniques
- Obesity

Q. 11. What are the maternal adaptations in twin pregnancy?

Most of the physiological changes of pregnancy are exaggerated in twin pregnancy. The main change is increased blood volume which is much more than in singleton. The colloid osmotic pressure is reduced causing edema of feet and increased susceptibility to pulmonary edema. This should be kept in mind while using tocolytics. Stroke volume and heart rate are increased with resultant increased cardiac output. The pregnancy hormone levels are markedly increased causing exaggerated pregnancy symptoms like vomiting and varicosities and conditions like GDM. These hormone levels may cause difficulty in interpretation of serum screening tests.

CASE 2

Mrs X1, 35 years age, W/o Mr Y1 hailing from ZZ1, gravida2 para 1 live1 diagnosed as twins in early pregnancy by USG presents at 32 weeks of gestation with:

C/o over distension of abdomen—10 days and swelling of feet—10 days.

She has been receiving iron and folic acid and got 2 doses of tetanus toxoid in 2nd trimester. She felt quickening at 18 weeks. She noticed swelling of feet of 10 days' duration marked at the end of the day which got relieved with night's rest. She noticed overdistension of abdomen for the last 10 days not associated with any pain. Fetal movements are perceived well. She had anomaly scan at 18 weeks and growth scan at 28 weeks and was told to be normal.

General examination revealed mild pallor, mild pitting pedal edema and BP 120/76 mm Hg. Abdominal examination revealed over distended uterus up to 36 weeks size, S-F height 36 cm and abdominal girth 96 cm. Multiple fetal parts with breech at fundus, two heads at the lower pole and two distinct FHS. Liquor appeared average.

Q. 12. What was the missing information?

It is not to enough to diagnose twins by USG. The chorionicity should have been established early in pregnancy and recorded so that appropriate counseling and followed up are done. If chorionicity is not established, monochorionicity should be assumed and surveillance for various complications should be in place.[2]

Q. 13. What is the schedule of antenatal care in twins?

Usually the antenatal visits are doubled so that complications are identified earlier. In first trimester, screening for Down syndrome is done by NT. In the second trimester, biochemical screening can be done. Anomaly scan is done between 18 weeks–22 weeks. Screening for diabetes mellitus should be done. At each visit special attention is paid to symptoms, edema, weight gain, hypertension, fundal height, abdominal girth, evidence of preterm labor, etc.

Advice regarding additional rest, diet (about 300 additional kcal daily), iron (100 mg elemental iron) and folic acid (5 mg) daily supplementation should be given. Liberal use of USG for growth monitoring is done. Fetal surveillance is started from 34 weeks unless the clinical condition warrants it earlier (care of MC twins is discussed below).

Q. 14. What are the problems in clinical examination and fetal surveillance in twins?

Unlike in singleton pregnancy, fundal height cannot be relied upon to estimate gestational age and growth of fetuses. It may not be possible always to know the fetal presentation as polyhydramnios is common. There may be difficulty in locating two FHRs. Same FHR may be heard at two places and wrongly interpreted. For fetal surveillance, DFMC cannot be relied. Estimation of amount of liquor and estimation of fetal weight is not possible. While performing NST, each fetus needs to be monitored separately. During USG estimation of liquor, AFI estimation of both may be difficult. Single deep pocket estimation for each fetus may be a better option.

Q. 15. What are the other applications of USG in twins?

Besides confirming the number of fetuses and establishing chorionicity, USG is used to rule out anomalies, assess growth of fetuses, diagnose the various complications of monochorionic twins and their management, confirm presentations, multifetal pregnancy reduction, selective feticide and assessment of cervical length in prediction of preterm labor.

Q. 16. At what frequency, USG is performed in twins?

After initial confirmation of twins, establishing zygosity and anomaly scan, Uncomplicated DC DA twins are followed with growth scans at 3–4 weeks intervals. In monozygotic twins follow up is done every 2–3 weeks starting from 16 weeks as there is higher fetal loss in 2nd trimester in MC pregnancies. If complications develop more frequent scanning may be needed.[3]

Q. 17. What are the antepartum complications of twins?

Maternal
- **In first trimester**
  - Hyperemesis gravidarum
  - Spontaneous miscarriage
- **In second and third trimesters**
  - Anemia
  - Antepartum hemorrhage—placenta previa and abruption
  - Preterm labor (50%), polyhydramnios (10%)
  - Hypertension (25%)
  - Gestational diabetes
  - Respiratory embarrassment
  - Malpresentations
  - Rarely acute fatty liver of pregnancy and peripartum cardiomyopathy

Fetal
- Congenital anomalies
- Prematurity
- Fetal growth restriction
- Discordant growth
- Demise of one or both twins.

Q. 18. What antenatal complications are specific to monochorionic twins?

Besides the complications mentioned above, monozygotic twins in addition are prone to develop the following:

- Twin-to-twin transfusion syndrome (TTTS)
- Twin reversed arterial perfusion (TRAP) sequence
- Twin oligohydramnios/polyhydramnios sequence (TOPS)
- Cord entanglement
- Conjoint twins.

Q. 19. What is the pattern of placental vasculature in monochorionic twins and its significance?

Placental anastomoses are of several types: superficial or deep. Superficial anastomoses are bidirectional, either arterioarterial or venovenous. These allow rapid flow from one fetus to its cotwin. Deep anastomoses (arteriovenous) represent a shared cotyledon, in which the arterial supply is derived from one twin, and the venous drainage is to the other; they are unidirectional and result in unequal distribution of flow. Twin-to-twin transfusion syndrome is associated with an absence of functional arterioarterial anastomoses in monochorionic twin pregnancies.[4]

Twin-to-twin transfusion syndrome

It may be seen in 10–15% of MC twins. Because of abnormal vascular communications of two placentae in MC twins, there is hemodynamic imbalance due to unidirectional blood flow from one to the other. This results in growth discordance and discrepancy in amniotic fluid volume. The donor twin is growth restricted and anemic with oligohydramnios. The recipient twin develops hydrops, cardiac failure and polydydramnios. This may also lead to preterm labor. USG criteria for diagnosis of TTTS are listed in the box. The treatment includes (i) repeated amnioreduction of recipient twin, (ii) septostomy of intertwine membrane to equalize pressure between two sacs, (iii) Laser photocoagulation of anastomotic vessels by fetoscopy, (iv) selective feticide by USG-guided bipolar coagulation of the cord. Laser ablation is preferred when severe TTT develops before 26 weeks rather than by amnioreduction or septostomy.[3]

Early USG signs of TTTS
1st trimester: CRL discrepancy and, nuchal translucency, reversal or absence of ductus A wave
2nd trimester: Discordant AC, membrane folding, velamentous cord insertion and hyperechoic donor portion of placenta. Fetal echo is a must for TTTS. (cardiac anomalies 6 times higher in MC)

USG criteria of TTTS
- MC twins
- Same sex
- Fetal weight discordance
- Oligohydramnios in one sac and polyhydramnios in the other

Quintero staging system[5]
Stage I: Oligo/polyhydramnios, bladder visible in donor twin
Stage II: Bladder not visible in donor twin
Stage III: Abnormal Doppler studies in either twin
Stage IV: Hydrops in one or both twins
Stage V: Demise of one or both twins

Twin reversed arterial perfusion sequence and acardiac twinning

This complication occurs in 1% of monochorionic pregnancies. In this the acardiac twin gets blood supply from the cotwin through arterioarterial anastomosis to the upper body resulting in nondevelopment of head, neck, heart, etc. The pump twin also develops cardiac failure, hydramnios and perinatal mortality is high. The treatment of TRAP is laser ablation of cord vessels of acardiac twin.

Acardiac twin has following types:
- Acardius acephalus
- Acardius myelacephalus
- Acardius amorphous

It is also classified as:
- Acephalus
- Anceps
- Acormus
- Amorphous

Twin oligohydramnios/polyhydramnios Sequence

In this complication (seen in MZ twins), there is deep AV anastomosis in placenta and gradual transfusion from one twin to the other. This results in weight discordance and amniotic fluid discordance with donor sac having oligo- and recipient polyhydramnios. The donor twin is hypovolemic, anemic and growth restricted. The recipient is larger, plethoric with hypervolemia. Doppler can be diagnostic. Treatment involves amnioreduction, amniotic septostomy and laser ablation of the anastomotic vessel.

Twin anemia polycythemia sequence (TAPS)

Another condition seen in MZ twins where there is inter twin hemoglobin difference but without TOPS. This is due to few AV anastomoses where blood from donor to recipient twin goes in low pace resulting in anemia of donor twin. Treatment includes intrauterine transfusion of anemic twin and laser coagulation of anastomotic vessel.

Q. 20. How is fetal anemia assessed?

Strong correlation was found between fetal anemia assessed by cordocentesis and fetal middle cerebral artery peak systolic velocity (MCA-PSV).[6]

Conjoint twins (Siamese twins)

This is a rare form of monozygotic twins. When division of embryo takes place after day 13 of fertilization, conjoint twins result. They have same karyotype and are of same sex. Depending on the site of union, they are thoracopagus (most common), omphalopagus, pygopagus, ischiopagus and craniopagus. Antenatal diagnosis is made, when there is no change of relative positions of the twins and repeated examinations show both heads at the same position. USG in 1st trimester shows bifid fetal pole. 3D ultrasound, fetal echo and MRI confirm the diagnosis and organ and vascular sharing by both the fetuses which decides the prognosis. Rarely, this may be diagnosed when it presents as obstructed labor or with one fetus partly delivered. Cesarean section is the safest option and survival of twins depends on the extent of sharing the organs by the twins.

Some of the common complications of twins are discussed below.

Miscarriage and vanishing twins

Miscarriage is more common than in singleton pregnancy, more so in monochorionic twins. Also, one of the two gestational sacs identified early in 1st trimester may disappear (vanishing twin). This may be seen in 20–30% of twins (it may be noted that very early USG may miss some gestational sacs which 'reappear' later).

Preterm labor

The mean gestational age at delivery in twins is 35.3 weeks, in triplets 32.2 weeks and for quadruplets 30 weeks. Preterm labor is seen in about 50% of twins and is the cause for increased perinatal mortality. The cause may be over distension, polyhydramnios, PROM and iatrogenic (due to premature induction of labor in monochorionic pregnancies). At risk patients can be identified by clinical examination of cervix, measurement of cervical length by TVS and maternal fetal fibronectin levels. If the cervical length at 24 weeks of gestation is >25 mm, the risk of preterm labor at 32 weeks is lower.

The prevention strategies may include restricted physical activity and serial measurements of cervical length. Prophylactic cervical cerclage, tocolytic therapy and progestogens have not proved to be effective. However, if a patient presents with preterm labor, corticosteroids are administered for fetal lung maturity.[2]

Congenital anomalies

Major malformations are doubled in twin pregnancy (2%) compared to singleton. It is mostly seen in monochorionic twins due to vascular complications or due to crowding. In

1st trimester aneuploidy screening is done by measuring NT (between 11 and 13 + 6 weeks gestation), maternal serum β hCG and PAPPA. For screening of NTD maternal serum AFP may be used keeping in mind that the values may be doubled.

Three categories of defects may be encountered.[7]

1. Conjoint twins and acardiac twins, sirenomelia, holoprosencephaly and anencephaly.
2. Vascular connections between MC twins or single fetal demise may produce microcephaly, porencephalic cysts, hydranencephaly, intestinal atresia, aplasia cutis, and limb amputation in the surviving twin.
3. Due to crowding in utero in late pregnancy. These may also occur in DZ twins. These include skull asymmetry, foot deformities, etc.

Q. 21. What is fetal reduction and what is selective termination?

Fetal reduction is to reduce the number of fetuses in early pregnancy (10–14 weeks) so that the complications are avoided. It involves reduction of triplets to twins or even to singleton. It may also be done for fetus with serious anomaly. This procedure is done abdominally by injecting KCl into the fetus which is away from the cervix, has lower CRL and easily accessible. This procedure is avoided in monochorionic twins. Selective termination later in pregnancy may be required to be done for a fetus which is abnormal.

The complications of selective termination include:

- Miscarriage of all the fetuses
- Termination of wrong fetus
- Preterm labor
- Complications in the surviving twin
- Coagulopathy.

Twin pregnancy with coexistent fetus and hydatidiform mole

This is extremely rare. This can be of two types: (i) twin gestation in which one twin is a diploid fetus with a normal placenta and the other twin is a complete hydatidiform mole, or (ii) singleton gestation consisting of a triploid fetus with partial hydatidiform mole placenta. The first one is associated with more of maternal complications (early onset preeclampsia, thyrotoxicosis and persistent trophoblastic disease) whereas the second one with fetal anomalies. Usually for the second variety termination of pregnancy is advocated. But for twins with one normal fetus and the other complete mole after proper counseling regarding the complications and bleeding, pregnancy can be carried forward to period of viability.[8]

Q. 22. How common is fetal growth restriction in twins?

FGR is common in twins (25%), more so in monozygotic. Serial USG measurements starting from 3rd trimester will identify the problem.

Q. 23. What are discordant twins?

Unequal growth of twins due to unequal division of zygote and placenta, placental insufficiency, TTT syndrome, etc. with resultant difference in birth weight of 25% or more is called discordant growth. The smaller twin is at increased risk of fetal death or long-term morbidity. In dizygotic pregnancy it may be due to genetically different growth potential whereas in monozygotic it is due to abnormal placental vascular anastomosis.

USG criteria for discordant growth
- Difference in HC >5%
- Difference in AC ≥20 mm
- Increased HC/AC or FL/AC ratio
- Difference in estimated fetal weight of >25%
Abnormal umbilical artery Doppler waveforms—S/D ratio difference >25%

Q. 24. How is pregnancy with single fetus demise managed?

Vanishing twin in 1st trimester does not have any effect on the pregnancy. However, if single fetal demise occurs in 2nd and 3rd trimesters, there is risk of death and neurological damage to surviving twin which is unpredictable. These risks are much higher in MC twins (12% and 18%, respectively) and include multicystic encephalomalacia, infarctions in brain, liver, spleen and kidney. This is the result of blood flowing from the surviving fetus to the dead one, and release of emboli and thromboplastins from dead fetus to the living one. Evaluation is usually done by ultrasound and MRI.[3] Mother also should have coagulation profile as prolonged retention of dead fetus may sometimes cause consumption coagulopathy. The management includes counseling regarding the risks to the fetus, a course of steroids (if preterm) and fetal monitoring till delivery which is carried out at the earliest period of viability.

Q. 25. At what gestational age should twins be delivered?

Fetal maturity in twins is hastened by 2 weeks compared to singletons (Table 1).
- Uncomplicated DCDA twins are delivered by 37–38 weeks
- MCDA twins by 36 weeks (unexplained demise common after this)[3]
- MCMA twins delivered by 32 weeks.

If complications develop, earlier delivery is planned accordingly. A course of corticosteroids should be given prior to delivery.

Table 1: Timing of delivery in multiple pregnancy

Pregnancy	Timing of delivery
Singleton—low risk	41 weeks to 42 weeks
Majority of twins	Spontaneous by 37 weeks
Majority of triplets	Spontaneous by 35 weeks
DCDA twins—uncomplicated	Preferably by 38 weeks

Contd...

Contd...

Pregnancy	Timing of delivery
Triplets	Preferably by 36 weeks
Monochorionic—Uncomplicated	36 weeks—with steroid coverage
Dichorionic-Uncomplicated	37 weeks
Triplets—uncomplicated	35 weeks—with steroid coverage
DCDA with FGR	36–37 weeks
MCDA with FGR, fetal compromise or with one fetal demise	32–34 weeks
Diamniotic with one fetal demise	38 weeks/DIC features any duration

Q. 26. What are the types of fetal presentations at term?
- VX-VX most common (40%)
- VX—breech (30%)
- Breech—VX (10%)
- Breech-breech (6%)
- VX-transverse (3%)
- Transverse-VX (1%)
- Both transverse (0.8%).

Q. 27. What are the indications for elective cesarean section in twins?
- First twin in transverse lie
- First twin breech (by majority obstetricians)
- Monoamniotic twins (because of risk of cord entanglement)
- In previous cesarean section (relative)
- Conjoint twins (which is rare)
- Severe fetal growth restriction
- Discordant twins
- Other obstetric complications warranting cesarean section.

Q. 28. How is the labor managed in twins?
- Adequate number of health professionals should be available—2 obstetricians, 2 neonatologists and also an anesthetist should be present to provide epidural analgesia
- Ambulation is restricted
- Oral fluids are allowed but IV line with wide bore needle should be in place

- Cross matched blood should be arranged
- CTG machines with dual recording for simultaneous monitoring of both the fetuses used.

Second stage is managed in the usual manner, cord of the first baby clamped at 2 places and baby handed over to the pediatrician and labeled. Uterotonic drugs like methylergometrine and oxytocin should not be given at this stage.

Q. 29. How is 2nd twin delivered?

An abdominal examination is performed to check for presentation and position of the 2nd twin and FHR verified. Vaginal examination will confirm the presentation and rule out cord presentation if any. In vertex presentation, ARM is performed.

If needed oxytocin augmentation may be started. If there is FHR abnormality or evidence of abruption (vaginal bleeding) delivery should be expedited using forceps/vacuum depending on the station and rotation of the fetal head. Very rarely LSCS will be required.

If it is breech, assisted-breech delivery can be conducted. For fetal distress/abruption, breech extraction can be done.

If it is transverse/oblique lie, external cephalic version (ECV) followed by ARM and vaginal delivery can be conducted. If ECV fails, ARM and internal podalic version (IPV) and breech extraction can be done. Rarely, LSCS will be needed for 2nd twin when ECV and IPV fail and cervix collapses or fetus is disproportionately large. The usual interval between deliveries is not more than 30 minutes. However, if fetal condition deteriorates early intervention will be needed.

If first baby delivers vaginally and second by cesarean section, it is called 'combined delivery'. It has been observed that when second twin presents by breech or transverse lie, the chances of successful vaginal delivery are better with IPV and breech extraction than ECV and vaginal delivery or failed ECV followed by IPV and breech extraction.

> 2nd twin: Indications for cesarean section
> - Abruptio placentae/cord prolapse with presenting part at or above pelvic brim/collapsed cervix
> - Transverse lie with failed ECV/IPV
> - 2nd twin size>1st → CPD
> - Interlocking of twins

Q. 30. How is third stage of labor managed in twins?

Active management of 3rd stage should be done (a) by giving oxytocin 10 units IM, (b) delivery of placenta by controlled cord traction after the signs of placental separation appear and (c) uterine massage.

Placenta is examined carefully to know if it is complete and to confirm chorionicity. In dichorionic placentation four layers of membranes and in monochorionic two layers of membranes will be present.

Q. 31. What are the intrapartum complications in twins?

- Hypotonic uterine inertia may lead to prolongation of labor. However, since the fetuses are small delivery is usually not prolonged
- PROM/early rupture of membranes
- Abnormal presentations—more common
- ↑ operative interventions
- Locked twins (extremely rare)
- Retained placenta
- Postpartum hemorrhage (mainly due to atonicity of over distended uterus, large placental bed and also ↑trauma due to interventions).

Q. 32. What is the role of intrapartum USG?

USG is useful in:
- Estimation of fetal weights
- Exact presentation/attitude of head in breech
- Identifying FHR in case of doubt while using CTG
- In assessing 2nd twin's weight
- Checking FHR after ECV of 2nd twin.

Q. 33. What is interlocked twins?

This is extremely rare. Here, the first baby presenting as breech delivers partially. The aftercoming head gets locked with the 2nd fetus presenting as cephalic causing arrest of delivery. The treatment involves pushing away the head of 2nd twin under general anesthesia and extraction of the first baby. However, an emergency cesarean may be the best option to save the 2nd fetus. In modern obstetrics as most breeches are delivered by cesarean section, one may not come across this complication in one's lifetime.

Q. 34. How is twins with previous CS managed?

Though most obstetricians prefer to do repeat CS, trial vaginal delivery is not contraindicated. Gentle manipulations like ECV/IPV can also be performed.

Higher order multiple gestations

Triplets and other higher order births have increased in the last two decades due to unregulated ART. These are associated with very high perinatal morbidity and mortality. Preterm labor occurs in 75% triplets. One option is multifetal pregnancy reduction where higher order pregnancies are reduced to twins or even singletons. If this is not done these pregnancies need more intense monitoring for complications and elective cesarean section performed by 34–36 weeks is the best option after a course of steroids.

Q. 35. What are the postnatal issues in twins?

Increased risk of puerperal sepsis, subinvolution of uterus and feeding problems due to inadequate milk. Rearing the twins can be very exhausting and stressful to the mother.

Q. 36. What is the perinatal outcome in twins?

Perinatal mortality in twins is 5 times more than singleton. This is due to congenital malformations, low-birth weight as a result of prematurity, growth restriction and discordancy, increased operative intervention due to abnormal presentations and fetal distress. Second twin is at much increased risk due to abnormal presentation, delay in delivery, placental abruption and cord complications. All the complications including cerebral palsy are more in monochorionic twins.

References

1. Wood SL, St Onge R, Connors G, et al. Evaluation of twin peak or lambda sign in determining chorionicity in multiple pregnancy. Obstet Gynecol. 1996;88:6-9
2. Institute of Obstetricians and Gynaecologists, Royal College of Physicians of Ireland.Clinical practice guideline- management of multiple pregnancy (guideline No.14). 2012.
3. Royal College of Obstetricians and Gynaecologists- Management of Monochorionic Twin Pregnancy. Green-top Guideline Number 51;2008.
4. Denbow LM, Cox P, Talbert D, et al. Colour Doppler energy insonation of placental vasculature in monochorionic twins: absent arterio-arterial anast ornoses in association with twin-to-twin transfusion syndrome. British J Obstet Gynaecol. 1998;105:760-5.
5. Quintero RA, Morales WJ, Allen MH, et al. Staging of twin- twin transfusion syndrome. J Perinatol. 1999;19:550-5.
6. Senat MV, Couderc S, Bernard J, et al. The value of middle cerebral artery peak systolic velocity in the diagnosis of fetal anemia after intrauterine death of one monochorionic twin. Am J Obstet Gynecol. 2003;189:1320-4.
7. Schinzel AGL A, W Smith WD, Miller RJ. Monozygotic twinning and structural defects. J Pediatrics. 1979;95:6:921-30.
8. Shazly M SAE, Ali KM, Badee A AY, et al. Twin pregnancy with complete hydatidiform mole and coexisting fetus following ovulation induction with a non-prescribed clomiphene citrate regimen: a case report. J Med Case Reports. 2012;6:95.

13
CHAPTER

Preterm Labor

S Vijayalakshmi

Preterm Labor

Definition

- Labor prior to 37 weeks of gestation[1]
- Extreme preterm (<28 weeks)
- Very preterm (28–31 weeks)
- Late preterm (32–37 weeks).

Diagnosis

- Preterm labor (PTL)
- Uterine contractions at least 2 in 20 min
- Cervical length <1 cm
- Cervical dilatation >2 cm.

Threatened preterm labor is diagnosed when there are documented uterine contractions but no evidence of cervical change.

Incidence

- Eleven percent of live-births
- One-third of preterm deliveries are due to spontaneous rupture of membranes
- One-third to obstetrical causes
- One-third due to idiopathic preterm labor.

A 26-year-old G2P1L1 belonging to low socioeconomic status presented with history of 7½ months of amenorrhea with crampy pain abdomen since 8 hours increasing in intensity, frequency and duration. Initially, pain was once in 20–25 minutes, later it progressed to once in 5–10 minutes. There is no history of leaking per vagina, bleeding PV or foul smelling discharge per vagina. Patient gives history of burning micturation and increased frequency since 3 days. Previously, it was spontaneous preterm vaginal delivery at 8 months-baby 2 kg at birth, now 1½ years alive and healthy.

General physical examination and systemic examination findings were normal. Obstetric examination revealed 28 weeks size uterus with 4 contractions in twenty minutes lasting 35 to 40 seconds, unengaged head in lower pole. Liquor volume appears adequate clinically. FHS 146/min, regular.

On per speculum examination, cervix and vagina healthy, no leaking, no bleeding. Cervical swab, high and low vaginal swab taken.

On per vaginal examination, cervix 3 cm dilated, 80% effaced, vertex at 2 station, membranes present, pelvis adequate.

All routine investigations were normal except urine routine examination which revealed 10–15 pus cells/HPF. Urine culture sensitivity showed *E. coli* growth sensitive to ampicillin, erythromycin, nitrofurantoin and cefixime. Anomaly scan was normal and cervical length at 20 weeks was 3.2 cm.

> **Indian scenario[2]**
> Globally every year 15 million babies are born preterm. India has highest number of preterm births of 3,519,100 per year. Out of 27 million births annually, 3,519,100 babies are born preterm and 3,00,000 of these preterm babies die each year because of prematurity and associated complications.

Q. 1. How will you confirm the diagnosis?

It is confirmed by typical history and the diagnosis is established in this case by the presence of (a) uterine contractions 4 in 20 minutes each lasting for 35–40 seconds, (b) cervical changes having cervical dilatation more than 2 cm and more than 80% effacement of cervix, (c) gestational age less than 37 completed weeks.

Q. 2. Tell the points which are specific to be noted in history?

We have to give importance to the following history:
- Persistent pain abdomen with increasing in intensity, duration and frequency
- Leaking, bleeding or foul smelling discharge per vagina
- Symptoms suggestive of UTI
- Fever, crampy abdominal pain, low backache.

We also have to give significance for the history of smoking or alcohol abuse, low socioeconomic status with poor nutrition, past history cervical conization, periodontal disease, genetic factors, psychological factors affecting the health, stress manual labor.

Q. 3. What are the causes of preterm labor?

- Idiopathic—40-50%
- Subclinical infection of fetal membranes with subsequent spontaneous rupture
- Amniotic fluid infection
- Cervical factors—incompetent cervix, cervical trauma or congenital anomalies
- Cervicovaginal infection—bacterial vaginosis, *N. gonorrhoeae*
- Uterine factors—anomalies, fibroids
- Trauma or surgery
- Antepartum hemorrhage—placenta previa or abruptio placenta
- Maternal factors—preeclampsia (iatrogenic prematurity)
- Fetal anomalies
  - Polyhydramnios
  - Multiple pregnancy
  - Congenital anomalies
  - Preterm premature rupture of membranes (PPROM)
  - Intrauterine fetal death
  - Iatrogenic causes.

Q. 4. Enumerate the risk factors for preterm labor.

- **There are previous history of preterm delivery**
  - Low socioeconomic status: Age less than 18 or more than 35 years
  - Prepregnancy weight less than 50 kg and prenatal weight gain less than 6 to 6.5 kg, smoking, uterine malformations, vaginal infection are nonpregnancy-related factors to be considered.
- **Obstetric related factors are** placenta praevia, placenta abruption, and polyhydramnios, multiple gestation and cervical changes
- Hypertension, diabetes mellitus, systemic lupus erythematosus, renal diseases and other maternal complications are to be considered under maternal factors.

Q. 5. What are risks for preterm birth in the present case at discussion?

The factors to be considered are:
- Low socioeconomic status with poor nutrition
- History of previous preterm birth
- Short interpregnancy interval
- Urinary tract infection.

Q. 6. Describe the pathogenetic factors involved in preterm labor.

Flowcharts 1A and B dipict the pathogenetic factors involved in preterm labor.[4]

Flowchart 1A: Pathogenesis of preterm labor

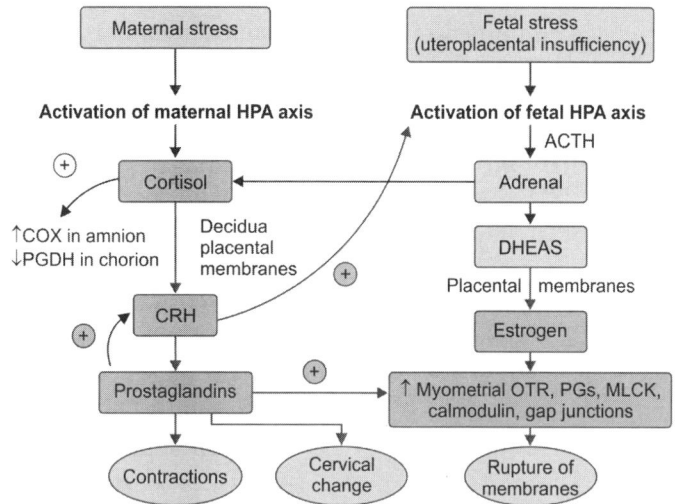

Flowchart 1B: Pathogenesis of preterm labor

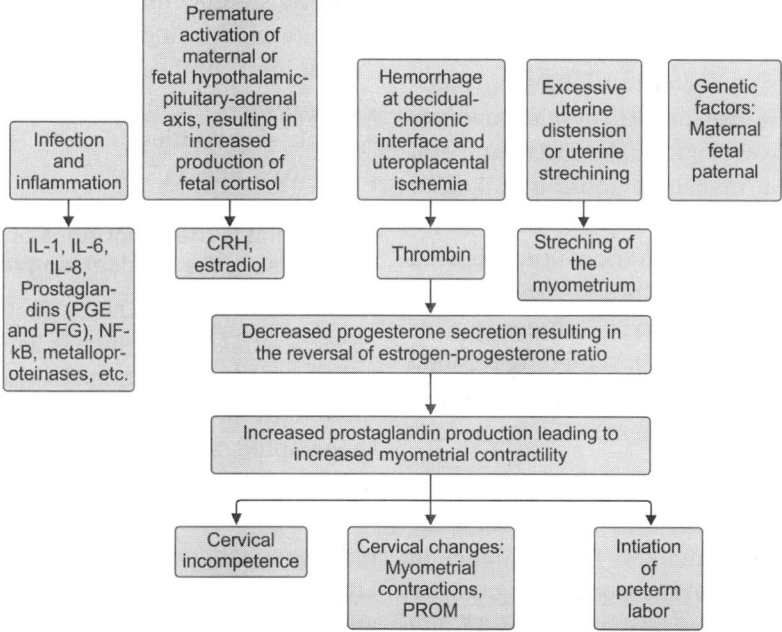

Abbreviations: OTR, oxytocin receptor; MLCK, myosin light chain kinase; CRH, corticotropin-releasing hormone; DHEAS, dehydroepiandrosterone sulfate; ACTH, adrenocorticotropic hormone; PG, prostaglandins; COX, cyclooxygenase; PGDH, prostaglandin dehydrogenase; HPA, hypothalamic-pituitary-adrenal; IL, interleukin; PGE, prostaglandin E; PGF, prostaglandin F

Q. 7. Could any preventive measures have helped in this case?

As the patient is at risk for preterm birth because of previous history of preterm labor, proper nutritional advice and progesterone therapy could have been started at 16 weeks as per ACOG guidelines.

Q. 8. What are the warning signs and symptoms of preterm labor?

- Crampy pain abdomen
- Low backache
- Bleeding or leaking per vagina
- Pressure symptoms
- Uterine hardening associated with contractions
- Cervical shortening with dilatation and effacement
- Descent of the presenting part.

Q. 9. Enumerate about the predictors of preterm labor.

Up to 75% of preterm labor occurs either spontaneously or following PPROM and many attempts have been made to develop methods that may help us to predict the onset of preterm labor so that measures could be taken to prevent its occurrence.

These include: Risk marker (enumerated below), home uterine activity monitoring (HUAM), salivary estriol, screening for bacterial vaginosis (BV), screening for fetal fibronectin (fFN), cervical ultrasonography (cervical length assessment).

Risk Markers

- A previous history of preterm labor is the strongest risk marker. The incidence of preterm labor in subsequent pregnancies after one preterm birth rises to 14.3% and after two preterm births to 28%
- Other risk markers include multiple pregnancy, cigarette smoking, cervical incompetence or uterine anomalies, uterine over-distension (polyhydramnios, macrosomia, fibroids), previous cervical surgery, using smokeless tobacco, bleeding in early pregnancy, bacterial vaginosis, poor socioeconomic or educational status, and young or advanced maternal age
- Preconceptional multivitamin treatment was inversely associated with both early and late preterm birth
- There is now evidence to support an association between severe periodontal disease and spontaneous preterm labor
- Short interval between pregnancies (less than 12 months) has been found to increase the risk of recurrent preterm birth
- Recently, domestic violence, especially injury due to physical abuse, was found to be significantly associated with both preterm birth and low birth weight.

But, most of these risk markers are poor predictors of preterm labor as they have variable sensitivities (35–60%) and positive predictive values (15–30%).

Q. 10. What is the importance of ultrasound in assessing the cervical length?

According to ACOG (Oct 2012), transvaginal cervical ultrasonography has been shown to be a reliable and reproducible way to assess the length of the cervix (Table 1). Routine sonographic measurement of cervical length helps in predicting preterm labor.[6]

ACOG and American Institute in Medicine recommends cervical length measurement at around 18–20 weeks at the same time for fetal anatomic survey. This is useful screening test for prediction of spontaneous preterm birth.

Table 1: Comparing the diagnostic modalities for cervical insufficiency

Manual examination	Transvaginal USG	Transabdominal USG	Translabial/transperineal USG
• Subjective • Interobserver variability 52% • Internal os not measurable	• TVS can detect shortening of cervical canal earlier • No significant inoculation with bacteria • Minimal discomfort • 99% agreed for similar procedure • Identify the presence of other ultrasound risk markers such as the presence of intra-amniotic debris and choriodecidual separation	• Fetal can obscure the cervix especially after 20 weeks • Requires UB filling which can elongate Cervix and mask funneling	• Fetal parts do not obscure vision • Bladder filling not required • No pressure exerted on cervix • Additional transducer not required • Well accepted

Home Uterine Activity Monitoring (HUAM)

HUAM is based on the principle of tocodynamometry and created a lot of interest and excitement among obstetricians when it was first introduced. Large randomized trials have showed no benefit of HUAM in predicting preterm labor. Hence, it cannot be recommended in routine clinical practice.

Q. 11. Explain what is fetal fibronectin and how to carryout screening of preterm labor?

- It is a basement membrane protein produced by the fetal membranes and functions as an **'adhesion binder'**
- It facilitates the attachment of the placenta and membranes to the uterine decidua
- Detectable in cervical secretions until 16–20 weeks of gestation
- Presence of fFN in cervical secretions after 24 weeks of gestation will point towards the disruption of the normal adhesion between chorioamnion and the underlying deciduas, thereby considered as diagnostic of inflammation of the fetal membrane/decidual interphase, which leads to the onset of preterm labor with or without infection
- Studies have shown if fFN is positive after 24 weeks it increases the risk of preterm birth and if this protein is negative in cervical secretion it is indicative of decreased risk.

Fetal fibronectin along with cervical length together is more valuable than each predictor alone.

A combination of fFN and USG measured cervical length has been effectively used as a predictor of preterm labor (Table 2).

Table 2: Combination of cervical length assessment and fetal fibronectin (fFN) in predicting recurrent risk of preterm delivery[5]

Cervical length	fFN Positive	fFN Negative
<25 mm	65%	25%
26–25 mm	45%	14%
>35 mm	25%	07%

Q. 12. Is there any role of screening for bacterial vaginosis and lower genital tract infection?

Bacterial vaginosis is a polymicrobial condition associated with preterm delivery and is an independent risk factor for prediction of preterm labor.

Screening of BV and lower genital tract infection may be investigated with following methods:
- Endocervical sampling for gonorrhea and Chlamydia
- Vaginal fluid pH
- Wet smear for BV and *Trichomonas* infection
- GBS culture
- Urine analysis and culture.

Positive result treated with appropriate treatment is likely to be beneficial in reducing preterm births. In women who are at high risk for preterm labor, treatment with clindamycin, metronidazole and erythromycin shows marked reduction in preterm delivery, but presently available studies are not sufficient to support screening of bacterial vaginosis.

Q. 13. Enumerate about role of routine screening in asymptomatic women.

Bacterial vaginosis testing, and home uterine activity monitoring although are predictors of preterm labor, these methods are not recommended as routine screening strategies as they have failed to demonstrate improved perinatal outcomes in studies which are based on the use of these tests in asymptomatic women.

Q. 14. What are the examinations and investigations considered necessary in case of preterm labor?

Confirmation of gestational age by menstrual history and available previous ultrasound report done at less than 14 weeks.

Examination
- General physical examination to look for nutritional status and periodontal disease
- Temperature to be recorded to rule out chorioamnionitis or other infections
- Obstetric examination: Liquor volume to be noted, multiple pregnancy and big baby to be ruled out, signs of abruption like hard, tense and tender uterus to be noted. Any palpable fibroid and tenderness over it to be ruled out
- A speculum examination with full aseptic technique and not touching the cervix with the speculum. Cervical swabs shall be taken for immediate bacteriological assessment. If the cervix is closed and there is no blood or amniotic fluid to be seen in the vagina, fetal fibronectin (fFN) test shall be performed
- Digital examination shall be avoided unless there is a possibility of cord presentation or prolapsed or when the cervix is not visualized properly.

Samples to be collected during vaginal examinations are:
- Endocervical sampling for gonorrhea and Chlamydia
- Vaginal fluid pH
- Wet smear for bacterial vaginosis and trichomonas infection
- Group B *streptococcus* (GBS) culture.

Other investigations are:
- **Complete hemogram**
- **C-reactive protein**
- **Nonstress test (NST)**
- **Electrolytes and RBS when tocolytics are used**
- **Urine microbiology**—mid-stream urine sample for microscopy and culture
- **Ultrasound**—to assess presentation, placental localization, gestational age, fetal well being (BPP), fetal weight and the possibility/advisability of amniocentesis.
- Transvaginal ultrasound is best for detecting early changes in the internal cervical os
- **Electronic fetal heart monitoring (EFM)**—shall be performed in case of viable fetus to assess fetal wellbeing. Ongoing continuous electronic fetal monitoring (EFM) is done at gestation age of more than 25 weeks

- **Amniocentesis**—to be made only whenever indicated to assess the presence or absence of intra-amniotic sepsis.

Q. 15. Brief about the precautions while collecting the sample for fFN and importance of fFN as a predictor of preterm labor.

Fetal fibronectin (fFN) test

It is a screening test used to assess the risk of preterm delivery within the next seven days (Table 3).

Table 3: Procedure for fetal fibronectin test

Indications	• Symptomatic preterm labor between 24 and 36 weeks gestation • Intact membranes and • Cervical dilatation less than 3 cm
Contraindications	• Ruptured membranes • Visual evidence of moderate or gross bleeding • Cervical cerclage *in situ*
Relative contraindications	• After the use of lubricants or disinfectants • Within 24 hours of coitus • Within 24 hours of vaginal examination
Procedure	• Performed using a sterile speculum examination prior to any examination or manipulation of the cervix or vagina • Use only sterile water as a lubricant • Obtain the sample for testing from the posterior fornix of the vagina • As per test instructions
Positive result	• Consider transvaginal ultrasound of cervical length • Admit for tocolysis and steroids • A false-positive result may occur as a result of recent coitus • Digital vaginal examination or transvaginal ultrasound
Negative result	• Low risk of delivery within 7 days • False-negative result may occur due to the use of a lubricant with • Speculum examination or intravaginal disinfectants

Contd...

Q. 16. Brief the preventive measures in the management of preterm labor.

Prevention of preterm labor is very important as the prematurity constitutes for majority of perinatal mortality.

Preventive measures include primary, secondary and tertiary prevention.

Primary prevention (prevention and risk reduction in the population)[8]

Primary prevention contributes significantly in reducing perinatal mortality incidences can be lowered by reducing the prevalence of smoking, counseling regarding nutrition, avoiding or lowering stressful jobs, education and awareness of preterm births in ARTs, advocating the usage of condoms to prevent in the transmission of STDs, and dealing appropriately psychological factors if any may also contribute in reducing preterm births.

Secondary prevention (Identification and treatment for individuals with increased risk).

The following steps can be initiated for prevention of preterm labor:

- Evaluating physical and psychological well being of pregnant women
- Proper dietary supplementation fulfilling macro and micronutrient requirement
- Preconceptional surgical correction of uterine anomalies if any
- Progesterone therapy
- Considering prophylactic or therapeutic cervical encirclage in cases of proven cervical incompetence
- Periodontal care.

Progesterone therapy

Current guidelines recommended by The Society for Maternal-Fetal Medicine (SMFM) regarding the progesterone therapy for prevention of preterm births (Table 4).[9]

Table 4: Current Society for Maternal-Fetal Medicine recommendations regarding use of progestogens for prevention of preterm birth

Population	Recommendation regarding use of progestogens
Asymptomatic	
Singletons without prior SPTB and unknown or normal TVU CL	No evidence of effectiveness
Singletons with prior SPTB	17-OH progesterone caproate 250 mg IM weekly from 16–20 weeks until 36 weeks
Singletons without prior SPTB but CL20 mm at24 weeks	Vaginal progesterone 90 mg gel or 200 mg suppository daily from diagnosis of short CL until 36 weeks
Multiple gestations	No evidence of effectiveness
Symptomatic	
PTL	No evidence of effectiveness
PPROM	No evidence of effectiveness

Abbreviations: CL, cervical length; IM, intramuscularly; PPROM, preterm premature rupture of membranes; PTL, preterm labor; SPTB, spontaneous preterm birth; TVU, transvaginal ultrasound
Source: SMFM. Progesterone and preterm birth prevention. Am J Obstet Gynecol. 2012.

Q. 17. Contraindications for progesterone therapy.

- Current or past history of thrombosis
- Thromboembolic disorders
- Known or suspected breast cancer
- Cholestatic jaundice in pregnancy
- Liver tumors—benign or malignant
- Active liver disease
- Uncontrolled hypertension.

Q. 18. What is the next step after confirmation of the diagnosis of preterm labor?

Tertiary Prevention (Treatment initiated after the parturition process has begun to limit perinatal morbidity and mortality)
Measures include:
- Establish the diagnosis of preterm labor
- Administration of corticosteroids to induce fetal lung maturity
- Tocolysis to halt the uterine contractions
- Usage of antibiotics to treat infections if any
- Hospitalization and bed rest.

Establish the diagnosis of preterm labor

Gestational age must be confirmed by menstrual history and any available previous ultrasound report done before 14 weeks of gestation.

Q. 19. Brief about the protocol for administration of corticosteroids. Is there a role in this patient?

As there is definite diagnosis of preterm labor in this case corticosteroids have to be administered in this case.

The beneficial effects of corticosteroids: Glucocorticoids act in fetus to promote maturation over growth. In the lung, it promote surfactant synthesis, increase lung compliance, reduce vascular permeability, and generates an enhanced response to postnatal surfactant treatment thus reducing the incidence of perinatal morbidity and mortality.

For prophylaxis against neonatal respiratory distress syndrome, a single course of steroids is given.

NIH Consensus Recommendations, 2000.[11]
- All fetuses 24–34 weeks at risk for preterm delivery should not be influenced by race or gender of fetus
- If patient eligible for tocolytics, she is eligible for corticosteroids
- Treatment recommendations are:
  - Betamethasone 12 mg intramuscular/24 h × 2 doses
  - Dexamethasone 6 mg intramuscular/12 h × 4 doses

In the event of maternal diabetes, endocrinologist shall be consulted regarding blood glucose level (BGL) control.

Benefit of repeated courses of steroids is doubtful and currently not recommended.

Q. 20. What is the role of tocolytics? Discuss briefly about tocolytics.

The goal by tocolytics is to prevent imminent preterm birth, to get sufficient time to administer steroids and if appropriate, to allow for in utero transfer to hospital with NICU. In this patient as the gestational age is 30 weeks and the diagnosis of preterm labor is established, tocolytics have definite role in the management.

Indications
- Considered for women with confirmed PTL between 24 and 34 weeks of gestation, where there is no contraindication to their use
- To gain time to allow for completion of course of corticosteroids
- To allow for safe in utero transfer to tertiary-level hospitals with appropriate NICU facilities.

Contraindications
- Chorioamnionitis/sepsis
- Significant antepartum hemorrhage, such as placental abruption/active vaginal bleeding
- Advanced cervical dilatation
- Abnormal CTG suggesting non-reassuring fetal status
- Placental insufficiency
- Preeclampsia/eclampsia
- Lethal congenital/chromosomal malformation
- Intrauterine fetal demise
- Maternal allergy to specific tocolytic agents, or where tocolytics are contraindicated with specific comorbidities (e.g. beta-agonists should not be given in case of cardiac disease)
- Gestational ages <24 weeks or >34 weeks.

Tocolytic drugs used in clinical practice (Table 5):
- Calcium agonists—nifedipine
- Oxytocin receptor agonists—atosiban
- Inhibitors of prostaglandin synthesis—indomethacin
- Nitric oxide donors—nitroglycerin
- Betamimetics—terbutalin and ritodrine
- Magnesium sulfate.

Atosiban can be given in the following condition:
- Diabetes
- Cardiac disease
- Multiple pregnancies
- More effective than other tocolytics both in prolonging the pregnancy with less side effects.

Table 5: Dosage and side effects of tocolytis

Drugs	Dosage	Contraindications	Side effects	
			Maternal	Fetal
Calcium channel blockers—nifedipine	30 mg loading dose, 10–20 mg 4–6 hourly for 24 hours	Cardiac diseases, Maternal hypertension, concomitant use of MgSO$_4$, renal disease	Flushing headache, transient hypotension, nausea	Sudden fetal death

Contd...

Contd...

Drugs	Dosage	Contraindications	Side effects	
			Maternal	Fetal
Oxytocin agonist—atosiban	Intial bolus dose 6.75 mg over one minute, followed by an infusion of 18 mg/h for 3 h and 6 mg/h up to 48 h	None	Nausea, allergic reaction, headache	None
Prostaglandin synthase inhibitors Indomethacin	Loading dose 50 mg per rectally or 50–100 mg orally then 25–50 mg orally every 6 h for 2 days	Renal and hepatic impairment, platelet dysfunction or bleeding disorders, asthma	Nausea, heart burn, postpartum hemorrhage, renal impairment, headache, dizziness	Constriction of ductus arteriosus, oligohydromnios—its use should be limited <32 weeks, hyperbilirubinemia, pulmonary hypertension, IVH, NEC
Nitric acid donors—nitroglycerine patch	10 mg patch 12 hourly until contraction ceases or 48 hours		Headache, hypotension	Neonatal hypotension
Betamimetics: • Terbutalin	0.25 mg subcutaneously every 20 min to 3 hours, limited to maximum of 2 dose	Tachycardia, thyroid disease, cardiac arrhythmias, diabetes mellitus	Tachycardia, hypotension, tremors, palpitations, hypokalemia, hyperglycemia, pulmonary edema	Fetal tachycardia
• Ritodrine	Initial dose of 50–100 µg IV later increased by 50 µg/min every 10 min until contraction cease or maximum 35 µg/min. Ritodrine help in lung maturity	Tachycardia, thyroid disease, cardiac arrhythmias, diabetes mellitus	Tachycardia, hypotension, tremors, palpitations, hypokalemia, hyperglycemia, pulmonary edema	Fetal tachycardia

Q. 21. Role of magnesium sulfate as neuroprotector in preterm labor. What are the guidelines for its administration? Is it advisable in this case?

Antenatal maternal treatment with magnesium has been inconsistently associated with reduced rates of IVH, cerebral palsy, and perinatal mortality in premature infants. Trials have showed that, women delivered before 30 weeks of gestation found significantly lower rates of gross motor dysfunction and nonsignificant trends of reduced mortality and cerebral palsy in surviving infants in the treated group at 2 years of age. Trials have failed to demonstrate significant pregnancy prolongation when magnesium sulfate was given. **Though the tocolytic action of magnesium is not useful for** pregnancy prolongation, the available evidence suggests that magnesium sulfate given before anticipated early preterm birth reduces the risk of cerebral palsy in surviving infants thus promoting its use as neuroprotector (BEAM Study).

Neuroprotective action of magnesium sulfate:

- Exerts a vasodilator effect in the fetal cerebral vessels mitigating hypoxia and/or ischemia induced brain damage
- Has an anti-inflammatory effect resulting in decreased production of pro-inflammatory cytokines and free radicals which ultimately decreases cerebral cell death secondary to inflammation
- It down regulates NMDA receptors for the neurotransmitter glutamate thereby decreasing calcium entry into the cell and modulating a protective mitigation of excitatory action potential propagation.

Guidelines for reduction of cerebral palsy

ACOG committee opinion, March 2010
- Magnesium sulfate can be given before early preterm birth reduces the risk of cerebral palsy in surviving infants is supported by the available evidence.

Modified beam trial protocol[12]

- Neuroprotection protocol is instituted for imminent delivery from 24–34 weeks with at least 2 hours. Magnesium infusion prior to delivery for benefit. Patients anticipated to deliver in <2 hours or contraindicated to $MgSO_4$ (e.g. myasthenia gravis or severe SIRS/sepsis) are excluded.
- Criteria to suspect delivery is **imminent** if delivery is anticipated within ~ 12–24 hours
- Regular contractions associated with advanced cervical dilation (3–4 cm) with either preterm rupture of membranes OR intact membranes,

OR
Clinical suspicion for imminent delivery with isolated premature preterm rupture of membranes
OR
Clinical suspicion of imminent delivery with antenatal bleeding
OR
Before an indicated preterm delivery.

Dosage

Neuroprotection protocol: $MgSO_4$ loading dose of 6 g followed by 2 g/h for 12–24 hours until delivery. $MgSO_4$ 2 g/h maintenance to be discontinued if delivery is imminent delivery is not anticipated after the initial 12 hours.

Calcium gluconate should be readily available to reverse the respiratory effects of magnesium.

Q. 22. Enumerate the role of antibiotics in PTL.

Antibiotic therapy in women with preterm labor and intact membranes is not effective to prolong pregnancy. The failure of antibiotics to prolong pregnancy may be attributed to treatment of women whose preterm labor did not result from infection, and to the timing of treatment relative to the infectious process. Antimicrobial therapy of women in preterm labor should be limited to GBS prophylaxis, women with preterm PROM, or treatment of a specific pathogen (e.g. urinary tract infection).

Screening for UTI, BV and lower genital tract infection and its treatment with antibiotics at midtrimester helps in reducing preterm births. But, ORACLE I and II trials have revealed the unlikely benefit of prophylactic outcomes with intact membranes, on neonatal outcomes. However, antibiotics may be used in women with PROM between 24 weeks and 32 weeks of gestation to prevent preterm births and it also helps in continuing the pregnancy thereby improving the neonatal outcome and reducing perinatal complications.

- **GBS (Group B Streptococci) prophylaxis:** Patients with preterm labor are all at high risk for neonatal GBS sepsis. Patients with imminent delivery with preterm labor should be given GBS prophylaxis unless it is proved to be GBS culture negative.
  GBS infection treatment requires IV benzyl penicillin prophylaxis in labor. IV benzyl penicillin 3 g loading dose to be given as soon as possible, then 1.2 g IV every 4 hours. If allergic to penicillin, lincomycin 600 mg IV every 8 hours, or azithromycin 500 mg IV once daily are alternatives, preferably prescribed based on sensitivity results from antenatal swabs
- **Urinary tract infections in pregnancy:** The antibiotic of choice should be based on sensitivity report and treatment should be according to bacterial sensitivity. The treatment is said to be satisfactory when the repeat culture yields no growth
- **Bacterial vaginosis:** *Recommended Regimens[13]*
- Metronidazole 500 mg orally twice a day for 7 days
  OR
- Metronidazole gel 0.75%, one full applicator (5 g) intravaginally, once a day for 5 days
  OR
- Clindamycin cream 2%, one full applicator (5 g) intravaginally at bedtime for 7 days. Studies have concluded that no antibiotic regimen prevented preterm birth (early or late) in women with BV (symptomatic or asymptomatic), though there are several regimens recommended for bacterial vaginosis.

Q. 23. How will you manage delivery when tocolysis fails or tocolysis is contraindicated?

In the absence of obstetric risk factors or complications, a preterm fetus with vertex presentation may be delivered vaginally however if the presentation is non vertex, delivery by cesarean section may be considered.

Principles of management of preterm labor

- To prevent birth asphyxia and development of RDS
- To prevent birth trauma.

First stage

- Patient to be confined to the bed to prevent early rupture of membranes
- Oxygen mask to mother to ensure adequate fetal oxygenation
- Avoid strong sedatives
- Epidural analgesia is preferred
- As preterm fetus is more prone for hypoxia and acidosis which increases the risk of intraventricular hemorrhage, continuous intrapartum fetal monitoring is required to ensure fetal well being
- Antibiotic prophylaxis against GBS
- Delivery must be conducted in presence of expert neonatologist
- NICU is a Sine-Qua-Non.

Second stage

- Delivery should be slow and gentle to avoid rapid compression and decompression of head
- Forceps delivery may be beneficial for the baby whereas ventouse is contraindicated
- Episiotomy to minimize head compression (if there is perineal resistance)
- Cord to be clamped quickly, cord length to be kept long (to prevent hypervolemia and hyperbilirubinemia
- The air passages to be cleared of mucus
- Avoid hypothermia
- Injection vitamin K 1 mg IM
- Shift the baby to NICU for observation and further management.

Q. 24. Summarize the management of this case.

As this case is diagnosed to have established preterm labor, there is definite role of corticosteroids, tocolytics and treatment of UTI as per culture sensitivity report. Magnesium sulfate for neuroprophylaxis has to be given as gestational age is 30 weeks when delivery is imminent.

Delivery to be conducted as per above mentioned protocol.

In general, the algorithm for screening and treatment of pregnant woman to reduce the risk of preterm birth is shown in Flowchart 2.

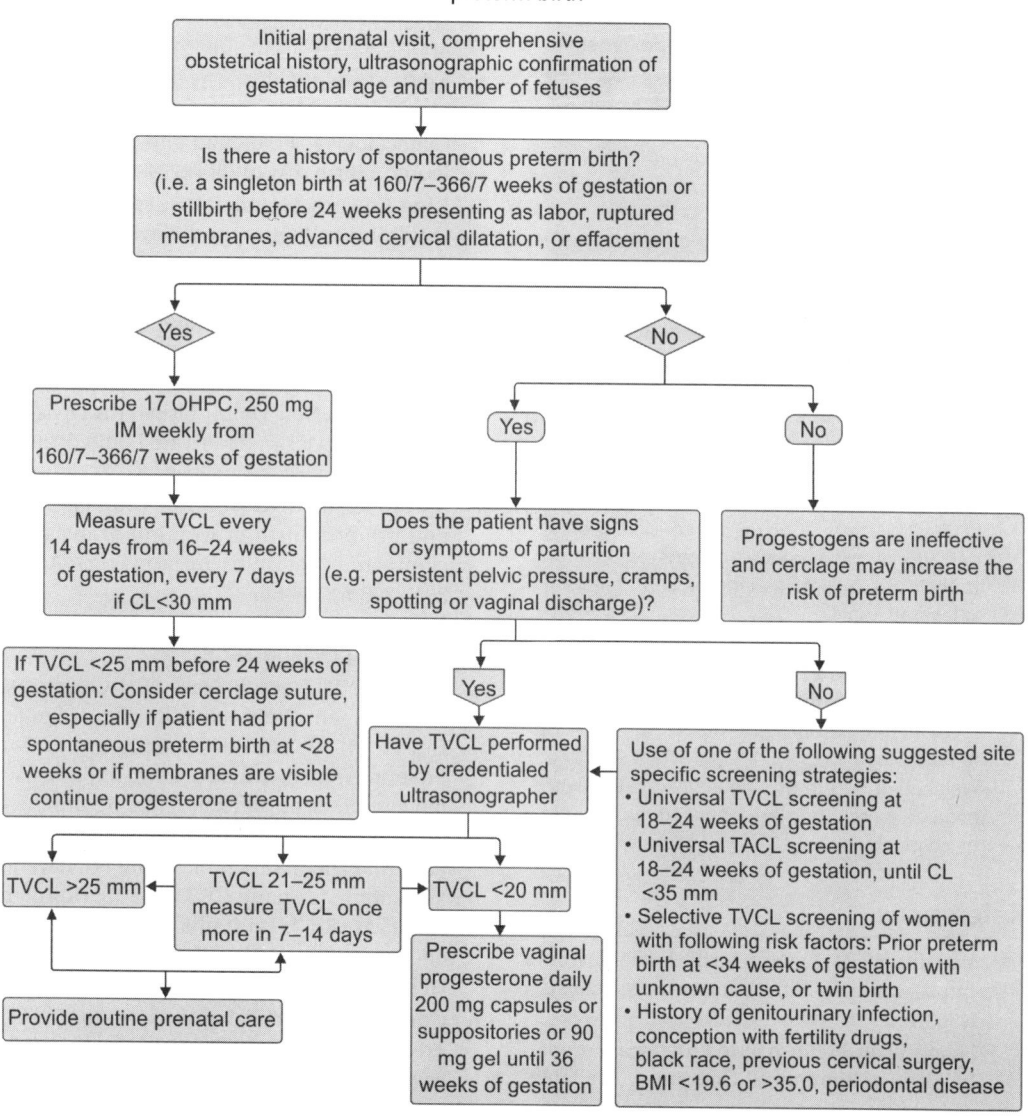

Flowchart 2: Algorithm for screening and treatment of pregnant woman to reduce the risk of preterm birth

Points to Remember

1. (a) Early detection of preterm labor, (b) Appropriate treatment of maternal and fetal conditions such as anemia, hypertension, asymptomatic bacteriuria, etc.
2. Educated patient to recognize the warning signs of preterm labor and approach for medical care at the earliest.
3. Cerclage is reserved for women with history of cervical injury, uterine anomalies and/or progressive shortening of cervix despite progesterone therapy. Prophylactic cerclage is not indicated for all asymptomatic women with short cervical length.
4. Patient with history of previous preterm birth, short cervix or both progesterone supplementation is recommended.
5. Combined assessment of fetal fibronectin and cervical length is better predictor than individually tested.
6. Compared to multiple courses of steroid therapy single course of antenatal corticosteroids are proven to be beneficial in reducing the incidence of perinatal complication associated with premature babies born before 34 weeks of gestation.
7. First line of tocolytic to be considered are calcium channel blockers based on due consideration of gestational age, etiology and contraindication to their use. Tocolytics are to be considered for at least 48 hours.
8. Uses of antibiotics are of definite value in chorioamnionitis and GBS infection.
9. Maternal magnesium sulfate administration is recommended in preterm birth <32 weeks as neuroprotector.
10. Well-equipped intensive neonatal care unit with neonatologist is the place where preterm should be conducted.

References

1. Who.int. WHO | Preterm birth. Available from: http://www.who.int/mediacentre/factsheets/fs363/en/
2. Nibmg.ac.in. Preterm Birth Program | National Institute of Biomedical Genomics. Available from: http://www.nibmg.ac.in/?q=content/preterm-birth-program.
3. Nichd.nih.gov. What are the risk factors for preterm labor and birth?. Available from: http://www.nichd.nih.gov/health/topics/preterm/conditioninfo/Pages/who_risk.aspx
4. Saxena R. Bedside Obstetrics & Gynaecology. 2nd edition. Kundli: Jaypee; 2014.
5. Chandraharan E, Arulkumaran S. Recent advances in Management of preterm labour. J of Obstet & gynaecol India. 2005;55(2):118-24.
6. ACOG Practice Bulletin No. 130: Clinical Management Guidelines for Obstetrician-Gynecologists. Prediction and prevention of Preterm Birth. 2012;120(4):964-73.
7. King Edward Memorial Hospital Clinical Guidelines: Women and Newborn Health Service, 2014;pp.1-7.
8. Simhan HN, Iams JD, Romero R. Preterm Birth. In:Gabbe SG, Niebyl JR, SimpsonJL, Landon MB, Galan HL, Jauniaux ERM, et al (Eds). Obstetrics Normal and Problem Pregnancies. 6th edition. New Delhi: Elsevier A Division of Reed Elsevier India Private Limited; 2012. pp.627-58.
9. SMFM Clinical Guideline Progesterone and preterm birth prevention: translating clinical trials data into clinical practice. AJOG. 2012;206(5):376-86.
10. Iams JD. Prevention of Preterm Parturition. NEJM. 2014;370(3):254-61.
11. Nih.gov. NIH News Release-NIH Consensus Development Conference Reaffirms Single Course of Antenatal Corticosteroids for Preterm Women; Available from: http://www.nih.gov/news/pr/aug2000/omar-18.htm.
12. Cunningham FG, Leveno KJ, Bloom SL, et al. Preterm Labour. In: Cunningham FG, Leveno KJ, Bloom SL, Spong CY, Dashe JS, Hoffman BL, et al (Eds). Williams Obstetrics. 24th edition. United States of America: McGraw Hill Education; 2014.pp.829-61.
13. Cdc.gov. Bacterial Vaginosis—2015 STD Treatment Guidelines. Available from: http://www.cdc.gov/std/tg2015/bv.htm.

14

CHAPTER

Case with Previous Aneuploidy

K Srinivas

Mrs X, G2P1L1, aged 21 years studies till 10th standard, husband a school teacher, presented with history of 2 months amenorrhea. She has come with history of having given birth to a live female baby 3 years ago who was diagnosed to be a Down syndrome baby 2 years ago. She has no other complaints

Obstetric History

She has been married for the past 5 years marriage being 2nd degree consanguineous.

First Pregnancy

Conceived at the age of 18, had ANC in her village PHC. She was a booked case. Had an anomaly scan done at 20th week. Full-term normal delivery of a live female baby weighing 3 kg. Baby cried immediately. Antenatal, intranatal and postnatal periods were uneventful.

> **Degrees of consanguinity and its significance**
> When a couple share at least one common ancestor their relation amounts to consanguinity.
> 1st degree is incest where the similarity of genetic constitution is 50%. 2nd and 3rd degree the genetic makeup is common to the extent of 25% and 12.5%

Because of the delayed milestones when she took the baby to a local doctor, she was referred to a medical college hospital and a diagnosis of Down syndrome was made.

> **Preconception counseling and its importance**
> Many genetic disorders, especially autosomal recessive disorders carry the risk of recurrence in subsequent pregnancies to the extent of 50%. Some anomalies, mental retardations, aneuploidy, etc. need counseling regarding the chances of recurrence. Periconceptional interventions, earlier diagnostic imaging/biochemical studies make early diagnosis possible. Strict control of precipitating factors also is possible in the preconceptional period

She used intrauterine contraceptive device (IUCD) for 2 years. Two months after removal of the IUCD, she conceived. No pre-conceptional counseling done.

Second Pregnancy

Patient confirmed her pregnancy by up to 2 weeks ago. She is eager to know the chances of this baby being born with similar problems like her first baby.

Menstrual History

- AOM—13 year
- Past cycles
- Regular LMP ....
- EDD ....

> **Importance of family history**
> Family history of mental retardation in 1st or 2nd degree relatives, in the siblings, aneuploidies raise the possibility of one of the parent with karyotypic abnormalities. And may warrant parental karyotyping

No other significant past history.

Family history: No history of birth of any baby with anomalies, mental retardation in the family. No history of any 1st degree or 2nd degree relatives with mental retardation in the family.

General Examination

Patient is moderately built and nourished.
- No pallor, cyanosis, jaundice, enlarged lymph nodes, pedal edema, etc.
- Pulse 92/min, regular
- BP 100/80 mm of Hg
- Afebrile
- Height—154 cm weight—54 Kg
- Breast, spine, thyroid examination—Normal
- Gait—Normal.

Signs of early pregnancy

Pregnancy diagnosis nowadays is based on biochemical and ultrasound evidences
But historically pregnancy was diagnosed by various vaginal, cervical and pelvic signs
Chadwick's sign: Dusky hue of vestibule and anterior vaginal wall and cervix
Goodell's sign: Softening of the cervix
Osiander's sign: Pulsations felt through the lateral vaginal fornices
Piskacek's sign: asymmetrical enlargement of uterus with lateral implantation
Hegar's sign: On bimanual examination the abdominal and vaginal fingers tend
To approximate below the body of the uterus
Palmer's sign: Regular rhythmic contractions of the uterus

- CVS: S1 S2 heard, no added sounds
- RS: normal vesicular breath sounds. No adventitious sounds
- CNS: Clinically normal
- P/A soft no significant inspector, palpatory, auscultatory findings
- P/S cervix and vagina appear healthy. Signs of early pregnancy seen
- P/V uterus bulky anteverted, fornices free.

Diagnosis

G2P1 L1, with 10 weeks of gestation with history of previous baby born with trisomy 21.

Discussion

Q. 1. How early in pregnancy can we proceed with diagnosis of chromosomal anomalies in the fetus?

Gestational age	
Estimated by	Importance
• LMP	• Assessment
• UPT	• Timing of tests
• Clinical	• Interpretation of tests
• USG	• Pregnancy termination
• Quickening	

Chromosomal abnormalities could be suspected with abnormal NT measurement as early as 11 weeks of pregnancy. Biochemical marker analysis may strengthen the suspicion. But definitive diagnosis is possible only with chorion villus biopsy (Even CVB can have false positivity and negativity rarely in cases of placental mosaicism).

NT and NB
- NT 11–13 weeks (CRL 45–85 MM)
- 2.5 to 3.4 mm 8% aneuploidy
- 3.5 to 4.4 27%
- 4.5 to 5.4 48%
- >6.5 87%

>4 MM go ahead with CVB and other anomaly detection
Note: Equal sign presence or absence of nasal bone

It becomes very important to clearly define the gestational age of the fetus as the marker values tend to vary with gestational age. There are other important issues too in relation to the gestational age.

Methods of genetic screening
- USG- NT and NB and others
- Serum markers
- Invasive methods

Abnormal NT with normal karyotyping could be associated with increased risk of IUD. Stillbirth, Pre-eclampsia, perinatal death.

Q. 2. What are the various screening strategies?

Methods available
- Triple test
- Quad test
- With/without ultrasound

T1 and T2 screening methods
- Ultrasound (genetic sonogram): NT, nasal bone, soft markers
- Biochemical markers: PAPP-A
  - Beta hCG
  - Unconjugated estriol
  - Inhibin-A
  - Maternal serum alpha-fetoprotein screening (MSAFP)
- Invasive procedures

Maternal age	Trisomy 21 detection	False positive
<35 years	66.7%	3.7%
>35 years	89.8%	15.2%

Screening could be individualized depending on the risk factors and the history. Maternal age, family history, sibling history, maternal disease like diabetes, twin pregnancy could be the confounding factors in interpretation of the results. Gestational age could be the single most strong confounding factor. As none of the strategies are diagnostic of the aneuploidy, various 1st trimester, 2nd trimester and combined screening strategies have evolved. But the BUN (Biochemistry, ultrasound nuchal translucency) study has proved the superiority of 1st trimester screening over other strategies.

Q. 3. How to proceed with abnormal values of double marker tests?

The following algorithm (Flowchart 1) could be used to proceed with the results of first trimester screening methods.

The BUN study (Biochemistry, ultrasound, nuchal translucency) was conceived to evaluate the performance of first trimester screening using PAPP-A, free beta hCG, and ultrasound measurement of the nuchal translucency when introduced into practice. Over a 4-year period, 13 prenatal diagnostic centers evaluated over 8500 patients and reported an 85.2% trisomy 21 detection rate with a 9.4% false positive rate.

Data from the FASTER Trial demonstrates that the contingent sequential test is the most cost-effective. This information can help shape future policy regarding Down syndrome screening

Flowchart 1: Algorithm for managing results of first trimester aneuploidy screening methods

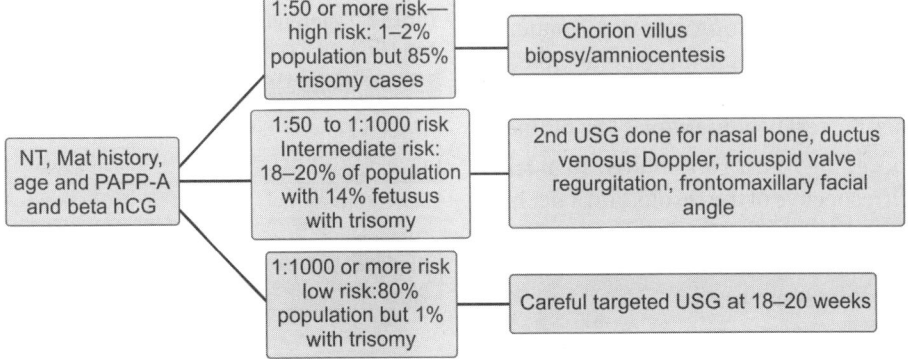

Q. 4. What is karyotyping?

Most cells in the human body have 23 pairs of chromosomes, or a total of 46 chromosomes. (The sperm and egg, or gametes, each have 23 unpaired chromosomes, and red blood cells have no nucleus and no chromosomes).

One copy of each pair is inherited from the mother and the other copy is inherited from the father. The first 22 pairs of chromosomes (called autosomes) are numbered from 1 to 22, from largest to smallest. The 23rd pair of chromosomes are the sex chromosomes. Normal females have two X chromosomes, while normal males have one X chromosome and one Y chromosome. The characteristics of the chromosomes in a cell as they are seen under a light microscope are called the karyotype.

Q. 5. What are the 2nd trimester screening tests?

> **Why so many tests?**
> **Sensitivity and false positivity**
> Example:
> - Test 83% sensitive 8% false +
> - If incidence of down's is 1 : 700
> - Population of 70,000
> - This test detects 830 out of 1000 cases
> - Unnecessary 5600 amniocentesis
> - 280 Normal babies lost!

2nd trimester screening tests once again consider the estimation of serum free beta hCG, estriol, alpha fetoprotein in the maternal serum (MSAFP). This test is called triple test and when serum inhibin is estimated along with this, the test becomes quad test (Table 1).

Proceeding with an anomaly scan at 18–20 weeks irrespective of the results and a decision could be taken whether or not to proceed with an invasive test, i.e. amniocentesis depending on the risk assessment.

Table 1: Sensitivity of various screening tests at different periods of gestation

T1 (Free beta hCG, NT, PAPP-A)	Trisomy 21 detection
11 weeks	87%
12 weeks	85%
13 weeks	82%
T2 (15–18 weeks)	
Triple test	69%
Quad test	81%
T1 and T2 combined test	
Disclosure of T1 results	95%
Nondisclosure group	96%
Serum screening only	88%

Q. 6. What is TIFFA scan?

TIFFA scan is the name given to 2nd trimester anomaly scan, anatomical survey and is targetted imaging for fetal anomalies.

It can pick up major anomalies associated with aneuploidy or other chromosomal abnormalities or can show soft markers which could raise the possibility of aneuploidy.

> **Markers**
> - Major cardiac anomalies
> - Diaphragmatic hernia
> - Exomphalos
> - Megacystis
> - Body stalk anomaly
> - Skeletal abnormality

Table 2: Differentiating the trisomies by biochemical and USG methods

Aneuploidy	Free beta hCG	PAPP-A
Trisomy21	Higher	Lower
13 and 18	Lower	Lower
Sex chromosomal	Normal	Lower
Triploidy Diandric Digynic	Very high Decreased	Mild decrease Decreased

Trisomy 13	Trisomy 18	Trisomy 21
• Holoprosencephaly • Corpus callosum agenesis • Midline cleft lip/palate • Arhinia (absent nose) • Fetal tachycardia • Cyclopia (single median eye) Proboscis • Polydactyly • VSD/ASD • Early IUGR	• Facial dysmorphism with micrognathia, low set abnormal ears, hirsutism • Spina bifida, omphalocele, heart defects, clubfeet and radial aplasia • A relative bradycardia • Early IUGR • Strawberry skull • Camptodactyly	• Duodenal atresia • Cardiac atrioventricular septal defect (AVSD), omphalocele and cerebral mild ventriculomegaly **Reversed ductus venosus a wave— more common** Frontomaxillary facial angle by 3D scan—>95th percentile for normal population

Tricuspid regurgitation: More frequently seen in aneuploidy.

Q. 7. Discuss the various ultrasound findings which may give a clue about aneuploidy.

Refer Tables 2 and 3.

Table 3: Soft markers and their significance for aneuploidy screening

Soft marker	Percentage
Nuchal fold thickness	38%
Short femur/humerus	36%
Pyelectasia	19%
Echogenic bowel	11%
Ventriculomegaly	6%
Ear length	78%
Short frontal bone	21%
5th Phalangeal hypoplasia	75%
Cardiac anomaly	50%

A detailed ultrasound examination is necessary to pick up the markers for aneuploidy.
- CNS markers: Ventriculomegaly (atrium >10 mm), Enlarged cisterna magna, choroid plexus cyst
- Head: Absent nasal bone, increased nuchal transluscency
- Long bones: Shortening <3rd percentile
- GIT: Omphalocele, echogenic bowel, single umbilical artery
- CVS: Echogenic focus in the cardia
- Kidney: Pyelectasia
- Feet: Sandal gap, Rocker bottom feet
- Hands—Clenched fist (Fig. 1)

- Final interpretation requires correlation with maternal age, other history and sometimes tests of serum markers.

Q. 8. Consolidate the sensitivity and false positivity of various screening tests.

Refer Table 4.

Table 4: Combined screening strategies-effectiveness

Screening 1st trimester	% detection	False positivity %
MA + MSAFP + free beta hCG Double test	55–60	5
MA + MSAFP + free beta hCG, uE3 triple test	65–70	5
MA + MSAFP + free beta hCG, uE3, inhibin A Quadruple test	70–75	5
MA + NT + PAPP-A (T1) and Quadruple test	90–94	5
Screening 2nd trimester	**% detection**	**False positivity %**
MA + MSAFP + free beta hCG Double test	55–60	5
MA + MSAFP + free beta hCG, uE3 triple test	65–70	5
MA + MSAFP + free beta hCG, uE3, inhibin A Quadruple test	70–75	5
MA + NT + PAPP-A (T1) and Quadruple test	90–94	5

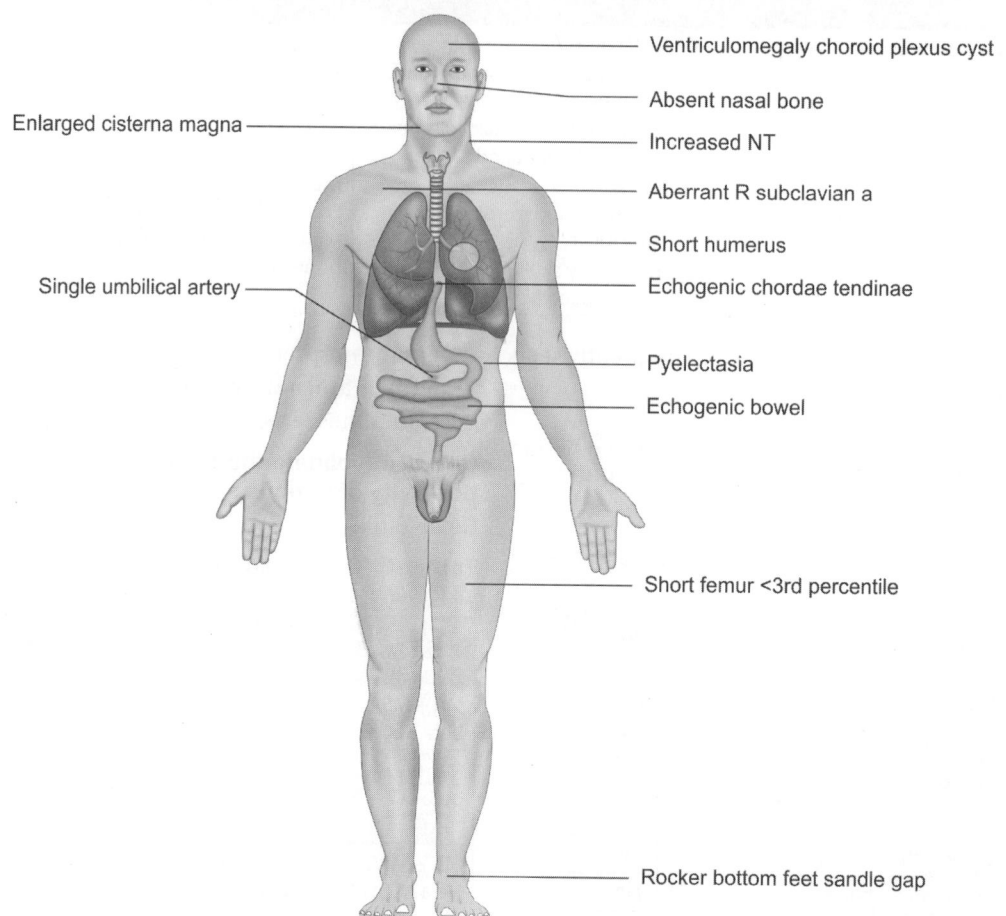

Fig. 1: Aneuploidy markers

Q. 9. What are the causes for chromosomal problems in the fetus?

The following are the causes for chromosomal abnormalities:
- Aneuploidy: Somatic or sex chromosome
- Mendelian disorders
- Multifactorial disorders
- Parental chromosomal abnormalities (translocations)
- Chromosomal inversions.

There are broadly three different types of non-disjunctional mechanisms:
- Nondisjunction that can affect any chromosome
- Ventriculomegaly and choroid plexus cyst affecting similar chromosomes: For example, acrocentric, 13, 14, 15, 21, and 23 trisomies happen because of similar mechanism
- That can affect only a single chromosome- trisomy 16 is almost always due to errors in meiosis.

Q. 10. How to proceed with abnormal soft markers on scan?

In presence of normal or low-risk value for trisomy, and no major abnormalities in the anomaly scan not much of importance is given to the soft markers. But though the probability of aneuploidy may be low, the choice of to proceed with or not to proceed with the invasive tests are given to the clients.

Q. 11. Comment on the recurrence of aneuploidy.

There is a 3% risk of aneuploidy recurrence in our population. Such data could modify counseling of these couples for invasive prenatal diagnosis.

Q. 12. What are the modes of definitive diagnosis of an aneuploidy baby?

Invasive procedure
- Chorionic villus biopsy
- Amniocentesis-routine/early
- Percutaneous umbilical blood sampling

Some tests to obtain fetal tissue for karyotyping may be the best available method to make a definitive diagnosis of chromosomal abnormality in the baby.

But in CVB, there may be fallacies as the mosaicism in placenta may give either a false positive or false negative result. FISH technique gives a quick result on some specific chromosomes, and a detailed karyotyping may take a few weeks.

Other Markers
Noninvasive
- Cell free fetal DNA in maternal plasma
- Intact fetal cells in maternal serum
- Fetal trophoblasts in cervix

Invasive
- Skin biopsy
- Muscle biopsy

Q. 13. What are the risks of invasive methods/ Any alternative noninvasive definitive diagnostic tool?

Obviously, invasive methods increase the risk of pregnancy loss.

Risk of abortion is about 1–2% with CVB, 0.5% with amniocentesis, 3–4% with cordocentesis.

Early amniocentesis and CVB are also associated with facial abnormality and limb defects in the baby.

The noninvasive method is looking for fetal cells in maternal blood and doing a karyotyping. There are other methods of obtaining fetal tissue from fetal liver, skin, etc., but they are invasive techniques. But the latter ones are definitive diagnostic tests.

Q. 14. What is NIPT? Discuss.

NIPT is noninvasive prenatal diagnostic technique.

The principle is that DNA of trophoblastic cells are circulating in maternal circulation which are identified, amplified and karyotyped.

As they are obtained from the maternal blood, it is a noninvasive test.

It is usually done after 10 weeks of gestation.

It has a very low false positive rate, but carries the same disadvantage of missing the cases in a rare situation of placental mosaicism.

Thus in cases who require invasive testing, NIPT could be the initial investigation followed by amniocentesis or cordocentesis for final confirmation.

NIPT can detect sex (Useful in X-linked disorder), it can know the Rh typing (Helps to determine the risk of isoimmunization).

It cannot be expanded for screening all as cost is its important limitation.

Q. 15. How do you manage an abnormal invasive test report?

Abnormal biochemical markers, ultrasound markers are usually followed by invasive testing. There is no much dilemma in taking a decision with abnormal karyotype reported by invasive tests. As most of the invasive procedures are done before 20 weeks (except cordocentesis) MTP could be offered to the patient in India which complies with the MTP Act 1971. Beyond 20 weeks, the patient has no choice other than to continue pregnancy.

Bibliography

1. Agathokleous M, Chaveeva P, Poon LC, et al. Meta-analysis of second-trimester markers for trisomy 21. Ultrasound Obstet Gynecol. 2013;41(3):247-61. doi:10.1002/uog. 12364.
2. American College of Obstetricians and Gynecologists Committee on Genetics: Committee Opinion No. 545: Noninvasive prenatal testing for fetal aneuploidy. Obstet Gynecol. 2012; 120:1532-4.
3. Bouhanna P, et al. Aneuploidy recurrence: New data. Ultrasound in Obstet & Gynecol. 2009;34(Suppl. 1):177-284.
4. Ball RH, Caughey AB, Malone FD. First and Second Trimester Evaluation of Risk (FASTER) Research Consortium First- and second-trimester evaluation of risk for Down syndrome. Obstet Gynecol. 2007;110(1):10-7.
5. Bugge M, Collins A, Hertz JM, et al. Non-disjunction of chromosome 13. Hum Mol Genet. 2007;16:2004-10.
6. Dan S, et al. Clinical application of massively parallel sequencing-based prenatal non-invasive fetal trisomy test for trisomies 21 and 18 in 11 105 pregnancies with mixed risk factors. Prenatal Diagnosis. 2012;32:1-8.
7. Cuckle HS, van Lith JMM. Appropriate biochemical parameters in first trimester screening for Down syndrome. Prenat Diagn. 1999;19:505-2.
8. Wapner RJ. First trimester screening: The BUN study. Semin Perinatol. 2005;29(4):236-9.
9. Hall H, et al. The origin of trisomy 13. Am J Med Genet. (in press).
10. Hall H, et al. The origin of trisomy 22: evidence for acrocentric chromosome-specific patterns of nondisjunction. Am J Med Genet. (in press).
11. Lamb NE, Sherman SL, Hassold TJ. Effect of meiotic recombination on the production of aneuploid gametes in humans. Cytogenet. Genome Res. 2005;111:250-5.
12. Larion S, Warsof SL, Romary L, et al. Association of combined first-trimester screen and noninvasive prenatal testing on diagnostic procedures. Obstet Gynecol. 2014;123:1303-10.
13. Non-invasive prenatal testing for aneuploidy and beyond: challenges of responsible innovation in prenatal screening. Semin Perinatol. 2005;29(4):236-9.
14. Sullivan AE, Silver RM, LaCoursiere DY, et al. Recurrent fetal aneuploidy and recurrent miscarriage. Obstet Gynecol. 2004;104(4):784-8.
15. Raniga S, Desai PD, Parikh H. Ultrasonographic soft markers of aneuploidy in second trimester: are we lost? Med Gen Med. 2006;8(1):9.
16. Recurrent F, et al. Aneuploidy and Recurrent Miscarriage Sullivan, European Journal of Human Genetics. 2015;23:1438-50; published online. 18 March 2015.
17. Society of Obstetricians and Gynaecologists of Canada. Canadian guidelines for prenatal diagnosis, techniques of prenatal diagnosis. JOGC Clinical Practice Guidelines No. 105; 2001 July.
18. Spencer K, Tul N, Nicolaides KH. Maternal serum free beta hCG and PAPP-A in fetal sex chromosome defects in the first trimester. Prenat Diagn. 2000b;20:390-4.
19. Tul N, Spencer K, Noble P, et al. Screening fortrisomy 18 by fetal nuchal translucency and maternal serum free beta hCG and PAPP-A at 10–14 weeks of gestation. Prenat Diagn. 1999;19:1035-42.
20. Van den hof MC, Wilson RD. Fetal soft markers in obstetric ultrasound. J ObstetGynaecol Can. 2005;27(6):592-636.
21. Wax JR, Cartin A, Pinette MG, et al. Does the frequency of soft sonographic aneuploidy markers vary by fetal sex? J Ultrasound Med. 2005;24(8):1059-63.

15

Case with Previous Cesarean Delivery

K Srinivas

CASE

A G2 P1 L1 aged about 28 years with LMP-....., EDD-...... belonging to class 3 socioeconomic status.

Admitted to the hospital with 9 months of amenorrhea for safe confinement. She is a booked case in a PHC and was referred to the tertiary care hospital for further management in view of previous delivery by cesarean section.

No history of (h/o) pain abdomen, leak per vaginum (PV), or bleeding P/V. She perceives the fetal movements. No h/o pedal edema, headache, blurring of vision, nausea, epigastric pain, giddiness, etc.

No h/o easy fatiguability or generalized weakness.

Table 1: History to be taken

Past cesarean details to be asked	Past cesarean details to be verified
Elective/emergency	Indication
Indication	Stage of labor
Outcome	Comorbid condition
Blood transfusion	Pelvic architecture
Postoperative period	Uterine incision
Discharge	Incision extension
Duration of gestation	Postpartum hemorrhage
Weight of the baby	Placental abnormalities
Thromboembolism	No. of layers closure
Any other surgery on the uterus	Suture material used
History of labor induction/failure	Postoperative complications
History of Post-datism	

Obstetric History

Married for the past 5 years, nonconsanguinous.

First Pregnancy

Conceived spontaneously 1 year after marriage. Booked case. All trimesters uneventful, went into spontaneous labor.

Managed at the PHC, but in view of meconeum stained liquor was referred to the major hospital where in view of fetal distress an emergency cesarean section was done.

Outcome was a 3.5 kg weighing live female baby which cried immediately after birth. Her postoperative period was uneventful. She breastfed the baby from 2 hours after birth to 9 months of age. She was discharged on the 6th postoperative day. She had opted for intracesarean Cu T insertion. Baby has been immunized till date and is healthy (Table 1).

Importance of first trimester scan
- Dating and to know EDD
- Confirm pregnancy
- Site of pregnancy
- Pathological pregnancy
- Confirm viability
- For multifetal gestation
- Some neural tube defect detection
- Nuchal transluscency/nasal bone
- Uterine pathology/anomalies
- Adnexal pathology

Second Pregnancy

She got her Cu T removed 1 year ago and she conceived 3 months after removal. Booked at the PHC

First Trimester

Pregnancy confirmed by UPT at 11/2 months in the primary health care (PHC). Was advised folic acid tablets after Cu T removal which she continued during 1st trimester. Got her scan done by 2½ months. No h/o excessive vomiting, bowel or bladder disturbances, bleeding PV, or pain abdomen. No h/o any other drug intake, radiation exposure.

Second Trimester

Had 3 antenatal care (ANCs). Initiated on 100 tabs of iron and folic acid. Took 2 doses of TT at an interval of 1 month. Felt quickening at 4½ months. Took an ultrasound scan at 5th month and was told that everything was normal. No other history suggestive of pre-eclampsia, bleeding PV, or any other ailment. Underwent blood sugar estimation also.

Third Trimester

Continued to have ANCs. No history suggestive of preeclampsia. Continued to perceive fetal movements. Was asked to go to the major hospital for safe confinement before the EDD.

Menstrual History

Age of menarchy—14 years
Past cycles—3-4/28, regular, moderate flow, no dysmenorrhea, no WDPV
LMP = ...

Past History

Not a known case of diabetes mellitus, epilepsy, hypertension, asthma or no h/o tuberculosis. Tonsillectomized at the age of 9 years.

Family History

No family history of hypertension, diabetes, twinning, or any other hereditary diseases. No h/o mental retardation in any of the family members on both her and her husband's side.

Personal history

Her appetite is normal, gets good sleep. Bowel habits are regular and bladder habits are normal. No h/o any addiction like tobacco chewing, coffee, alcohol, or smoking. H/o passive smoking present.

General Examination

Body mass index (BMI) is not calculated for the pregnant lady unless the pre-pregnancy weight is known. First trimester weight can be considered for BMI calculation. It becomes important especially when weight gain recommendations are to be made for the pregnant mother

The lady aged about 28 years, moderately built and nourished.

No pallor, no cyanosis, no jaundice, no lymphadenopathy, pedal edema on both feet below the ankle present.
- Pulse—90/min, regular, volume good
- Breast—normal
- BP—124/82 mm Hg
- Spine—normal

- Temperature—normal
- No thyromegaly
- Height—153 cm
- Weight—66 kg
- Gait—waddling gait of pregnancy
- Cardiovascular system
- S1, S2 heard, no murmurs
- RS
Normal vesicular breath sounds heard. No Added sounds.

Central Nervous System

No clinically detectable abnormalities.

> **Inspectory findings to be looked for:**
> - Degree of distension
> - Flank fullness
> - Umbilicus everted/transversely stretched,
> - Linea nigra, striae gravidarum
> - Movement of the quadrants with respiration
> - Scars, how healed
> - Visible and engorged veins
> - Visible pulsations
> - Visible peristalsis
> - Skin discolorations
> - Herneal orifices
> - Fetal movements visibility
> - Any other mass
> - Any visible signs of inflammations on the skin

Per Abdomen

Inspection

- Abdomen uniformly distended
- Flanks full, linea nigra and striae gravidarum present
- A suprapubic transverse scar healed by primary intension seen.

Palpation

- Uterine height 32 weeks
- Fundal grip—breech felt
- Lateral grip—back to the left and limb buds to the right
- 1st pelvic grip—head, unengaged and mobile

> **Palpatory characteristics**
> **Breech:** Soft, irregular, wide, non independently ballotable part
> **Head:** Round and globular, hard, smooth ballotable independent of the body
> **Back:** Smooth curved part offering uniform resistance
> **Limbs:** Multiple nodular structures

- 2nd pelvic grip—may not give any extra-information and may not be necessary as the head is mobile

> Uterine height—Bladder should be empty, Patient supine with semiflexed hips and knees, Dextrorotation of the uterus corrected by the palm of the right hand, ulnar border of left hand moved downwards from the xiphisternum

> Symphysiofundal height, abdominal girth are useful in estimating the gestational age, fetal weight and management formulation

- Symphysiofundal height—32 cm
- Abdominal girth—98 cm
- Uterus is relaxed
- Clinically liquor appears adequate.

> It is unlikely for the uterine scar to give way during pregnancy in cases of previous LSCS. Hence, unless the patient c/o pain or on examination uterus is found to be acting, it is unnecessary to look for scar tenderness. Rarely, silent ruptures are also known but scar tenderness is not a feature in them too.
>
> *While looking for scar tenderness, patient is placed in supine position with hips and knees semiflexed after she empties the bladder, and her attention is diverted by some queries. The tips of the fingers of the right hand are moved with moderate pressure across a curvilinear line joining the two anterior superior iliac spines with its convexity toward symphysis, in the suprapubic area and her reaction is observed*

Auscultation

FHS heard best medial to the left spinoumbilical line—144/min regular.

Diagnosis

A 28-year-old G2P1L1 with term pregnancy with EDD on ....

With previous cesarean delivery with a single live intrauterine gestation in longitudinal lie with a mobile head in the lower pole not in labour admitted for safe confinement.

Investigations

- Hb%, RBS, TSH urine routine (RFT, LFT, platelet count if necessary)
- VDRL, HIV I and II, HBsAg
- Blood grouping and Rh typing, BT, CT
- Obstetric ultrasound
- NST and if necessary proceed with BPP, umbilical artery Doppler.

Discussion

Q. 1. What are the factors influencing the management options for such patients?

- Maternal comorbid conditions
- Fetal well-being
- Pelvic architecture
- Details of the previous section, including indication
- Postoperative morbidity
- Other conditions warranting cesarean delivery now.

Q. 2. When would you terminate pregnancy?

In case of previous LSCS where in termination by cesarean is decided upon for comorbid conditions, timing of terination is dictated upon by the comorbidity (e.g. severe preeclampsia, uncontrolled DM may require immediate termination). In case vaginal trial has been decided, spontaneous labor onset is most ideal. If elective LSCS is decided upon, 39 completed weeks would be ideal for the baby.

NICU admissions, TTN, RDS, 24-hour ventilatory support, sepsis, hypoglycemia, >5 days hospitalization for the baby has been found to be least when elective LSCS is done after 39 weeks

Q. 3. How to terminate?

Termination by operative delivery is essentially by repeat LSCS. Very rarely if the lower segment is highly masked by adhesions classical may have to be done.

If vaginal trial has been planned, spontaneous onset of labor gives the best prospects for a successful trial.

Induction is a controversial issue in view of various studies reporting an increased risk of rupture with pharmacological methods and by augmentation also.

Q. 4. How do you counsel a patient for TOLAC?

Counseling for trial of labor after cesarean (TOLAC) requires the patient to be aware of the following:

- Success of TOLAC
- Determinants of success
- In her case what is the possibility of success
- Risk of rupture
- Risk of hysterectomy
- Risk of emergency cesarean delivery
- Need for blood transfusion
- Other risks of vaginal delivery like episiotomy, instrumental delivery, perinatal risks, asphyxia, brain damage associated with it, etc.

Q. 5. What are the criteria for selecting a patient for TOLAC (Trial of Labor after cesarean)?

Selection criteria for TOLAC
- Previous 1 lower segment cesarean
- No other scar on the uterus
- No previous rupture uterus
- Clinically adequate pelvis
- Facility for emergency LSCS round the clock

Q. 6. What are the determinants of success and failure of TOLAC?

Determinants of failure
- Induced labor
- LSCS done for dystocia
- No previous vaginal deliveries
- Delivery after 41 weeks

Contd...

Contd...
- Baby weight >4 kg
- Past preterm LSCS
- Male baby, non-white race
- LSCS done within the past 2 years
- Short stature of the mother

When the first four features coexist, success of TOLAC is about only 40%

Determinants of success are:
- Age of the patient elderly and teenage unfavorable
- BMI—normal 85% success, 30–40—70% success
- Previous vaginal delivery also
- Post-cesarean vaginal delivery
- Recurrent indication during past LSCS

Q. 7. What is the role of scar assessment?

Various methods have been described for assessment of the scar.

In the nonpregnant state, hysteroscopy and hysterography could be used.

Oblonsky criteria
By hysterography,
Undulant deformity = Grade 1 deformity
Small spicule + Sacculation <6 mm = Grade 2
Spicules + Sacculation >6 mm + Grade 3
Large saccules-Worm eaten look = Grade 4

Definition of Uterine Scar Defects with Imaging Techniques
In 1966, Waniorek described uterine scar defect as a small deformity (wedge shape, spicule, or convexity 5 mm or less in depth) or as a large deformity (6 mm or more in depth, or with a sacculation, bursa or pocket shape).
Subsequently, others defined scar defects as concavity with a depth of more than 1–6 mm or as remaining myometrium thickness equal to or less than 2.2 or 2.5 mm.
Recently, Osser et al. proposed the evaluation of uterine scar defect according to the ratio between the remaining myometrium over the defect and myometrium thickness at the cesarean scar site.
Currently, there is no consensus on the exact definition of uterine scar defect assessed by imaging.

During Pregnancy
Scar thickness is assessed by ultrasound scan.

But none of the methods have been proved to be effective in predicting the successful conduct of TOLAC.

USG assessment of scar
- Rozenburg: At 37 weeks by abdominal scan scar should be >3.5 cm
- Fukuda-TAS: <2 mm is risky
- Gotoh-TVS: <2 mm is risky
- Michaels. Looking at the symmetry, thickening, ballooning and movement of the scar wedge defect is diagnosed and grouped into 3 classes.
- Herneation of the amniotic sac and transmission of fundal pressure to it is also studied
- Scar vascularity is studied by color Doppler and fibrosis is diagnosed.

Echogenic outer wall with underlying myometrial thickness is the landmark

Q. 8. What are the complications of TOLAC?

As a successful TOLAC could bring smiles on the faces of the client and the obstetrician, it has its own inherent problems (Table 2).

A multicentric study by Landon et al. comparing 18,000 women who attempted a VBAC, and 15000 patients opting for elective section saw some significant complications.

Table 2: Risks associated with attempted VBAC and elective repeat cesarean section

Complications	Attempted VBAC(%)	Elective LSCS (%)
Rupture uterus	0.7	Nil
Thromboembolism	0.04	0.1
Blood transfusion	1.7	1
Infection	2.9	1.8
Stillbirth (antepartum)	0.2–0.4	0.1
Intrapartum stillbirth	1	0
Term HIE/neonatal death	0.08	0–0.05

Maternal death, incidence of hysterectomy, scar dehiscence didnot show statistically significant difference.

Q. 9. Discuss the conduct of TOLAC under the headings—induction, augmentation 2nd stage, 3rd stage.

Essentially, TOLAC is to be conducted in an institution with all facilities for emergency LSCS. All criteria to be fulfilled.

> Forceps delivery could be a better choice than ventouse, as ventouse delivery requires maternal efforts, which could be detrimental to the scar

Induction—ACOG discourages the use of prostaglandins. Though earlier studies showed a higher rates of rupture in induced cases later reports have brought in controversy.

Mechanical Methods of Induction may be safer

In selected cases induction may be attempted. Use of oxytocin and amniotomy in the 1st stage may be carefully done, partographic management is to be made a must. Continuous fetal monitoring is very essential.

> Scar tenderness is elicited after diverting patient's attention, by pressing with the tip of the three or four fingers of the right hand along a curvilinear line probably corresponding to the uterine scar over the abdomen in the supra pubic area between the two anterior superior iliac spines

2nd stage is cut short in the interest of the scar as the maximum intrauterine pressure is reached during the expulsive phase of this stage.

3rd stage management is as usual, AMTSL. Scar exploration is advocated by some. But some would not want to disturb a scar after a successful delivery if there is no PPH arousing the suspicion of rupture.

Q. 10. Comment on cases with >1 LSCS, ECV in Previous LSCS, labor analgesia during TOLAC, multiple pregnancy in previous LSCS.

More than 1 LSCS though the rupture incidence is not alarmingly high, TOLAC is not recommended by ACOG.

> **RCOG 2015 (ACOG and NICE concensus)**
> Can women with two or more prior cesareans be offered planned VBAC?
> Women who have had two or more prior lower segment cesarean deliveries may be offered VBAC after counseling by a senior obstetrician. This should include the risk of uterine rupture and maternal morbidity, and the individual likelihood of successful VBAC (e.g. given a history of prior vaginal delivery). Labor should be conducted in a centre with suitable expertise and recourse to immediate surgical delivery

>1 LSCS increases the risk of placenta praevia and morbidly adherent placenta, hence should be discouraged.

Labor analgesia is safe and noncontroversial during TOLAC.

ECV in patients with Previous LSCS could be risky, but in carefully selected cases may be attempted. It is a relatively contraindicated. Attempting ECV in patients with previous LSCS in labor may increase the risk of rupture. Otherwise determinants of successful ECV are:

- Good scar
- Healed by first intention
- Average size of the baby
- Liquor in good quantity
- No uterine contraction, relaxed uterus.

If the patient is in labor chances for rupture are very high.

Multiple pregnancy with previous LSCS per se does not contraindicate TOLAC. But the cumulative weight of the babies, 2nd baby in breech or transverse lie may pose dilemmatic situation.

Q. 11. How do you manage a case of suspected rupture uterus during a TOLAC?

> - Buhimachi et al. have made an interesting observation in 2005
> - Prostaglandin usage has resulted in rupture mostly at old scar site whereas oxytocin usage at a different site other than scar

Once there is a suspicion of rupture by any of the signs, patient is to be taken up for laparotomy.

Diagnosis of rupture
- Fetal distress
- A screaming parturient becomes silent, momentary relief of pain
- Tachycardia
- Hypotension
- Fresh bleeding from vagina
- Hematuria
- Loss of uterine contour
- Superficially felt fetal parts
- Recession of the presenting part in PV
- Scar tenderness

The scar rupture is usually managed with repair in majority of the cases.

If there is extension to the upper segment, irrepairable rupture, hysterectomy may have to be done.

In multiparous women, it is advisable to combine sterilization operation along with repair of rupture.

While scanning the location of the placenta in a case of previous section; care should be taken to exclude placenta acreta. If the placenta is adherent to the scar then it is called as placenta previa cesarean

Q. 12. How do you diagnose adherent placenta?

- Normal hypoechoic boundary between the placenta and urinary bladder serosa is lost.
- Placenta appears to be contiguous with bladder wall
- Sonolucent spaces are visible within the placenta adjacent to the uterine wall
- Color Doppler reveals persistent blood flow between the basal placenta and myometrium
- Scanning and locating the placenta are very imporatant
  1. To give TOLAC
  2. If placenta is adherent then blood can be kept ready and urologist can be informed.

Q. 13. How to categorize the urgency of indications of cesarean section?

Ranzcog Classification of Indications for LSCS

Category 1: Urgent threat to the life or the health of a woman or fetus
Category 2: Maternal or fetal compromise but not immediately life-threatening
Category 3: Needing earlier than planned delivery but without currently evident maternal or fetal compromise
Category 4: At a time acceptable to both the woman and the cesarean section team, understanding that this can be affected by a number of factors

Q. 14. What are the scoring systems to predict the success of VBAC?

To determine the success of vaginal delivery after cesarean section (VBAC: vaginal birth after cesarean), in an observational study involving 5022 patients, Bruce L. Flamm, MD, and Ann M. Geiger, PhD create Admission Scoring System as follows (Tables 3 and 5):

Table 3: Scoring for predicting VBAC success

No.	Criteria	Value
1.	Under 40 years of age	2
2.	History of vaginal delivery:	
	• Before and after cesarean section	4
	• After the first cesarean section	2
	• Before the first section	1
	• Has never been	0
3.	Cesarean section is not the first indication of failure of labor progress	1
4.	Cervical effacement at the time of hospital admission	
	->75%	2
	- 25–75%	1
	- <25%	0
5.	The opening of the cervix at the time of hospital admission ≥4 cm	1

Interpretation:

Score 0–2: 49% chance of vaginal delivery

3–8: 50–94% chance of vaginal delivery

8–10: 95% chance of vaginal delivery

(Quoted from: Klein GH. Commentary and reviews: vaginal birth after cesarean delivery: an admission scoring system).

Q. 15. What are the advantages and disadvantages of elective vs emergency LSCS?

When cesarean section is done after the onset of labor or due to any complications (maternal–fetal), it is referred to as emergency cesarean (Table 4).

Q. 16. Discuss the Robson's 10 group classification of indications.

High cesarean birth rates are an issue of international public health concern. Worries over such increases have led the World Health Organization to advise that cesarean section (CS) rates should not be more than 15%, with some evidence that CS rates above 15% are not associated with additional reduction

Table 4: Differences between elective and emergency cesarean section and their advantages and disadvantages

Elective LSCS	Emergency LSCS
Advantages • Patient is well-prepared • Anemia/infection and other comorbidities corrected • A team is ready to attend if there are complications • Blood may be kept ready	**Disadvantages** • Patient is not well-prepared • Anemia/infection and other comorbidities may complicate the surgery and postoperative period • Senior consultant's availability may not be there • Arranging blood may be difficult • Drained liquor, deeply engaged head may result in extraction difficulties • Litigation possibility may be more for all the above reasons
Disadvantages • Lower segment not formed • Bleeding may be more • Thick lower segment may lead to defective healing • Extraction may be difficult • If not assessed properly a preterm baby may be delivered	**Advantages** • Well-formed lower segment, easy approximation of edges, less bleeding, better healing of uterine scar

Table 5: Weinstein score for successful prediction of VBAC

Parameter	Score 0	Score 1	Score 2
VBAC history	Nil	FTND before CS	VBAC
Bishop's score	0–3	4–5	6–10
Indication for Prev LSCS	Non-progress of labour (NPOL)	Twin pregnancy or post-dates or intrauterine growth retardation (IUGR) or placental abruption or oligohydraminios	Breech presentation or fetal distress
Age	>30	25–30	<25
Gestational age	<39 weeks	39–40	>40
BMI in kg/M^2	>30	25–29.9	<25

Total score	Success rate
>4	58%
>6	67%
>8	78%
10	85%

in maternal and neonatal mortality and morbidity. Analyzing CS rates in different countries, including primary *vs.* repeat CS and potential reasons of these, provide important insights into the solution for reducing the overall CS rate. Robson, proposed a new classification system, the Robson Ten-Group Classification System to allow critical analysis according to characteristics of pregnancy.

The Robson ten-group classification system.

Group 2 and 4 are subclassified as A and B for induced labor and cesarean done before labor.

Group 5 to 10 are subgrouped as A, B and C for spontaneous labor, induced labor and cesarean done before labor. This is a modification on Robson's criteria.

1. Nulliparous, singleton, cephalic, ≥37 weeks' gestation, in spontaneous labor.
2. Nulliparous, singleton, cephalic, ≥37 weeks' gestation, induced labor or cesarean section before labor.
2a. Nulliparous, singleton, cephalic, ≥37 weeks' gestation, induced labor.
2b. Nulliparous, singleton, cephalic, ≥37 weeks' gestation, cesarean section before labor.
3. Multiparous (excluding previous cesarean section), singleton, cephalic, ≥37 weeks' gestation, in spontaneous labor.
4. Multiparous without a previous uterine scar, with singleton, cephalic pregnancy, ≥37 weeks' gestation, induced or cesarean section before labor.
4a. Multiparous without a previous uterine scar, with singleton, cephalic pregnancy, ≥37 weeks' gestation, induced labor.
4b. Multiparous without a previous uterine scar, with singleton, cephalic pregnancy, ≥37 weeks' gestation, cesarean section before labor.
5. Previous cesarean section, singleton, cephalic, ≥37 weeks' gestation.
6. All nulliparous with a single breech.
7. All multiparous with a single breech (including previous cesarean section).
8. All multiple pregnancies (including previous cesarean section).
9. All women with a single pregnancy in transverse or oblique lie (including those with previous cesarean section).
10. All singleton, cephalic, <37 weeks' gestation pregnancies (including previous cesarean section).

Q. 17. Complications of repeat LSCS.

Peroperative:
- Difficult access
- Bladder injury
- Bowel injury
- Extraction difficulties
- Increased bleeding
- Hysterectomy
- Prolonged surgery

Postoperative
- ICU care
- Ventilation
- Transfusion
- Ileus
- Prolonged hospital stay

Long-term
- Placenta previa
- Morbidly adherent placent
- Hysterectomy/injuries during next pregnancy
- Mortality.

In a study, there were 6,201 first (primary), 15,808 second, 6,324 third, 1,452 fourth, 258 fifth, and 89 sixth or more cesarean deliveries. Placenta accreta was present in 15 (0.24%), 49 (0.31%), 36 (0.57%), 31 (2.13%), 6 (2.33%), and 6 (6.74%) women undergoing their first, second, third, fourth, fifth, and sixth or more cesarean deliveries, respectively. Hysterectomy was required in 40 (0.65%) first, 67 (0.42%) second, 57 (0.90%) third, 35 (2.41%) fourth, 9 (3.49%) fifth, and 8 (8.99%) sixth or more cesarean deliveries.

In the 723 women with previa, the risk for placenta accreta was 3%, 11%, 40%, 61%, and 67% for first, second, third, fourth, and fifth or more repeat cesarean deliveries, respectively

Classical section
1. Perimortem CS
2. CS in Ca cervix
3. *Unapproachable lower segment due to adhesions/fibroids
4. Rarely placenta previa
5. Planned cesarean hysterectomy

*Even if the UV fold is not possible to be opened, an incision may be taken on the fold over probably the lower segment, which yields after baby's extraction

Q. 18. Maximum number of LSCS possible/recommended.

There are no recommendations for the maximum number of cesarean sections a woman may undergo.

Other than placental issues like placenta previa and morbidly adherent placenta and its associated complications, no major maternal or perinatal complications are reported.

The risk of hysterectomy increases with each cesarean for various indications

Five or more cesareans also has been found to increase the risk of preterm delivery in subsequent pregnancy. Thus empirically a woman may be counseled about not going beyond 4 cesarean sections.

Concurrent sterilization needs to be considered in repeat cesarean sections, but patient needs to be counseled and her opinion documented a week before the planned caesarean section as per NICE guidelines.

Q. 19. What is the contraceptive counseling required in a case of previous LSCS?

The following methods can be used in a case of previous cesarean patient:
- Spacing methods: PPIUCD (intracesarean), Interval IUCD, Hormonal contraception following MEC, barrier methods. Interval insertion of IUCD to be done with care
- Limiting methods: Concurrent tubectomy, Interval tubal ligation, laparoscopic or minilap method/husband may under go vasectomy
- Except for considering the options strongly with an intention to have a spacing of Birth to Birth of 3 years, and a limiting method at the earliest possible delivery is the idea
- Indications and contraindications do not differ much in view of a scarred uterus.

Bibliography

1. Althabe F, Belizán JM. Caesarean section: the paradox. (comment). Lancet 2006;368(9546): 1472-1473 10. 1016/S0140-6736(06)69616-5 [PubMed] [Cross Ref]
2. Bret AJ, Sanchez Ramos J. Histerographic, clinical and histological study of transverse and longitudinal segmental cesarean scars. Rev Fr Gynecol Obstet. 1968;63:573-600.
3. Buhimschi CS, Buhimschi SP, Malinow A, et al. Rupture of the uterine scar during term labour: contractility or biochemistry? BJOG. 2005;112:38-42.
4. Camilleri AP, Busuttil T. "Twice a saesarean." J Obstet Gynaecol Br Commonw. 1968;75:1305-8.
5. Categorisation of urgency for caesarean section, The Royal Australian and New Zealand College of Obstetricians and Gynaecologists.
6. Hayakawa H, Itakura A, Mitsui T, et al. Methods for myometrium closure and other factors impacting effects on cesarean section scars of the uterine segment detected by the ultrasonography. Acta Obstet Gynecol Scand. 2006;85:429-34.
7. Juntunen K, Makarainen L, Kirkinen P. Outcome after a high number (4–10) of repeated cesarean sections. BJOG. 2004;111: 561-3.
8. Landon MB, Hauth JC, Leveno KJ, et al. maternal and perinatal outcomes associated with a trial of labour after prior caesarean delivery. N Engl J Med. 2004;351:2581-9.
9. Jastrow N, Vikhareva O, Gauthier RJ, et al. Third trimester assessment of the uterine scar in women with prior caesarean: what is the evidence? Ultrasound in Obstetrics and Gynaecology.
10. Osser OV, Jokubkiene L, Valentin L. Cesarean section scar defects: agreement between transvaginal sonographic findings with and without saline contrast enhancement. Ultrasound Obstet Gynecol. 2010;35:75-83.

11. Osser OV, Jokubkiene L, Valentin L. High prevalence of defects in Cesarean section scars at transvaginal ultrasound examination. Ultrasound Obstet Gynecol. 2009;34:90-7.
12. Rashid M, Rashid RS. Higher order repeat cesarean sections: how safe are five or more? BJOG. 2004;111:1090-4.
13. RCOG greentop guidelines October 2015.
14. Robson MS. Can we reduce the caesarean section rate? Best Pract Res Clin Obstet Gynaecol. 2001;15(1):179-194 10.1053/beog.2000.0156
15. Silver RM, Maternal morbidity associated with multiple repeat cesarean deliveries. Obstet Gynecol. 2006;107(6):1226-32.
16. Tita AT, landonMB, Spong CY, et al. timing of elective cesarean delivery at term and neonatal outcome. N Engl J Med. 2009;360:111-20.
17. Van Roosmalen J, van der Does CD. Caesarean birth rates worldwide. A search for determinants. Trop Geogr Med. 1995;47(1):19-22 [PubMed]
18. Vikhareva Osser O, Valentin L. Clinical importance of appearance of cesarean hysterotomy scar at transvaginal ultrasonography in nonpregnant women. Obstet Gynecol. 2011; 117:525-32.
19. Vikhareva Osser O, Valentin L. Risk factors for incomplete healing of the uterine incision after caesarean section. BJOG. 2010;117: 1119-26.
20. Waniorek A. Hysterography after cesarean section. With special reference to the effect of subsequent delivery on the hysterographic findings. Am J Obstet Gynecol. 1966;94:42-4922.
21. Weinstein D, Benshushan A, Tanos V, et al. Predictive score for vaginal birth after caesarean section. Am J Obstet Gynecol. 1996; 174:192-8.
22. World Health Organization. Monitoring emergency obstetric care: a handbook. Geneva, Switzerland; 2009.

16

Retropositive Pregnancy

K Srinivas

A G2P1L1 aged about 25 years with LMP-....., EDD-...... belonging to class 4 socioeconomic status.

Admitted to the hospital with 9 months of amenorrhea for safe confinement.

She is a booked case in a primary health center (PHC) and was referred to the tertiary care hospital for further management in view of retropositive status.

No history of pain abdomen, leak pervaginum, or bleeding pervaginum. She perceives the fetal movements. No history of pedal edema, headache, blurring of vision, nausea, epigastric pain, giddiness, etc.

No history of easy fatiguability or generalized weakness.

No history of cough, cold, symptoms suggestive of UTI, skin lesions, etc.

Patient gives history of being on antiretroviral drugs from the 4th month of her pregnancy, her CD4 count being 650 cells.

Obstetric History

Married for the past 6 years, nonconsanguineosus.

First Pregnancy

Conceived spontaneously 2 years after marriage. Booked case. All trimesters uneventful. Went into spontaneous labor.

Managed at the PHC, had a vaginal delivery of a live male baby weighing 3.1 kg following which she had retained placenta for which she was referred to a major hospital. There under anesthesia manual removal of placenta (MRP) was done and was transfused with 2 units of blood because of postpartum hemorrhage (PPH).

She was in the hospital for 3 days. Baby has been immunized till date and is healthy. She was breastfed for 1½ years. She used OC pills for 2 years.

Second Pregnancy

She conceived spontaneously after 1 year. During her antenatal workup she was found to be retropositive, and on testing her husband, he was also found to be retropositive.

Counseled and they decided to continue their pregnancy and the lady was started on ART.

She is a booked case. Ultrasound done twice.

> HIV counseling protocols
> OPT In
> OPT Out
> PPTCT and VCTC have been merged and now called Integrated counseling and testing centers (ICTC)

1st trimester: Pregnancy confirmed by UPT at 1 1/2 months in the PHC. She was advised folic acid tablets. Got her scan done by 3 months. No history of excessive vomiting, bowel or bladder disturbances, bleeding PV, or pain abdomen. No history of any other drug intake, radiation exposure.

2nd trimester: Had 4 ANCs. Initiated on 100 tabs of iron and folic acid. Took 2 doses of TT at an interval of 1 month. Felt quickening at 4½ months. Took an ultrasound scan at 5th month and was told that everything was normal. No other history suggestive of pre-eclampsia, bleeding PV, or any other ailment.

3rd trimester: Continued to have ANCs. No history suggestive of pre-eclampsia. Continued to perceive fetal movements was asked to go to a major hospital for safe confinement.

Menstrual History

- *Age of menarche:* 12 years
- *Past cycles:* 3–4/30–32, regular, moderate flow, no dysmenorrhea, no WDPV
- *LMP:* ....

Past History

Not a known case of diabetes mellitus, epilepsy, hypertension, asthma or no history of tuberculosis.

Family History

No family history of hypertension, diabetes, twinning, or any other hereditary diseases. No history of mental retardation in any of the family members on both her and her husband's side.

Personal History

Her appetite is normal, gets good sleep. Bowel habits are regular but on and of she gives history of bleeding per rectum. Bladder habits are normal. No history of any addiction like tobacco chewing, coffee, alcohol, or smoking.

General Examination

> Pregnancy can cause congestion in the pelvic veins due to compression on the Inferior vena cava by the gravid uterus. This can present as hemorrhoids, varicose veins, pelvic thrombophlebitis, increased predilection for thromboembolic complications.

The lady aged about 25 years, moderately built and nourished.

No pallor, no cyanosis, no jaundice, no lymphadenopathy, no pedal edema.
Pulse: 90/min, regular, volume good
Breast: Normal
BP: 110/70 mm Hg
Spine: Normal
Temp: Normal
No thyromegaly
Height: 148 cm
Weight: 70 kg
Gait: Waddling gait of pregnancy
CVS
S1, S2 heard, no murmurs
RS
Normal vesicular breath sounds heard. No added sounds.

> **Breast Examination**
> - Nipple: Look for cracked nipples, retracted nipples any abnormal discharge
> - Discharge is not a definitive sign of pregnancy
> - Color of areola and nipple, increased size, tingling sensation in the breast, prominent vessels and discharge may be the probable signs of pregnancy in a primigravida.

> Measurements to be made while examining a pregnant woman
> - Height and weight
> - BMI if pre-pregnancy weight is known or even earliest pregnancy weight may be taken
> - Abdominal girth
> - Symphysiofundal height.

Central Nervous System

No clinically detectable abnormalities.

Per Abdomen Inspection

- Abdomen uniformly distended
- Flanks full, linea nigra and striae gravidarum present.

Palpation

- Uterine height: 32 weeks
- Fundal grip: Breech felt
- Lateral grip: Back to the left and limb buds to the right
- 1st pelvic grip: Head, engaged
- 2nd pelvic grip: Engaged head
- Symphysiofundal height: 32 cm
- Abdominal girth: 96 cm
- Uterus is relaxed
- Clinically liquor appears adequate.

> Importance of SFH and abdominal girth
> SFH in cm corresponds to gestational age in weeks till 36 weeks
> Abdominal girth in inches corresponds to gestational age in weeks.

Auscultation

FHS heard best medial to the left spinoumbilical line: 144/min regular

PV cervix firm, posterior 3 cm long admits tip of the finger pelvis adequate.

Diagnosis: A 28-year-old G2 P1 L1 with term pregnancy with retropositive status with EDD on ....

With previous vaginal delivery with a single live intrauterine gestation in longitudinal lie with engaged head in the lower pole not in labor admitted for safe confinement.

Investigations

- Hb%, RBS, TSH urine routine, (RFT, LFT, platelet count, if necessary)
- VDRL, HIV I and II, HBsAg (already done)
- Bl. Gp and Rh Typing, BT, CT, CD4 count
- Obstetric ultrasound
- NST and if necessary proceed with BPP, umbilical artery Doppler.

Q. 1. What is PPTCT program?

Prevention of parent to child transmission interventions are included in PPTCT programme. It is a national program which is aiming at reducing the vertical transmission from mother to child during pregnancy, childbirth and postnatal period.

The program is important in preventing the country's future generation from being burdened with retropositive population.

Q. 2. What steps are taken to prevent the mother to child transmission?

The first step is to screen all pregnant mothers for the detection of retropositive status, if found to be positive, it is important to determine the status of the spouse. This is the intervention for primary prevention.

If found positive, the woman needs to be counseled and if the pregnancy is unwanted or the couple wants termination, the services need to be provided (secondary prevention).

If the mother desires to continue pregnancy, the ART interventions, follow-up, ANC care, intranatal services, postnatal care along with newborn care and breastfeeding options need to be considered.

Q. 3. What is antenatal care to be offered to a retropositive pregnant woman?

She needs to be taken care for her retropositive status and routine pregnancy care.

Retropositivity Management

- When a pregnant woman is found to be retropositive, spouse status is determined.
- Her wishes to continue/terminate pregnancy need to be honored.
- Her condition is staged (WHO staging).
- She is linked to an ICTC for advise and follow-up of lifelong ART and CD4 monitoring.
- She needs to be screened for other STIs, tuberculosis (TB needs to be screened for in each visit).

- Weight gain needs to be monitored as a failure to gain may give a clue about progress of the disease.

Routine Pregnancy Care

- Routine antenatal visits as with any other pregnancy.

> ECV should be offered to woman with a viral load <50 copies/mL and a breech presentation at > 36 + 0 in the absence of obstetric contraindications.

- Two doses of tetanus toxoid
- Iron and folic acid tablets
- Antenatal USG
- Other investigations like Hb%, urine routine, RBS, HBsAg, blood group and Rh typing, TSH and any other, as per institutional protocol
- Nutritional advise
- Institutional delivery
- Breastfeeding counseling.

> T1 NT and PAPP-A are the best parameters to screen for aneuploidy as, T2 triple screening test may show false positive result (beta-hCG, alpha-FP are increased and uE3 decreased in HIV + population) and increase the rate of unnecessary invasive procedures. Non-invasive prenatal diagnostic technique may be used.

Q. 4. How does the interventions reduce the transmission rate?

The interventions start from screening, and screening finds out the status and when the woman opts for termination, obviously the issue is sorted out.

When the woman continues pregnancy, if no interventions are done, the transmission rate could be to the tune of 20–45%. Some of this occurs during antenatal period, around 5–10% transmission, which is taken care by 3 drug ART started as early as possible in pregnancy to a large extent.

Intranatal transmission is 10–15% and this is prevented by antenatal ART and this 3 drug ART has even decreased the need for elective cesarean delivery in this woman.

Postnatally, breastfeeding can cause transmission to the tune of 5–20% and nevirapine for the baby, continued breastfeeding exclusively and infant diagnostic algorithms have helped in early diagnosis, effective treatment and prevention of MTCT.

By all the interventions the transmission has been found to be as low as 1–2% if effectively followed.

All antenatal interventions should aim at reducing viral load to <50 copies/mL by 36 weeks. Vaginal delivery is safe with <50 copies, but when >499 copies/mL is the viral load, LSCS is recommended. This is applicable when viral load can be determined which may not be the situation in every center.

> There are two different ways to approach pregnant women about HIV testing:
> 1. **Opt-in:**
>   - Pregnant women are given pre-HIV test counseling.
>   - They must agree to receiving an HIV test, usually in writing.
> 2. **Opt-out:**
>   - Pregnant women are told that an HIV test will be included in the standard group of prenatal tests (that is to say, tests given to all pregnant women), and that they may decline the test.
>   - Unless they decline, they will receive an HIV test.

Thus cesarean is considered only for obstetric indications.

> In the 2006 *revised recommendations for HIV testing of adults, adolescents, and pregnant women in healthcare settings*, CDC recommended the opt-out approach to testing for all adult and adolescent patients in healthcare settings, including pregnant women.

Q. 5. What are the NACO guidelines in the management of HIV positive pregnancy?

- Screen all the pregnant mothers after counseling (Opt-in/Opt-out).
- Initiate all retropositive mothers on lifelong ART at the earliest possible opportunity.

- Those on ART needs to continue them.
- Triple drug regime needs to be used (Tenofavir, Lamivudine and Efavirenz).
- Routine antenatal care and ICTC linkage to be done.
- If CD4 count is <250 co-trimoxazole prophylaxis to be started to the mother (160 mg Trimethoprim + 800 mg Sulfamethoxazole once a day) throughout pregnancy and postnatal period.
- Iron, folic acid, calcium intake needs to be assured.

Q. 6. What are the methods to diagnose and to know the severity of HIV infection?

Whole blood finger prick test-rapid tests (ELISA) done at periphery. When the report is positive, the client needs to be referred to ICTC.

Three rapid tests (antibody) are done at ICTC.

If all the three are positive the report is given as positive otherwise any other situation with one or two tests being positive is taken as indeterminate.

All three negative is taken as negative.

Western blot test is one of the confirmatory tests but not mandatory.

Indeterminate tests could be repeated with repeat 3 rapid tests after 3 months or with PCR tests by HIV RNA or branched DNA.

In infants early infant diagnosis involves PCR on dry blood sample (DBS) at 6 weeks age. If positive, whole blood HIV 1 PCR is done and if still positive, ART is initiated, otherwise the baby is followed for the next 18 months with periodic testing.

To know the severity of infection:
- CD4 count can be done
- Viral load estimation
- Detection of other opportunistic infection
- Clinical evaluation.

The aim of all the antiretroviral therapy is to bring down the viral load to between 20 and 75 copies/ml which amounts to negligible load.

Q. 7. Discuss the management of discordant couple.

- One of the spouse is retropositive and the other negative form a discordant couple. It is a delicate issue during counseling but is to be done effectively.
- Discordant couples form a special group during management of HIV. The possibilities are that the negative spouse is in the window period is to be kept in mind.
- The partner should be offered HIV testing.
- Counseling is important especially for disclosures.
- Seronegative partner would also be benefitted by antiretroviral therapy as this reduces transmission.
- If the CD4 count is >350, in spite of it, seropositive partner needs to take ART.

If pregnant, further sexual intercourse, barrier method needs to be used.

If wants to become pregnant:
- Timed intercourse only at the time of ovulation
- IUI (H) with washed sperms (When husband is +ve, otherwise routine IUI).
- IVF with washed husband's sperms (When husband is +ve).
- IUI with donor insemination (When husband is +ve).

Use of washed specimen does not guarantee total elimination of transmission.

Q. 8. Contraception for PLHIV and double protection.

Retropositive women unless have AIDS related complex or in the 4th stage, can use most of the contraception methods.

Women on ART need to be cautious about the increased failure of hormonal contraception.

Limiting methods (Tubectomy) can be used by them.

In spite of using any of the spacing or limiting methods, they need to use condom consistently for preventing other STIs and to prevent cross infection to the partner although both of them are positive for the retrovirus. This is called double or dual protection.

Individual Methods

Lactational amenorrhea method (LAM): If properly used in the first 6 months offers a good protection. If for some reasons mother is not breastfeeding, not a good method.

Limiting methods: Any method of tubal ligation, vasectomy, NSV can be used as a contraception in PLHIV. But HIV status and health of the baby is to be confirmed at 18 months of age of the baby before adopting a limiting method.

Hormonal method: Most of the hormonal methods fall under MEC category 1 or 2 in women on ART, hence can safely use COC, POP, injectable, implants LNG/etonogestrel implants.

Intrauterine contraceptive device (IUCD) is a good contraceptive method for retropositive women. Copper T 380A/Cu T 375 may be adopted immediately after delivery except in women who have AIDS and are not on ART. It can be used immediately after delivery, after abortion, as an interval method. But additional use of condoms needs to be stressed to them.

Q. 9. Discuss the breastfeeding recommendations for a HIV exposed infant.

Every mother needs to be counseled regarding the importance of breastfeeding. Non-breast-fed babies are more prone for diarrheal diseases and pneumonia. The mortality due to which is far higher than the risk of HIV transmission due to breastfeeding. At the same time adopting 3 drug ART for mothers, infant prophylaxis with nevirapine for the first 6 weeks substantially reduces the transmission in spite of breastfeeding.

> Interventions for infants at 6 weeks:
> - Do re-inforcement for exclusive breastfeeding for the first 6 months (Continuation of breastfeeds with introduction of complementary feeds thereafter)
> - Do EID testing
> - Do immunization
> - Do CPT initiation and continue until baby is 18 months old or longer if baby is confirmed positive
> - Do stop NVP Prophylaxis for baby at 6 weeks

Hence, the mother need to exclusively brest feed for first 6 months, wean from 6 months.

Continue breastfeeding for 1 year, if the baby is negative with early infant diagnosis algorithm.

Continue breastfeeding for 2 years if the baby is positive with Early infant diagnosis algorithm.

> If the mother strongly denies to breastfeed, consider exclusive replacement feeds. Never mix both which increases the transmission possibility because of gut fragility and damage due to replacement food. The replacement is considered if there is assurance regarding affordability, feasibility, safety, sustainability and acceptability by family (AFASS criteria)

Q. 10. Comment on CD4 monitoring.

Baseline CD4 count needs to be determined to decide upon the need for ART but in a pregnant mother irrespective of her CD4 count ART is initiated.

A CD4 count decides about the need for CPT prophylaxis (Initiated at CD4 <250).

Viral load determination and monitoring may be better and have implications on the management options (LSCS *vs* vaginal delivery, etc.) but may not be available at every center.

Otherwise CD4 are monitored once in 6 months at the ART centers and cost is a limiting factor today and more frequent monitoring may not be feasible.

Q. 11. Drug regime of NACO in pregnant women.

Three drug regime is the preferred ART in antenatal retropositive women.

Tenofovir (TDF) (300 mg) + Lamivudine (3TC) (300 mg) + Efavirenz (EFV) (600 mg).

This needs to be initiated as early as possible in pregnancy, at the earliest opportunity. Those who are already on ART need to continue.

> Safety is a critical issue for pregnant (Risk of teratogenicity) and breastfeeding women and infants (Secretion in milk and any adverse effects on the baby) and women planning pregnancy (Teratogenicity). Data provide increased assurance for recommending TDF+3TC+EFV as the first-line ART regimen for pregnant and breastfeeding women EFV also may be used in first trimester. Women on EFV already need not terminate their pregnancy for this reason.

Viral load is an important determinant of transmission to the baby and thus reducing the viral load is very critical in reducing the transmission to the baby. This is achieved by this three drug regime effectively. The viral load when reduced to <1000 copies/mL transmission is <1%.

If the patient is exposed to antiretroviral drug neviripine in the previous pregnancy then cross resistance with efavirenz is common as they belong to the same group and thus in these women efavirenz is replaced with lopinavir or ritonavir.

Q. 12. What are the other measures to be taken in retropositive pregnant mother.

- Screen for STIs.
- Screen for Tuberculosis in each visit, start the ATT if positive and postpone the initiation of ART by 2 weeks after initiating ART.

Table 1: Estimated HIV transmission risk per exposure for specific activities and events

Activity	Risk
Vaginal sex female to male	1 in 263
Male to female	1 in 333

Contd...

Contd...

Activity	Risk
Receptive anal sex from unknown	1 in 370
Receptive anal sex from HIV +	1 in 123
MTCT with viral load <50	1 in 1000
Injecting drug	1 in 41 to 1 in 150
Needle stick	1 in 769
Blood transfusion	9 in 10
Heterosexual unsafe sex = 1 L breast milk consumption of HIV + mother	

Neviripine is not preferred to be used with Rifampicin, Efavirenz may be used. If EFV is not tolerated, NVP or a boosted PI regimen is to be given, but rifampicin needs to be changed to Rifabutin.

Q. 13. What are the risk factors that increase the rate of vertical transmission?

The following factors are associated with increased risk of mother to child transmission.

> Expanded rescreening in the third trimester for women who test negative for HIV early in pregnancy especially with high-risk behavior or with strong clinical suspicion.

- Antenatal transmission is less before 36 weeks, whereas it could be around 50% of the total transmission during antenatal period.
- Vaginal delivery poses increased risk-effectively reduced by 3 drug ART.
- Breastfeeding risk which is substantial is also reduced by maternal ART and NVP to baby for 6 weeks.
- Preterm labor increases the risk by 4 times.
- Viral load is an important risk factor.
- PROM >4 hours risk is around 25%, 1 hour PROM 2% increase.

A fall in CD4 to <15% of normal causes FGR in about 20–25% and preterm labor in 20%, 3 drug ART and cesarean delivery together reduce the risk by about 90%.

Q. 14. What are the opportunistic infections encountered in PLHIV?

A person with HIV due to immunocompromise is predisposed to various uncommon infections which are not commonly found in other negative population. This is to say the infections are found in immunocompromised individuals who cannot immunologically fight against these. They are:

- Tuberculosis
- Oropharyngeal candidiasis
- Herpes-zoster-dissemination also
- Cryptococcal meningitis
- Bacterial pneumonia
- Cryptosporidiosis
- *Pneumocystis jiroveci (carinii)* pneumonia
- Toxoplasmosis.

If the above infections are found in a pregnant woman, HIV needs to be considered.

Q. 15. Discuss the strategies for prevention of HIV transmission (primary, secondary, tertiary) personal protection, PEP.

Primary Prevention

To prevent infection from occurring. Table 1 gives the risk associated with various ways by which HIV may be transmitted. Very important for health care personnel and the other patients who are cared for in the same health care facility:

- Disposable latex gloves
- Disposable laboratory gowns
- Disposable plastic aprons
- Disposable face mask/goggles
- Disposable caps
  - Shoe covers
  - Rubber boots
  - Hand rubs/disinfectant solution for hand wash
  - Needle destroyer
  - Sharp disposal containers
  - 1% sodium hypochlorite.

Secondary Prevention

If a person accidentally gets exposed to the risk of HIV infection, he needs to take post-exposure prophylaxis preferably initiated within 3 days of exposure. It could be an injury with needle, scalpel, exposure to body fluids, etc. The severity is graded. The treatment is to be taken for 4 weeks. It also needs to be considered in unprotected sex and sexual assault victims. It may not be 100% effective.

Administering Neviripine to the baby is a secondary preventive strategy.

Tertiary Prevention

Screening a pregnant woman—could be a secondary preventive strategy with respect to the baby if she continues pregnancy, primary for the baby (not allowing a positive baby to be born at all!), if she wants to terminate, but tertiary for her if found positive.

Other interventions in the ART center aims at tertiary prevention which is prevention of progression and complications.

Q. 16. Drug classification and mode of action.

The life cycle of the HIV virus dictates the classification of drugs to know at what level in the cycle the drug interferes the progression (Flowchart 1).

- NRTIs (Nucleoside reverse Transcriptase Inhibitors)
  - Zidovudine (AZT)
  - Stavudine
  - Lamivudine (3TC)
  - Tenofovir (TDF)
  - Combination of some of the above drugs
- NNRTIs (Non-nucleoside reverse transcriptase inhibitors)
  - Nevirapine (NVP)
  - Efavirenz (EFV)
  - Etravirine (ETR)
  - Rilpivirine (RPV)
- Protease inhibitors
  - Indinavir (IDV)
  - Ritonavir (RTV)
  - Lopinavir (LPV)
  - Tipranavir (TPV)
  - Darunavir (DRV)

- Entry inhibitors
  - Enfuvirtide
  - Maraviroc
- Integrase inhibitors (some are on trial as once a month injections)
  - Raltegravir
  - Elvitegravir
  - Dolutegravir
  - Cabotegravir

*Dual therapy with 3TC and integrase inhibitor has been found to be coming with remarkable results

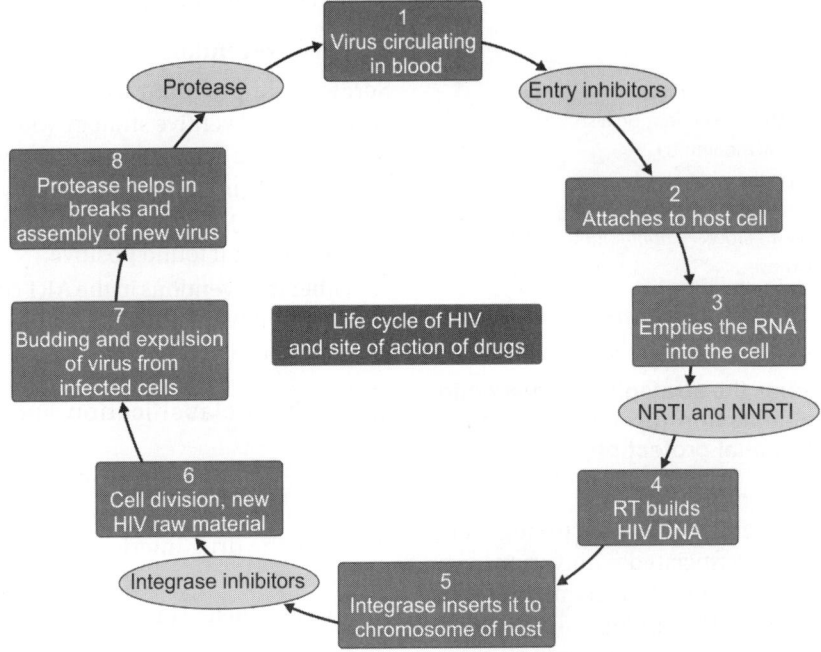

Flowchart 1: Site and mechanism of action of antiretroviral drugs.

Q. 17. Comment on HIV 2 infection.

- HIV 2 is a less severe infection
- Progression to AIDS is slow
- MTCT is less around 0–4%
- Some pockets of western India, it is found
- Transmission is similar to HIV 1
- ELISA test that is done to screen for HIV is the method for HIV 2 also
- It can sometimes co exist with HIV 1. In this the treatment is as it is for HIV 1
- HIV 2 is not acted upon by NNRTI (NVP/EFZ) hence a combination of 2 NRTIs and a protease inhibitor (LPR) is preferred.
- Infant prophylaxis is with ziduvidine.

Q. 18. What measures need to be taken during delivery of a retropositive parturient?

- Vaginal delivery is the preferred mode as protection from cesarean against MTCT is almost half of the protection offered by 3 drugs ART
- Take universal precautions when the status is known (even when not known)
- Except in suspected fetal distress do not rupture the membranes
- Avoid frequent internal examination (P/V)
- Prefer non-invasive fetal monitoring over invasive procedures

- Avoid episiotomy, instrumental deliveries especially ventouse, as ventouse is known to be more traumatic to fetus than forceps.
- Routine newborn care, try to avoid suctioning of the newborn.

> PPH is managed with oxytocin and PGs, as ergots can interact with reverse transcriptase inhibitors and protease inhibitors (PIs) to cause severe vasoconstriction.

Q. 19. Discuss the measures to be taken during cesarean section in a retropositive mother.

- Cesarean delivery is done only for obstetric indications
- Universal precautions
- Better to be done a senior person
- Follow surgical planes to minimize bleeding
- Blunt dissection is preferred to use of knives and scissors
- Cautery use may be good for hemostasis
- 'Caul delivery' with intact membranes at least till the head comes out is desirable
- Practice early cord clamping
- Effective measures to be taken to prevent PPH/manage energetically PPH
- Long sturdy, blunt needles are preferred for suturing
- Transfer the sharps placing them in a kidney tray instead of handing over directly
- Use forceps or other instruments while handling the needles (No touch)
- Follow proper tissue, instrument, soiled cloth disposal and OT disinfection procedures.

Q. 20. Discuss the lab diagnosis of HIV infection and tests available for HIV testing.

The tests for diagnosing HIV are classified as antibody tests and antigen tests.

Antibody Tests

- **ELISA test**: ELISA test is done as the first screening test at the primary level. This is an antibody test. It is done 3 times and if all are positive then the case is reported as positive. It is a highly sensitive test.
- **Western blot test**: This is usually done to confirm a positive ELISA. But nowadays it is not mandatory, three ELISAs are the routinely followed method.
- **Saliva tests**: Buccal swab is being used to look for HIV infection, but needs confirmation by blood tests.

Antigen Tests

- **Viral load**: It is a quantification test. It is important to know the severity of infection, response to treatment and to decide about certain obstetric management like, route of delivery, ECV, etc.
  It may look for reverse transcription PCR (RT-PCR), branched DNA (bDNA), nucleic acid sequence-based amplification (NASBA).
- **HIV RNA test (PCR)**: It can detect the virus in the blood within 9 days of infection.
- **Antigen p24 test**: p24 is a protein antigen present on the cell surface of the virus which can be detected by ELISA accurately.

Q. 21. Discuss the early infant diagnosis algorithms.

Early infant diagnosis follows two algorithms:
1. Within 6 months
2. 6–18 months

Infant is tested at:
- 6 weeks
- If symptomatic at any time
- 6 weeks after last breastfeeding
- 6 months
- 12 months
- 18 months
- From 6 weeks to within 6 months antigen test, i.e. dry blood spot (DBS) for HIV DNA PCR is done. If positive, confirmed by whole blood DNA PCR and initiated on infant ART.
- From 6 months to 18 months, rapid test is done if positive DNA PCR is done on

DBS, followed by whole blood PCR, if DBS is positive. If rapid test is negative, if breastfed in the last 6 weeks, repeat test at 12 months/after 6 weeks of cessation of breastfeeding. If not breastfed in the last 6 weeks, baby is preferably not put to breast anymore and CPT is stopped.
- In all the negative cases, 3 rapid tests are done at 18 months and if found negative then the baby is declared as non-infected.

Bibliography

1. Baggaley RF, et al. Risk of HIV-1 transmission for parenteral exposure and blood transfusion. AIDS. 2006;20:805-12.
2. Boily MC, et al. Heterosexual risk of HIV-1 infection per sexual act: systematic review and meta-analysis of observational studies. Lancet Infect Dis. 2009;9(2):118-29.
3. Branson B. Current HIV epidemiology and revised recommendations for HIV testing in health-care settings. J Med Virol. 2007;79(Suppl)1:S6-10.
4. British HIV Association (BHIVA) guidelines for the management of HIV infection in pregnant women 2012 (2014 interim review) (UPDated May 2014).
5. CDC. Detection of acute HIV infection in two evaluations of a new HIV diagnostic testing algorithm—United States, 2011- 2013. MMWR Morb Mortal Wkly Rep. 2013;62:489-94.
6. Cunningham FG, Leveno KJ, et al. William's Obstetrics, 24th edn.
7. Current progress in obstetrics and gynaecology, John Studd, Vol 2.
8. Del Romero J, et al. Evaluating the risk of HIV transmission through unprotected orogenital sex. AIDS. 2002;16(9):1296-7.
9. Ford N, Ekouevi DK, et al. Use of Efavirenz during pregnancy: a public health perspective, technical update on treatment optimisation, Geneva, World Health Organization, 2012.
10. Forsgren A, Nordstrom K. Protein A from *Staphylococcus aureus*: the biological significance of its reaction with IgG. Ann N Y Acad Sci. 1974;236(0):252-66.
11. Garcia PM, Kalish LA, Pitt J, et al. Maternal levels of plasma human immunodeficiency virus type 1 RNA and the risk of perinatal transmission. Women and Infants Transmission Study Group. The New England Journal of Medicine. 1994;341(6):394-402.
12. Gross S, Castillo W, Crane M, et al. Maternal serum alpha-fetoprotein and human chorionic gonadotropin levels in women with human immunodeficiency virus. Am J Obstet Gynecol. 2003;188:1052-6.
13. Gupta A, Bhosale R, Kinikar A, et al. For the Six Week Extended-Dose Nevirapine (SWEN) India Study Team. Maternal Tuberculosis: A Risk Factor for Mother-to-Child-Transmission of Human Immunodeficiency virus. JID 2011:203 (1 February).
14. Key tests to monitor HIV – CD4 and viral load aidsmap.com, 2013.
15. Laboratory Testing Plasma HIV-1 RNA (Viral Load) and CD4 Count Monitoring; AIDS info, 2014.
16. Ly TD, Ebel A, Faucher V, Fihman V, Laperche S. Could the new HIV combined p24 antigen and antibody assays replace p24 antigen specific assays? J Virol Methods. 2007;143(1):86-94. Laboratory Testing for the Diagnosis of HIV Infection: Updated Recommendations Published June 27, 2014 CDC.
17. Masciotra S, McDougal JS, Feldman J, Sprinkle P, Wesolowski L, Owen SM. Evaluation of an alternative HIV diagnostic algorithm using specimens from seroconversion panels and persons with established HIV infections. J ClinVirol. 2011;52(Suppl 1):S17-22.
18. McDonagh EM, Thorn CF, Bautista JM, et al. PharmGKB summary: very important pharmacogene information for G6PD. Pharmacogenet Genomics. 2012;22(3):219-28.
19. MEC for Contraceptive Use, 5th edn WHO.
20. Minkoff Howard. Human immunodeficiency virus infection in pregnancy. Obstetrics and Gynecology. 2003;101(4):797-810.
21. Mother-to-child transmission of HIV infection in the era of highly active antiretroviral therapy. Clinical Infectious Diseases: An Official Publication of the Infectious Diseases Society of America. 2005;40(3):458-65.

22. Nasrullah M, Wesolowski LG, Meyer WA, et al. Performance of a fourth-generation HIV screening assay and an alternative HIV diagnostic testing algorithm. AIDS. 2013;27(5):731-7.
23. Savvidou MD, Samuel I, Syngelaki A, et al. First-trimester markers of aneuploidy in women positive for HIV. Br J Obstet Gynecol. 2011;118:844-8.
24. Ford N, et al. The future role of CD4 cell count for monitoring antiretroviral therapy. Lancet Infectious Diseases. 15(2):131-24. (AIDS infonet .org)
25. The World Health Organization release "Guidance on couples HIV testing and counselling, including antiretroviral therapy (ART) for treatment and prevention in serodiscordant couples: Recommendations for a public health approach" conception in HIV-discordant couples 2nd edn J. T. Wilde.
26. Townsend C, et al. Low rates of mother-to-child transmission of HIV following effective pregnancy interventions in the United Kingdom and Ireland, 2000-2006. AIDS. 2008;22:973-81.
27. Tzong-Hae L, Daniel MC, Robert JB, et al. The role of transplacental microtransfusions of maternal lymphocytes in in utero HIV transmission. J Acquir Imm Deficien Syndrom. 1999;55(2):143-7.
28. Vittinghoff E, et al. Per-contact risk of human immunodeficiency virus transmission between male sexual partners. American Journal of Epidemiology. 1999;150:306-11.

17
CHAPTER

Recurrent Pregnancy Loss

Ratnamala Desai

CASE

Mrs X a 28-year-old woman wife of Mr Y comes to the OPD with history of amenorrhea from three months. She is a gravida IV, para 0, miscarriages III.

She gives history of amenorrhea from three months. She has no other complaints. She is very anxious because she has had three spontaneous miscarriages and has come to the hospital for further evaluation. This is her first antenatal visit.

History of Present Pregnancy

First Trimester

- Patient has conceived spontaneously
- No history of vomiting
- No history of fever or rashes
- No history of burning micturition
- No history of bleeding or discharge per vaginum
- No history of radiation or any teratogen exposure.

Menstrual History

- Past menstrual cycles are regular
- LMP
- EDD

Obstetric History

- Married life from 4 years
- Gravida IV para 0 miscarriages III
- Patient gives history of three consecutive missed miscarriages. All three pregnancies were spontaneous conceptions. Each time the pregnancy was confirmed by urinary pregnancy test. The patient gives history of cardiac activity being confirmed on ultrasonography for every pregnancy. However, the patient had consecutive miscarriages at about 12 weeks.
- Last miscarriage was eight months back.
- No history of the abortuses being subjected for examination.

Past History

No history of diabetes mellitus, hypertension, hypothyroidism, tuberculosis or any other chronic illness in the past. No history of any bleeding disorders.

Personal History

- Patient is a vegetarian.
- Her bowel and bladder habits are regular.
- She has no addictions.

Family History

- No family history of diabetes or hypertension.
- There is no history of recurrent pregnancy loss in the family.

Recurrent Pregnancy Loss

Socioeconomic History
Patient belongs to class II according to modified Kuppuswamy classification.

Dietary History
Patient takes 2,000 calories per day. Her protein and mineral intake is adequate.

On Examination
Patient is conscious and well oriented to time, place and person. Patient is moderately built and nourished. Her height is 155 cm. Her weight is 54 kg.

Vitals
- Her pulse rate is 80/min regular, good in volume, bilateral synchronous without any radiofemoral delay
- Her BP is 120/80 mm Hg
- Her JVP is not raised. She is afebrile
- Her respiratory rate is 20/min.

General Physical Examination
- On general physical examination, there is no pallor, icterus, cyanosis, clubbing, lymphadenopathy or pedal edema.
- Breasts, spine and thyroid examination are normal.

Systemic Examination
Cardiovascular system: S1 and S2 heard. No murmurs heard.
Respiratory system: Air entry equal on both the sides. No added sounds or crepitations heard.
Central nervous system: No abnormality detected.
Abdominal examination
Inspection:
- Abdomen is scaphoid in shape
- Umbilicus is normal
- No scars or visible veins
- Hernial orifices are normal
- No hepatosplenomegaly.

Palpation:
- Uterus is just palpable in the suprapubic region.
- No other mass felt.

Per speculum examination:
- Cervix is healthy, no discharge.

Bimanual pelvic examination:
- Uterus is 12–14 weeks size, soft globular
- No adnexal masses.

Final Diagnosis
A 20-year-old woman gravida IV para 0 missed miscarriages III with 12 weeks gestation for evaluation.

Q. 1. What is the incidence of spontaneous miscarriage?
The incidence of spontaneous miscarriages is about 15% amongst clinical pregnancies. Many miscarriages occur before pregnancy is diagnosed. Only one third of all pregnancies end in live births.[1]

Q. 2. What is the definition of RPL?
Recurrent pregnancy loss (RPL), recurrent miscarriage (RM) or recurrent abortion or habitual abortion is defined as three or more consecutive miscarriages occurring before twenty weeks of gestation. The Practice Committee of the American Society for Reproductive Medicine defines RPL as two or more miscarriages.[2]

Q. 3. What is the incidence of RPL?
Only 1–2% women experience recurrent miscarriage.

Q. 4. What are the risks of miscarriage after two or three miscarriages?
The risk of having a recurrent miscarriage after 2 miscarriages is 30%, whereas the

risk of having a recurrent miscarriage after 3 miscarriages is 33%.

Q. 5. What are the risk factors for RPL?

- Maternal age >35 years
- Paternal age >40 years
- Number of previous pregnancy losses
- Cigarette smoking
- Alcohol consumption
- Caffeine intake
- Polycystic ovarian syndrome (PCOS)
- Maternal obesity.

Q. 6. What are the causes of RPL?

The accepted causative factors for RPL include parental chromosomal abnormalities, uterine abnormalities, and antiphospholipid antibody syndrome. Other possible causes include endocrine disorders, thrombophilias, immunologic abnormalities, infections, and environmental factors. In about 50% of the cases no definite causative factor can be detected.[3]

Though the cause for RPL is unexplained in 50% of the cases, the likelihood of a live birth is 50–80%, without any interventions with evidence-based treatment and supportive care.[4]

Q. 7. What is the incidence of chromosomal abnormalities in sporadic miscarriages, and RPL?

Approximately, 50–60% of spontaneous first trimester miscarriages are due to chromosomal abnormalities. Fetal aneuploidy is the most common cause of sporadic first trimester pregnancy loss. Chromosomal abnormalities are seen in about 2–4% of the couples suffering from recurrent pregnancy loss. The chromosomal abnormalities commonly associated with recurrent pregnancy loss are balanced reciprocal or Robertsonian translocations. Chromosomal abnormalities such as mosaicism, insertions and inversions are also associated with recurrent pregnancy loss.

Q. 8. What are the anatomical factors which cause RPL?

Anatomical abnormalities account for 15% of the cases of RPL. Congenital abnormalities of the uterus that cause RPL are bicornuate uterus, unicornuate uterus, septate uterus, uterus didelphys, arcuate uterus and cervical insufficiency. Acquired conditions causing RPL are intrauterine adhesions, uterine fibroids, cervical insufficiency and polyps. The miscarriage is caused by interruption of the vascular supply resulting in abnormal placentation. Septate uterus has 76% risk of miscarriage.[5] While septate uterus causes first trimester pregnancy loss, arcuate uterus and cervical insufficiency cause second trimester pregnancy loss.

Q. 9. What are the causes of cervical insufficiency?

Cervical insufficiency can be congenital or acquired.

- *Congenital:* Mullerian anomalies—uterus didelphys, bicornuate uterus, unicornuate uterus.
- *Acquired:* Cervical amputation, conization, large loop excision procedure of the transformation zone and trachelectomy.

Q. 10. What are the endocrine causes for RPL?

Endocrine disorders account for about 8–12% of recurrent pregnancy losses. The common endocrine disorders which may cause recurrent pregnancy loss are diabetes mellitus, thyroid disorders, polycystic ovarian disease, hyperprolactinemia and luteal phase defect.[6]

Polycystic ovarian syndrome is likely to cause RPL. The causative factors being hyperinsulinemia and hyperandrogenemia.

However, uncontrolled diabetes mellitus and hypothyroidism are known to cause spontaneous miscarriage. There is no evidence to show that they cause RPL.

Q. 11. What are the immunological causes for RPL?

Immunological factors account for 15% of RPL. Immune factors can be autoimmune or alloimmune. Autoimmune causes are systemic lupus erythematosis (SLE) and antiphospholipid antibody syndrome (APLA syndrome).

Alloimmune factors: Conception and pregnancy being carried to term is dependent on the mother's immune tolerance. Immunological imbalance has been demonstrated where the fetus and placenta are affected by maternal autoantibodies or autoreactive cells leading to infertility or RPL. Alloimmune rejection-type activity of maternal humoral or cellular immunity is responsible for RPL.[7]

Q. 12. What is APLA syndrome?

APLA syndrome is an important cause for RPL. APLA syndrome is an autoimmune disease with antiphospholipid antibodies produced against one's own tissues. These antibodies interfere with blood coagulation. APLA syndrome is associated with antiphospholipid antibodies and adverse pregnancy outcome or vascular thrombosis. Antiphospholipid antibodies are found in 2–5% of uncomplicated pregnancies. However, antiphopholipid antibodies are found in 5–15% of women with recurrent pregnancy loss. The antiphospholipid antibodies cause a procoagulant phenotype in the blood vessels. They also cause changes in placenta, like abnormalities in proliferation and differentiation of the cells. These changes are responsible for the vascular and placental complications associated with the syndrome.[8]

Q. 13. What is the role of inherited thrombophilias in RPL?

Several inherited and acquired thrombophilias, such as Factor V Leiden mutation, prothrombin gene mutation, hyperhomocysteinemia, protein C/S and antithrombin deficiencies III are causative factors for systemic thrombosis. In inherited thrombophilas thrombosis of the uteroplacental vasculature may cause recurrent pregnancy loss.

Q. 14. What are the complications of thrombophilias in pregnancy?

- Recurrent pregnancy loss
- Intrauterine growth restriction
- Intrauterine death
- Preeclampsia
- Preterm labor
- Abruptio placentae
- Venous thromboembolism.

Q. 15. What is the role of infections in causing RPL?

Severe infections can cause spontaneous miscarriage. Infections like Listeria monocytogenes, TORCH infections and coxsackie virus infections cause spontaneous miscarriage. Bacterial vaginosis is a risk factor for preterm births and late miscarriages.[9] Immune-compromised patients with chronic infections may have recurrent pregnancy loss.

Q. 16. What are the environmental factors which cause RPL?

Exposure to environmental factors such as ionizing radiation, toxins and chemicals may result in spontaneous miscarriage or recurrent pregnancy loss. The risk of spontaneous miscarriage and recurrent pregnancy loss may increase with alcohol, caffeine and nicotine consumption by the mother.

Q. 17. What are the epidemiological factors which cause RPL?

Maternal age is an important determinant of pregnancy outcome. As the maternal age increases the risk of pregnancy loss increases. A history of prior miscarriage predisposes the woman to a recurrence of miscarriage.

Increased body mass index above the normal range may cause spontaneous miscarriage as well as recurrent pregnancy loss.

Q. 18. When do you start investigations in a case of RPL?

A couple should be investigated for recurrent pregnancy loss after two consecutive miscarriages, particularly if the couple do not have a living child. Investigations should be initiated early without waiting for the third miscarriage to recur if the couple are subfertile or the woman is aged more than 35 years.

Q. 19. What are the investigations recommended for RPL?

Apart from the routine investigations done for all antenatal cases, the following investigations need to be done:
- Complete blood count
- Serological tests for syphilis
- Thyroid function test
- Glucose tolerance test
- Karyotyping of the couple
- Indirect Coomb's test
- Antiphospholipid antibodies
- Anti-beta-2 glyoprotein I antibodies
- Serum prolactin
- Serum insulin
- Cytogenetic studies of the products of conception
- Transvaginal ultrasonography
- Three-dimensional (3D) ultrasound
- Magnetic resonance imaging (MRI)
- Screening for thrombophilias
- Vaginal swab for culture sensitivity.

Q. 20. What are the indications for fetal/parental karyotyping?

Fetal
- Chronic villus biopsy (CVB), amniocentesis, cordocentesis, noninvasive prenatal testing (NIPT)
- Abnormal biochemical/combined screening test—high risk
- Other risk factors like previous children with aneuploidy, siblings of the parents with mental retardation, aneuploidy, abnormal markers on fetal USG, family history of chromosomal abnormality and cansanguinous marriage.

During the Perinatal Period
- *Abortus:* If more than 2 unexplained abortions
- *Stillbirth:* When the cause cannot be established or in suspected chromosomal abnormality, can be done from umbilical cord, muscle fibroblasts, etc.

Postnatally
Anomalies, dysmorphology or ambiguous genitalia.

Parental
- Fetus/infant has chromosomal abnormality
- RPL in whom other causes are ruled out.

Q. 21. What is the importance of cytogenetic studies in RPL?

Cytogenetic studies of the products of conception is indicated in RPL. Chromosomal abnormalities are detected in 50-60% of spontaneous miscarriages. More than 50% of these are autosomal trisomies. Routine karyotyping of the couples with recurrent miscarriage is not recommended. A strong family history of RPL or a chromosomal abnormality in one of the partners indicates parental karyotyping. Parental karyotyping is indicated in unbalanced chromosomal abnormality in the products of conception.

Q. 22. What are the different methods employed for chromosomal analysis

The various methods may be classified as direct and indirect methods:
- Cytotrophoblastic culture and mesenchymal cell culture and karyotyping—2-3 weeks
- Flourescent in situ hybridization (FISH) can be done quickly and needs specific

probes for each chromosome. Hence, a few selected chromosomes like X, Y, 13, 18 and 21 may be studied by this—2-3 days
- Quantitative fluorescent PCR: Used similar to FISH, but it reduces contamination chances due to maternal tissues.
- Chromosom microarray analysis (CMA): No need for cell culture. Failure rates are less. Works on formalin fixed tissue. Rules out maternal contamination. Sub-microscopic copy number variants (CNV) are detected. Neither ACOG nor European best practice guidelines recommend its routine use in prenatal diagnostic tests. But some CNV of unknown significance if detected, it creates parental anxiety which cannot be clarified.
  - Single nucleoside polymorphism array
  - Array CGH (comparative genomic hybridization)
    - Helps to detect small amount of excess or defect in chromosomes. It can be done fast.
    - Eight hours as it can be done on uncultured cells. May miss balanced translocations and triploidy.

Q. 23. What are the investigations done for anatomic defects?

All women with RPL must undergo a transvaginal sonography to assess the uterine anatomy. Sonohysterography is a simple noninvasive method with 95% accuracy in identifying uterine anomalies. Suspected cases may require further evaluation with hysteroscopy, laparoscopy, 3D ultrasound or MRI.

Q. 24. How is luteal phase defect (LPD) diagnosed?

LPD is diagnosed when there is a lag in histological dating of endometrium by two days or mid-luteal phase serum progesterone level is less than 10 ng/mL.

Q. 25. How do you diagnose APLA syndrome?

All women with RPL should be investigated for the presence of anticardiolipin antibodies, lupus anticoagualant and anti-β2GP-1 (anti-β2 glycoprotein-1). Presence of anticardiolipin antibodies is not diagnostic of APLA syndrome. Antiphospholipid antibody syndrome is diagnosed when antiphopholipid antibodies are found in moderate to high titers on two occasions twelve weeks apart. Antiphospholipid antibodies may be found in infections such as syphilis, lyme disease, viral infections caused by hepatitis C, human immune deficiency virus and cytomegalovirus. The anti-β2GP-1 immunoassay is more specific but not as sensitive as anticardiolipin antibody assays for the diagnosis of antiphopholipid antibody syndrome.[10]

APLA Syndrome is characterized by the presence of at least 1 clinical and 1 laboratory criterion.[11,12]

- Clinical
  - 1 or more confirmed episodes of vascular thrombosis (venous, arterial, or small vessel)
  - Pregnancy complications, including:
    - Either 3 or more consecutive pregnancy losses at less than 10 weeks of gestation
    - 1 or more fetal deaths at greater than 10 weeks of gestation
    - At least 1 preterm birth (<34 weeks) due to severe preeclampsia or placental insufficiency
- Laboratory (repeated at least 2 times, more than 12 weeks apart)
  - Positive plasma levels of the anti-cardiolipin antibodies (IgG or IgM) at medium to high levels
  - Positive plasma levels of the lupus anti-coagulant
  - Positive plasma levels of anti-β2 GP1 antibody of IgG and/or IgM at medium or high titer.

Q. 26. What is seronegative APLA and what is resistant APLA?

When a lady presents with history strongly suggestive of APLA but serological tests show no positive results, the situation is called seronegative APLA. They respond to low molecular weight heparin and aspirin as any other seropositive case.

Resistant APLA is one in which in spite of treating with low dose aspirin and low molecular weight heparin, patient may abort. This may be treated with double dose of aspirin (150 mg), chloroquine or therapeutic dose of low molecular weight heparin.

Q. 27. Should screening for thrombophilias be done routinely?

There is a weak association between thromophilias and recurrent pregnancy loss. Some studies show a stronger relation between thrombophilias and stillbirth rather than RPL. Screening for thrombophilias is not cost effective and should be done under research settings.[13,14]

Q. 28. Should screening for TORCH infections be done in RPL?

TORCH infection screening is not indicated in RPL as TORCH infections cause sporadic abortions and do not cause RPL.

Q. 29. What preconceptional counseling should be done for RPL?

Couples with RPL need to counseled by an experienced obstetrician. They should be preferably managed in a dedicated RPL clinic.

Women should be counseled regarding high rates of successful pregnancies with supportive treatment.

Lifestyle modifications should be advised. Women should be advised to stop smoking and alcohol consumption. Caffeine should be taken in moderation. Women who are overweight should reduce their weight. Environmental and occupational toxins, if any, should be avoided.

Preconceptional folic acid should be started.

Q. 30. What are the treatment options for RPL?

As this is high-risk pregnancy, such cases are better treated in tertiary care centers.

Treatment options depend on the etiology that has been worked up.

Q. 31. What are the options for women with RPL caused by genetic factors?

If the parental karyotyping is abnormal, the couple need to be referred to a geneticist for counseling. Couples with translocations must be offered preimplantation genetic diagnosis, gamete donation or adoption. For conditions that cause embryonic aneuploidy like Robertsonian translocation the couple may be offered conception with donor gametes.[15]

Q. 32. What is the treatment for RPL caused by anatomical factors?

Anatomical causes for RPL include septate uterus, bicornuate uterus, intrauterine adhesions, fibroids and polyps. Surgical treatment is beneficial in all these lesions except bicornuate uterus.[16]

The live birth rates increased after septal resection to 81.3% as compared to 61.5% in those who did not undergo septal resection. Hysteroscopic septal resection has shown good results. The live birth rates after hysteroscopic septal resection is as high as 85%.[17]

In women who had a bicornuate uterus surgery reduced the preterm deliveries and low-birth weight.[18]

Myomectomy should be offered for women with submucosal fibroids or any fibroid more than 5 cm. The live birth rates increase from 57 to 93%.[19]

Women with history suggestive of cervical insufficiency are likely to benefit with cervical encerclage. Cervical encerclage is not without risks. It can stimulate uterine contractions, and cause miscarriage. Cervical encerclage has proven to be beneficial in women when cervical length was less than 25 mm before 24 weeks of gestation.[20]

Q. 33. What are the indications for cervical encerclage?

- History compatible with incompetent cervix
- Sonogram demonstrating funneling
- Clinical evidence of cervical trauma.

Q. 34. What are contraindications for cerclage?

- Uterine contractions
- Bleeding per vagina
- Premature rupture of membranes
- Chorioamnionitis
- Cervical dilatation more than 4 cm.

Q. 35. What are the complications of cervical encerclage?

- Rupture of membranes
- Infection
- Hemorrhage
- Cervical tears
- Preterm labor
- Cervical dystocia.

Q. 36. What is the role of hormonal treatment in RPL?

Progesterone is an essential hormone for implantation and maintenance of pregnancy. Progesterone is an immunomodulator and induces anti-inflammatory Th-2 cytokine response which protects pregnancy and down regulates Th-1 cytokines which cause termination of pregnancy. *There is no evidence for routine supplementation of progestogen for prevention of miscarriage.* There seems to be evidence to support progesterone supplementation for prevention of RPL.[21]

The role of human chorionic gonadotropin supplementation in prevention of RPL is also unclear.

Miscarriage in women with PCOS is caused by insulin resistance. However, there is no evidence to use metformin for prevention of RPL.

Q. 37. What is the treatment of APLA syndrome?

Low dose aspirin and heparin should be considered for the treatment of APLA syndrome to prevent recurrent pregnancy loss. Low dose aspirin can be administered before pregnancy or after the pregnancy test becomes positive. Unfractionated heparin or low molecular weight heparin can be started after the pregnancy test is positive. Heparin is safe in pregnancy as it does not cross the placenta because of the large molecule. The risk of thrombocytopenia and osteopenia is less with low molecular weight heparin compared to unfractionated heparin.[22] Intravenous immunoglobulins and corticosteroids have not shown any benefit compared to heparin and low dose aspirin. Corticosteroids may cause fetal and maternal complications.[23,24]

Q. 38. What is the pregnancy outcome in APLA syndrome?

The pregnancy outcome in women with APLA syndrome is very poor if treatment is not initiated. Pregnancy loss is as high as 90% with a successful outcome of only 10%. Heparin and low dose aspirin administered to women with APLA syndrome reduces the pregnancy loss rate by 54%.[23]

Q. 39. What is immunotherapy?

Various immunotherapies like intravenous immunoglobulin, third-party donor leukocytes, trophoblast membranes and paternal cell immunization have not shown any benefit.[26] In a large trial intravenous immunoglobulin did not improve the live birth rates, hence, it is not recommended for prevention of RPL in clinical practice.[27]

Further research is needed to know if immunological treatment modalities using natural killer cells, tumor necrosis factor α, regulatory T-cells, cell derived microparticles leptin, some glycoproteins and cytokines will improve the outcome in recurrent pregnancy loss.[28]

Q. 40. How do you treat hyperhomocysteinemia?

Supplementation with folate, vitamin B_6 and vitamin B_{12}.

Q. 41. How do you treat inherited thrombophilias?

There is no evidence to show that anticoagulation improves live birth rates. Studies in women with unexplained RPL and inherited thrombophilias has not shown any beneficial effects with either aspirin and/or heparin.[29]

Further research is needed to know if low molecular weight heparin improves live birth rates in women with thrombophilia.

Q. 42. Can low molecular weight heparin be used for the treatment of unexplained RPL?

As there is lack of evidence to support the use of low molecular weight heparin for the treatment of unexplained RPL it should not be offered routinely.[30,31]

Q. 43. What is the prognosis for women with RPL?

The prognosis will depend on the cause and the number of losses. Correction of anatomic defects and treatment of endocrinal disorders and APLA syndrome will result in a 60–90% success rate. Patients with genetic disorders have a success rate of 20–80%.

Q. 44. What is the prognosis for RPL with unexplained pregnancy loss?

In more than 50% of RPL, a definite cause may not be detected. Supportive care in a dedicated clinic improves the outcome by 75%. However, prognosis worsens with advanced maternal age and number of pregnancy losses. The overall prognosis is encouraging.

Q. 45. What are the methods of chromosome/gene analysis?

The following are the methods:
- *Fluorescent in situ hybridization (FISH):* It is a cytogenetic technique that uses fluorescent probes that bind to only those parts of the chromosome with a high degree of sequence complimentary. There are limited probes. It can detect chromosome 13,16, 18,21,XO. Time required 72 hours. False reports possible.
- *Karyotype:* It is a test to identify and evaluate the size, shape, and number of chromosomes in a sample of body cells which detects extra or missing chromosomes, or abnormal positions of chromosome pieces. Time required for test is one to 2 weeks. Draw backs of the test are small abnormality cannot be detected and the procedure requires cell culture.
- *Microarray:* No need for cell culture. Failure rates are less. Works on formalin fixed tissue. Rules out maternal contamination. Detects submicroscopic rearrangement.
- *New CGH array (comparative genomic hybridization):* It is a method of genetic testing that may identify small deletions and duplications of the subtelomers, each pericentromeric region and other chromosome regions. Can detect abnormal embryo fast. Time required for the test is 8 hours.
- *SNP array (Single nucleotide polymorphisms):* It is the most common type of genetic variation among people. Each SNP represents a difference in a single DNA building block, called a nucleotide. Most commonly, these variations are found in the DNA between genes.
- *NGS (Next growth sequencing):* NGS is cost effective sequencing of complex samples at remarkable scale and speed.

Low cost, less DNA, fast run and results in informative data by simultaneously evaluating variation in several genes in a single experiment. Large genomic deletions of exons or whole genes and rearrangements such as inversions and translocations can be derived from NGS data directly. NGS is applied in preimplantation, genetic screening for screening aneuploid embryos, etc.

References

1. Macklon NS, Geraedts JPM, Fauser BCJM. Conception to ongoing pregnancy: the "black box" of early pregnancy loss. Hum Reprod Update. 2002;8:333-43.
2. Practice Committee of the American Society for Reproductive Medicine. Evaluation and treatment of recurrent pregnancy loss: A committee opinion. Fertil Steril. 2012;98:1103-11.
3. Ford HB, Schust DJ. Recurrent Pregnancy Loss: Etiology, Diagnosis, and Therapy. Reviews in Obstetrics and Gynecology. 2009;2(2):76-83.
4. Shahine L, Lathi R. Recurrent pregnancy loss: evaluation and treatment. Obstet Gynecol Clin North Am. 2015;42(1):117-34.
5. Lin PC. Reproductive outcomes in women with uterine anomalies. J Womens Health. 2004;13:33-9.
6. Smith ML, Schust DJ. Endocrinology and recurrent early pregnancy loss. Semin Reprod Med. 2011; 29(6):482-90.
7. Zarnani AH. Recurrent Pregnancy Loss through the Lens of Immunology. J Reprod Infertil. 2015;16(2):59-60.
8. Willis R, Gonzalez EB, Brasier AR. The journey of antiphospholipid antibodies from cellular activation to antiphospholipid syndrome. Rheumatol Rep. 2015;17(3):16.
9. Leitich H, Kiss H. Asymptomatic bacterial vaginosis and intermediate flora as risk factors for adverse pregnancy outcome. Best Pract Res Clin Obstet Gynaecol. 2007;21:375-90.
10. Amengual O, Atsumi T, Khamashta MA, et al. Specificity of ELISA for antibody to beta 2-glycoprotein I in patients with anti-phospholipid syndrome. Br J Rheumatol. 1996; 35:1239-43.
11. Derksen RH, de Groot PG. The obstetric antiphospholipid syndrome. J Reprod Immunol. 2008;77(1):41-50.
12. American College of Obstetricians and Gynecologists Committee on Practice Bulletins-Obstetrics. ACOG Practice Bulletin No.118: Antiphospholipid syndrome. Obstet Gynecol. 2011;117:192-9.
13. Lopes L, Jacob GP. Thrombophilia testing in pregnancy: should we agree to disagree? J Perinat Med. 2015;43(2):269-72.
14. de Jong PG, Goddijn M, Middeldorp S. Testing for inherited thrombophilia in recurrent miscarriage. Semin Reprod Med. 2011;29(6):540-7.
15. The Investigation and Treatment of Couples with Recurrent First trimester and Second trimester Miscarriage. Green top guidelines No: 17 April 2011.
16. Bailey AP, Jaslow CR, Kutteh WH. Minimally invasive surgical options for congenital and acquired uterine factors associated with recurrent pregnancy loss. Womens Health (Lond Engl). 2015;11(2):161-7.
17. Grimbizis GF, Camus M, Tarlatzis BC, et al. Clinical implications of uterine malformations and hysteroscopic treatment results. Hum Reprod Update. 2001;7:161-74.
18. Sugiura-Ogasawara M, Lin BL, Aoki K, et al. Does surgery improve live birth rates in patients with recurrent miscarriage caused by uterine anomalies? J Obstet Gynaecol. 2015;35(2):155-8.
19. Bajekal N, Li TC. Fibroids, infertility and pregnancy wastage. Hum Reprod Update. 2000;6:614-20.
20. Berghella V, Odibo AO, To MS, et al. Cerclage for short cervix on ultrasonography: Meta-analysis of trials using individual patient-level data. Obstet Gynecol. 2005;106:181-9.
21. Haas DM, Ramsey PS. Progestogen for preventing miscarriage. Cochrane Database Syst Rev. 2013 Oct 31;10:CD003511.
22. Greer IA, Nelson-Piercy C. Low-molecular-weight heparins for thromboprophylaxis and treatment of venous thromboembolism in pregnancy: a systematic review of safety and efficacy. Blood. 2005;106:401-7.
23. Empson M, Lassere M, Craig JC, Scott JR. Recurrent pregnancy loss with antiphospholipid antibody: a systematic review of therapeutic trials. Obstet Gynecol. 2002;99(1):135-44. Review

24. Dendrinos S, Sakkas E, Makrakis E. Low-molecular-weight heparin versus intravenous immunoglobulin for recurrent abortion associated with antiphospholipid antibody syndrome. Int J Gynaecol Obstet. 2009;104:223-5.
25. Empson M, Lassere M, Craig J, et al. Prevention of recurrent miscarriage for women with antiphospholipid antibody or lupus anticoagulant. Cochrane Database Syst Rev. 2005;(2):CD002859.
26. Wong LF, Porter TF, Scott JR. Immunotherapy for recurrent miscarriage. Cochrane Database of Systematic Reviews 2014, Issue 10. Art. No.: CD000112.
27. Christiansen OB, Larsen EC, Egerup P, et al. Intravenous immunoglobulin treatment for secondary recurrent miscarriage: a randomised, double-blind, placebo-controlled trial. BJOG. 2015; 122(4):500-8.
28. Garrido-Gimenez C, Alijotas-Reig J. Recurrent miscarriage: causes, evaluation and management. Postgrad Med J. 2015;91(1073):151-62.
29. de Jong PG, Kaandorp S, Di Nisio M, et al. Aspirin and/or heparin for women with unexplained recurrent miscarriage with or without inherited thrombophilia. Cochrane Database of Systematic Reviews 2014, Issue 7. Art. No.: CD004734.
30. Rodger MA. Recurrent pregnancy loss: drop the heparin needles. Blood. 2015;125(14):2179-80.
31. Pasquier E, Martin L, Bohec C, et al. Enoxaparin for prevention of unexplained recurrent miscarriage: a multicenter randomized double-blind placebo-controlled trial. Blood. 2015;125(14).

18
Case-based Approach to Thyroid Disorders in Pregnancy

Padma Balasubramanyam

Thyroid in Pregnancy

Thyroid hormone synthesis is regulated by thyroid stimulating hormone (TSH), a glycoprotein released by the anterior pituitary gland. TSH has an alpha and beta subunit, the alpha subunit is shared with human chorionic gonadotropin (hCG), luteinizing hormone (LH) and follicle stimulating hormone (FSH). TSH stimulates the thyroid hormone receptor on the thyroid follicular cells which results in the production of two hormones—thyroxine (T4) and triiodothyronine (T3) by the thyroid gland. Thyroxine binding globulin (TBG) is a glycoprotein that binds to most of the circulating T4 and T3. Thyroid hormone synthesis increases by 50% during the first trimester of pregnancy. Not only is there an increased demand but the deiodinases produced in the placenta breakdown T4 and T3 to inactive forms. TBG levels in pregnancy are increased by estrogen's stimulating effect on its synthesis in the liver. Estrogen also increases the half life of TBG by decreasing its catabolism. The increase in TBG concentration in pregnancy results in an increase in T4 and T3 levels in the first trimester of pregnancy, these levels plateau around 16 weeks of pregnancy. Free T4 and T3 levels have been the subject of controversy with some studies showing no change while others showed mild increase or decrease. hCG levels peak between 9 and 11 weeks of pregnancy and stimulate thyroid hormone production by acting on the TSH receptor and can lower TSH levels in the first trimester. The fetus depends on the mother for thyroid hormone until about 20 weeks of pregnancy although it starts to produce thyroid hormone from 10 weeks of gestation.[1,2] Iodine is an essential component of thyroid hormone and is needed for its synthesis. There is increase in iodine excretion in pregnancy alongside an increase in requirement. World Health Organization (WHO) recommends 250 µg per day iodine supplementation in pregnant and lactating women.

In this chapter, the common thyroid disorders encountered in pregnancy will be addressed through case discussions.

Hypothyroidism Cases

1. A 22-year-old female calls you on the phone, reports she is pregnant, her last menstrual cycle was 8 weeks ago. She was diagnosed with primary hypothyroidism 3 years ago when her TSH was elevated at 24 mIU/L (reference range 0.34–4.8 mIU/L). She takes levothyroxine, 75 µg daily. Her TSH was evaluated 6 months ago and was normal at 2.2 mIU/L. What is the best next step?

A. Continue levothyroxine, 75 µg once daily
B. Increase levothyroxine to 150 µg once daily
C. Increase levothyroxine to 75 µg tablets, taking nine tablets per week and obtain laboratory data including TSH and confirmatory tests for pregnancy.

The correct answer is C—increase levothyroxine to 75 µg tablets, take nine tablets per week and obtain laboratory data including TSH and confirmatory tests for pregnancy.

2. A 30-year-old slender built female who is generally healthy reports history of ectopic pregnancy in August of 2014. In January of 2015, she had a miscarriage at 7 weeks of gestation. Family history was noteworthy for autoimmune thyroiditis in her mother and one sister. She is very concerned that she may have a miscarriage again. Her thyroid gland is 3 times normal in size on examination without any nodules. Her TSH is 3.3 mIU/L (reference range 0.34–4.8 mIU/L). Free T4 is within the normal range. Thyroid peroxidase antibodies (TPOAb) are 332 IU/mL (normal <9.0 IU/mL). What would you recommend now?
   A. Reassure her that her TSH is within the normal range for the laboratory and that you will repeat TSH after 6 weeks
   B. Start her on 50 µg daily of levothyroxine and repeat TSH after 4–5 weeks
   C. Start her on 100 µg of levothyroxine and repeat her TSH and anti TPO antibodies after 6–8 weeks.

The correct answer is B—start her on 50 µg daily of levothyroxine and repeat her TSH in 4–5 weeks.

3. All of below are causes for primary hypothyroidism except for which one?
   A. Iodine deficiency
   B. Chronic autoimmune thyroiditis (Hashimoto's thyroiditis)
   C. Surgical or radioactive iodine treatment for hyperthyroidism
   D. Drugs such as lithium
   E. Radiation treatment for pituitary disease.

The correct answer is E—radiation treatment of the pituitary gland can lead to secondary or central hypothyroidism but is not a cause for primary hypothyroidism.

Discussion

Thyroid disorders are the most common endocrine disorders in pregnancy after diabetes. Primary hypothyroidism is defined as inadequate thyroid hormone synthesis due to disorder of thyroid gland. Secondary or central hypothyroidism which is rare is due to disease in the pituitary gland or hypothalamus which results in inadequate production of thyrotropin or thyroid stimulating hormone. Hypothyroidism is more common than hyperthyroidism and in this chapter, we will be discussing primary hypothyroidism. Overt hypothyroidism in pregnancy is defined as a TSH greater than trimester and population specific range. If trimester specific ranges for the population are unavailable, TSH greater than 4.0 mU/L as per the 2017 American Thyroid Association (ATA) guidelines is defined as hypothyroidism.[6] In pregnant women with TSH greater than 2.5, thyroid peroxidase antibodies (TPOAb) must be obtained.[4]

In a multicenter cross-sectional study in secondary and tertiary hospitals in India from 2011–2012, hypothyroidism was detected in 13.13% in their study population with the upper end of normal for TSH being 4.5 µIU/mL, majority had subclinical hypothyroidism. A significant number of these women had underlying autoimmune disease.[5] Other causes of primary hypothyroidism in pregnancy include iodine deficiency, thyroidectomy for hyperthyroidism, multinodular goiter and thyroid cancer, radioactive iodine treatment for hyperthyroidism, radiotherapy to the head and neck for cancer and congenital hypothyroidism. Secondary hypothyroidism can result from lymphocytic hypophysitis from pituitary disease and after pituitary surgery for a pituitary tumor.[3]

Maternal hypothyroidism prior to conception is associated with decrease in fertility rates and an increase in the incidence of miscarriage. During pregnancy, maternal hypothyroidism is associated with an increased prevalence of gestational hypertension, preeclampsia, anemia, placental abruption and postpartum hemorrhage. On the fetal side fetal distress, low birth weight and risk of developing neurocognitive defects show a significant increase. One large retrospective study showed higher rates of placental abruption and preterm birth in women with subclinical hypothyroidism. However, there are other studies that have not showed adverse outcomes.

The best test to evaluate the thyroid function in pregnancy is a serum TSH. In the earlier guidelines from the ATA, the reference ranges for TSH for first trimester was 0.1–2.5 mU/L, for the second trimester of pregnancy—0.2–3.0 mU/L, and for the third trimester of pregnancy—0.3–3.0 mU/L. The 2017, ATA Thyroid and Pregnancy guidelines, recently released, recommends "the lower reference range reduced by 0.4 mU/L and upper reference range by 0.5 mU/L". The optimal method to measure free T4 (FT4) is by liquid chromatography/tandem mass spectrometry (LC/MS/MS). Free T4 assays by immunoassay are not always reliable in pregnancy due to elevated levels of TBG.

The American Thyroid Association and American Association of Clinical Endocrinologists (AACE/ATA) guidelines recommend that pregnant woman with hypothyroidism should increase the dosage of levothyroxine as soon as possible. Physicians caring for these patients should aim for a serum TSH less than 2.5 mIU/L and total T4 in the normal reference range for pregnancy. Hypothyroid patients on levothyroxine treatment who have a positive pregnancy test should have TSH checked as soon as possible and in the interim increase the dose by 25–30% or take 2 additional doses per week.[2] Pregnant women are recommended to take antenatal multivitamin which contains iodine, calcium and iron which can interfere with absorption of levothyroxine; therefore, they should be advised to take this in the evening if they are taking the levothyroxine in the morning or at least 4 hours after levothyroxine. After delivery these individuals may be able to go back on the dose they were taking prior to the pregnancy.

The American Thyroid Association (ATA) recommends treatment with levothyroxine in pregnancy in women with positive thyroid peroxidase antibodies (TPOAb) and subclinical hypothyroidism (SCH). European Thyroid Association and Endocrine Society (US) recommend treatment even in women with SCH who are Ab negative. The guidelines recommend that TSH and free T4 measurements should be checked every 4 weeks until 16–20 weeks of gestation and at least once between 26 and 32 weeks of gestation. In patients with Hashimoto's thyroiditis, there is no need for any other testing like serial fetal ultrasounds unless there are other comorbidities.

In pregnant women with normal thyroid function and positive TPOAb who have had recurrent spontaneous miscarriages, one could consider treating with a small dose of levothyroxine although there are no robust studies to support this. After delivery, levothyroxine can be stopped in these individuals and a TSH checked after 6 weeks. In women who are being evaluated for infertility measurement of TSH should be part of the investigations as hypothyroidism is associated with increased risk of infertility. Based on current evidence, overt hypothyroidism in women with history of infertility should be treated with levothyroxine. There is no hard evidence to treat women with subclinical hypothyroidism who have infertility with levothyroxine if they do not have TPOAb.

Indian Thyroid Society guidelines recommend measuring TSH levels of all pregnant women at their first antenatal visit. However, Endocrine Society of America does not recommend universal screening at this time and recommends screening only high-risk pregnant women at their first antenatal visit.

Hyperthyroidism Case

1. A 28-year-old woman 10 weeks of gestation comes to your clinic complaining of fatigue, impaired sleep and intermittent palpitations. She has not gained or lost any weight. She has no family history of thyroid disorders. She reports nausea and has been vomiting once in a while. On physical examination, she has a pulse of 90/minute, blood pressure of 100/80. She looks well hydrated, does not have proptosis and her thyroid gland is twice normal in size without any nodules. Her TSH is 0.09 (reference range 0.34–4.8 mIU/L), free T4 and free T3 are normal.
   You recommend the following:
   A. Fluids and supportive measures and repeat TSH, free T4 after 4 weeks
   B. Start propranolol
   C. Start PTU
   The correct answer is A—fluids and supportive measures and repeat TSH, free T4 after 4 weeks.

2. A 34-year-old woman 11 weeks of gestation with a history of weight loss of 1.5 kg in the preceding 2 weeks is concerned that her thyroid is 'overactive'. She has palpitations, diarrhea and an increased appetite and is surprised she has lost weight. She reports nausea but no vomiting. Her family history is significant for a brother with type 1 diabetes mellitus and first cousin with Crohn's disease. On physical examination, she has a mild stare and lig lag, her pulse is 100/minute, blood pressure is 110/80. Thyroid gland is 3 times normal in size and is diffusely enlarged with a bruit. She has fine tremors in her hands and has moist palms.
   Her TSH is suppressed at less than 0.01, free T4 is 3.2 ng/dL (range 0.8–1.8 ng/dL), free T3 is 6.0 pg/mL (range 2.3–4.2 pg/mL). What is the diagnosis? What will be your next steps?
   A. Reassure her that her thyrotoxicosis is transient from pregnancy and repeat thyroid tests after 4 weeks
   B. Treat her with propranolol and avoid any other medications as she is in her first trimester of pregnancy
   C. Give her propylthiouracil (PTU) during the 1st trimester and then treat her with methimazole
   D. Treat with RAI
   The correct answer is C—treat her with PTU during the first trimester and then switch to methimazole and monitor her thyroid tests closely.

Discussion

Hyperthyroidism in pregnancy can be caused by toxic multinodular goiter, solitary autonomously functioning nodule and Graves' disease. Graves' disease is an autoimmune disease and is the most common etiology for overt hyperthyroidism. High serum levels of human chorionic gonadotropin (hCG) during the first trimester can lead to gestational hyperthyroidism or gestational transient thyrotoxicosis (GTT) and present with subclinical or mild overt hyperthyroidism.

Patients with hyperemesis gravidarum have severe nausea and vomiting resulting in 5% or more weight loss. The high circulating concentration of hCG stimulates the TSH receptor and leads to overt hyperthyroidism. This hyperthyroidism is transient in nature with improvement in thyroid tests by 14–18 weeks of gestation when serum hCG concentration falls. Other causes include destruction of thyroid follicles from thyroiditis-silent which is autoimmune in etiology, subacute thyroiditis which may be viral or acute thyroiditis from a bacterial infection. Hyperthyroidism rarely can be caused by trophoblastic disease—molar pregnancy or choriocarcinoma. The level of hCG and disease burden will determine the development of hyperthyroidism. A minority are clinically hyperthyroid and require treatment.[7,8]

The prevalence of hyperthyroidism in pregnancy is from 0.1–0.4% with the vast majority of cases from Graves' disease.[11] Graves' disease in pregnancy that is untreated or inadequately treated can cause congestive heart failure, preeclampsia and also lead to the life-threatening emergency of thyroid storm. There is increased risk of miscarriage, placental abruption and preterm delivery. Fetal complications include goiter, growth retardation, malformations, death or stillbirth. In the neonates, there is risk of transient hyperthyroidism.

It is important to distinguish between Graves' hyperthyroidism and gestational transient thyrotoxicosis (GTT). Family history of thyroid disorders or other autoimmune disorders is usually seen in Graves' disease. Patient may have had symptoms before pregnancy. Thyroid eye disease can be present in Graves' disease with complaints of diplopia, foreign body sensation, photophobia, redness and tearing. Proptosis may be present. Patients with Graves' disease can present with a bruit on auscultation and a palpable thrill over a diffusely enlarged goiter.

Gestational transient thyrotoxicosis (GTT) is seen in the first trimester, there is no specific association with family history of thyroid disorders or autoimmune diseases. Most often these women have only mild or absent signs of hyperthyroidism. GTT is typically associated with hyperemesis gravidarum or multiple gestation. These patients do not have an underlying autoimmune thyroid disease, TPOAb and TRAb are negative.[7,8]

Laboratory data in hyperthyroidism in pregnancy will reveal a suppressed TSH which is less than 0.1 mU/L, levels can be lower than 0.01 mU/L. In addition, the patient will have high levels of serum free T4 and/or free T3 or total T4 and/or total T3 measurement that is above the normal range for pregnancy. Patients with Graves' disease will typically have elevated T4 and T3 concentrations. In GTT, TSH is suppressed with usually normal serum T3 or free T3 concentrations. Occasionally mildly elevated levels are encountered.

Patients with overt hyperthyroidism from Graves' disease, toxic multinodular goiter (toxic MNG) or solitary autonomously functioning thyroid nodule/hot nodule are treated with antithyroid drugs (ATD) like propylthiouracil (PTU), methimazole (MMI) or its derivative carbimazole. These drugs decrease the synthesis of thyroid hormone. PTU has an additional benefit in blocking the conversion of T4 to T3 which is the active thyroid hormone. Use of both PTU and MMI are associated with birth defects. MMI in the first trimester of pregnancy has been associated with a higher incidence of teratogenic effects like scalp defects—aplasia cutis and more serious defects including choanal atresia, developmental delays and tracheoesophageal atresia.[4] The ATA recommends PTU through 16 weeks of pregnancy.[4] Patients can be treated with a starting dose of 100 mg of PTU 3 times a day. Hepatic enzymes may be monitored every 3 weeks as PTU has been associated with acute liver failure/fulminant hepatotoxicity. ATDs can be associated rarely with agranulocytosis. Patients have to be advised to report any mouth ulcers, fevers or sore throat and if they experience any of these symptoms, a complete blood count must be obtained. PTU should be stopped and patient should be placed on methimazole after 16 weeks of pregnancy. In order to avoid hypothyroidism in the fetus, the lowest dose of antithyroid drug possible should be used, aiming for a maternal free T4 concentration at the upper end of normal for non-pregnant women. At least one-third of women will not need the ATD after the first trimester due to fall in the concentration of TRAb.

If a patient develops a serious adverse reaction to ATD, has a large goiter with compressive symptoms, or requires persistently high doses of ATD thyroidectomy may be indicated. The optimal time for surgery would be in the 2nd trimester. Radioactive iodine treatment is contraindicated in pregnancy. Beta-blockers like propranolol or atenolol may be given for moderate to severe hyperthyroidism in pregnant women if they report palpitations and have tachycardia. Beta-blockers should be stopped when patients no longer have palpitations.

TRAb cross the placenta and can lead to fetal hyperthyroidism. These antibodies should be measured between 20 and 24 weeks of gestation in women currently being treated for Graves' disease, those with a history of radioactive iodine treatment or thyroidectomy before pregnancy for Graves' disease. Fetal ultrasound to screen for goiter should be obtained in the 18th–22nd week if the TRAb or thyroid-stimulating immunoglobulin are elevated 2-3 times the upper end of normal and in women treated with ATD, and repeated every month if necessary.[3,4]

Gestational transient thyrotoxicosis is usually transient and is treated symptomatically. Women with severe hyperemesis should be treated with intravenous fluids and other supportive measures. Beta-blockers such as metoprolol may be helpful in very symptomatic patients and may be used after consultation with the obstetricians if they are in agreement.

Thyroid Nodule Case

A 29-year-old woman who is 12 weeks gestation' comes to the clinic and complains of a swelling in the neck that she noticed 10 days prior to her visit. Family history is noteworthy for her maternal grandmother with a goiter. The nodule measures 2.5 cm in the right lobe of the thyroid gland on palpation. It moves up with swallowing and is firm in consistency. There is no cervical lymphadenopathy. Rest of her exam is unremarkable. TSH is normal. What would be the next step in her evaluation?

A. Reassure her that the TSH is normal and she can wait until she delivers for further investigations
B. Obtain a RAI scan to see if it is a functioning nodule
C. Perform a fine needle aspiration biopsy (FNA biopsy) of the right thyroid nodule
D. Follow her with serial thyroid ultrasounds.

The correct answer is C—perform a fine needle aspiration biopsy (FNA biopsy) of the right thyroid nodule.

Discussion

Thyroid nodules are lesions in the thyroid gland which can be identified as separate from the surrounding thyroid tissue. The prevalence of thyroid nodules in pregnant women in studies from Brussels, China and Germany based largely on thyroid ultrasound varied between 3% and 21%. The vast majority of the nodules are benign. Less than 10% of thyroid nodules in the general population are malignant and the incidence of malignancy in thyroid nodules in pregnant women is also low.[10]

In a pregnant woman with thyroid nodule, obtain a TSH first. If TSH is low or suppressed and stays suppressed after the first trimester of pregnancy, the nodule can be followed and further evaluation performed after delivery.[4]

In women with normal TSH, thyroid fine needle aspiration biopsy/cytology (FNA) is a safe and reliable procedure to evaluate thyroid nodules. US-guided FNA biopsy is better than palpation-guided biopsy as it has lower non-diagnostic cytology rates. Nodules greater than 1 cm in size with suspicious features such as microcalcifications should be biopsied. If there are no suspicious features, FNA of nodules greater than 1.5 cm is recommended. FNA can be delayed until after delivery in the last few weeks of pregnancy.[4,10]

Of the less than 10% of thyroid nodules that are malignant, the vast majority are papillary thyroid cancer (PTC). If PTC is diagnosed in the first trimester of pregnancy and the patient does not have any suspicious lymph nodes on US, surgery can be postponed until after delivery with close monitoring of the nodule. If the nodule shows significant growth, surgery should be considered in the second trimester. Thyroid hormone may be administered to achieve a low but detectable TSH in pregnant women with an FNA positive for or suspicious for cancer, or in those who elect to delay surgical treatment until postpartum.[4,8,10]

Postpartum Thyroiditis Case

A 33-year-old woman, 4 months postpartum, is referred for further evaluation of fatigue, intolerance to heat, irritability and palpitations. She denies any loss of weight, neck pain or diarrhea. She is breastfeeding her child. There was no previous history of thyroid disease. Her blood pressure is normal but she has tachycardia with a resting heart rate of 100/minute. She does not have any proptosis. Neck exam does not reveal tenderness, thyroid gland is twice normal in size and is diffusely enlarged. Blood tests reveal a suppressed TSH at 0.01 and elevated free T4 at 3.4 ng/dL (range 0.8-1.8 ng/dL). Free T3 is normal. Thyroid peroxidase antibodies (TPOAb) are elevated at 280 IU/mL (normal <9.0 IU/mL). What would be the next step?

A. Start her on an ATD like methimazole
B. Order radioactive iodine scan
C. Treat her with a beta-blocker such as atenolol, metoprolol or propranolol.

The correct answer is C—treat with a beta-blocker.

Discussion

Postpartum thyroiditis (PPT) is an autoimmune thyroid disorder that presents during the first postpartum year. PPT is characterized by lymphocytic infiltration of the thyroid gland. The classical course of PPT seen in less than a third of cases has the thyrotoxic phase followed by the hypothyroid phase. This is followed by recovery. The thyrotoxic phase can occur between 2 and 10 months after delivery. Hypothyroid phase presents usually at 6 months postpartum but can occur between 2 and 12 months after delivery.[9] Most of the women who experience PPT have normal thyroid function one year postpartum. A third of patients develop permanent hypothyroidism. Patients with type 1 diabetes mellitus which is an autoimmune disorder have a higher prevalence of PPT.

Patients who have a history of Hashimoto's thyroiditis have a higher incidence of developing PPT, these women also have an increased risk of developing permanent primary hypothyroidism in the 5-10 years period after the episode of PPT. TSH should be performed once a year in these patients.

Inflammation of the thyroid gland in PPT damages thyroid follicles and results in release of large amounts of thyroxine (T4) and triiodothyronine (T3) into the circulation, and clinical features of hyperthyroidism. The differential diagnosis is with Graves' disease. Patients with Graves' disease may have eye symptoms and signs like proptosis, a more significant thyroid enlargement with a bruit due to increased vascularity. Radioiodine uptake values are low in postpartum thyroiditis and high in Graves' hyperthyroidism. However, radioactive iodine testing should be avoided in women who are breastfeeding their infants.

PPT is treated symptomatically with beta-blockers in patients who have palpitations. ATDs are not necessary as patients with PPT do not have increased synthesis of thyroid hormones as is seen in patients with Graves' disease. Patients should be advised that they are at increased risk for recurrence of PPT in subsequent pregnancies.

References

1. Glinoer D. The regulation of thyroid function in pregnancy: pathways of endocrine adaptation from physiology to pathology. Endocrine Reviews. 2013;18(3).
2. Cignini P, Cafa EV, Giorlandino C, et al. Thyroid physiology and common diseases in pregnancy: review of literature. J Prenat Med. 2012;6(4):64-71.
3. De Groot L, Abalovich M, Alexander EK, et al. Management of thyroid dysfunction during pregnancy and postpartum: an Endocrine society clinical practice guideline. J Clin Endocrinol Metab August. 2012;97(8):2543-256.
4. Alexander EK, Pearce EN, Brent GA, et al. 2017 Guidelines of the American Thyroid Association for the diagnosis and management of thyroid disease during pregnancy and the postpartum. Thyroid. 2017;27(3):315-89.doi 10.1089/thy.2016.0457.
5. Dhanwal DK, Bajaj S, Rajput R, et al. Prevalence of hypothyroidism in pregnancy: An epidemiological study from 11 cities in 9 states of India. Indian J Endocrinol Metab. 2016;20(3):387-90. doi:10.4103/2230-8210.179992.
6. Teng W, Shan Z, Patil-Sisodia K, et al. Hypothyroidism in pregnancy. The Lancet Diabetes & Endocrinology. 2013;1(3):228-37.
7. Cooper, DS, Laurberg P. Hyperthyroidism in pregnancy. The Lancet Diabetes & Endocrinology. 2013;1(3):238-49.
8. Walkington L, Webster J, Hancock BW, et al. Hyperthyroidism and human chorionic gonadotrophin production in gestational trophoblastic disease. Br J Cancer. 2011;104(11):1665-9.
9. Popoveniuc G, Jonklaas J. Thyroid Nodules. Med Clin North Am. 2012;96(2):329-49.
10. Stagnaro-Green A. Postpartum thyroiditis. The Journal of Clinical Endocrinology & Metabolism. 87(9):4042-7.
11. Haugen BR, Alexander EK, Bible KC, et al. 2015 American Thyroid Association Management Guidelines for Adult Patients with Thyroid Nodules and Differentiated Thyroid Cancer: The American Thyroid Association Guidelines Task Force on Thyroid Nodules and Differentiated Thyroid Cancer Thyroid. 2016;26(1):1-133.

CHAPTER 19

Abnormal Uterine Bleeding

Sunanda R Kulkarni

Patient by name A aged 46 years, came with the history of spotting for 20 days, preceded by amenorrhea of 3 months duration.

Since one year her cycles were once in 2 to 3 months and bleeding used to last for 10–15 days. No dysmenorrhea. She underwent D & C for the same complaint and histopathological report was hyperplasia without atypia. She was advised medroxyprogesterone acetate 10 mg/day for 9 months. She took MPA for 9 months and had stopped. She did not come for follow-up during her treatment. After stopping the tablets she had again amenorrhea of 3 months followed by spotting for 20 days.

History

Gynecology History

Menarche 14th year. Past cycles regular and normal flow.

Obstetric History

- Married life—25 years. Non-consanguineous marriage.
- P2L2. Both were FTND. Alive and healthy.
- Last delivery—22 years back.

Family History

No history of diabetes or hypertension or cancer in the family.

Personal History

Diet vegetarian, bowel and bladder were regular.

Q. 1. What is your diagnosis based on her history?

Based on her history probable diagnosis is—AUB-H.

Q. 2. What are your examination findings?

On examination

- Patient aged 46 years, well-built, conscious and cooperative.
- Pulse rate—96/minute, regular
- BP—110/70 mm of Hg, BMI—24
- Mild pallor +
  CVS } NAD
  RS
- PA> Soft, no mass palpable
- PV—cervix hypertrophied. Uterus bulky anteverted, fornixes free. No tenderness
- Based on examination, the diagnosis is AUB (O).

Investigations

- Hb%—10 g.
- Urine routine—NAD
- Blood group—A+ve
- RBS—129 mg%
- Urea—28 mg%
- Creatinine—0.6 mg%

- TSH—2.35 MIU/mL
- Transvaginal Scan—Uterine size—10.1 × 5.9 × 3.6 cm and right ovary 31 × 17 and left ovary 3.2 × 1.8 endometrium 1.2 cm.
- Ovaries normal
- BT—CT- normal limits
- Chest X-ray–NAD
- D & C
- Pap smear—Negative for intraepithleal lesions and malignancy.

Q. 3. How will you manage this patient?

I will do hysteroscopic-guided endometrial biopsy. If her report says persistence of hyperplasia, I will do hysterectomy and type of hysterectomy depending on her choice (Table 1).

Table 1: Old and new terminology for AUB

Recommendations for discarding terminology	Accepted abbreviations describing menstrual symptoms
• Menorrhagia • Hypermenorrhea • Hypomenorrhea • Menometrorrhagia • Polymenorrhea • Polymenorrhagia • Epimenorrhea • Epimenorrhagia • Uterine hemorrhage • Dysfunctional uterine bleeding • Functional uterine bleeding • Metropathia hemorrhagica • Oligomenorrhea Amenorrhea	• AUB—Abnormal uterine bleeding • HMB—Heavy menstrual bleeding • HPMB—Heavy and prolonged menstrual bleeding • IMB—Intermenstrual bleeding • PMB—Postmenopausal bleeding

Q. 4. What is dysfunctional uterine bleeding (DUB)?

DUB is defined as abnormality in the normal cyclic menstrual flow, where in the amount, duration or interval is altered due to endocrine mechanism that controls menstruation in the absence of pathology, pregnancy, systemic and iatrogenic cases. However, this term DUB is obsolete. This is classified by FIGO as AUB(O).

Q. 5. How DUB is diagnosed?

DUB is diagnosed by exclusion—exclusion by history, exclusion by examination and exclusion by investigations.

By history of pregnancy, abortion, ectopic pregnancy, blood dyscrasias, endometriosis, IUCD, etc. by examination carcinoma cervix, polyp, fibroid, PID, IUCD, ovarian tumors, splenomegaly, petechial hemorrhages, acanthosis nigricans, etc. and by investigations—scan blood, etc.

Q. 6. What are the investigations for AUB?

- Hematological—Hb%, blood group, platelet count, coagulation factor, Glanzmann's disease, von Willebrand disease, ITP, ESR, hematological indices, insulin levels.
- Hormonal—prolactin, FSH, LH, TSH, testosterone, DHEA, cortisol, dexamethasone suppression test.
- Scanning—fibroid, endometrial thickness, IUCD, adenomyosis, polyp, PCO, endometriosis.
- Saline infusion sonography if hysteroscopy is not available.
- Hysteroscopy—to locate the lesion, polyps, and to take biopsy.
- Laparoscopy—adnexal masses, ovarian tumors, cysts, endometriosis, PID, when there is doubt after other investigations are equivocal.
- MRI—adenomyosis, fibroid location, before planning for surgery of myomas and MRGFUS, after treatment of embolization.
- CT scan—in suspected malignancy
- X-ray—suspected tuberculosis
- Arteriography, venography and Doppler- if there is suspicion of hemangioma, or suspected deep venous thrombosis and AV malformation.
- Endometrial biopsy—genital TB, malignancy premalignant condition, ovulatory disorders.
- Pipelle—to know the endometrial pathology, phase of the endometrium.

Q. 7. How do you diagnosis adenomyosis?

- By history—triple dysmenorrhea
- Examination—enlarged uterus, tenderness
- Investigations—Sonographic appearance of adenomyosis
- Uterus may be enlarged, thickening of transitional zone, heterogeneous echo texture, subendometrial echogenic endometrial striations, thickened uterine wall, cystic anechoic lakes in the myometrium.
- MRI—thickened junctional zone, sub endometrial cysts, myohyperplasia especially on posterior wall.

Q. 8. What are causes of HMB ?

HMB means heavy menstrual bleeding. It may be in the form of duration or amount.

Causes are:
- Hormonal imbalance
- Growth—Fibroids and polyps
- Bleeding disorder—von Willebrand disease, ITP, pancytopenia
- Adenomyosis
- Genital malignancy
- Medications—anticoagulants, anti-inflammatory drugs, etc.
- Contraception—IUCD
- Systemic disease—thyroid, liver, kidney diseases
- Infection—PID
- Rarely uterine AV malformation.

Q. 9. What are the causes of oligomenorrhea?

Oligomenorrhea, epimenorrhea and hypomenorrhea are no longer recommended by FIGO classification, but it is better to be aware of these old terms also.

Thyroid disease, hyperprolactinemia, obesity, PCOS, androgen producing tumors,

Causes of Hypomenorrhea

Uterine synechiae, tuberculosis, OC pills, thyroid diseases.

Q. 10. What are the causes of epimenorrhoea?

When cycle is <21 days it is called epimenorrhea

Causes are—PID, ovarian endometriosis. Some cases of tubectomy status.

Q. 11. What are the causes of AUB in adolescents?

- Hematological causes—coagulation disorders, leukemia, ITP, von Willibrand factor, platelet dysfunction, hemophilias, deficiency of factor V, X, XI etc.
- Hypothalamic causes—immature HPO axis, increased exercise, stress, eating disorders, psychological, low body fat
- Endocrinal dysfunction—thyroid, adrenal, PCO
- Anatomical causes—uterus didelphys
- Pregnancy complications—abortion, ectopic
- Systemic causes—tuberculosis, liver disorder, diabetes, renal disease
- Iatrogenic causes—OC pills
- Pelvic tumors—estrogen-producing tumors, fibroid uterus
- Miscellaneous causes—trauma, sexual abuse
- Immunological—ovarian antibodies
- Refer Flowchart 1.

Flowchart 1: Classification of pubertal menorrhagia after excluding pregnancy

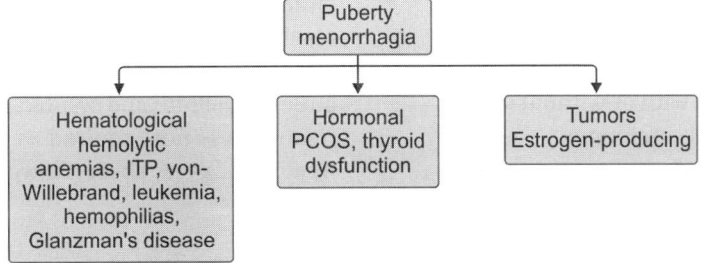

Abbreviations: ITP, Immune thrombocytopenic; PCOS, polycystic ovary syndrome.

Q. 12. How do you assess bleeding?

- Subjective—number of pads, days, amount of clots, etc.
- Semiobjective—menstrual calendar, **Higham's chart**, anemia
- Laboratory—alkali hematin
- Clinical—pallor, heart rate, nails, tongue, conjunctiva, etc.

Menstrual dimensions

	Normal	Abnormal cycles	Short cycles
Frequency	24–28 days	>38 days	<24 days
Duration	7 days	>8 days	<2 days
Volume	5–80 mL	>80 mL	<5 mL

USG in normal cycle

In the menstrual and early proliferative phase— endometrial thickness will be 6–7 mm. It appears echogenic due to the growth of glands and blood vessels, it is a thin, brightly echogenic strip comprising of the basal layer in the late proliferative phase, it develops a trilaminar appearance: outer echogenic basal layer, middle hypoechoic functional layer, and an inner echogenic strip at the central interface.

Secretory phase—more echogenic, 12–16 mm in the secretory phase it is at its thickest and becomes uniformly echogenic, as the functional layer becomes edematous and isoechoic to the basal layer.

Q. 13. What are the histopathological findings in endometrial biopsy?

- Proliferative
- Secretary
- Discordant endometrium
- Atrophic
- Hyperplasia with or without atypia
- Endometrial carcinoma
- TB endometrium.

Q. 14. Describe Pipelle biopsy.

Pipelle is a polypropylene suction cannula with diameter of 3.1 mm, can be used in outpatient as it is safe and cost effective. It is not helpful in detecting submucous fibroid and endometrial polyps. It can be used for follow-up. It is useful only when an adequate sample is obtained.

Q. 15. What are the advantages of D & C?

It shows:

- Phase of endometrium
- Diagnosis of TB, carcinoma of endometrium
- Control bleeding temporarily
- Also acts as therapeutic in case of abortion, polyp and IUCD and in some cases of AUB also.

Q. 16. How do you treat based on endometrial biopsy?

In young girls and near menopause either there will be anovulation or there will be deficiency of progesterone. In young girls endometrial biopsy is rarely indicated.

Histopathology picture may be proliferative or mixed. In these cases MPA 10 mg/day or norethisterone 5 mg/day from 5th to 25th day is given or low dose oral pills also can be given 3–6 months.

If there is bleeding in secretory phase the progesterone secreted may not be sufficient hence low dose oral pills are given or dydrogesterone 10 mg/day from 5th to 25th day can be given for 3 cycles.

Atrophic endometrium: Most of the atrophic endometritis do not require treatment as they resolve spontaneously. Premarin 0.625 daily once for eight weeks is given if associated with atrophic vaginitis and cystitis and progesterone treatment is not required as the duration of treatment is very short (Flowchart 2).

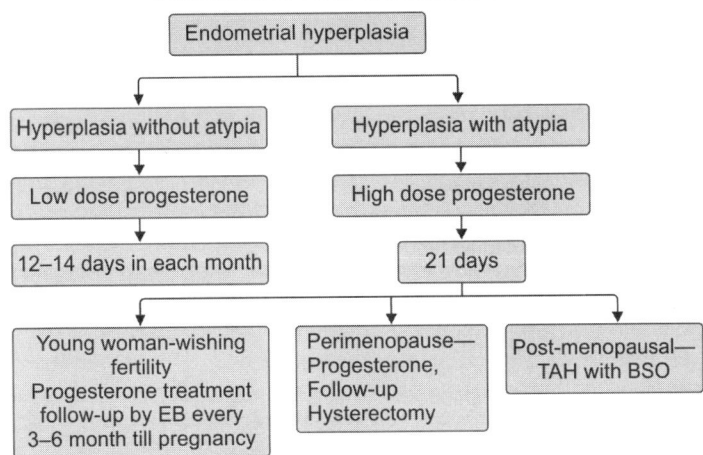

Flowchart 2: WHO classification 2014

Abbreviations: TAH, total abdominal hysterectomy; BSO, bilateral salpingo-oophorectomy

Q. 17. How do you treat endometrial hyperplasia?

Treatment depends upon the etiology and potentiality of cancer, whether patient wishes fertility, and presence or absence of comorbidities and patients preference.

LNG is the first line of treatment. It also acts as contraceptive in perimenopausal age.

Low dose 12 months	High dose 12 months
• MPA 10–20 mg • Norethindrone acetate 5 mg/day • Micronized progesterone 200 mg • Megestrole acetate 20–40 mg/day	• Medroxyprogesterone acetate 40–100 mg/day • Micronized progesterone 300–400 mg/day • Megestrol acetate 80–160 mg/day

Follow up is with endometrial biopsy every 3–6 months.

Hysterectomy should be considered in the following conditions: Progression to atypical hyperplasia occurs during follow-up, there is no histological regression of hyperplasia despite 12 months of treatment, there is relapse of endometrial hyperplasia after completing progestogen treatment and there is persistence of bleeding symptoms.

Hysterectomy can be considered as a first line of treatment in the following condition also:

- Non-compliant patient in perimenopausal age
- Postmenopausal patient without atypia
- Perimenopausal patient and not ready for LNG or progesterone.

RCOG 2016-recomends LNG-IUS and oral progesterone continuously for the hyperplasia without atypia as the first line of treatment and continuous progesterone those who decline for LNG-IUS. For hyperplasia with atypia total hysterectomy is advised unless the woman wants the uterus for pregnancy. If the uterus is retained risk of malignancy, progression of the disease and hysterectomy after fertility is over should be explained.

Q. 18. What are the causes of anovulatory cycles?

- Hypothalamic dysfunction—athletes, anorexia, stress
- Age—adolescent, perimenopuase
- Endocrine—thyroid, hyperprolactinemia PCO, increased androgen syndromes
- Chronic diseases.

Drug	Dosage	Mechanism of action	Effectiveness	Side-effects	Contraindications
Mefenamic acid	500 mg TID	Prevents PG's formation	20%	Rash, swelling, liver problems	IBS, gastric ulcer, renal damage
Tranexemic acid	1 g/QID	Blocks plasminogen, causes fibrin degradation	54–60%	Nausea, vomiting, DVT	Allergy thrombosis
Ethamsylate	250–500 mg, 4–6th hourly	Increases platelet aggregation, angioprotective, PG inhibitor	Minimal	Head ache, skin rash	Pregnancy
EACA	10 mg/kg body weight TID/QID	Plasminogen inhibitor	Minimal	Hypotension	DVT history

Q. 19. What drugs which cause AUB?

Refer Flowchart 3.

Flowchart 3: Drugs caused for AUB

- Antineoplastic drugs
- Anticoagulants like heparin, aspirin
- Antiepileptic drugs
- Drugs history in AUB
- Antidepressants/antipsychotics
- Herbs: Ginseng, chasteberry, danshen
- Hormones/depo-provera, tamoxifen
- Corticosteroids

Q. 20. What are types of surgery for AUB?

- Hysteroscopic polypectomy or myomectomy
- Endometrial ablation
- Myomectomy
- Hysterectomy.

Q. 21. What are the newer modalities of endometrial ablation?

They are classified into heading:

- *1st generation*—is ablative surgery with hysteroscope—TCRE, ND: YAG laser and roller ball.
- *2nd generation*—without hysteroscope-hydrothermal ablation, cryoablation, diode laser, microwave endometrial ablation, unipolar electrodes, bipolar electrodes, nova sure, radiofrequency probes, cavetrerm ablation system (glycine).

Q. 22. What are the prerequisites for minimal ablative surgery?

Young patient, obese patient, medical contraindication, those who have completed their family.

Abnormal Uterine Bleeding

Failure of medical line of treatment, benign endometrial biopsy.

Q. 23. What are the key points for counseling of women planned for endometrial ablation?

- Confirm childbearing is complete
- Need for contraception
- Rule out underlying uterine pathology (i.e. hyperplasia or malignancy)
- Clearly outline expectations (patient satisfaction, not amenorrhea)
- Possibility of hysterectomy in the future.

Q. 24. What are the criteria for transcervical endometrial resection (TCRE)?

- Abnormal or bleeding justifying hysterectomy
- Failure of medical treatment
- Benign endometrial histology
- Uterine size <10 cm
- Completed family.

Q. 25. What are the exclusion criteria for endometrial ablation?

- Large cavity >12 cm
- Malformed uterus
- Malignancy
- Age <40 years (more likely to fail)
- Genital tract infections
- Scarred uterus (classical)
- Transmural myomectomy
- Fibroid
- Patient who wants pregnancy
- Postmenopausal woman
- Previous failed endometrial ablation.

PALM-COEIN Classification of AUB

A. *Structural causes:* Polyps, adenomyosis, leiomyomas—Submucosal, malignancy and hyperplasia, Iatrogenic

B. *Non-structural causes:* Coagulopathy, ovulatory dysfunction, other endometrial (primary disorder of mechanisms regulating local endometrial "hemostasis")

C. Not yet specified

Newer Classification (AUB modalities)

P—Polyp
A—Adenomyosis
L—Leiomyoma
M—Malignancy
C—Coagulopathy
O—Ovular causes
I—Iatrogenic causes
E—Endometrial causes
N—Not classified

Q. 26. How do you treat von Willebrand disease?

- Decompression (DDAVP) or nasal spray.
- Antifibrinolytic or clot stabilizing medications like tranexemic acid
- Contraception are useful in controling heavy bleeding during menstruation
- Replacement therapy—von Willebrand factor VIII is needed in severe form of the disease.

Q. 27. What is the role of role of hysteroscopy in AUB?

- Intrauterine lesions—malignancy, tuberculosis
- Growth—fibroid polyp, submucous myoma
- Can locate exact site of biopsy
- Can treat at the same time
- Forgotten IUCD.

Q. 28. What are the indications for hysteroscopy?

- Intermenstrual spotting
- In a regularly menstruating woman sudden menorrhagia
- Persistence of symptoms despite medical treatment
- Uncertain diagnosis
- TVS suggestive of polyp, submucosal fibroid
- Even after D&C bleeding persists
- Peri and postmenopausal AUB.

Q. 29. What are the indications for giving gonadotropin in fibroid?

- To reduce the operating time
- To reduce bleeding
- To improve anemia
- They also decrease the size of the fibroid and endometrium becomes atrophic
- Alters the route of surgery. Abdominal hysterectomy could be converted to vaginal.

Q. 30. What are the prerequisites for TCRE?

- Endometrial sampling
- Pregnancy test
- Scan anomalies
- Culture and sensitivity
- GnRh analogs to reduce the thickness of endometrium.

Q. 31. What are the indication for hysterectomy?

- Failure of medical line of treatment
- Definitive treatment for those who want permanent cure
- Coexistence of adnexal pathology
- Postmenopause—hyperplasia, infection, fibroid
- Infections, fibroid
- Premalignant conditions with family completed
- Failure following other modalities like balloon, TCRE
- Noncompliant patient, due side effects of drugs, cost of the drug, etc.

Q. 32. Can you tell in nut shell the treatment of AUB?

- Near menopause—hysterectomy, if patient wants definitive treatment
- High risk patient—hysterectomy
- Peri menopausal—refuses surgery → Mirena, progesterone ormiloxiphene SERMS
- Mirena—non-tubectomized perimenopausal with small fibroids and endometriosis, added contraceptive effect.
- Ablative procedure—low risk patients
- Balloon therapy—IHD, high BP, mental retardation, where drugs like antifibrinolytic drugs cannot be given.

Treatment Options—*For Fibroid:*

- Medical management
- Surgical
- Miscellaneous
- Embolization.

Medical Management of AUB(O)

Nonhormonal

- Non-steroidal anti-inflammatory drugs
- Capillary wall stabilizers—Ethamsylate
- Antifibrinolytics.

Hormonal

GnRh is given to those patients who are not fit for surgery and also as a preoperative in case of ablation therapy. If the treatment is prolonged more than 6 months, then add back therapy is advised.

Other therapies are LNG-IUS, oral progesterone, DMPA, testosterone, high dose of estrogen, SERMs, etc.

Q. 33. What is the medical management of acute uterine bleeding?

Medication	Description	Dose	Frequency
Estrogen	Conjugated estrogen	25 mgIV	6th hourly
Oral pills	Monophasic pill	35 µg of ethinyl estradiol	TID for 7 days
Progesterone + pills	MPA	10–20 mg TID for 7 days	
	Megestral	20–60 mg	TID for 7 days
Tranexamic acid	Hemostatic	1.3 g orally or 10 mg/kg max 600 mg	TID for 5 days

Role of LNG-IUS

It is an intrauterine system, which releases progesterone continuously. It acts as contraception and the life span is for 5 years.

- LNG-IUS is now recommended as first line ot treatment as it is found to be more effective in treating endometrial hyperplasia with lower recurrence rate thus reducing the need for hysterectomy.
- Suspect endometrial cancer if there is recurrence of symptoms or hyperplasia inspite of LNG-IUS.
- LNG is effective in treating inherited bleeding disorders causing menorrhagia.
- Is better than continuous oral or local progesterone's for endometrial hyperplasia without atypia.
- Cyclic progesterone are less effective in inducing regression of the hyperplasia than LNG-IUS.
- The strong antiproliferative effect of levonorgestrel is because of reduced PR expression which results in suppression of estrogen activity and thus the endometrial thickness.

Medical line of treatment for DUB

Treatment	Dosage	Mechanism	Contraindication	Side effects	Benefits	Contraception
Hormonal	OC pills X 21 days, continuous, a patch or ring	HPO axis suppression	Brest cancer, liver, disuses, migraine, HTN	Breast tenderness, water retention	50% reduction in PMS and MBL, regularity	yes
Cyclic oral progesterone	MPA 5–10 mg × 10–14 days	Inhibits endometrial proliferation	Breast CA, Liver and renal diseases	Breast tenderness, mood changes	Bleeding reduced by 87%	Decrease ability to conceive
Injectable progesterone DMPA	150 mg IM X 90 days	Inhibits steroids genesis	Same as above	Irregular bleeding BMD decrease	60% amenorrhea at 12 months	Yes
LNG-IUS	50 mg releasing 20 µg/day	Local suppression	Intra cavity fibroids, past PID	Same as above	70–90% reduction MBL	Yes
GnRH agonists Leuprolide	3.75 mg/month IM	Decreases steroids-genesis— endo atrophy	Allergy	Hot flashes, dry vagina	89% MBL stops, amenorrhea	No
Danazol	100–400 mg/daily	Endometrial atrophy	Liver disease	Wt gain, hirsutism	81% reduction in MBL	No
Ormiloxiphene	60 mg bd/3 months 60 mg wkly/yr	SERMs	Liver disease	Amenorrhea, wt gain	Decreases MBL	Yes
Gestrinone	2.5–5 mg/day orally	Endometrial atrophy		Deepening of voice	Reduction in MBL	No

Comparison of hysterectomy with ablative procedures

	Hysterectomy	Ablation 1st generation	2nd generation
Anesthesia	GA/Spinal	GA	Local
Visualization of cavity	Not possible	Yes	Not possible
Duration of surgery	More	May be same	Less
Stay in hospital	+++	++	+
Complications during surgery	Injury to viscera, hemorrhage	Perforation, electric trauma, embolism, fluid over load	Cervical laceration
Remote complication	Hernia	Postablation syndrome	
Menstruation	No	Possible	Possible
Satisfaction	+++	++	+
Need for hysterectomy		May need	May need
Pregnancy	No	Yes	Yes
Endometrial cancer	No	Yes	Yes
Instruments	Routine	Hysteroscope + accessories	No hysteroscope, specific instrument
Skill	Required	Required	Not required
Size of the uterus	Any size	<10–12 cm	<10–12 cm in general
Fitness for surgery	Fit	Fit	Not fit for surgery
Uterine anomalies	Possible to do	No	No
Any other unexpected pathology	Possible to do	Not possible	Not possible
Psychological impact of loosing uterus	Yes	No	No
Presence of lower genital infection	Possible to do	Not recommended	Not recommended
Perforated/missing IUD	Possible to do	Not recommended	Not recommended

Comparison of 1st and 2nd generation ablation

1st/2nd	Technique		Advantages	Disadvantages	Complications
1st	TCRE	Resectoscope	Polypectomy possible Endometrial sample for HPE Success rate 80%	Hysteroscope, anesthesia, skill required	Peroration Electrical burns
1st	Roller ball	Roller ball – 2 mm and 4 mm moving up and down	Less time and perforation, less absorption of fluid	Same as above	Electrical burns

Contd...

Contd...

1st/2nd	Technique		Advantages	Disadvantages	Complications
2nd	Thermal balloon ablation (hydro)	Duration 8 min Temp 87° C Pressure 160–180 mm of Hg	TBEA is effective, safe, and cost-effective for patients with DUB. For women who are not worried about amenorrhea	Cannot be used in irregular cavity. In the treatment of menorrhagia, bipolar radiofrequency endometrial ablation system is superior to hydrothermablation	Cramps, infection, pain
2nd	Microwave	Duration 3 min Cervix dilatation up to 8 mm	83% satisfaction		Perforation Pain—analgesics
2nd	Cryoablation	−90°C 2 mins cool f/b 2 mins thaw Done for 10 mins Ablates up to depth 4–5 mm	50–70% amenorrhea, no complications of distension of uterus	Vaginal watery discharge for a week	Cramping, requires analgesics, takes to time to act
2nd	Photodynamic	Time = 60 mins, 5-Aminolevulinic acid Light WL635 nm Intensity 300 MW	No fibrosis, No adhesions	Feasibility and clinical usefulness not established	Photodynamic endometrial ablation is selective
2nd	Bipolar radiofrequency ablation (Nova sure)	Procedure time 4 minutes Treatment cycle time 90 sec	Can be done at anytime of the menses. Rapid recovery. Excellent success rate, superior to hydrothermal	Bipolar radio-frequency and microwave ablative devices are more effective than thermal balloon and free fluid ablation in the treatment of heavy menstrual bleeding	Bipolar radiofrequency impedance-controlled system is associated with increased rates of amenorrhea at 12-months post-treatment as compared to the MEA method. MEA group required more analgesiscs than Nova sure group
2nd	Cavaterm ablative system [Glycerin]	Glycerin 1.5 % T : 75oC P: 180 mm Hg, 200 mm of Hg, 15 Time-minutes Cervix 6–8 mm dilatation	40% amenorrhea		

Contd...

Contd...

1st/2nd	Technique		Advantages	Disadvantages	Complications
1st	Laser Nd-YAG	Cx 7 mm, dilatation, device opens inside light absorbed by Hb, temp 102°, 1–3.5 mm of myometrium also destroyed	No distension of cavity		
2nd	Radiofrequency	Time = 20 mins electromagnetic radiations 27 MHz Power 550 W		Abandoned due to high complication rate	
2nd	Unipolar electrodes [Vesta]	----	---------	---------------	----------------

Polyps
- Polyp—sessile, pedunculated
- Fibroid polyp—benign and malignant can cause menorrhagia, metrorrhagia
- Placental polyp—formed by retained placental tissue, causes postpartum bleeding
- Small polyps can be removed by rescetoscope along with ablative procedure
- Larger one—operating hysteroscope.

Points to Remember
- Postnatal, post abortion, post IUCD—cycles will be most of the time irregular in rhythm and flow. Hence Hb% should be checked and anemia should be treated.
- Perimenopausal bleeding—Diagnostic hysteroscopy and guided EB is required.
- If no malignancy—and only symptom of menorrhagia then 1st or 2nd generation of endometrial ablation can be advised.
- If there is family history endometrial carcinoma then hysterectomy is justified
- Defer hysterectomy and advise for LNG-IUS unless there is strong indication for hysterectomy.
- In NHEA (non-hysteroscopic endometrial ablation) are effective ,safe, can be done under local anaesthesia and bleeding is less.

Bibliography

1. ACOG-committee opinion. Management of acute abnormal uterine bleeding in non-pregnant reproductive-aged women. 2013;557.
2. Angioni S, Pontis A, Nappi L, et al. Endometrial ablation: first- vs. second-generation technique. 2016;68(2):143-53. Epub 2016 Feb 29.
3. Athanatos D, et al. Department of uterine bleeding: a double-blind, randomized controlled trial of obstetrics and gynecology. J Am Assoc Gynecol Laparosc. 2003;10(1):17-26.
4. Baskett TF, Clough H, Scott TA. NovaSure bipolar radiofrequency endometrial ablation: report of 200 cases. J Obstet Gynaecol Can. 2005;27(5):473-6.
5. Billow MR, El-Nashar SA. Management of Abnormal Uterine Bleeding with Emphasis on Alternatives to Hysterectomy. Obstet Gynecol Clin North Am. 2016;43(3):415-30. doi: 10.1016/j.ogc.2016.04.002.
6. Bonnar J, Sheppard BL. Treatment of menorrhagia during menstruation: randomised controlled trial of ethamsylate, mefenamic acid, and tranexamic acid. BMJ. 1996;313(7057):579-82.

7. Chuong CJ, Brenner PF. Management of abnormal uterine bleeding. 1996;175(3):787-92.
8. Cooper JM, Anderson TL, Fortin CA, et al. Microwave endometrial ablation vs. rollerball electroablation for menorrhagia: a multicenter randomized trial. Indications and options for endometrial ablation. J Am Assoc Gynecol Laparosc. 2004;11(3):394-403.
9. Daniels JP, Middleton LJ, Champaneria R, et al. Second generation endometrial ablation techniques for heavy menstrual bleeding: network meta-analysis. IPD meta-analysis Collaborative Group BMJ. 2012;344:e2564. Published online 2012 Apr 23.doi: 10.1136/bmj.e2564PMCID: PMC3339574.
10. Duleba AJ, et al. A randomized study comparing endometrial cryoablation and rollerball electroablation for treatment of dysfunctional uterine bleeding. Lasers Surg Med. 2003;32(4):305-9.
11. Fernandez H, Capella S, Audibert R. Thermal balloon ablation for the treatment of menorrhagia in an outpatient setting. Oxford Journals Medicine & Health Human Reproduction. 14;11:2743-7.
12. Fraser IS, Critchley HO, Broder M, et al. The FIGO recommendations on terminologies and definitions for normal and abnormal uterine bleeding. Semin Reprod Med. 2011;29(5):383-90. doi: 10.1055/s-0031-1287662. Epub 2011 Nov 7.
13. Gallos ID, Krishan P, Shehmar M, et al. LNG-IUS versus oral progestogen treatment for endometrial hyperplasia: a long-term comparative cohort study. Hum Reprod. 2013;28(11):2966-71. https://doi.org/10.1093/humrep/det320.
14. Gallos ID, Shehmar M, Thangaratinam S, et al. Oral progestogens vs levonorgestrel-releasing intrauterine system for endometrial hyperplasia: a systematic review and metaanalysis. Am J Obstet Gynecol. 2010;203(6):547.e1-10. doi: 10.1016/j.ajog.2010.07.037.
15. Gervaise A, Fernandez H, Capella-Allouc S, et al. Gomel thermal balloon ablation versus endometrial resection for the treatment of abnormal uterine bleeding. Hum Reprod. 1999; 14(11):2743-7.doi: 10.1093/humrep/14.11.2743
16. Goldfarb HA. A review of 35 endometrial ablations using the Nd:YAG laser for recurrent menometrorrhagia 60% had amenorrhea. Obstet Gynecol.1990;76(5 Pt 1):833-5.
17. Green-top Guideline No. 59. March 2011.
18. Green top guidelines- No 67. February 206. Management of endometrial hyperplasia, RCOG/BSGE joint guidelines, Feb 2016.
19. Hajiali F, Nassiri M. Report of severe menorrhagia following the maximum amount of lamotrigine overdose. Iran J Pharm Reas. 2015;14(4):1289-93.
20. Hawe J, Abbott J, Hunter D, et al. A randomised controlled trial comparing the Cavaterm endometrial ablation system with the Nd:YAG laser for the treatment of dysfunctional uterine bleeding. Nd:YAG laser and carter are comparable results. BJOG. 2003;110(4):350-7.
21. Kabalak AA, Soyal OB, Urfalioglu A, et al. Menometrorrhagia and tachyarrhythmia after using oral and topical ginseng. J Womens Health (Larchmt). 2004;13(7):830-3.
22. Kingman CE, Kadir RA, Lee CA, et al. The use of levonorgestrel-releasing intrauterine system for treatment of menorrhagia in women with inherited bleeding disorders. BJOG. 2004 Dec;111(12):1425-8.
23. Lee SY, Kim MK, Park H, et al. The effectiveness of levonorgestrel releasing intrauterine system in the treatment of endometrial hyperplasia in Korean women. J Gynecol Oncol. 2010;21(2):102-5. doi:10.3802/jgo.2010.21.2.102
24. Leminen H, Hurskainen R. Tranexamic acid for the treatment of heavy menstrual bleeding: efficacy and safety. Int J Women's Health. 2012;4:413-21.
25. Management of endometrial hyperplasia, Green top Green-top Guideline No. 67 RCOG/BSGE Joint Guideline. February 2016.
26. Moore E, Shaf M. Endometrial hyperplasia review article. Obstetrics, Gynaecology and Reproductive Medicine. 23(3):89-93.
27. Rao S, Pawar V, Badhwar VR, et al. http://www.bhj.org.in/journal/2004_4602Medical Interventions in Puberty Menorrhagia_april/html/medical_interventions_121.htm Genital tuberculosis causing puberty menorrhagia

28. Ray S, Ray A. Non-surgical interventions for treating heavy menstrual bleeding (menorrhagia) in women with bleeding disorders. Cochrane Database Syst Rev. 2016; 11:CD010338.
29. Shanti SA, Jehon A. Pubertal Menorrhagia: Evaluation and Management. Journal of Clinical and Biomedical Sciences.
30. Thermal balloon endometrial ablation for dysfunctional uterine bleeding: an evidence-based analysis. Ont Health Technol Assess Ser. 2004;4(11):1-89. Epub 2004 Sep 1. Health Quality Ontario.
31. van Eijkeren MA, Christiaens GC, Geuze HJ, et al. Effects of mefenamic acid on menstrual hemostasis in essential menorrhagia, Am J Obstet Gynecol. 1992;166(5):1419-28.
32. Wildemeersch D, Janssens D, Pylyser K, et al. Management of patients with non-atypical and atypical endometrial hyperplasia with a levonorgestrel-releasing intrauterine system: long-term follow-up. Maturitas. 2007;57(2): 210-3. Epub 2007 Jan 31.
33. Wyss P, et al. Photodynamic endometrial ablation: morphological study. Obstet Gynecol. 2010;116(4):819-26.

20
CHAPTER

Benign Ovarian Tumors: A Clinical Approach

HR Damayanthi

Main Objective of Study of Benign Ovarian Tumors

- Age—for assessment distribution of tumor by decades of life is important
- Method (s) of presentation—clinical approach and assessment
- Laboratory methods to add and support clinical diagnosis.

Management Guidelines

- Risk assessment
- Observation/expectant
- Medical management
- Surgical—elective/emergency
- Follow-up
- Special problems
- Final diagnosis—(clinical + histopathological)
- Communication/counseling.

Note: Many procedures do not replace a careful medical history and thorough physical and pelvic examination.

Benign Ovarian Tumors: A Clinical Approach

Ovarian masses are a common finding in general gynecology. Neoplasms constitute a significant number and most are benign. Diagnosis of a pelvic mass in adolescent age group is a challenge. Age group needs to be considered because the likelihood of functional masses increases after menarche.

It is entirely possible that the different types of ovarian neoplasms have differing etiologies, particularly as germ cell tumors, which account for 25% of ovarian neoplasms occur in younger women than do the epithelial ovarian tumors, which account for 75% seen in the reproductive age group.

Unlike cervical cancer there is no clearly defined preinvasive ovarian lesion. Benign, borderline and malignant tumors are distinct pathological entities.

CASE

A 35-year-old parous woman presents with occasional vague abdominal discomfort. On pelvic examination, a 6 × 6 cm cystic, non-tender left adnexal mass was felt. How is this case to be managed?

Q. 1. What are the specific points to be noted in history?

- *Reproductive history:* It is an important determinant of epithelial ovarian cancer risk. Risk is inversely correlated with parity—number of ovulation events is the main risk factor. Improvements in diagnostic methods have contributed a great deal in establishing an accurate diagnosis. Occasionally or often, it is difficult to differentiate a benign from a malignant tumor clinically.

During the reproductive years, ovarian masses are generally benign. They can be functional or neoplastic. Neoplastic tumors can be benign or malignant. Neoplasia can arise from any of the elements of a mature ovary—serosal, mucosal and stromal elements.

- *Age:* Most ovarian tumors are benign— 80–85%. About 75% of these tumors occur between 22 years and 44 years. Risk of ovarian malignancy is 1 in 15 in these women less than 45 years.
- *Symptoms:* In most of the cases, neoplasm is asymptomatic/never painful. Without any accident they are amazingly quiet excluding those who have an endocrine function. Mechanical symptoms are due to the size of the mass and its location. Important age groups to be remembered are prepubertal, reproductive age group— women who present with menorrhagia and postmenopausal women where hormonal disruption is suspected.
- *History of infertility and whether being investigated.*
- *Previous surgeries*
- *Drug history:* If a woman is on oral contraceptive pills, functional cysts should not be present.
- *Menopausal status:* About 70–80% of neoplasia arise from primary epithelial structures, 10% from stromal, 5% germ cell origin. 2–3% of the tumors are seen during pregnancy which requires careful evaluation and planning.

Q. 2. How should such a patient be examined?

- General physical examination—built, pallor, signs of distress, edema, lymph nodes
- Examination of thyroid, breast
- Respiratory and cardiovascular examination
- Abdominal examination (Fig. 1):
  - Location of mass (pelvic/abdominal)
  - Size, mobility, consistency, tenderness, bilaterality, whether lower border made out or not
  - Associated ascites or any other organomegaly.

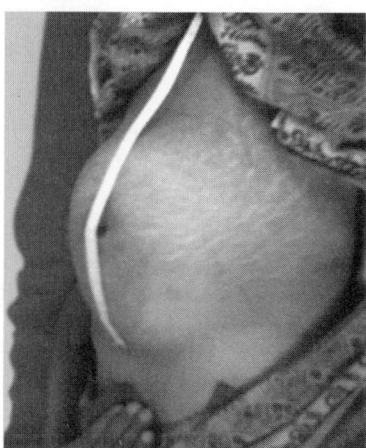

Fig. 1: Mass being measured

Important Clues:
- 75% of all tumors occur in younger age—mostly benign (80–85%), 75% are seen between 22 years and 44 years of age.
- 70–80% of neoplasia arise from primary epithelial structures, 10% from stromal, 5% germ cell origin. 2–3% of the tumors are seen during pregnancy which requires careful evaluation and planning.
- More than 75% of adnexal masses are functional (not true neoplasms).
- Among the 25% of true neoplasms—10% are malignant.
- Epithelial tumors comprise the largest group.
- Most common tumor of reproductive age group is cystic teratoma.
- History with clinical assessment are sufficient to make a clinical diagnosis supported by sonographic studies—CT/MRI have limited value in asymptomatic women.
- Tumor markers are important for suspected and specific tumors (CA125, CEA, AFP, LDH etc.)
- Every adnexal mass requires individual assessment and management. Generally. Expectant management for functional cysts.
- More than 6 cm—thorough evaluation mainly to rule out malignancy.

Benign Ovarian Tumors: A Clinical Approach

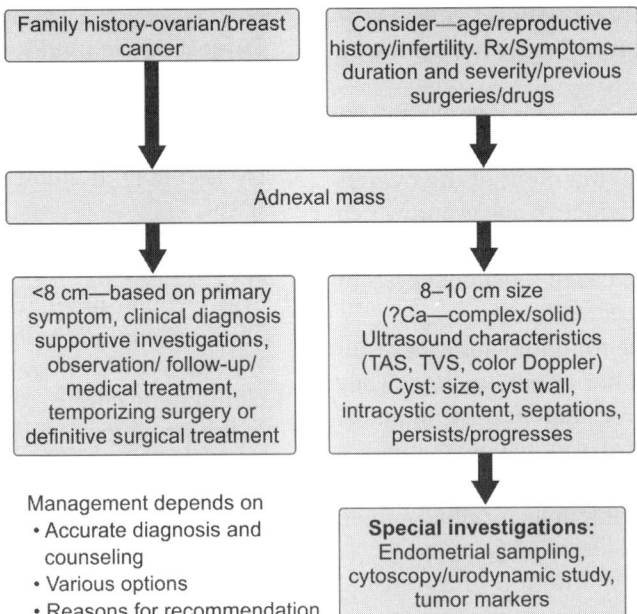

Flowchart 1: Evaluation of an adnexal mass

Pelvic examination: Speculum examination (including Pap smear), bimanual examination to confirm details of adnexal mass and its various characteristics
Per rectal examination
Management depends on (Flowchart 1):
- Accurate diagnosis and counseling
- Various options
- Reasons for recommendation.

Q. 3. What are the differential diagnoses that need to be considered?

Differential Diagnoses
- Acute appendicitis with or without abscess formation
- Ectopic pregnancy
- Encysted ascites
- Degenerating fibroid
- Ruptured corpus luteum
- Tubo-ovarian abscess
- Less commonly (nongynecological pelvic pathology)—pelvic kidney/GI abnormalities

Critical value(s) in assessment
- Age of the patient
- Methods of presentation
- Physical and pelvic examination
- Most probable nature of tumor—benign/malignant or functional cyst
- Management guidelines after relevant laboratory assessment—Doppler study, tumor markers
- Documentation

Give a brief note on pregnancy associated with ovarian tumor
- Incidentally recognized during pregnancy or exists prior to it
- Symptomatic/asymptomatic
- Most probable nature of tumor, anticipated complications to plan intervention
- Incidence is 2–3%
- Often require surgical intervention
- Thorough assessment of fetal status and optimal time of intervention are crucial
- Generally intervention during the second trimester is favored after counseling regarding risks and benefits

- Rate of torsion is 1%
- The most common tumor is benign cystic teratoma followed by serous cysts and endometrioma.

Q. 4. What are functional cysts of ovaries?

Non-neoplastic enlargement of the ovaries usually in the reproductive age group which are dependent on the hormones or dysfunction of the HPO axis are called functional cysts or physiological cysts of the ovaries.

- These cyts arise from follicles as a result of alteration of hormonal function. They are related to ovulation and are the most common cause of ovarian enlargement
- Masses arise due to collection or accumulation of intrafollicular fluid—there is no cellular proliferation
- Anovulation, dysfunction or abnormal gonadotropic stimulus result in expansion of the follicular antrum
- Hence, follicular cysts are non-neoplastic in nature, can be single or multiple, 3–5 cm in size and regress on their own
- However, following ovulation or hemorrhage in to the corpus luteum—results in the formation of a corpus luteal cyst (5–6 cm) which are often symptomatic
- Risk factors associated are:
  - Smoking (cause is not clear)
  - Women on progestin only pills (2–9%)
  - LNG-IUDs
  - Tamoxifen therapy (30%) which increases to 80% in premenopausal women
- About 95% of the cysts resolve with observation, occasionally emergency situations may be seen with rupture of corpus luteal cyst, mimicking ruptured ectopic pregnancy.
- Important functional cysts of the ovary are:
  - Follicular cysts—most common
  - Corpus luteal cyst/hemorrhage
  - Theca lutein cysts
  - Luteoma of pregnancy
  - Hyperreactio luteinalis.

Briefly explain the features of theca lutein cysts

- Largest of the functional cysts, but less common than follicular or corpus luteal cysts
- More often bilateral, multicystic, 25–30 cm
- Cysts contain multiple solid foci of luteal tissue
- Excessive levels of βhCG is responsible for stimulation and formation of these cysts—molar pregnancy, invasive mole, choriocarcinoma, multiple pregnancy
- Use of ovulation inducing drugs like clomiphene citrate, gonadotropins result in the formation of these cysts
- When primary lesion is treated they often regress
- Large cysts develop torsion, hemorrhage and rupture.

Q. 5. What do you mean by luteoma of pregnancy?

- Rare, benign process unique to pregnancy
- Represents a hyperplastic condition
- Spontaneous resolution is known to occur after delivery
- Luteinized stromal cells become hormonally active and result in the secretion of androgens—normal ovarian parenchyma is replaced
- In 30% of cases virilization may be seen; in 50% of the cases there is risk of virilization of the female fetus also
- Sonography reveals a nonspecific hypoechoic mass which is highly vascular.

Think of possibility of luteoma with signs of virilization in pregnancy

Hyperreactio luteinalis also could be found in pregnancy:
- No history of ovulation induction
- Increased incidence in PCOS
- Seen as an abnormal response to βhCG
- In 60% of cases seen in singleton pregnancies

- Often asymptomatic, maternal virilization in 25%
- Shifts in body fluids are rare
- Ovaries are enlarged, self limiting and resolves on its own.

Q. 6. What are hemorrhagic cysts? What are their sonological features?

Subclass of functional cysts have been recognized as hemorrhagic cyst (acute):
- Sonography reveals a hyperechoic lesion
- It mimics a solid mass—usually has a smooth posterior wall with acoustic enhancement (indicating cystic nature) with diffuse low level echoes
- After hemolysis attains a reticular pattern with interdigitating strands due to fibrin, later to have a concave margin
- There if fluid in pouch of Douglas
- No flow on colour Doppler
- Accuracy of the diagnosis of this type of cyst is 90%
- In contrast corpus luteal cyst contains low level echoes with thicker wall, unilateral and crenulated appearance. Color Doppler reveals a peripheral rim of color, larger than 6-7 cm and often symptomatic.

Theca lutein cysts, corpus luteal cysts, hyperreactio luteinalis and luteoma are all related to pregnancy.

Q. 7. What is the origin of ovarian tumors?

Neoplasms can arise from any of the element that comprise a normal ovary including surface epithelial (serosal) or mucosal elements. 70-80% of tumors arise from epithelial elements. 10% belong to the stromal category, 5% are germ cell in origin and the rest belong to other groups.

- Sonography in their evaluation during preoperative period is an important tool
- Emergency situations, such as torsion, hemorrhage, associated pregnancy can happen
- Tumor markers need to be estimated occasionally with high index of suspicion
- Management guidelines dictate surgical intervention (laparotomy/laparoscopy)
- In majority of ovarian tumors careful analysis of clinical data, supported by sonographic evaluation, the most probable histopathological nature of lesion can also be known in the preoperative period
- However, the final word of histopathology reveals the diagnosis

Q. 8. What is the most common of benign tumors?

Among germ cell tumors, 90-95% are benign, the commonest being benign cystic teratoma often called dermoid (Figs 2 and 3).

Benign Cystic Teratoma
- Benign teratomas comprise 10-25% of all ovarian neoplasm, only 1-2% become malignant

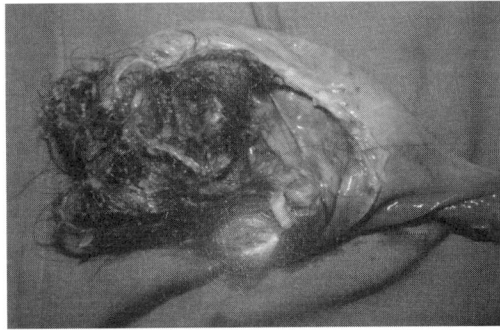

Fig. 2: Dermoid cyst with ectodermal derivatives

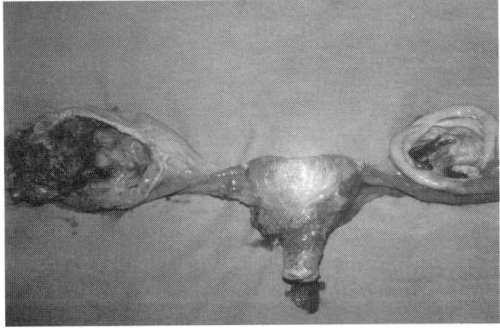

Fig. 3: Bilateral dermoid cyst

- It belongs to the germ cell family, arises from a single germ cell—asexual reproduction. In mammals, it falls short of normal embryonal development. Almost all mature teratomas have 46XX as chromosomal pattern
- Generally slow growing, size varies between 5-10 cm, less than 10 cm on 80% of cases
- Age: Any age more often seen in 3rd/4th decade of life. 91% occur between 20-40 years of age
- The term dermoid is a misnomer (because of prevalence of dermal elements), it contains tissues arising from all 3 elements. Occasionally, thyroid tissue may be seen. When it comprises more than 75% of the tumor it is called as strumaovarii (2-3%) (signs of hyperthyroidism with adnexal mass, strumaovarii should be suspected)
- Bilateral in 10% of cases
- More often associated with pregnancy—25-50% of all pregnancy associated with ovarian tumors
- Cut section of the tumor reveals Rokitansky's protuberances also called dermoid plug/process/mamilla or embryonal rudiment. Varied tissue types may be present but ectodermal elements predominate. Carcinoma may develop—squamous cell carcinoma
- Mature teratoma is subclassified into:
  - Mature cystic teratoma (benign/dermoid)
  - Mature solid tumor—elements form a solid mass
  - Fetiform tumor or homunculus: Which is doll-shaped consisting of germ cell layers
  - Monodermal tumor—tissues are arranged in normal spatial differentiation, solely or predominantly contains only one type of highly specialized tissue type, e.g. thyroid tissue when it is called struma ovarii.
- Cyst is lined by keratinized squamous epithelium; contents are sebaceous material, sweat glands, fatty tissue, hair, teeth, bone, cartilage
- Often asymptomatic or present with signs and symptoms of abdominopelvic mass. In 15% of cases torsion is seen. Thyroid storm can occur in about 12%; carcinoid syndrome is rare
- Pelvic examination reveals a mass more often anterior to the uterus; because of fat content floats in the abdominal cavity and likely to rest in uterovesical pouch
- Sonographic evaluation:
  - Signs of complete cystic mass with mural nodules to solid mass. Anechoic to hyperechoic due to hair and sebum. Cystic component is purely due to sebum which is liquid at body temperature
  - Dermoid plug (creates an acute angle with cyst wall) contains hair, teeth and fat, 1-4 cm in size—creates an acoustic shadow.
  - Because of multiple tissue interfaces, poorly defined acoustic shadow obscures the posterior wall of the lesion. Acoustic shadowing is due to attenuating mass. This is called " tip of iceberg" sign
  - Teeth and bone are seen as highly echogenic foci with acoustic shadowing
  - Hair is seen as linear hyperechogenic interfaces floating is a specific sign called as dermoid mesh
  - Fat fluid with hair form a dependent layer is more echogenic. In 30% of tumors nondependent layer will be more echogenic
  - When there is a large cystic pelvic mass (rare but characteristic feature)—multiple, mobile, spherical echogenic structures are seen floating as pellets. Microscopic examination reveals the presence of keratin, fibrin and hair
  - Two or more characteristic ultrasound findings when present—100% positive predictive value

- Color Doppler study reveals central blood flow is absent
- Role of CT/MRI is limited.

X-ray abdomen reveals pelvic calcification, possibilities are:
* Benign cystic teratoma
* Calcified uterine fibroid
* Papillary serous cystadenoma—Psammoma bodies

- *Management:* Surgical intervention should be planned. During pregnancy unless there is an emergency suggestive of torsion or rupture of the tumor which requires immediate intervention, Surgical intervention is carried out during the 2nd trimester. Surgery is for relief of symptoms, to prevent complications and to retain or preserve ovarian function. In nonpregnant women, laparoscopic procedure is an option.

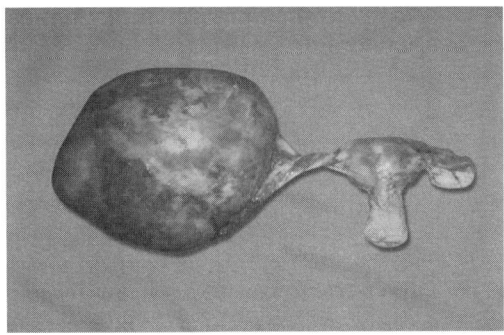

Fig. 4: Huge unilateral cystic mass with torsion.

Final word: Regardless of Doppler findings if ovary is morphologically normal, there is no torsion

Q. 9. What are the features of torsion of ovarian tumor?

- Fallopian tube and ovary along with the tumor rotate as a single entity around the broad ligament (Fig. 4)
- Commonly seen in the age group of 20–40 years, however, can also occur in post menopausal period
- Incidence of torsion in pregnancy with ovarian tumor is 15%
- When the size of the cyst is more than 6 cm with a long pedicle the risk of torsion increases
- Pathophysiology reveals that low pressure veins are compressed initially, later flow gets arrested which is followed by arterial compression. Adnexal structures become congested and edematous and progressive stromal swelling is observed. Arterial compression results in infarction and necrosis resulting in acute severe abdominal pain with nausea, vomiting and syncopal attacks. Pain is also felt in the sacroiliac region and upper medial thigh (referred pain).
- Sonographic findings depend on the duration of torsion, degree of vascular compression and extent of involvement of the adnexal mass
  - Ovary is enlarged on the ipsilateral side or multiple cortical follicles in an enlarged ovary which is a specific sign. There is transudation of fluid into the cortical follicles due to circulatory impairment
  - Presence of arteriovenous flow does not exclude torsion. On color Doppler absent flow is seen. Absence of internal ovarian flow is not specific to torsion
  - Twisted ovarian pedicle appears like a round hyperechoic structure with multiple concentric hypoechoic stripes
  - Ovarian mass anterior to the uterus and cephalad to the bladder should lead to the suspicion of torsion
  - The appearance of ovarian pedicle is called as target appearance or ellipsoid structure with heterogeneous internal echoes
  - *Whirlpool sign:* Color Doppler study reveals the presence of circular or coiled twisted vessel within the vascular pedicle. Absence of blood flow suggests nonviable ovarian tissue. Most constant sign is unilateral enlargement of the ovary.

Q. 10. What are the differential diagnoses for ovarian torsion?

- Acute salpingitis
- Acute appendicitis
- Hemorrhage or rupture of ovarian cyst
- Ectopic pregnancy
- Intestinal obstruction
- Renal colic
- *Treatment:* Surgical intervention (either laparotomy or laparoscopy). Confirmation of intraoperative findings, extent of torsion, viability of organ, presence or absence of necrosis/infarction, conservative or extirpative procedure is done. Ovarian cystectomy is reasonable procedure. Proper patient selection is critical for laparoscopic management and also depends on surgical expertise.

Q. 11. What are epithelial ovarian tumors?

Features of Serous Cystadenoma

- Commonly seen during the reproductive age group—4th and 5th decade of life—risk increases with age
- 20–25% of all benign ovarian tumors
- 10–20% are bilateral, generally benign, unilocular or multilocular, 20–30 cm in size
- Women present with mass or pelvic pain or heaviness
- 5–10% belong to low malignant potential group (borderline malignant)
- 20–25% become malignant; hence, availability of frozen section biopsy is important
- Multilocular tumors have papillary components or projections, the cavity is lined by columnar or cuboidal epithelium. These may be cystic, papillary, adenofibromatous on microscopic examination
- The intracystic content is thin, clear or light yellow-straw colored
- Psammoma bodies are fine calcific granulations scattered within the tumor seen on X-ray—concentrically laminated calcified concretions

- *Sonography* reveals the origin, size, consistency and echogenic characteristics of the mass. Solid components, mural nodules, papillary excrescences and ascites increase the suspicion of malignancy. TAS and TVS enhance interpretation and accuracy of diagnosis.

Features of Mucinous Cystadenomas

- Account for 20% of all ovarian tumors and 50% of all benign ovarian tumors.
- Seen during 30–50 years of age
- 5% are bilateral, usually multiloculated, 30–40 cm in size
- Incidence of malignancy is 5–10% (Fig. 5)
- The site of continued growth of cyst is marked by a mass of small locule. Inner wall is smooth and occasionally intracystic papillae are seen. The thickness of outer wall varies, white or gray in color. Generally adhesions to surrounding structures are not seen.

> Authors share the experience of having seen a woman at 58 years of age, not attained menopause, presenting with cyclical menorrhagia. Endometrial study revealed evidence of hyperplasia. LAVH with BSO done. Cut section of the ovary revealed a circumscribed lesion 1–1.5 cm, histology proved as benign Brenner's tumor. The lady had an uneventful recovery

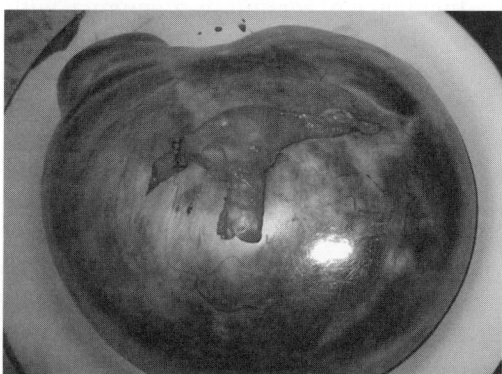

Fig. 5: Uterus placed over a huge tumor: Mucinous cystadenoma

- Columnar cells line the cyst wall and secrete a glycoprotein with a high content

of neutral polysaccharide. Intracystic content is thick and often colorless. If the cyst ruptures though rare it results in pseudomyxoma peritoneii resulting in intraperitoneal adhesions
- Similar situation is also seen with mucocele of the appendix, and it can coexist with ovarian pathology
- Generally present as an abdominopelvic mass.

Q. 12. What are Brenner's tumors?

- Generally these tumors are small, solid, smooth, <5 cm in size and are recognized during histological examination
- Columns of squamous or transitional celled with coffee bean nucleus lie in the stroma
- Maybe seen along with mucinous cystadenoma or fibroma
- Most often benign, 2–3% of epithelial tumors
- May present with menorrhagia due to endometrial hyperplasia probably as a result of theca cell activity
- 1% of epithelial cancer is due to Brenner's tumor.

Q. 13. What are paraovarian cysts?

- The cyst arises from epithelial remnants, usually the epoophoron or as a true neoplasm. It is located in the mesovarium, while it increases in size the ovary and tube are separated. The tube and fimbriae remain stretched over the superior surface of the cyst
- Constitutes 5% of adnexal cysts, most are non-neoplastic
- Generally small in size (<5 cm), but occasionally they attain huge sizes becoming abdominopelvic
- Even though benign occasionally papillary growths can be seen inside the cyst
- These cysts when neoplastic resemble cystadenoma/cystadenofibroma
- Generally unilocular with a thin cyst wall, containing colorless fluid with cholesterol crystals
- Anechoic on ultrasonography
- These cysts are seen in younger age groups when compared to ovarian tumors, often asymptomatic but may present with features of torsion, hemorrhage or rupture
- They are fixed in the pelvis displacing the uterus to the opposite side (unlike a freely mobile ovarian tumor)
- Broad ligament fibroid and pelvic kidney should be kept in mind as possible differential diagnosis
- Malignancy is rare
- Sonography can delineate the characteristics of the cyst in addition to which the ipsilateral ovary can also be seen which is of diagnostic significance
- Treatment is surgical. During the procedure typical stretching of tube over the upper pole of the cyst is seen. The presence of vessels crossing each other in the capsule provides clue to the diagnosis that the tumor is extraperitoneal. The vessels belong to the peritoneum and to the true capsule. Cyst is shelled out. Displaced ureter with large cysts needs attention to avoid injury.

Q. 14. Comment on ovarian endometriosis.

- Predominantly seen in women of the reproductive age group. Occasionally, seen in adolescents and postmenopausal women on hormone therapy
- It is perceived as a chronic disease
- The objective of consideration of this condition is manifold. Though, it is not considered under tumors, cystic enlargement of the ovary can be seen measuring 10–12 cm
- Incidence—10%
- It is prudent to remember a few important risk factors in women presenting with infertility or subfertility.

- Dysmenorrhea, dyspareunia
- Chronic pelvic pain
- Short cycle length, menorrhagia
- Family history of endometriosis (1st degree relative).

However, they may be asymptomatic even with advanced disease. Gastrointestinal symptoms can coexist and quality of life is affected. The time interval from the onset of pain to establishment of diagnosis is around 8 years.

- In endometrioma, the tube and ovary are distorted, and there is ovulatory dysfunction with abnormal follicular growth and development. There is alteration in the hormonal milieu
- Clinically signs may not be obvious however on examination, uterosacral nodularity and scarring, painful swelling in rectovaginal septum, presence of unilateral ovarian cyst and a retroverted uterus with fixed adnexa help in diagnosis
- Sonography and estimation of CA-125 levels are important in confirmation of diagnosis. The role of laparoscopy is invaluable in confirming diagnosis and various treatment modalities
- Ultrasound findings:
  - Endometrioma is usually located over the anterior surface of the ovary. A well defined uni- or multilocular cyst of the ovary with retraction, pigmentation and adhesion to the posterior peritoneum
  - It is predominantly cystic with diffuse homogeneous low level internal echoes (seen diffusely throughout the mass or in a dependent position). The accuracy of diagnosis is 95%, with 97% positive predictive value
  - Small linear hyperechoic foci may be present in the wall of the cyst (cholesterol deposits in the cyst wall), occasional foci of calcification are also seen
- Endometrioma is seen rarely in pregnancy. If decidualisation of wall of endometrioma occurs results in a solid vascular mural mass that cannot be differentiated from carcinoma
- Endometroid and clear cell cancer can occur in endometrioma
- Principles of management focus on prevention, individualized treatment and assessment of impact of the disease or quality of life, its outcome following treatment. The various treatment options are:
  - Vaporization of surface lesions of ovary
  - Extirpation of the lesion—removal of the cyst capsule, drainage, electrocauterization of cyst wall with maximum preservation of ovarian tissue.
  - If the size of the cyst is more than 3 cm removal is recommended with GnRH analogs.
- Histologically, presence of endometrial glands with stroma with or without hemosiderin proves the diagnosis. Negative histology does not rule out the disease. Visual and histological confirmation of atleast one lesion is ideal. Varying degrees of proliferative and secretory activity with smooth muscle tissue are seen. If the endometrioma is more than 4 cm or infiltrating – carcinoma to be ruled out.

Large endometrioma is a marker of extensive disease, including intestinal disease. In 1% only endomterioma is seen and other organs are not affected.

Q. 15. Discuss the differential diagnosis for solid ovarian tumors.

Completely solid ovarian masses are benign. Removal of the mass is indicated because malignancy cannot be ruled out. Solid ovarian masses may represent sex cord stromal tumors, ovarian fibroma, fibrothecoma, carcinoid tumor, etc.

- **Granulosa and theca cell tumors**
  - These tumors are composed of granulosa cells, theca interna cells in varying proportion. Fibrous tissue predominates in thecoma

- Majority are pure tumors, mixed variety is also seen
- These tumors are solid, round, yellowish-white, 5–6 cm in size
- Degenerations are seen
- 70% of these tumors occur in postmenopausal age and present with post menopausal bleeding
- They are unilateral, almost always benign and secrete estrogen
- Histological patterns described in granulosa cell tumor are folliculoid or cylindromatous. Secretory activity and fluid collection which creates the appearance of Call–Exner bodies
- Recurrence is less common and occurs locally in the pelvis
- Theca cell tumor contains more of fibrous elements (stromal) and are rarely malignant.

- **Fibroma**
  - Comprise 3–5% and generally occur in the 5th decade of life
  - Solid white in color and cut section reveals a whorled appearance/spherical/lobulated
  - Size: 12–15 cm
  - Both hyaline and cystic degenerations are seen
  - When there is calcification it is called a calcified fibroma
  - The tumor can also contain adenomatous structures called as adenofibroma
  - The tumor should arise from the ovary, is solid in appearance and benign in character—it is a fibroma, though there are schools of thought that say presence of ascites and hydrothorax (20%) are essential in the diagnosis. After removal of the tumor ascites and hydrothorax resolve.
- On ultrasound—tumor appears hypoechoic with posterior attenuation of sound
- Differential diagnosis—Brenner's tumor, Pedunculated fibroid

- Surgery is removal combined with hysterectomy.

Referral to gynecologic oncologist
1. Premenopausal age:
   - Family history of ovarian malignancy or breast cancer
   - Abdominal mass + ascites
   - Abdominal or distant metastases
   - Levels of CA-125 >200 IU/L
2. Postmenopausal age:
   - Nodular or fixed pelvic mass
   - Family history of ovarian or breast cancer
   - Abdominal or distant metastases
   - CA125 >35 IU/L

Q. 16. How do you differentiate a benign tumor from malignancy by USG.

Sonographic evaluation of pelvic mass is shown in Table 1.

Table 1: Sonographic evaluation of a pelvic mass

Feature	Benign	Malignant
Age	Younger age	Older age
Size	<6–8 cm	>10 cm
External contour	Unilateral, thin wall, well defined, unilocular, cystic	Maybe bilateral, thick walled, irregular borders, solid/complex, fixed
Internal consistency	Purely cystic, thin septae	Thick irregular septae, echogenic solid nodule, papillary projections +
Doppler study	High resistance, no flow	Low resistance flow
Associated finding	Avascular nodule	Vascular nodule, ascites with peritoneal implants

Q. 17. Critically evaluate the methods used for calculating the risk of malignancy in a pelvic mass.

- To quantify the risk of ovarian malignancy ROMA scoring systems are used.

- Age
- Menopausal status (pre/post menopausal)
- CA-125 level >35 IU/L postmenopausal and >200 IU/L premenopausal
- USG findings
- CA 125 and HE4 are two markers approved by FDA for monitoring ovarian cancer progression.

FDA approved two algorithms, ROMA and OVA1, to estimate the risk of ovarian cancer in women with pelvic mass.

Risk of ovarian malignancy algorithm (ROMA)
- A quantitative serum test that combines **HE4**, **CA-125** and **menopausal status** into a numerical score
- To assess whether a woman who presents with an ovarian adnexal mass is at high or low likelihood of finding malignancy on surgery
- Calculation:

Premenopausal:
Predicative index (PI) = $-12.0 + 2.38 * LN[HE4] + 0.0626 * LN[CA-125]$
Postmenopausal:
Predicative Index (PI) = $-8.09 + 1.04 * LN[HE4] + 0.732 * LN[CA-125]$
ROMA = $\exp(PI)[1+\exp(PI)] * 10$
- A cut off of ≥1.31 and ≥2.77 were used for pre- and postmenopausal women with an ovarian adnexal mass, respectively, to provide a specificity level of 75%.

OVA1
Combine 5 serum markers **CA-125, transthyretin (prealbumin), apolipoprotein A1, β2-microglobulin, transferrin and menopausal status** into a numerical score.

- *Morphology index:* Relative risk of malignancy to specific morphologic finding. Both morphologic complexity and tumor volume are directly related to the risk of cancer. Score of 0–10 are observed.
  Risk of malignancy (study of 442 cases)
  i. 0.3% is MI is < or = 5
  ii. 84% is MI is > or = 8

ROCA-test: The ROCA® test is a quantitative algorithm that uses a woman's age, menopausal status, personal ovarian cancer risk status and serum CA125 levels. The ROCA® test compares a woman's individual longitudinal profile of the CA125 results over time, with the known profiles of women prior to diagnosis of ovarian cancer and women without ovarian cancer, to provide an accurate risk of having the disease.

OVA 1—better than ROMA. OVA1 (MIA) score determines if your mass is at lower risk for ovarian cancer or at a higher risk. Patients with elevated cancer risk may benefit from treatment by a gynecologic oncologist who specializes in the diagnosis and treatment of cancer in the reproductive organs. If cancer is present, getting to a specialist for the first surgery increases a woman's chance of survival up to 40 percent.

OVA 2—includes HE4. Draw back -waiting period for 8–10 days.

CA125- is not specific.

HE 4 is reliable, not increased in endometriosis. ROMA better than RMI.

RMI—USG X CA 125 X menopausal status.

Bibliography

1. Agarwal N, Kriplani A, Bhatla N, et al. Management and outcome of pregnancies complicated with adnexal masses. Archives of gynecology and obstetrics. 2003;267(3):148-52.
2. Bayer AI, Wiskind AK. Adnexal torsion: can the adnexa be saved?. Am J Obstet Gynecol. 1994;171(6):1506-11.
3. Berek, Jonathan S, Neville F. Hacker (Eds). Berek and Hacker's Gynecologic Oncology. Lippincott Williams & Wilkins; 2010.
4. Berek, Jonathan S. Berek and Novak's Gynecology.Wolters Kluwer Health/Lippincott Williams and Wilkins; 2012.
5. Bradshaw KD, Santos-Ramos R, Rawlins SC, et al. Endocrine studies in a pregnancy complicated by ovarian theca lutein cysts

and hyperreactioluteinalis. Obstetrics and Gynecology. 1986;67(3):66S-9S.
6. Bromley B, Benacerraf B. Adnexal masses during pregnancy: accuracy of sonographic diagnosis and outcome. J Ultrasound Med. 1997;16(7):447-52.
7. Carter JR, Lau M, Fowler JM, et al. Blood flow characteristics of ovarian tumors: implications for ovarian cancer screening. Am J Obstet Gynecol. 1995;172(3):901-7.
8. Christensen JT, Boldsen JL, Westergaard JG. Functional ovarian cysts in premenopausal and gynecologically healthy women. Contraception. 2002;66(3):153-7.
9. DePriest PD, Shenson D, Fried A, et al. A morphology index based on sonographic findings in ovarian cancer. Gynecologic oncology. 1993;51(1):7-11.
10. Di-Xia CH, Schwartz PE, Xinguo L, et al. Evaluation of CA 125 levels in differentiating malignant from benign tumors in patients with pelvic masses. Obstetrics & Gynecology. 1988;72(1):23-7.
11. Early Detection and treatment monitoring of Ovarian cancer, Zengliu (Leo) Su Clinical Chemistry Postdoctoral Fellow, Department of Pathology & Laboratory MedicineMedical University of South Carolina.
12. Hogston P, Lilford RJ. Ultrasound study of ovarian cysts in pregnancy: prevalence and significance. BJOG. 1986;93(6):625-8.
13. Jacobs I, Oram D, Fairbanks J, et al. A risk of malignancy index incorporating CA 125, ultrasound and menopausal status for the accurate preoperative diagnosis of ovarian cancer. BJOG. 1990;97(10):922-9.
14. Malhotra N, Kumar P, Malhotra J, et al. Jeffcoate's Principles of Gyneacology. Jaypee Brothers; 2014.
15. Modesitt SC, Pavlik EJ, Ueland FR, et al. Risk of malignancy in unilocular ovarian cystic tumors less than 10 centimeters in diameter. Obstet Gynecol. 2003;102(3):594-9.
16. Outwater EK, Siegelman ES, Hunt JL. Ovarian Teratomas: Tumor Types and Imaging Characteristics 1. Radiographics. 2001;21(2): 475-90.
17. Rock John A. TeLinde's operative gynecology. Lippincott Williams and Wilkins; 2003.
18. Rufford BD, Jacobs IJ. Ovarian cysts in postmenopausal women. RCOG Green Top Guideline. 2003;34:1-8.
19. Chang HC, Bhatt S, Dogra VS. Pearls and Pitfalls in Diagnosis of Ovarian Torsion 1. Radiographics. 2008;28(5):1355-68.

21
CHAPTER

Cervical Cancer

Michael George Muto

CASE

Chief Complaint

Postcoital bleeding.

History of Present Illness

The patient is a 40-year-old G5 P5 with a last menstrual period 2 weeks prior to presentation who comes to gynecology clinic complaining of a 12-week history of postcoital bleeding. She was in her usual state of good health until approximately 3 months ago when, following an episode of vaginal intercourse with her husband, she noted the onset of vaginal spotting. This spotting has continued to occur with each episode of intercourse and is becoming increasingly significant. She denies any pelvic pain or pain with intercourse. She denies back, flank pain, or a change in bowel or bladder function. She has had no unexpected weight loss. She presents today accompanied by her sister.

History of Past Illness

Past Gynecologic History

The patient had menarche at the age of 14 and has had regular menses her entire reproductive life. She reports that shortly after her marriage at the age of 18, she suffered an outbreak of vulvar herpes but she has had no recurrent infections. She denies a history of other sexually transmitted diseases, including gonorrhea, syphilis or vulvar condyloma. She has been screened with Pap smears infrequently and thinks her last Pap was prior to the birth of her youngest child 13 years ago.

Past Obstetrical History

The patient has five living children born by normal spontaneous vaginal delivery. They range in age from 13 to 19 years of age. Following the delivery of her youngest child, she underwent a postpartum tubal sterilization procedure.

Past Medical History

The patient denies any history of chronic medical conditions.

Past Surgical History

The patient denies any history of surgery other than her sterilization procedure.

Allergies

The patient has no known drug allergies.

Medications

The patient denies the use of any prescription medications.

Family History

The patient's sister was diagnosed and treated for cervical cancer three years ago. There are no other cases of cancer of any type in her immediate family.

Social History

The patient has been married for 22 years. She considers this a stable monogamous relationship. She does not drink, smoke or use other illicit medications. She is a homemaker and her husband is employed as a factory floor supervisor.

Screening Studies

The patient has not had a mammogram or colonoscopy. Her Pap smear history is noted in the history of present illness.

Review of Systems

The patient denies any symptoms other than those listed in the history of present illness.

Physical Examination

The patient is a healthy appearing middle-aged woman in no apparent distress.

Vital Signs

- Pulse—68 beats per minute
- Respiratory rate—14 per minute
- Blood pressure—130/76 mm Hg
- Weight 155 lbs
- Height—5.1 feet.

There is no supraclavicular or cervical adenopathy. Her lungs are clear to auscultation and percussion. Her heart has a regular rate and rhythm without murmurs, rubs or gallups.

Her abdomen is soft and nontender without hepatosplenomegaly or masses. She has no inguinal or femoral lymphadenopathy.

Her extremities were without cyanosis clubbing or edema.

Upon pelvic examination, she is found to have normal external genitalia. With placement of a vaginal speculum, the vaginal canal is noted to contain a modest amount of clotted blood. The vaginal mucosa appears grossly normal. The cervix appears enlarged and inflamed. There is a region of exophytic growth on the cervical portio, which measures 2 cm in diameter. A Pap smear was performed inducing brisk bleeding, which is controlled with direct pressure with a sponge.

A bimanual and rectovaginal examination are attempted but were felt to be suboptimal due to patient discomfort and a fear of inducing further bleeding.

Case Summary

This is a 40-year-old woman with symptoms, signs and physical findings suggestive of cervical carcinoma.

Q. 1. What are risk factors for the development of cervical cancer?

Risk factors for the development of cervical cancer include age at onset of sexual activity, multiple sexual partners, exposure to a high-risk sexual partner, a history of sexually transmitted disease, and a history of human papillomavirus (HPV) associated preinvasive vulvar or vaginal lesions.

Women who begin having sexual intercourse under the age of 18 are twice as likely to develop cervical cancer as those women who have first coitus over the age of 21.[1]

Women who have six or more lifetime partners are three times more likely to develop cervical cancer than a woman with one lifetime partner.

Not all partners carry the same degree of risk. Partners who are high risk by virtue of known HPV infection or who have had multiple sexual partners are considered high-risk males. If a man has had a prior wife who developed or died of cervical cancer, this also establishes the male as high risk. There is also data to suggest that the noncircumcised male may be a higher risk partner than the circumcised male.[2]

Women with chronic immunosuppressive disease like human immunodeficiency virus patients are at significantly increased risk.

Women with more than three children, with the first born by the age of 18 are also at increased risk.[3] Finally, a failure to comply with recommended screening is also significant risk factor (Table 1).

All of these risk factors have one common denominator. They are associated with an increased risk of HPV infection, or a decreased ability to clear HPV infection.

There is some data to suggest that a woman's capacity to clear an HPV infection may be genetically determined; however, this data is not conclusive at this time.[4]

Q. 2. What is the differential diagnosis for this patient?

In cases of postcoital bleeding, one must always be careful to consider benign etiologies. These include chronic cervicitis associated with chlamydial, viral or bacterial infections. Bleeding may also be caused by an exaggerated ectropion or granulation tissue resulting from prior birth trauma. The cervical portio may be irritated by tampon use, douching and the use of certain sexual appliances.[5]

Great care must be taken to distinguish primary cervical neoplasia from benign and malignant conditions, which masquerade as cervical cancer. For example, a prolapsing leiomyoma may present as a cervical mass. These tumors may appear eroded and my bleed heavily. If inflamed, these partially necrotic tumors may fuse to the cervical portio and give the false impression of primary cervical cancer on pelvic examination.

Table 1: Cervical Cancer Screening Guidelines 2012 (Healthy low-risk women).

<21	None
21–29	Pap smear every three years
30–65	Pap smear every three years or
	Pap smear every 5 years with HPV cotesting
>65	None

Note:
1. This only applies to healthy, well screened women (defined as women with at least three documented negative smears or two documented negative cotests within the prior ten years).
2. Women who have had a hysterectomy for benign disease do not require further smears.
3. Healthy women under 21 should not be screened regardless of sexual history.
4. HPV cotesting should not be performed under the age of 29.

The cervix may be involved with metastatic disease from other sites. The most common primary cancer to secondarily involve the cervix is endometrial cancer. Colorectal cancer, breast cancer and lymphoma have all been reported to metastasize to the cervix. (Table 1).

Q. 3. What is the next step in evaluation of this patient?

In cases of suspected cervical cancer, it is of paramount importance to obtain sufficient tissue to establish a definitive diagnosis. Remember that a Pap smear is not a tissue diagnosis. The smear may be read as "consistent with" a malignancy but a biopsy is the only way to determine the true histology of the lesion. Additional cultures may also be obtained to exclude an infectious etiology. In selected cases a pelvic ultrasound examination may help delineate the source of the cervical mass. When advanced disease is suspected, an intravenous pyelogram may be ordered. Advanced pelvic imaging with CT, MRI or PET scanning is rarely indicated at this point.[6]

Q. 4. How does one perform a proper examination under anesthesia (EUA)?

Cervical cancer is the only gynecologic malignancy, which is clinically, rather than surgically staged. The FIGO staging system for cervical cancer is included (Table 2). The key to the proper EUA is to measure the diameter of the cervical lesion and to assess the uterosacral and cardinal ligaments for nodular involvement of disease. The examination begins with observation. With the placement of the speculum one may accurately assess the diameter of the lesion and whether or not there is visible extension to the vaginal mucosa. If the cervix is deviated to one side, this may be indicative of cancer invasion into the parametrial tissues on that side. Remember, parametrial invasion foreshortens the parametrium, thereby resulting in the cervix being pulled toward the diseased side. This may be the first clue of more advanced disease.

Following observation, one moves to palpation beginning with a two finger vaginal exam. It is important to assess the cervix for mobility and to compare the right and left vaginal fornix for symmetry. This will also help the gynecologic surgeon assess surgical resectability. Care should be taken to note any subvaginal induration. In some cases, vaginal involvement may be submucosal. This cannot be seen on speculum examination, but can be appreciated upon palpation. Finally, one performs the rectovaginal examination. This allows for palpation of the uterosacral and cardinal ligaments. Asymmetry, nodularity and fixation are important findings and suggest tumor extension. Women with advanced pelvic endometriosis may have similar findings on this portion of the exam, but endometriosis is more often symmetrical.

When performing the cervical biopsy, every attempt must be made to avoid necrotic tissue. The more generous the biopsy and the more sites sampled the less likely a nondiagnostic specimen will be obtained. In cases of extreme necrosis, a frozen section can be employed to insure a diagnostic specimen. Topical agents to stem bleeding including silver nitrate or ferrous subsulfate should be readily at hand.

In cases where advanced disease is suspected, a cystoscopy and proctoscopy may be added to the EUA. At the time of cystoscopy it is not uncommon to see bladder base elevation and bullous edema of the bladder mucosa. It is important to remember that these findings do not upstage the patient to stage IV disease unless there is biopsy proven cancer in the bladder.

There is one clinical scenario in which even the most experienced clinician may under stage a cervical cancer patient. This is the case of the barrel-shaped cervix. Most squamous cell carcinomas, will grow in an exophytic growth pattern from the face of the cervical portio. Adenocarcinoma of the endocervix, on the other hand, is more likely to demonstrate endophytic growth. This expands the diameter of the cervix greatly while sparing the cervical portio. It is very easy to be mislead by the rectovaginal examination. If surgery is elected, it is often not until the case is well underway

Table 2: Differential diagnosis of postcoital bleeding

Benign neoplasms   • Endometrial polyp   • Cervical polyp   • Prolapsing uterine leiomyoma
Infectious conditions   • Chronic cervicitis   • *Chlamydia*   • Herpes simplex virus   • Lymphogranuloma venereum   • Condyloma accuminatum
Malignant neoplasia   • Primary cervical cancer   • Metastatic endometrial cancer   • Metastases from other locations
Other sources   • Trauma   • Vaginal atrophy   • Foreign body

that this underestimate of tumor diameter is recognized.

Q. 5. What are the common histopathology types of cervical cancer?

More than 70% of women with cervical cancer will develop squamous cell carcinoma.[7] These often arise on the cervical portio in areas of high-grade squamous intraepithelial neoplasia and are therefore amenable to early detection with the Pap smear. Squamous cancers are most commonly associated with HPV 16. Adenocarcinoma of the cervix represents 25% of all cervical cancer.[8] The precursor lesion, adenocarcinoma in situ, occurs in a multifocal pattern along the endocervical canal. These lesions are more likely associated with HPV 16 and 18. Because they are multifocal and deep within the endocervical canal, adenocarcinoma and its precursors are more difficult to detect with traditional Pap tests. The introduction of the cervical brush and the advent of thin prep liquid cytology were introduced in hopes of improving detection of adenocarcinoma. Recent data suggest that HPV testing, as a primary screen, may be more sensitive than cytology for detecting adenocarcinoma precursors.

Presentation of Case Continued

The patient's Pap smear obtained at the initial visit revealed cells suspicious for squamous cell carcinoma. Due to her lack of concerning symptoms, no advanced pelvic imaging was performed. During her EUA a 2 cm exophytic cervical lesion was noted. The cervix was centered within the vaginal canal and there was no evidence of extension to the vaginal mucosa. On bimanual and rectovaginal examination, the cervix was mobile and the vaginal fornices were symmetrical. There was no nodularity in the cardinal or uterosacral ligaments. The cystoscopy and proctoscopy were normal.

The cervical biopsy result was squamous cell carcinoma of the cervix.

FIGO stage was stage IB1 (TNM = T1b1).

Q. 6. What are the treatment options for cervical cancer?

Options for the treatment of cervical cancer include fertility sparing surgery, simple extrafascial hysterectomy, radical hysterectomy with pelvic lymphadenectomy and chemo-irradiation. Many factors must be considered when selecting the optimal treatment option. These include the age of the patient, desire for fertility, the stage and histologic type of cervical cancer and the resources available for treatment.[9]

Fertility sparing surgeries include conization and radical trachelectomy. A conization is the removal of the central portion of the cervix. This tissue can be removed with an electrosurgical instrument called a loop electrosurgical device, or by scalpel (the so called cold knife cone). Because the loop procedure can sometimes render margins difficult to interpret, the cold knife procedure is preferred. Conization has historically been offered to women who wish to preserve fertility and have stage IA1 disease and squamous or adenocarcinoma. If the cone margins are negative for invasive cancer, the cure rate is well over 95%. Recent data suggest a conization can be safely performed in some cases of IA2 and highly selected IB1 cancers, but this is considered investigational at this time. At higher stage, the cone is coupled with sampling of the regional lymph nodes.[10]

The radical trachelectomy and pelvic nodal dissection may be performed transvaginally or via laparoscopy. This procedure allows for the removal of larger stage I lesions, while still preserving the uterus. The lower uterine segment and residual upper endocervix is sutured to the top of the vagina after placement of an abdominal cerclage.[11]

When fertility is not desired, some form of hysterectomy is preferred. For early lesions, a simple extrafascial hysterectomy and bilateral salpingectomy is an excellent option. Ovaries may be spared in younger patient with squamous carcinomas.[12]

For women with stage IA2 through IB1 disease, the radical hysterectomy with pelvic lymphadenectomy is the best surgical option. If the surgeon can achieve negative margins and the nodes are uninvolved the cure rate approaches 90%. For patients who cannot tolerate this type of operation, primary chemoirradiation is an excellent alternative.[13]

The use of chemoirradiation in patients fit for radical hysterectomy is discouraged for three compelling reasons. Radiation may cause permanent changes in the lower genital tract, which may affect sexual function. Radiation may increase the risk of secondary pelvic malignancies. Finally, radiation will result in loss of ovarian function.

For patients with stage IB2 disease and above, radical chemoirradiation is the preferred treatment. Lesions in excess of 4 cm have a high risk of locoregional nodal spread and a high risk of close or positive surgical margins. Radiation therapy, when properly administered, results in greater likelihood of cure with lower risk of long-term complications.[14]

The treatment involves two phases. Phase one is treatment by external beam therapy to the entire pelvis. Phase two involves the placement of brachytherapy devices within the endocervical cancel and vagina. These instruments can then be loaded with either low dose rate or high dose rate sources thereby delivering a very high dose to the tumor, whilst sparing bladder and rectum.[15] It is very common to administer a weekly dose of cisplatin during the 6 weeks of radiation therapy. Cisplatin functions as a radiation sensitizer and results in improved overall survival when compared with radiation therapy alone. Decisions regarding the use of surgery versus chemoirradiation are very dependent upon the resources available to the clinician.[16]

Presentation of Case Continued
The patient, having had a prior tubal ligation, has no interest in future fertility. She is slender and fit for surgery. She has a squamous carcinoma. Therefore, after careful consideration, she has elected to proceed with a radical hysterectomy with bilateral salpingectomy and bilateral pelvic lymph node dissection.

Q. 7. How does a radical hysterectomy differ from a simple extrafascial hysterectomy?

A simple extrafascial hysterectomy removes only the uterus and cervix. A radical hysterectomy removes not only the uterus and the cervix, but also all parametrial tissue on either side of the cervix, along with a portion of the uterosacral ligaments, cardinal ligaments and the upper 1-2 cm of vagina (Fig. 1). In order to accomplish this, the ureter must be dissected along its entire length and reflected laterally. The operation may be performed via an abdominal incision, through the vagina or by straight stick or robotic laparoscopy. The procedure is commonly coupled with lymph node assessment via bilateral pelvic lymphadenectomy or sentinel node biopsy.[17]

The classic pelvic lymphadenectomy involves the removal of all nodal tissue from

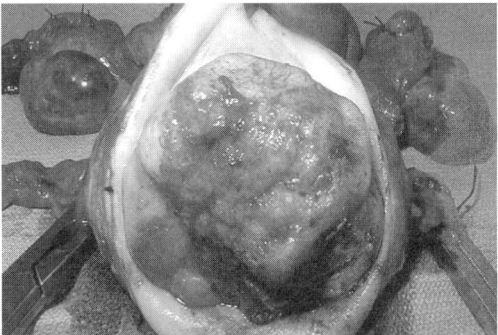

Fig. 1: Radical hysterectomy specimen (This is a radical hysterectomy specimen revealing a stage IB1 squamous cell carcinoma of the cervix. Note the wide vaginal margin and parametrial tissue marked by the surgical clamps. In this case, both ovaries have also been removed)

the internal and external iliac nodal chain and all nodes in the obturator space. Sentinel node dissection involves the preoperative injection of dye or radioactive tracer into the cervical stroma. These agents localize in the first node in the chain draining the cervix. These nodes are most often intra-iliac or obturator nodes. Sentinel node biopsy is associated with a lower risk of lymphedema than classic lymphadenectomy.[18]

Q. 8. What are the complications of radical hysterectomy?

A radical hysterectomy affects the innervation of the bladder and may result in temporary urinary retention. A Foley catheter or supra-pubic catheter are placed at the time of surgery and are continued until documented return of normal bladder function. The larger the primary lesion the more extensive the radical hysterectomy needs to be to obtain negative margins. Extensive radical surgery is associated with a higher risk of bladder dysfunction. A nerve sparing radical hysterectomy may reduce the risk of prolonged loss of bladder sensation. Constipation is a less likely consequence of the surgery.[19]

Because the genitourinary tract is dissected extensively, there is a 1–3% risk of ureterovaginal or vesicovaginal fistula formation. These fistulae often occur a few weeks following surgery and are preceded by pain and fever. Once a fistula forms and urinary incontinence begins, these symptoms often resolve. Repair may be undertaken after the acute inflammation has subsided.

It is uncommon for women to notice a loss of vaginal length given the normal elasticity of the vagina. Sexual dysfunction has been reported after all gynecologic cancer surgery and is multifactorial. It is critical to anticipate this during preoperative counseling and to address the issues during postoperative visits.[20]

Lymphedema may occur in up to 25% of patients. Some of this will improve in the ensuing postoperative year. The postoperative administration of radiation therapy because of positive nodes or close surgical margins will dramatically increase the risk of lymphedema.[21]

Presentation of Case Continued

The patient underwent an uncomplicated robotic radical hysterectomy, bilateral salpingectomy and pelvic lymphadenectomy. She was discharged from hospital on postoperative day number one with a supra-pubic catheter in place. Normal bladder function, assessed by post-void residuals resumed on postoperative day 14. The catheter was removed. On postoperative day 21, he was seen for a postoperative exam. All her port sites were well healed and she had returned to most normal activities. She was instructed to abstain from sexual intercourse for a total of 8 weeks to allow for vaginal cuff healing.

Her final pathology report revealed a well differentiated squamous cell carcinoma invasive to a depth of 5 mm (<30% of the cervical stromal thickness), with no evidence of lymphovascular invasion and widely negative margins. Thirty bilateral pelvic nodes were negative for metastatic disease.

Q. 9. Is additional therapy required at this time?

No, the patient has negative nodes and margins. In addition to this the cancer was invasive to less than 30% of the cervical stroma. Based upon criteria defined by Sedlis, this patient should have a 90% probability of cure with no further adjuvant radiotherapy required.[22] Had the cancer been invading more than 66% of the cervical stroma, or if margins or nodes were positive, adjuvant radiation with or without chemosensitization may have been required.[23]

Q. 10. How does management differ in patients with locally advanced disease?

Locally advanced cervical cancer (stage IB2-stage IVA) is more commonly treated with radiation therapy rather than surgical resection. Larger lesions are more likely to demonstrate deep cervical stromal invasion, surgical resection margins are more likely to be positive and the probability of metastatic disease to regional nodes rises sharply. Given these facts, it is no surprise that surgery for locally advanced lesions results in higher local failure rates than primary radiation therapy.[24]

For stage IB-IIB there is strong level I evidence that supports the use of radiation with concurrent chemotherapy. The benefit of concurrent chemotherapy is less pronounced in more advanced stages; however, it is common practice to treat stage III and IVA cases with concurrent chemotherapy as well. When compared to radiation therapy alone, concurrent chemotherapy results in up to a 10% improvement in survival, a 13% improvement in progression free survival and much better rates of local control. Depending upon the agents used, there may be an increased risk of serious side effects, predominantly gastrointestinal toxicity. Use of single agent chemotherapy regimens with cisplatin or carboplatin results in lower toxicity and have become the standard.

Chemotherapy is administered once a week during radiation treatment. Typically, cisplatin is administered intravenously at a dose of 40 mg/m^2 during both external beam and brachytherapy phases of treatment. Every effort is made to complete all treatment on schedule and within a period of 8 weeks. More protracted treatment results in increased loco regional failure.[25]

Overall five-year survival rates are highly dependent upon stage at presentation (Tables 3 and 4).

Table 3: Revised FIGO Staging of Cervical Carcinoma 2009

Stage I: Confined to cervix
  Ia: Invasive carcinoma only diagnosed by microscopy
  Ia1: Stromal invasion <3 mm in depth and <7 mm in extension
  Ia2: Stromal invasion >3 mm depth and not >5 mm and extension <7 mm
  Ib: Clinically visible lesions limited to the cervix or preclinical cancers >stage 1a
  Ib1: Clinically visible tumor <4 cm in greatest dimension
  Ib2: Clinically visible tumor >4 cm in greatest dimension

Contd...

Contd...

Stage II: Beyond cervix though not to the pelvic sidewall or lower third of the vagina
  IIa: Involves upper 2/3rd of vagina without parametrial invasion
  IIa1: Clinically visible tumor <4 cm in greatest dimension
  IIa2: Clinically visible tumor >4 cm in greatest dimension
  IIb: With parametrial invasion

Stage III
  IIIa: Tumor involves the lower third of the vagina with no extension to pelvic side-wall
  IIIb: Extension to pelvic side-wall or causing obstructive uropathy

Stage IV: Extension beyond true pelvis or biopsy proven to involve the mucosa of the bladder or the rectum
  IVa: Extension beyond true pelvis or rectal/bladder invasion
  IVb: Distant organ spread

Table 4: Five-year survival rate by cervical cancer stage

Stage IB	80%
Stage IIA	63%
Stage IIB	58%
Stage III	30%
Stage IVA	16%

Source: American Cancer Society 2012.

Q. 11. What is brachytherapy and why is it used?

Brachytherapy is a radiation therapy technique that places the radiation source in direct contact with the tissues to be treated. This allows the radiation oncologist to deliver very high doses to the epicenter of the tumor while sparing surrounding non-target tissues. When treating a locally advanced cervical cancer, external beam therapy is employed first (Figs 2A to H). During the first 3–4 weeks of treatment, most cervical cancers will shrink resulting in normalization of the anatomy. Once a local response has been documented, the patient is brought to the treatment room and brachytherapy applicators

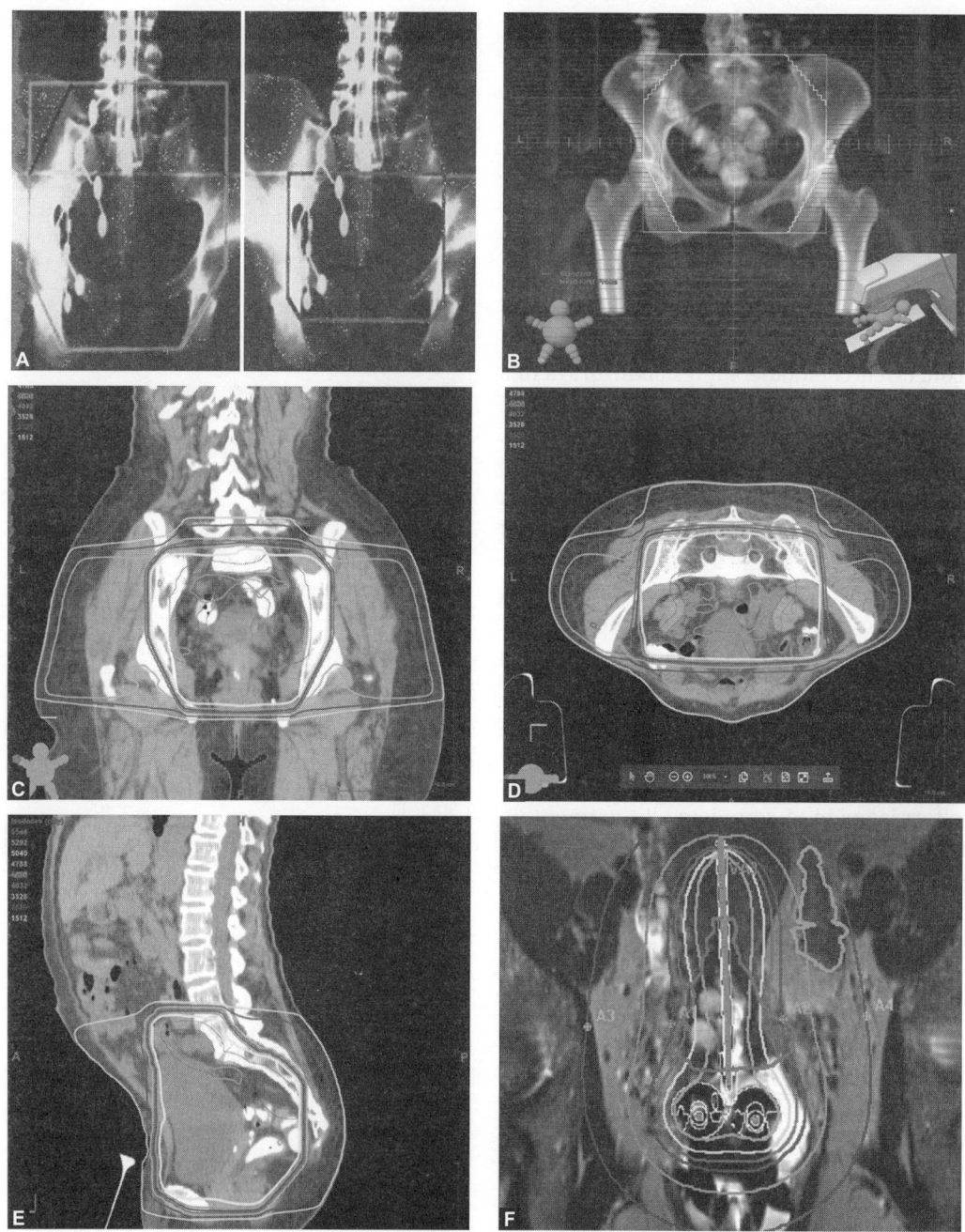

Figs 2A to F

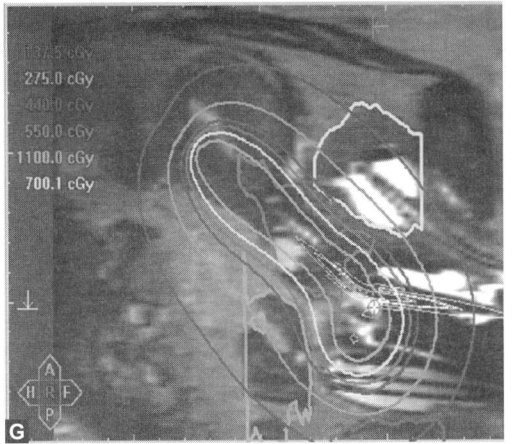
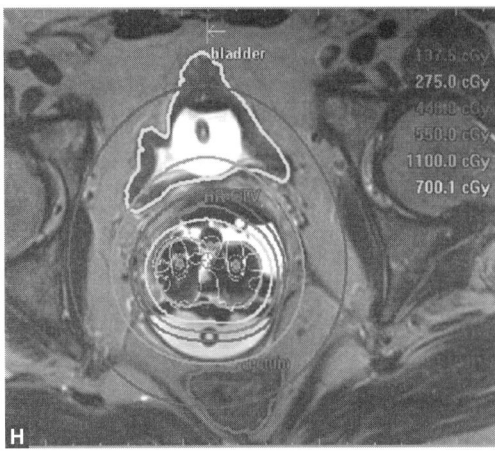

Figs 2G and H

Figs 2A to H: External beam therapy: (A) Pelvic radiation fields; (B) Alternative standard pelvic external beam radiation therapy; (C) Coronal view; (D) Axial view; (E) Sagittal view; (F) Coronal view of tandem and ovoids; (G) Sagittal view of tandem and ovoids; (H) Axial view of tandem and ovoids

are placed within the cervix and vagina. The applicators are subsequently loaded with radioactive sources, which are left in place for a prescribed period of time. There are many ways of delivering brachytherapy including both low dose rate and high dose rate protocols. In addition, there are a very wide variety of brachytherapy applicators including intracavitary and interstitial devices (Figs 3A to C). This allows the radiation oncologist and physicist to tailor the therapy to the patient's specific needs.

The use of brachytherapy significantly reduces local failure rates and improves overall survival.[26]

Q. 12. What is neoadjuvant chemotherapy?

Neoadjuvant chemotherapy is administered prior to definitive surgery for locally advanced cervical cancer. The therapy is administered in the hope that the tumor will regress sufficiently to allow resection to negative nodes and negative margins, thereby reducing the costs and complications associated with primary radiation therapy. In regions of the world where radiation therapy options are limited, this is a very attractive mode of therapy. Unfortunately, there is no prospective data comparing neoadjuvant chemotherapy to primary radiation therapy for locally advanced cervical cancer; however, there is an ongoing prospective trial designed to address this question. Until this trial is completed, the treatment should be considered investigational.[27,28]

Q. 13. What is the recommended follow-up?

The patient should be followed with a pelvic examination and vaginal cytology at 3-6 month intervals for two years, then at 6-month intervals for an additional three years. She is then a candidate for vaginal cytology on an annual basis for the foreseeable future. Because of her prior exposure to HPV and her history of cervical cancer, she is at risk for the development of vulvar of vaginal disease. In addition to this, a central recurrence of cervical cancer following primary surgery may be treatable and curable by radiation therapy. Therefore, it is very important these patients be followed postoperatively.

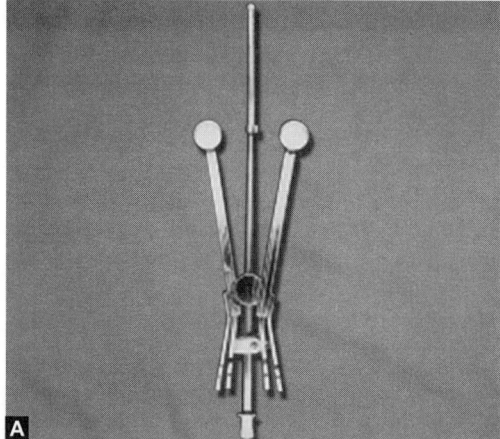

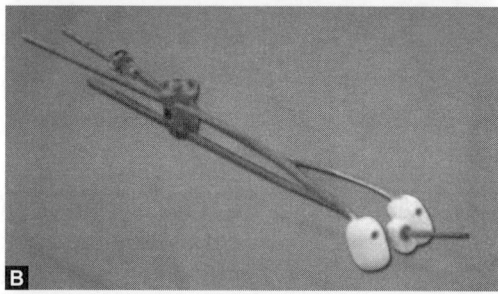

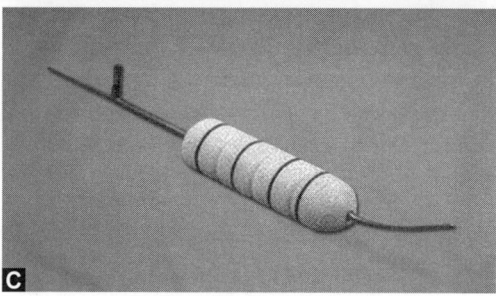

Figs 3A to C: Low and high dose rate brachytherapy devices: (A) Tandem and ovoids for low dose rate applications; (B) Tandem and ovoids for high dose rate applications; (C) Vaginal colpostat for high dose rate applications

References

1. International Collaboration of Epidemiological Studies of Cervical Cancer. Comparison of risk factors for invasive squamous cell carcinoma of the cervix and adenocarcinoma of the cervix: collaborative reanalysis of individual data on 8,097women with squamous cell cancer and 1,374 women with adenocarcinoma from 12 epidemiological studies. Int J Cancer. 2007; 120:885.
2. Castellsague X, Bosch FX, Munoz N, et al. Male circumcision, penile human papillomavirus infection, and cervical cancer in female partners. N Engl J Med. 2002;120:1105.
3. Munoz N, Francheschi S, Bosetti C, et al. Role of parity and human papillomavirus in cervical cancer: the IARC multicentric case-control study. Lancet. 2002;118:1481.
4. Hemminki K, Chen B. Familial risks for cervical tumors in full and half siblings: etiologic apportioning. Cancer Epidemiol Biomarkers Prev. 2006;15:1413
5. Tarney C, Han J. Postcoital Bleeding: A review on etiology, diagnosis and management. Obstet Gynecol Int. 2014; http://dx.doi/10.1155/2014/192087
6. Follen M, Levenback CF, Iyer RB, et al. Imaging in cervical cancer. Cancer. 2003;98:2028.
7. Look, KY, Brunetto VL, Clarke-Pearson DL, et al. An analysis of cell type in patients with surgically staged IB carcinoma of the cervix: a Gynecologic Oncology Group study. Gynecol Oncol. 1996;63:304.
8. Kurman RJ, Norris HJ, Wilkinson EJ. Atlas of tumor pathology: Tumors of the cervix, vagina and vulva, 3rd. Armed Forces Institute of Pathology, Washington, DC; 1992.
9. National Comprehensive Care Network (NCCN). NCCN Clinical practice guidelines in oncology. http://www.nccn.org/professionals/physician_gls/f_guidelines.asp
10. Mota F. Microinvasive squamous carcinoma of the cervix: treatment modalities. Acta Obstet Gynecol Scand. 2003;82:505.
11. Plante M. Evolution in fertility preserving options for early-stage cervical cancer: radical trachelectomy, simple trachelectomy, neoadjuvant chemotherapy. Int J Gynecol Cancer. 2013;23:982.
12. Sutton GP, Bundy BN, Delgado G, et al. Ovarian metastases in stage IB carcinoma of the cervix. A Gynecologic Oncology Group study. Am J Obstet Gynecol. 1992;166:50.
13. Bansal N, Herzog TJ, Shaw RE, et al. Primary therapy for early-stage cervical cancer: radical hysterectomy vs radiation. Am J Obstet Gynecol. 2009;201:485.e1.

14. Rotman M, Sedlis A, Piedmonte MR, et al. A phase III randomized trial of postoperative pelvic irradiation in Stage IB cervical carcinoma with poor prognostic features: follow-up of a Gynecologic Oncology Group study. Int J Radiat Oncol Biol Phys. 2006;65:169.
15. Han K, Milosevic M, Fyles A, et al. Trends in the utilization of brachytherapy in cervical cancer in the United States. Int J Radiat Oncol Biol Phys. 2013;87:111.
16. Chemoradiotherapy for Cervical Cancer Meta-analysis Collaboration (CCCMAC). Reducing uncertainties about the effects of chemoradiotherapy for cervical cancer: individual patient data meta-analysis. Cochrane Database Syst Rev 2010; CD008285
17. Lee YN, Wang KL, Lin MH, et al. Radical hysterectomy with pelvic lymph node dissection for treatment of cervical cancer: a clinical review of 954 cases. Gynecol Oncol. 1989;32:135.
18. Cibula D, Abu-Rustum NR, Dusek L, et al. Bilateral ultrastaging of sentinel lymph nodes in cervical cancer: Lowering the false-negative rate and improving the detection of micrometastasis. Gynecol Oncol. 2012;127:462.
19. Brooks RA, Wright JD, Powell MA, et al. Long-term assessment of bladder and bowel dysfunction after radical hysterectomy. Gynecol Oncol. 2009;114:75.
20. Ye S, Yang J, Cao D, et al. A systematic review of quality of life and sexual function of patients with cervical cancer after treatment. Int J Gynecol Cancer. 2014;24:1146.
21. Ferrandina G, Mantegna G, Petrillo M, et al. Quality of life and emotional distress in early stage and locally advanced cervical cancer patients: a prospective longitudinal study. Gynecol Oncol. 2012;124:389.
22. Sedlis A, Bundy BN, Rotman MZ, et al. A randomized trial of pelvic radiation therapy versus no further therapy in selected patients with stage IB carcinoma of the cervix following radical hysterectomy and pelvic lymphadenectomy. A Gynecologi Oncology Group study. Gynecol Oncol. 1999;73:177.
23. Rogers L, Siu SS, Luesley D, et al. Radiotherapy and chemoradiation after surgery for early cervical cancer. Cochrane Database Syst Rev. 2012;5.
24. Chemoradiotherapy for Cervical Cancer Meta-analysis Collaboration (CCCMAC). Reducing uncertainties about the effects of chemoradiotherapy for cervical cancer: individual patient data meta-analysis. Cochrane Database Syst Rev; 2010.
25. Perez CA, Grigsby PW, Castro-Vita H, et al. Carcinoma of the uterine cervix. Impact of prolongation of overall treatment time and timing of brachytherapy on outcome of radiation therapy. Int J Radiat Oncol Biol Phys. 1995;2:1275.
26. Viswanathan AN, Beriwal S, De Los Santos JF, et al. American Brachytherapy Society consensus guidelines for locally advanced carcinoma of the cervix. Part II: high dose rate brachytherapy. Brachytherapy. 2012;11:47.
27. Rydzewska L, Tierney J, Vale CL, et al. Neoadjuvant chemotherapy plus surgery versus surgery for cervical cancer. Cochrane Database Syst Rev; 2012.
28. EORTC Protocol 55994 at http://www.eortc.be/protoc/details.asp?protocol

Bibliography

1. American Society for Colposcopy and Cervical Pathology. Management and screening guidelines. www.asccp.org/Guidelines.
2. Frederick P, Whitworth J, et al. Radical hysterectomy for carcinoma of the uterine cervix. Glob. libr. women's med., (ISSN: 1756-2228) 2011; DOI 10.3843/GLOWM.10232
3. Frumovitz M. Invasive cervical cancer: Epidemiology, risk factors, clinical manifestations and diagnosis. In: Post TW (Ed): UpToDate, Waltham, MA; 2015.
4. Plante M. Fertility—sparing surgery for cervical cancer. In: Post TW (Ed). UpToDate, Waltham, MA; 2014.
5. Straughn, JM, Yashar C. Management of early-stage cervical cancer. In: Post TW (Ed). UpToDate, Waltham, MA; 2015.
6. Straughn JM, Yashar C. Management of locally advanced cervical cancer. In: Post TW (Ed). UpToDate, Waltham, MA; 2015.

22

Epithelial Ovarian Cancer

UD Bafna

CASE

A 64-year-old woman presented with the complaints of bloating of abdomen since two months. She also complained of feeling of fullness after eating. There were no urinary complaints. She was multiparous woman and had attained menopause 15 years ago. There was no family history of any malignancy.

Physical Examination

She was of moderate built and nourishment. She was slightly pale. Abdominal examination revealed distended abdomen with moderate amount of free fluid. There was a palpable mass of about 16–18 weeks gestation size. It was mainly cystic to palpate and was extending into the pelvis. Bimanual bi-digital pelvic examination revealed a mass felt in the right lateral fornix fixed to the uterus and extending into the abdomen. The parametrium appeared to be nodular on the right side. The rectal mucosa was free.

Investigations

- Complete blood count (CBC)
- Serum urea, creatinine
- Liver function test (LFT)
- Chest X-ray
- Tumor markers—serum Ca 125 and carcinoembryonic antigen (CEA)
- Ultrasonography (USG) of abdomen and pelvis
- Ascitic fluid cytology for acid fast bacilli (AFB) and malignant cells
- CT scan of abdomen and pelvis with contrast
- Diagnostic laparoscopy SOS.

Treatment Plan

A provisional diagnosis of epithelial ovarian cancer was made and based on the investigations and surgical fitness for a staging laparotomy, surgery was planned.

A generous midline incision extending from the symphysis pubis to 1" above the umbilicus was taken. Ascitic fluid was sent for cytological examination. All the abdominal organs were systematically inspected and palpated and were found to be free of gross disease. Right-sided ovarian tumor with intact capsule but densely adherent to the uterus and pelvic floor, was removed by opening up the retroperitoneal spaces, ligating the infundibulopelvic ligament and separating it from the uterus and pelvic floor by sharp dissection. It was sent for frozen section which revealed serous adenocarcinoma. A full staging laparotomy was then performed—total abdominal hysterectomy, bilateral salpingo-oophorectomy, infracolic omentectomy, appendicectomy, bilateral pelvic and aortic lymphadenectomy and multiple random peritoneal biopsies.

Postoperative histopathology revealed high-grade serous adenocarcinoma of the ovary with breached capsule and microscopic aortic lymph node metastasis.

Stage and Adjuvant Treatment

A pathological diagnosis of high-grade epithelial serous adenocarcinoma FIGO stage IIIa was made and six cycles of adjuvant chemotherapy with Paclitaxel 175 mg/sqm and Carboplatin with a dosing of AUC 6 were administered once in every three weeks.

Q. 1. What is the differential diagnosis?

1. Benign ovarian neoplasm
2. Malignant ovarian neoplasm
3. Meigs' syndrome
4. Primary ca colon with metastasis to ovary
5. Krukenberg tumor
6. Uterine sarcoma
7. Abdominal tuberculosis.

Q. 2. How to differentiate benign from a malignant ovarian tumor?

- Clinical history
- Imaging
- Ultrasound of abdomen and pelvis
- MRI scan of abdomen and pelvis with IV contrast.

Frankly malignant tumors are easily detected by ultrasound. Any irregular solid area; thick and irregular septae within a cystic adnexal mass are indicative of malignancy. The Doppler scan usually reveals pulsatility index of <1 and resistance index of less than 0.4 indicating low resistance to blood flow due to abnormal vasculature.

In small cystic adnexal masses with solid areas which are suspicious on ultrasound, MRI scan with IV gadolinium contrast is useful. The contrast gets enhanced and rapidly cleared from the solid areas in malignant tumors.[1-13]

Tumor Markers

Serum CA 125, CEA and HE4 Markers:
Serum CA 125 is elevated in 90% of malignant epithelial ovarian tumors. It is elevated in only 50% of malignant epithelial ovarian cancers when the tumor is confined to the ovary and the capsule is intact.

Serum CA 125 is not a specific marker. It is also elevated in any condition which stimulates the coelomic epithelium like normal pregnancy, uterine fibroids, gastrointestinal (GI) cancers, abdominal tuberculosis, pancreatitis, endometriosis, etc.

It is especially elevated to very high levels in common conditions like abdominal tuberculosis and endometriosis.

Serum CEA is a non-specific marker of colonic cancer. If both CA 125 and CEA are elevated and their ratio is >25 then GI malignancy must be ruled out by colonoscopy.

Serum HE4 is a recent marker with more sensitivity and specificity than CA 125. It is especially useful in differentiating malignancy from endometriosis during the reproductive age. This marker is usually not raised in endometriosis.[14]

Diagnostic laparoscopy may be useful in diagnosing abdominal tuberculosis which is a difficult condition to diagnose as PCR of the ascitic fluid may be falsely positive or negative for *Mycobacterium tuberculosis.*

Differentiating Nonovarian Malignancies

Bilateral solid adnexal masses on ultrasound point towards Krukenberg tumors with usual primary being stomach. The gallbladder and pancreatic cancers are readily diagnosed by good ultrasound/CT scan, whereas stomach cancer is difficult to diagnose without upper GI endoscopy.

Lower GI symptoms like altered bowel habits, bleeding, etc. point towards colonic malignancy and should be investigated by colonoscopy.

Differentiating Different Types of Ovarian Malignancies

There are mainly three different types—Epithelial (Serous, mucinous, endometrioid, clear cell and undifferentiated), stromal (Granulosa cell and Sertoli Leydig cell tumors) and malignant germ cell tumors (Dysgerminoma, embryonal, endodermal/Yolk sac tumor, immature teratoma, choriocarcinoma and mixed germ cell tumors).

The following Table 1 shows the differentiating features.

Q. 3. What are the risk factors?

Risk Factors[16-20]

Age—adolescent age and postmenopausal women are likely to have malignant tumors.

Lifestyle Factors (attributable in 21% cases) like smoking (2% cases), sedentary lifestyle, talcum powder use, high fat diet, etc.

Obesity—increased risk

Family History—first degree relative with cancer increases the risk by 3-4 times.

Obstetric and Menstrual Factors

- Infertility and nulliparity
- Use of ovulation inducing drugs
- Early menarchy and late menopause
- Breastfeeding protects against ovarian carcinoma.

Contraception

- OC pills—decrease by >50% if used for >5 years
- Tubectomy also protects against epithelial ovarian cancers
- Hysterectomy too confers protection.

Genetic Factors

- BRCA1 and 2 gene mutations increase the risk of ovarian cancer. Lynch II syndrome too increases the risk
- ARID 1A gene mutation may cause increased risk of clear cell carcinoma in patients who had ovarian endometriosis
- Asbestos exposure—can cause epithelial cancer and peritoneal carcinoma

Table 1: Differentiating features of different types of ovarian malignancy

	Malignant epithelial tumors	Stromal tumors	Malignant germ cell tumors
Usual age at presentation	Sixth decade	Third decade/ Peri-menopause	<30 years
Growth pattern	Moderate growth rate Nonspecific symptoms	Slow May produce androgens/estrogens	Fast to rapid
Nature	Mainly cystic tumors with solid ingrowths	Mainly solid with cystic areas within, sometimes mainly cystic	Usually solid
Tumor marker	CA 125, HE4	Inhibin in granulosa cell tumors	Serum AFP, hCG, LDH depending on the type of tumor
Usual stage at presentation	Stage III–70–80%	Stage I–80%	Any
Prognosis	25–30% five year survival in advanced stages after conventional treatment	Most of them do well as they present in early stage	Five year survival 85–90% even in advanced stages

- Previous PID (pelvic inflammatory disease) increases the risk.

Hormone Replacement Therapy (HRT)
- Small increased risk of serous cystadenocarcinoma is found when taken for >5 years though the incidence of other tumors may be less. The risk is present with current usage of HRT
- In general, anything that leads to prolonged period of ovulation or multiple ovulation increases the risk whereas anovulation offers protection
- High gonadotropin levels may predispose
- Blocking ascending carcinogens by tubal ligation or hysterectomy offers protection.

Q. 4. What are methods to screen for ovarian cancers?[21,22]

Screening is a very important intervention in the early diagnosis of cancers and aims at early treatment, near cure and long survivals.

An ideal screening method should be cheap, freely available, easy-to-do, mass screening should be feasible, sensitivity and specificity should be high and acceptable to the people.

Though various methods are available like:
- Periodic clinical examination
- Transvaginal scan
- Tumor markers
- Doppler study
- Genetic studies
- None of them work out to be an ideal screening method for ovarian cancer screening for the entire population
- The strategy may be restricted to high-risk population
- Some of the studies support the fact that universal screening is not only not feasible but also does not reduce the mortality due to ovarian cancer
- UKCTOS study—UK Collaborative Trial of Ovarian Cancer Screening.

A large trial in the USA in 2011 based on Hyperlink "http://patient.info/doctor/cancer-antigen-125-ca-125"CA-125 (cancer antigen 125) levels and ultrasound scan 2013 Scottish Intercollegiate Guidelines Network (SIGN) guidelines.

High-risk women are with:
- Family history
- Cancer gene mutations
- 1st or 2nd degree relative with mutation
- Two family members who are 1st degree relative to each other have Ca ovary
- One family member with both breast and ovarian cancer
- A family member who has Ca ovary at any age and is a 1st degree relative of someone who developed Ca breast under the age of 50 >/= 3 family members with colon cancer; or 2 with colon cancer and 1 with stomach, ovarian, endometrial, small bowel or urinary tract cancer in 2 generations.

Intervention planned in the above high-risk women
- Genetic screening
- Prophylactic salpingo-oophorectomy around 35 years.

Q. 5. What are the common well-known hereditary ovarian syndromes?[23-26]

Many hereditary syndromes are associated with ovarian cancers which prove the genetic predisposition/basis of the pathogenesis:

- Epithelial cancers (5-10%) are associated with nonpolyposis colon cancer syndrome (Colon, endometrium and ovary)
- Breast and ovarian cancer syndrome
- Site specific cancer—only ovarian
- Sex cord stromal tumors—Peutz-Jegher, Meig's, Cushing's and Gorlin's syndromes
- Some fibromas may affect >1 family member.

Q. 6. What is the molecular classification of the epithelial tumors?

There are two types—Type I and type II tumors
- Type I tumors are associated with kras and braf mutations are generally do not respond to chemotherapy
- Type II tumors are more aggressive and are associated with Tp53 mutations.

The Table 2 shows molecular characteristics of epithelial ovarian cancers.[27]

Table 2: Precursors and molecular features of different types of cancers

Type	Histology	Precursor	Molecular features
I	Low-grade serous carcinoma	Cystadenoma borderline tumor-carcinoma sequence	Mutations in KRAS and/or BRAF (≥60%)
I	Low-grade endometrioid carcinoma	Endometriosis and endometrial cell-like hyperplasia*	Mutations in CTNNB1, PTEN and PIK3CA with microsatellite instability
I	Mucinous carcinoma	Cystadenoma borderline tumor-carcinoma sequence; metastases from bowel	Mutations in KRAS; TP53 mutation associated with transition from borderline tumor to carcinoma
I	Clear cell carcinoma	Endometriosis	PTEN mutation or loss of heterozygosity; PIK3CA mutation‡
II	High-grade serous carcinoma	Denovo in epithelial inclusion cysts; fallopian tube	TP53 mutation (up to 80%) and BRCA1 dysfunction
II	High-grade endometrioid carcinoma	Epithelial inclusion glands or cysts	TP53 mutation and BRCA1 dysfunction; PIK3CA mutation

*Endometriosis and adjacent low-grade endometrioid carcinoma share common genetic events such as loss of heterozygosity at the same loci involving the same allele (for example, PTEN). By contrast, high-grade and poorly differentiated endometrioid carcinomas are similar to high-grade serous carcinomas.‡ PIK3CA at 3q26 encodes the p110α catalytic subunit of p13k.[19]

Q. 7. How is ovarian cancer staged?[28]

2014 FIGO ovarian, fallopian tube, and peritoneal cancer staging system and corresponding TNM (Table 3).

Table 3: Staging of ovarian cancer

Stage I. Tumor confined to ovaries or fallopian tube(s)

IA: Tumor limited to one ovary (capsule intact) or fallopian tube; no tumor on ovarian or fallopian tube surface; no malignant cells in the ascites or peritoneal washings
IB: Tumor limited to both ovaries (capsules intact) or fallopian tubes; no tumor on ovarian or fallopian tube surface; no malignant cells in the ascites or peritoneal washings
IC: Tumor limited to one or both ovaries or fallopian tubes, with any of the following:
    IC1: Surgical spill
    IC2: Capsule ruptured before surgery or tumor on ovarian or fallopian tube surface
    IC3: Malignant cells in the ascites or peritoneal washings

Stage II. Tumor involves one or both ovaries or fallopian tubes with pelvic extension (below pelvic brim) or primary peritoneal cancer
IIA: Extension and/or implants on uterus and/or fallopian tubes and/or ovaries IIB: Extension to other pelvic intraperitoneal tissues

Contd...

Contd...

Stage III. Tumor involves one or both ovaries or fallopian tubes, or primary peritoneal cancer, with cytologically or histologically confirmed spread to the peritoneum outside the pelvis and/or metastasis to the retroperitoneal lymph nodes

IIIA1: Positive retroperitoneal lymph nodes only (cytologically or histologically proven):
    IIIA1(i) Metastasis up to 10 mm in greatest dimension
    IIIA1(ii) Metastasis more than 10 mm in greatest dimension
IIIA2: Microscopic extrapelvic (above the pelvic brim) peritoneal involvement with or without positive retroperitoneal lymph nodes
IIIB: Macroscopic peritoneal metastasis beyond the pelvis up to 2 cm in greatest dimension, with or without metastasis to the retroperitoneal lymph nodes
IIIC: Macroscopic peritoneal metastasis beyond the pelvis more than 2 cm in greatest dimension, with/without metastasis to the retroperitoneal lymph nodes (includes extension of tumor to capsule of liver and spleen without parenchymal involvement of either organ)

Stage IV. Distant metastasis excluding peritoneal metastases
IVA: Pleural effusion with positive cytology IVB: Parenchymal metastases and metastases to extra-abdominal organs (including inguinal lymph nodes and lymph nodes outside of the abdominal cavity)

Q. 8. What is the pattern of spread?[29]

Ovarian tumor spreads by:
- Lymphatic spread (Pelvic and para-aortic)
    - Stage 1   24
    - Stage 2   50
    - Stage 3   73
    - Stage 4   74
- Local spillage
- Transperitoneal
- Transdiaphragmatic (Ascitis, Pl Effusion)
- Hematogenous.

Q. 9. What are the treatment options in the management of epithelial ovarian cancers?

Early stage ovarian cancer is managed by a thorough staging laparotomy which includes generous mid line incision, total abdominal hysterectomy, bilateral salpingo-oophorectomy, infracolic omentectomy, appendicectomy, multiple random peritoneal biopsies, pelvic and aortic lymph node biopsies. It is especially important to remove the upper aortic nodes below the renal hilum as the metastasis to this area is seen in about 10% of clinical stage I cases.

Advanced stages (III and IV, some include stage II also under advanced category) are managed with the aim of optimal debulking which is defined as <1 cm individual residual deposits. The ideal aim would be to have no macroscopically visible residual deposits (R0 resection) which gives tremendous survival advantage as compared to any residual disease. The debulking surgery may involve total omentectomy, small and large bowel resection, splenectomy, diaphragm resection and sometimes liver resection.

Q. 10. What are the indications for chemotherapy? What are the different chemotherapy regimens?

All type II—high-grade serous and carcinosarcoma need adjuvant chemotherapy.

Adjuvant chemotherapy is administered with the purpose of eradicating presumed are actual microscopic or minimal residual disease after primary debulking surgery or interval debulking surgery.

The standard chemotherapy consists of intravenous paclitaxel 175 mg/sqm and carboplatin calculated to achieve an area under curve of 6 mg/mL/h in the serum (AUC 6) as carboplatin is mainly excreted by the kidneys within first 24 hours. Therefore, the dosing is adjusted depending on the renal function.

Cockcroft-Gault formula is used to calculate the creatinine clearance which gives an approximate idea of the renal function. The formula is (140-age in years) X weight in kg/72X serum creatinine. This gives an estimate of creatinine clearance/GFR in men. This value is multiplied by 0.8 to get the creatinine clearance/GFR in women.

To achieve the target AUC dose Calvert's formula is used which is:
- Carboplatin dose in mg = (GFR + 25) X target AUC.

For example of the GFR is 75 then the carboplatin dose would be (75 + 25) × 6 = 600 mg for a target AUC of 6.

An alternate regimen which is not inferior to the combination of paclitaxel and carboplatin is combination pegylated liposomal doxorubicin (PLD) 30 mg/sqm + Carboplatin AUC 6 administered once every four weeks for six cycles. It has been found to have an overall better toxicity profile.

Q. 11. What is the role of neoadjuvant chemotherapy?[30]

Neoadjuvant chemotherapy has been shown to be equally effective as compared to the primary surgical debulking (EORTC RCT). It can be used as a treatment approach in all patients who are thought to have Stage III C and Stage IV disease especially when the patient's performance status is not suitable to undergo aggressive debulking surgery or when the tumor is infiltrating into the surrounding soft tissue structures grossly.

Neoadjuvant chemotherapy is administered after confirming the diagnosis of malignancy either by peritoneal fluid cytology or by a FNAC. Two to three cycles are given before interval debulking surgery which is followed by adjuvant chemotherapy so that total 6–8 cycles are administered.

Q. 12. What is the role of intraperitoneal chemotherapy?[31]

A meta-analysis of three large randomized controlled trial (Alberts 1996, Markman 2001 and Armstrong 2006) showed a 12-month increase in median overall survival with intraperitoneal chemotherapy. Despite these results IP chemotherapy has not yet been consistently used due to various logistic issues and toxicity.

Heated intraperitoneal chemotherapy (HIPEC) has shown encouraging results in the recurrent ovarian cancer settings.

Q. 13. What is the role of molecular targeted biological therapy in epithelial ovarian cancer?[32]

Bevacizumab which is a monoclonal antibody against vascular endothelial growth factor (VEGF) prevents formation of new blood vessels and controls cancer cell growth. Polymerase inhibitors (PARP) like Olaparib target only cancer cells and spares normal cells.

Q. 14. How do you follow-up these patients?

The risk of recurrence is highest within the first two years and hence generally the patients are followed up once in three months for two years. Later the follow-up interval may be increased to once in six months for at least three more years.

The follow-up includes:
- Clinical examination
- Serum CA125
- Ultrasound or CT scan of the abdomen and pelvis
- Biochemical recurrence is diagnosed when only serum CA 125 is elevated. There is no proven benefit of treating these patients with only biochemical recurrence with second line chemotherapy
- Second line chemotherapy is reserved for clinical recurrence which is symptomatic or which is increasing not in its dimension.

Q. 15. What is the prognosis?[34-47]

Overall, five-year survival in ovarian epithelial carcinoma is 35%. This low rate occurs because of the preponderance of late-stage disease at diagnosis.

Five-year survival rates drop as follows with stage:[6]

- Stage I: 92%
- Stage II: 55%
- Stage III: 21.9%
- Stage IV: 5.6%.

Bad prognostic factors
- Higher grade tumors
- Massive ascitis
- Dense adhesions
- Clear cell histology
- High-grade serous tumors favorable factors: 37–40
- Younger age
- Good physical status
- Cell type other than mucinous and clear cell
- Lower stage
- Well-differentiated tumor
- Smaller disease volume prior to any surgical debulking
- Absence of ascites
- Smaller residual tumor following primary cytoreductive surgery
- CA-125 as a prognostic factor-
- At the time of diagnosis, it is not significant as a prognostic factor
- Postchemotherapy (3 Cycles) in 3rd and 4th stage disease
- Increase in a priorly normalized CA 125 is significant.[42,43]

References

1. Gadducci A, Capriello P, Bartolini T, et al. The association of ultrasonography and CA-125 test in the preoperative evaluation of ovarian carcinoma. Eur J Gynaecol Oncol. 1988;9:373-6.
2. Salem S, White LM, Lai J. Doppler sonography of adnexal masses: the predictive value of the pulsatility index in benign and malignant disease. AJR. 1994;163:1147-50.
3. Kawai M, Kikkawa F, Ishikawa H, et al. Differential diagnosis of ovarian tumors by transvaginal color-pulse Doppler sonography. Gynecol Oncol. 1994; 54:209-14.
4. Levine D, Feldstein VA, Babcook CJ, et al. Sonography of ovarian masses: Poor sensitivity of resistive index for identifying malignant lesions. AJR. 1994;162:1355-9.
5. DePriest PD, Varner E, Powell J, et al. The efficacy of a sonographic morphology index in identifying ovarian cancer: A multi-institutional investigation. Gynecol Oncol. 1994;55:174-8.
6. Stein SM, Laifer-Narin S, Johnson MB, et al. Differentiation of benign and malignant adnexal masses: Relative value of gray-scale, color Doppler, and spectral Doppler sonography. AJR. 1995;164:381-6.
7. Rehn M, Lohmann K, Rempen A. Transvaginal ultrasonography of pelvic masses: Evaluation of B-mode technique and Doppler ultrasonography. Am J Obstet Gynecol. 1996;175:97-104.
8. Tingulstad S, Hagen B, Skjeldestad FE, et al. Evaluation of a risk of malignancy index based on serum CA125, ultrasound findings and menopausal status in the pre-operative diagnosis of pelvic masses. Br J Obstet Gynaecol. 1996; 103:826-31.
9. Buy JN, Ghossain MA, Hugol D, et al. Characterization of adnexal masses: Combination of color Doppler and conventional sonography compared with spectral Doppler analysis alone and conventional sonography alone. AJR. 1996; 166:385-93.
10. Valentin L. Gray scale sonography, subjective evaluation of the color Doppler image and measurement of blood flow velocity for distinguishing benign and malignant tumors of suspected adnexal origin. Eur J Obstet Gynecol Reprod Biol. 1997;72:63-72.
11. Aultman CJ, Feller JF, Jain KA, et al. MR imaging of sonographically indeterminate adnexal masses: Cost-benefit study (abstr). Radiology. 1995;197(P):354.

12. Medl M, Kulenkampff KJ, Stiskal M, et al. Magnetic resonance imaging in the preoperative evaluation of suspected ovarian masses. Anticancer Res. 1995; 15:1123-5.
13. Yamashita Y, Torashima M, Hatanaka Y, et al. Adnexal masses: Accuracy of characterization with transvaginal US and precontrast and postcontrast MR imaging. Radiology. 1995;194:557-65.
14. Van Gorp T, Cadron I, Despierre E, et al. HE4 and CA125 as a diagnostic test in ovarian cancer: prospective validation of the Risk of Ovarian Malignancy Algorithm. 14. Br J Cancer. 2011;104(5): 863-70.
15. Sutcliffe S, Pharoah PD, Easton DF, et al. Ovarian and breast cancer risks to women in families with two or more cases of ovarian cancer Int J Cancer. 2000;87(1):110-7.
16. Tan DS, Rothermundt C, Thomas K, et al. "BRCAness" syndrome in ovarian cancer: a case-control study describing the clinical features and outcome of patients with epithelial ovarian cancer associated with *BRCA1* and *BRCA2* mutations. J Clin Oncol. 2008;26(34):5530-6.
17. Tworoger SS, Gertig DM, Gates MA, et al. Caffeine, alcohol, smoking, and the risk of incident epithelial ovarian cancer. Cancer. 2008;112(5):1169-77.
18. Tung KH, Goodman MT, Wu AH, et al. Reproductive factors and epithelial ovarian cancer risk by histologic type: a multiethnic case control study. Am J Epidemiol. 2003; 158(7):629-38.
19. Titus-Ernstoff L, Perez K, Cramer DW, et al. Menstrual and reproductive factors in relation to ovarian cancer risk. Br J Cancer. 2001; 84:714-21.
20. Scottish Intercollegiate Guidelines Network (SIGN). Management of epithelial ovarian cancer. Edinburgh: SIGN; 2013. (SIGN publication no. 135). [November 2013]. Available from URL: http://www.sign.ac.uk
21. Ovarian cancer screening and mortality in the UK Collaborative Trial of Ovarian Cancer Screening (UKCTOCS): A randomised controlled trial, Lancet, Dec 2015.
22. Piver MS, Goldberg JM, Tsukada Y, et al. Characteristics of familial ovarian cancer: A report of the first 1,000 families in the Gilda Radner Familial Ovarian Cancer Registry. Eur J Gynaecol Oncol. 1996;17(3):169-76.
23. Miki Y, Swensen J, Shattuck-Eidens D, et al. A strong candidate for the breast and ovarian cancer susceptibility gene *BRCA1*. Science. 1994;266(5182):66-71.
24. Easton DF, Bishop DT, Ford D, et al. Genetic linkage analysis in familial breast and ovarian cancer: results from 214 families. The Breast Cancer Linkage Consortium. Am J Hum Genet. 1993;52(4):678-701.
25. Steichen-Gersdorf E, Gallion HH, Ford D, et al. Familial site-specific ovarian cancer is linked to BRCA1 on 17q12-21. Am J Hum Genet. 1994; 55(5):870-5.
26. Wooster R, Neuhausen SL, Mangion J, et al. Localization of a breast cancer susceptibility gene, BRCA2, to chromosome 13q12-13. Science. 1994;265(5181):2088-90.
27. Bast RC, Hennessy B, Gordon B, et al. The biology of ovarian cancer: new opportunities for translation. Nature Reviews Cancer. 2009;9: 415-28.
28. FIGO's staging classification for cancer of the ovary, fallopian tube, and peritoneum: abridged republication. Jaime Prat and FIGO Committee on Gynecologic Oncology. J Gynecol Oncol. 2015;26(2):87-9.
29. Burghardt E, Girardi F, Lahousen M, et al. Patterns of pelvic and paraaortic lymph node involvement in ovarian cancer. Gynecol Oncol. 1991;40(2):103-6.
30. Vergote I, Amant F, Kristensen G, et al. Primary surgery or neoadjuvant chemotherapy followed by interval debulking surgery in advanced ovarian cancer. Eur J Cancer. 2011 Sep;47Suppl 3:S88-92. doi: 10.1016/S0959-8049(11)70152-
31. Chan DL, Morris DL, Rao A, et al. Intraperitoneal chemotherapy in ovarian cancer: a review of tolerance and efficacy. Cancer Manag Res. 2012;4:413-22.
32. Coward JIG, Middleton K, Murphy F. New perspectives on targeted therapy in ovarian cancer. Int J Womens Health. 2015;7:189-203.
33. Dembo AJ, Davy M, Stenwig AE, et al. Prognostic factors in patients with stage I epithelial ovarian cancer. Obstet Gynecol. 1990;75(2):263-73.

34. Schueler JA, Cornelisse CJ, Hermans J, et al. Prognostic factors in well-differentiated early-stage epithelial ovarian cancer. Cancer. 1993;71(3): 787-95.
35. Young RC, Walton LA, Ellenberg SS, et al. Adjuvant therapy in stage I and stage II epithelial ovarian cancer. Results of two prospective randomized trials. N Engl J Med. 1990;322(15):1021-7.
36. Gershenson DM, Silva EG, Mitchell MF, et al. Transitional cell carcinoma of the ovary: a matched control study of advanced-stage patients treated with cisplatin-based chemotherapy. Am J Obstet Gynecol. 1993;168(4):1178-85; discussion 1185-7.
37. Omura GA, Brady MF, Homesley HD, et al. Long-term follow-up and prognostic factor analysis in advanced ovarian carcinoma: the Gynecologic Oncology Group experience. J Clin Oncol. 1991;9(7):1138-50.
38. van Houwelingen JC, ten Bokkel Huinink WW, van der Burg ME, et al. Predictability of the survival of patients with advanced ovarian cancer. J Clin Oncol. 1989;7(6):769-73.
39. Neijt JP, ten BokkelHuinink WW, van der Burg ME, et al. Long-term survival in ovarian cancer. Mature data from The Netherlands Joint Study Group for Ovarian Cancer. Eur J Cancer. 1991;27(11):1367-72.
40. Hoskins WJ, Bundy BN, Thigpen JT, et al. The influence of cytoreductive surgery on recurrence-free interval and survival in small-volume stage III epithelial ovarian cancer: A Gynecologic Oncology Group study. Gynecol Oncol. 1992;47(2):159-66.
41. Thigpen T, Brady MF, Omura GA, et al. Age as a prognostic factor in ovarian carcinoma. The Gynecologic Oncology Group experience. Cancer. 1993;71(2 Suppl): 606-14.
42. Mogensen O. Prognostic value of CA 125 in advanced ovarian cancer. Gynecol Oncol. 1992; 44(3):207-12.
43. Högberg T, Kågedal B. Long-term follow-up of ovarian cancer with monthly determinations of serum CA 125. Gynecol Oncol. 1992;46(2):191-8.
44. Rustin GJ, Nelstrop AE, Tuxen MK, et al. Defining progression of ovarian carcinoma during follow-up according to CA 125: a North Thames Ovary Group Study. Ann Oncol. 1996;7(4):361-4.
45. Vencken PM, Kriege M, Hoogwerf D, et al. Chemosensitivity and outcome of BRCA1- and BRCA2-associated ovarian cancer patients after first-line chemotherapy compared with sporadic ovarian cancer patients. Ann Oncol. 2011;22(6):1346-52.
46. Safra T, Borgato L, Nicoletto MO, et al. BRCA mutation status and determinant of outcome in women with recurrent epithelial ovarian cancer treated with pegylated liposomal doxorubicin. Mol Cancer Ther. 2011;10(10):2000-7.

23

Invasive Procedures in Obstetrics and Gynecology Practice

Radhakrishnan P

CASE

Prenatal diagnosis is an essential part of obstetric care. It includes all diagnostic methods by which it is possible to detect structural defects, chromosomal abnormalities and genetic syndromes.[1] High resolution ultrasound enables us to estimate an empiric risk for certain chromosomal abnormalities by modifying the maternal age related risk.[2]

"Fetal interventions" is a branch of fetal medicine where a single or a series of interventions are performed on the placenta, uterine cavity or the fetus. There have been immense advances in the field of fetal medicine and fetal interventions in the past few years. These interventions may either be for diagnostic purpose or a therapeutic one depending on the indication. In the past two decades, the goal of prenatal diagnosis has changed from merely deciding about terminating the pregnancy to possible active intervention for improving the long-term outcome for the fetus. Recently, medical and surgical fetal therapy has emerged as an option for the management of various fetal malformations. Rh immune prophylaxis is administered to Rh negative women after any invasive procedure.

Fetal Diagnostic Procedures

Amniocentesis, chorionic villus sampling (CVS) and fetal blood sampling (FBS) where the placental/fetal cells are analyzed directly and hence the diagnosis is confirmed. As the fetoplacental unit is invaded and hence, there is a procedure-related risk of miscarriage.[3]

Fetal Therapeutic Procedures

Primarily there are four modalities of fetal therapeutic procedures.
- **Ultrasonography-guided procedures,** e.g. intrauterine blood transfusions, thoracoamniotic shunt placements, etc.
- **Fetoscopic techniques** being minimally invasive have a clinical application in complications of monochorionic pregnancies as in twin to twin transfusion syndrome (TTTS) where laser ablation of placental anastomotic vessels is performed. In monochorionic twin pregnancies with selective fetal growth restriction (sFGR), bipolar cord coagulation is done, which is combination of both ultrasound and fetoscopic guidance. In fetal megacystis, laser fulguration of posterior urethral valves may be performed fetoscopically.[4]

In fetuses diagnosed to have congenital diaphragmatic hernia, in view of the poor development of the lungs resulting in severe pulmonary hypoplasia, Fetal endoscopic tracheal occlusion is performed under fetoscopic guidance.
- **Open fetal surgery** is currently performed at selected centers when the risk of the procedure to the mother and fetus is overridden by a diagnosis is made that is known to have a poorer outcome. Complications such as chorioamnionitis, preterm labor, bleeding, and direct trauma to the fetus are risks in most of these procedures.
- **Ex utero intrapartum treatment (EXIT) procedure** is performed at the time of delivery where the fetal airway is expected to be compressed and hence hinder in the breathing process.

Diagnostic Invasive Tests

Amniocentesis and chorionic villous sampling are the two most widely performed invasive procedures for diagnostic purposes. Both the procedures should be performed under continuous ultrasound visualization of the needle to minimize complications during the procedures. Although the risk of miscarriage quoted with a CVS is relatively higher, most studies from experienced centers suggest the same "procedure related" risk of miscarriage of about 1:250 for both procedures.

Indications for Diagnostic Invasive Procedures

- Fetal abnormalities
- Positive maternal screening tests
- Fetal markers
- Previous sibling with chromosomal abnormality
- Parental-balanced translocation
- Certain genetic syndromes where gene mutation analysis has been done from index child
- Confirm fetal infections.

Fetal DNA can be extracted and appropriately stored from the samples in special cases where the karyotype of the fetus is likely to be normal and if any further investigations are required, where cause for abnormalities cannot be ascertained.

Chorionic Villus Sampling (CVS)

Chorionic villous sampling (CVS) is a test performed between 11–15 weeks of pregnancy. CVS includes introduction of the needle through the mother's abdomen into the placenta and a sample of placental villi is obtained (Fig. 1). In majority of the cases, the placenta shares the same genetic information as the fetus. The risk of miscarriage is about 1:250–300 with experienced operators. The results of the culture karyotype are expected in 2–3 weeks. Limb reduction and oromandibular defects are known to occur if CVS is performed before 11 weeks. Rh immune prophylaxis is administered to Rh negative women.

Amniocentesis

This test is performed after 16 weeks. This includes introduction of the needle through

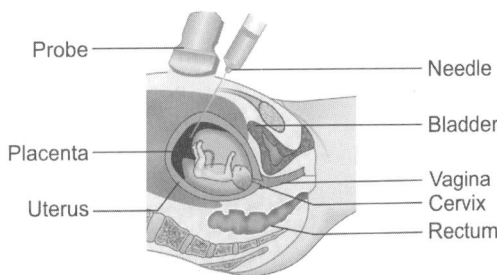

Fig. 1: Chorionic villous sampling: Needle inserted into placenta at 45° angle with the probe and continuous ultrasound guidance

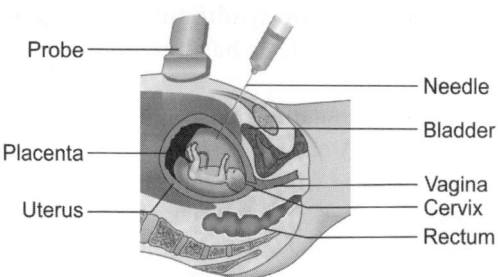

Fig. 2: Amniocentesis: Needle inserted into the amniotic cavity at 45° angle with the probe and continuous ultrasound guidance

the mother's abdomen into the amniotic cavity and withdrawing of about 20–30 mL of the amniotic fluid (Fig. 2). The sample is usually sent for fluorescent in situ hybridization (FISH) for major chromosomes–13, 18, 21 and the sex chromosomes which is expected in about a weeks' time. The complete karyotype result is available in 3 weeks. The risk of miscarriage because of the procedure is 1:300 in experienced operator's hands.

Fetal Reduction

Fertility treatment has significantly contributed to the increase of multiple pregnancy. First trimester multifetal pregnancy reduction can be given as an option to the parents to decrease the risk of perinatal mortality and morbidity. The termination of one normal fetus in a triplet pregnancy or two embryos in a quadruplet pregnancy is an alternative to either abortion of all the fetuses or acceptance to preterm delivery. With today's perinatal and neonatal care the outcome of triplet pregnancy has improve considerably. The higher the order of pregnancy, the higher is the risk of miscarriage. To avoid unselective fetal reduction, nuchal translucency measurement and detailed first trimester anomaly scan have to be completed as a prerequisite before fetal reduction. If any of the babies are diagnosed with abnormalities, then the abnormal one is reduced else the one which is technically easier to perform is reduced.[5]

Fetal reduction is performed by a transabdominal route after the labeling of the fetuses is done. It includes introduction of potassium chloride into the heart of the targeted fetus. The preterm delivery rate in a triplet pregnancy reduces from 25 to 10% with a procedure related risk of miscarriage of about 5%. The procedure has been shown to be relatively safe and results in improved pregnancy outcome, with a decrease in morbidity and mortality rates of the surviving fetuses. Successful outcome of the pregnancy is also dependent on initial number of fetuses.[6] The higher the number of initial fetuses requiring more than 1 fetus to be reduced, the higher would be the risk of miscarriage.

Fetal Therapeutic Interventions: Minimally Invasive Therapeutic Techniques

Intrauterine Fetal Blood Transfusion

Fetal anemia is one of the most serious fetal complications in pregnancy and associated with perinatal mortality and morbidity. When left untreated fetal anemia may result in cardiac failure, hydrops, hypovolemic shock, fetal or neonatal death, neurological injury or cerebral palsy. Timely intervention will save fetal lives. Fetal blood transfusion (FBT) is performed to correct fetal anemia from any cause.[7,8]

Diagnosis of Fetal Anemia on Ultrasound

The advent of middle cerebral artery Doppler has revolutionized the management of fetal anemia. Fetal anemia is diagnosed by performing the MCA Doppler of the fetus. If the MCA PSV is more than the 95th centile

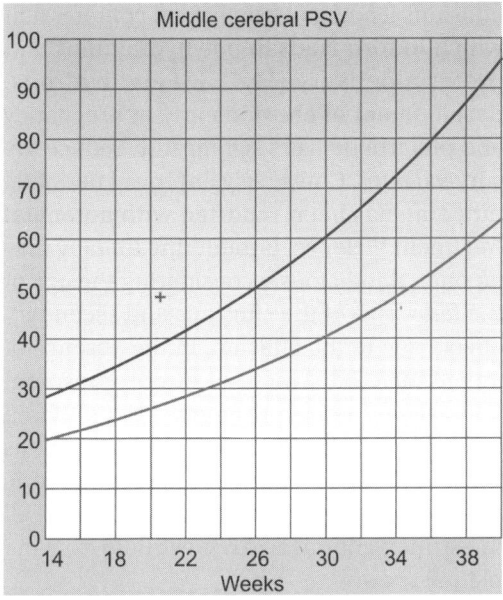

Fig. 3: Middle cerebral artery (MCA) Doppler peak systolic velocity above the 95th centile indicates fetal anemia

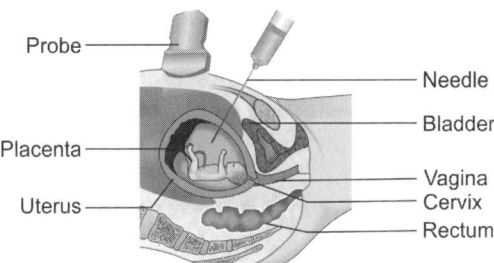

Fig. 4: Fetal blood sampling needle inserted into the umbilical cord from the placental insertion under continuous ultrasound guidance

then it is suggestive of fetal anemia (Fig. 3). MCA Doppler has 100% sensitivity with a 12% false positive rate.

Indications

- Red cell isoimmunization—remains the main indication for intrauterine FBT
- Fetomaternal hemorrhage
- Parvovirus B19 infection
- Twin anemia polycythemia syndrome (TAPS)—a complication of monochorionic twin pregnancy where one twin is anemic and the other is polycythemic
- Fetomaternal alloimmune thrombocytopenia
- Fetal intracranial hemorrhages
- Placental and fetal tumors (Chorioangiomas and sacrococcygeal teratomas).

Technique of FBT

This is usually a transplacental procedure done at the placental cord insertion (Fig. 4). FBT can also be performed into the intrahepatic portion of the umbilical vein, in particular when the placental cord insertion is difficult to access. Intraperitoneal transfusion has also considered to be an effective method for slow correction of fetal anemia. Fresh O-negative, irradiated packed cells are transfused after calculating the hemoglobin percentage in the fetus and amount required to correct the same. There are softwares available for correct calculation of amount of donor blood to be transfused depending upon the gestational age and weight of the baby. The procedure-related risk of miscarriage is about 1:100. Most of the times, in isoimmunized pregnancies, fetuses will require multiple transfusions.

FBT is generally considered to be a safe method to correct fetal anemia. However, procedural complications do occur sometimes that may affect the outcome of the pregnancy. Intrauterine bleeding due to cord accidents which leads to fetal distress, preterm labor, preterm premature rupture of membranes, chorioamnionitis are some of the commonest complications.[9]

Perinatal loss due to fetal anemia is about 3%, mostly being in hydropic fetuses. The presence of hydrops is also one of the main prognostic factors affecting the survival of the fetus. Outcome of the fetuses post-blood transfusion is significantly dependent on the gestational age, condition of the fetus at diagnosis and more importantly on the experience of the operator. It has been proved beyond doubt that FBT is a safe and successful method to treat fetal anemia of different indications. Early and timely detection, referral and treatment may prevent hydrops and improve long-term outcomes. There long-term neurodevelopment of babies that have been transfused in utero is not affected by FBT.

Pleural Drainage/Pleuro-amniotic Shunt

Primary hydrothorax is an uncommon complication in the fetus which has an unpredictable clinical course. It is due to lymphatic leakage which generates an increased intrathoracic pressure. It may resolve spontaneously, remain stable or may progress to fetal hydrops. The diagnosis of primary hydrothorax is made by exclusion of all structural and karyotypic abnormalities. Secondary effusions are a part of generalized fluid retention in nonimmune hydrops.[10] Smaller effusions may resolve spontaneously, however the larger ones will cause fetal hydrops, lung hypoplasia and mediastinal shift. Mediastinal compression occurs with bilateral effusions leading to esophageal compression which in turn leads to polyhydramnios and preterm delivery (Fig. 5). Fetal hydrops, development of effusion early in pregnancy and preterm delivery significantly reduce the survival rates. Conversely improved perinatal outcome has been reported with antenatal treatment.[11] Hence, intrauterine therapy may be offered judiciously considering the age of the fetus, size of the effusions and secondary effects due to the effusion, in the absence of any associated structural or chromosomal anomalies. Therapeutic interventions offered in a primary hydrothorax include thoracentesis may be single or multiple, thoracoamniotic shunting and pleurodesis. The main aim of all these interventions is to remove fluid from the pleural space.

Technique of Pleuro-amniotic Shunting

Thoracocentesis is performed under continuous ultrasound guidance (Fig. 6). Thoracocentesis may be single or multiple as in some fetuses the effusion resolves with a single drainage. Pleuro-amniotic shunting is done with a double pig tail catheter which is inserted through a Harrison/Rocket cannula depositing

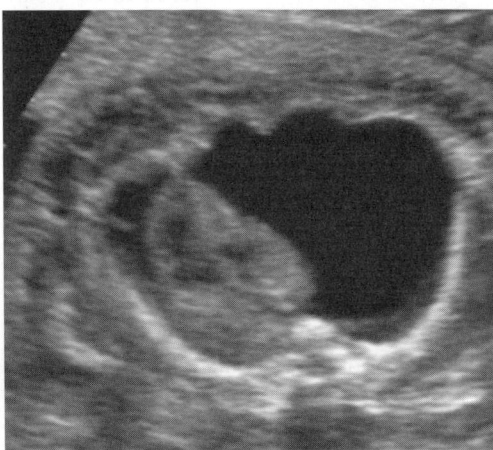

Fig. 5: Pleural effusion causing mediastinal shift to the opposite side

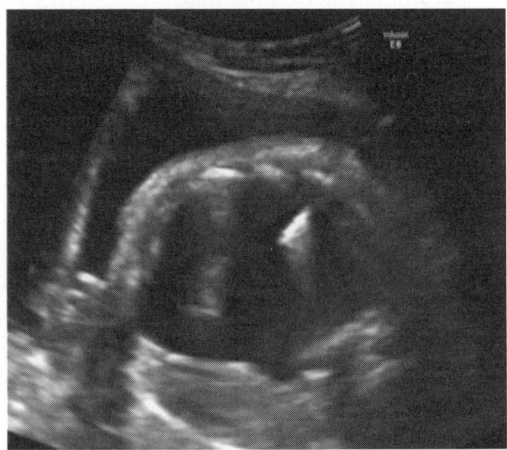

Fig. 6: Thoracentesis under continuous ultrasound guidance

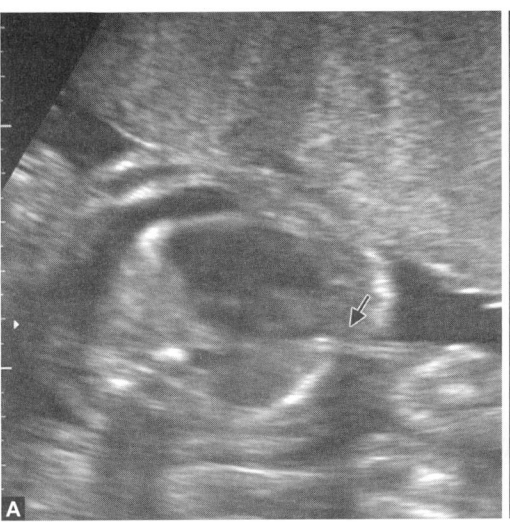 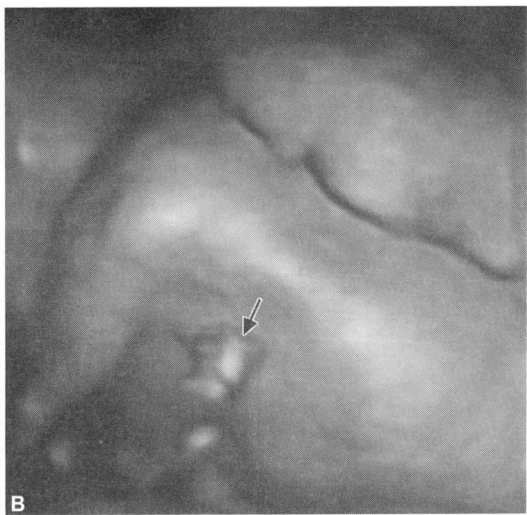

Figs 7A and B: Thoracoamniotic shunt

the distal end in the effusion and proximal end in the amniotic cavity (Figs 7A and B). The fetus needs to be followed up as occasionally the shunt might get displaced owing to the high intrathoracic pressures. Unilateral or bilateral shunting may be performed depending upon the need for the same.

One of the most difficult challenges, we come across in a hydropic fetus with pleural effusion, is the inability to ascertain whether the effusion is primary or a part of generalized hydrops. In summary, a fetus with primary hydrothorax can benefit from pleuro-amniotic shunting with good perinatal and neonatal outcomes, in the absence of associated anomalies and normal karyotype.

Fetoscopic LASER ablation (FLA)

Monochorionic pregnancies pose challenging therapeutic problems when only one fetus is in distress as delivery of both the twins is not an option. Complications in monochorionic pregnancies may present as twin-to-twin transfusion syndrome (TTTS), selective fetal growth restriction (sFGR) and twin reversed arterial perfusion (TRAP).

Approximately about 15–20% of the monochorionic diamniotic twin (MCDA) pregnancies have complications of which 50% of them would require interventions.[12]

Twin-to-twin transfusion syndrome (TTTS) is a complication of MCDA pregnancies which is a result of unbalanced unidirectional flow in the placental vascular anastomoses. The accuracy of the diagnosis depends on the determination of the chorionicity in the first trimester, demonstration of polyhydramnios (DVP >8 cm) in the recipient sac and oligohydramnios in the donor sac (DVP <2 cm).[13]

Quintero Staging of TTTS

Stage 1—Oligohydramnios in the donor sac and polyhydramnios in the recipient sac

Stage 2—Donor bladder absent

Stage 3—Abnormal Doppler

Stage 4—Fetal hydrops

Stage 5—Demise of 1 or both twins.

Follow-up of MCDA pregnancies:

Once the chorionicity is diagnosed in the first trimester, MCDA pregnancies have to be

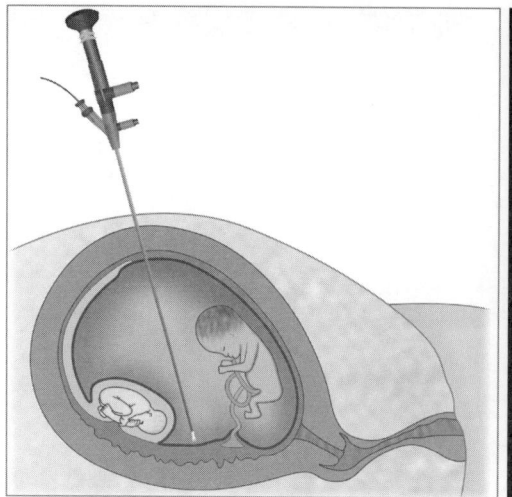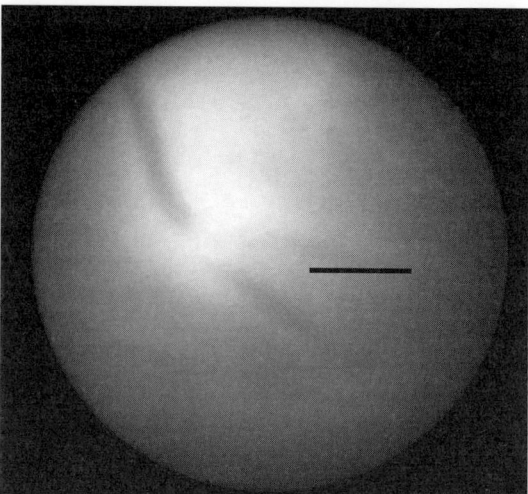

Fig. 8: Fetoscopic view of the placenta anastomoses

followed up every 2 weeks from 6 weeks to look for any evidence of TTTS. If there is any evidence of TTTS, fetoscopic LASER can be offered depending upon the severity of the condition. Surveillance in MCDA pregnancies is very important as early referral enables timely therapy and hence potentially decreases perinatal morbidity and mortality. Currently, fetoscopic LASER ablation of the anastomotic vessels on the placenta is indicated from Quintero stage II to stage IV TTTS. This is essentially a fetoscopic procedure done along with ultrasound guidance (Fig. 8). A thorough study of the placental site and position, both the cord insertions donor sac and position is a prerequisite as the entry point into the uterus is decided based on the placental position and both the cord insertions.

Outcome of FLA

With the performance of the laser coagulation of the placental anastomoses, the survival rates for a single fetus is about 80% and both fetuses is 50%. The larger Eurofetus trial comparing the efficacy of serial amnioreduction versus laser coagulation favored the latter with a high rate of single and double survival and lower incidence of morbidity from leukomalacia.[14]

Bipolar Cord Coagulation

Bipolar cord coagulation (BCC) is offered in:

i. **Selective fetal growth restriction (sFGR)** with abnormal umbilical artery Doppler in the smaller twin

   Type II sFGR fetuses have a high risk of further deterioration and death. About 15% of the sFGR twins die unexpectedly and 20% of the larger twins suffer from brain lesions, probably related to feto-fetal transfusion via large arterio-arterial vascular anastomosis.[15,16]

ii. **Discordant anomaly**, both, for parental decision to terminate and for the impending damage to the normal fetus.

   This is a fetoscopic procedure done along with ultrasound guidance.

iii. **Twin reversed arterial perfusion (TRAP)** sequence is a rare complication of MCDA pregnancies that is characterized by the presence of an acardiac mass perfused by an apparently normal (pump twin). Acardiac twins can be diagnosed antenatally on ultrasound scan by absence of identifiable cardiac pulsation and poor definition of the head, trunk and upper extremities, deformed lower extremities, and usually marked tissue edema.[17] In order to improve the outcome of the normal "pump twin" treatment approaches that aim to discontinue the perfusion to the TRAP twin have been introduced. TRAP sequence should be evaluated weekly by serial ultrasound examinations, when a rapid growth of the recipient twin is noticed, intervention is offered to the parents. The only successful method to interrupt the blood flow to the perfused twin is by vascular occlusion by laser coagulation or radiofrequency ablation. The former is achieved by ultrasound-guided interstitial laser therapy to the perfused twin (Figs. 9A and B). Positioning of the laser fiber within the body of the perfused twin rather than the cord diminishes the risk of hemorrhage secondary to vessel rupture and confines the laser to within the body the acardiac twin preventing inadvertent damage to the pump twin or the amnion.[18]

It is very important to accurately document the chorionicity in all multiple pregnancies. One must be aware about the potential complications of MCDA twins and it is also important to educate the patients regarding the complications. Fortnightly scans have to be performed to detect oligopoly sequence, differences in the bladder sizes and cardiac changes typical of TTTS. Patients have to be referred to a center performing fetoscopic procedures once complications of MCDA twin pregnancy is diagnosed.

Fetal Endoscopic Tracheal Occlusion (FETO)

Congenital diaphragmatic hernia (CDH) is a sporadic defect with a prevalence of 1:4000 (Figs 10A and B). About 30% of them are associated with chromosomal problems or other associated defects. It is associated with a high postnatal mortality rate due to pulmonary hypoplasia and pulmonary hypertension. Prenatal prediction of lethal pulmonary hypoplasia is based on assessment of the lung compression due to the hernia. The most widely used technique is ultrasonographic measurement of lung area to head circumference ratio.[19,20] Fetal endoscopic tracheal occlusion (FETO) is performed between 26 and 30 weeks has shown to increase the lung size and improve the pulmonary vascularization and

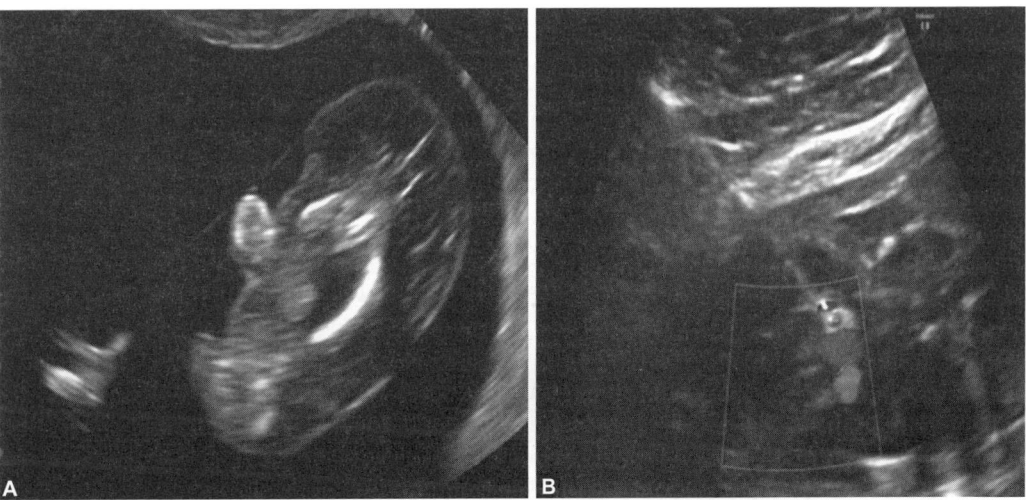

Figs 9A and B: (A) Acardiac fetus; (B) Interstitial laser coagulation of the acardiac fetus

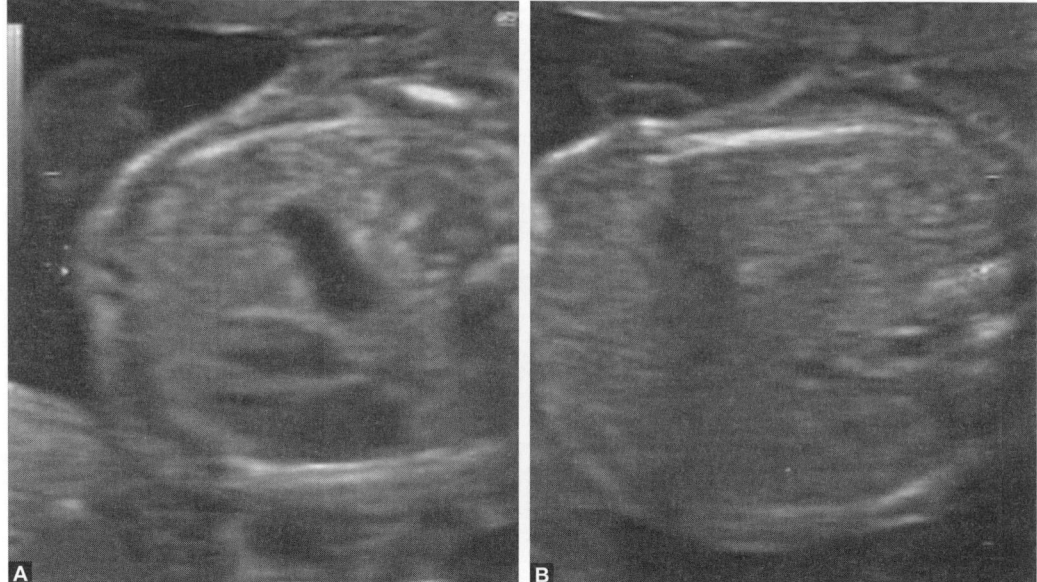

Figs 10A and B: Congenital diaphragmatic hernia with stomach and intestines in the fetal chest

hence improve the perinatal mortality and morbidity.[21,22] This allows the secretions of the lungs to stay within and helps in inflation and development of the lungs.

Currently, FETO is performed in very few centers across the world which are participating in the randomized control trial to assess the efficacy of FETO in severe forms of CDH, the TOTAL trial.

Technique of FETO

FETO is performed under spinal/epidural anesthesia. The fetus is also anesthetized with fentanyl by intramuscular injection to the thigh. Ultrasound examination is done to determine the fetal and the placental position. A gentle external podalic version of the fetus is performed if required to achieve better access to the trachea and the entry of the trocar being in the upper part of the uterus. Breech presentation is an ideal position for FETO. Tracheal occlusion is done by inflating the balloon just above the carina. This is achieved by passing the fetoscope through the mouth of the baby. The balloon is removed at 34 weeks by fetoscopic procedure or by puncturing the balloon by ultrasound guidance which avoids the need for delivery by cesarean section. Postnatal surgery is delayed till the baby is stabilized. Though FETO still remains an investigational procedure it has shown a substantial increase in the survival rates. However, FETO has to be performed in a highly specialized center and requires a lot of expertise.

Open Fetal Surgery

Spina bifida occurs when the neural tube fails to close. The commonly accepted two main categories of spina bifida are (i) open spina bifida (OSB)—Neural tissue/and or meninges are exposed to the surrounding environment and (ii) closed spina bifida—skin is seen covering the defect. OSB is a devastating congenital abnormality and is associated with significant disability, high morbidity and mortality. Closed spina bifida, however have a favorable outcome. The most valuable marker to detect closed from an open spina bifida is absence of cranial signs.[4]

Typically open spina bifida is treated by postnatal surgery with the closure of the defect. However, the MOMS (Management of myelomeningocele study) trial has shown that fetal surgical procedures both open and fetoscopic can be performed relatively safely for the closure of the defect. This can result in significant benefit to the child. The skin covering the defect, absence of the cranial signs and kyphosis are excluded from the fetal surgery. Data from MOMS also suggest that prenatal surgical repair offer significant benefit compared to postnatal surgery. Open fetal surgeries/fetoscopic techniques bifida are performed only in a few licensed centers and still in the experimental stage.[23]

Ex utero Intrapartum Treatment (EXIT)

The EXIT procedure is done in cases where difficulty is anticipated in the neonatal airway establishment at delivery and is done at the time of cesarean section. EXIT to airway is done in fetuses with neck masses, fetal oral and facial tumors, chest masses, CHAOS, etc. These babies have a high mortality following delivery due to difficulties related to ventilation, intubation and tracheostomy.[24]

Technique of EXIT

EXIT procedure requires a multidisciplinary approach which includes fetal medicine specialists, obstetricians, pediatric surgeons, anesthesiologists and neonatologists. The baby is anesthetized in utero by intramuscular injection with appropriate agents. The cesarean section is carried out under general anesthesia for the mother. The fetus is partially delivered (head and neck) and the fetal circulation is maintained on uteroplacental support while the newborn's airway is established. This allows careful laryngoscopic exploration of the upper airways. Once the baby is stabilized, the umbilical cord is cut and the baby is transferred to the care of neonatologist and the pediatric surgeon.[25] The combination of intensive maternal and fetal monitoring, cesarean section with maximal uterine relaxation and maintenance of intact fetoplacental circulation provides a controlled environment for securing airway in babies with prenatally diagnosed airway obstruction.

Conclusion

In utero interventions have progressed a long way in the last 2 decades with the advent of high resolution ultrasound machines. In addition, training for such procedures is being offered at various centers. Improvement in skills, technique, and development of instruments for minimally invasive procedures have in addition contributed to making most procedures relatively safe. However, interventions should be performed in **specialized multidisciplinary fetal treatment centers** within **strict protocols** and with the approval of the local **ethics** committee when necessary. **Informed consent, verbal and written** of the mother or parents must be obtained after thorough counseling about the pros and cons of all the available options. Interventions are performed to improve the fetal and the neonatal outcomes. The parents must also be counseled about the effects of not doing the procedure. Fetoscopic procedures are minimally invasive which show less maternal morbidity when compared to the open procedures. However, premature rupture of the membranes and pretermdelivery remain as the complications of fetal therapy. Further research in order to minimize this is necessary.

References

1. European Study Group Prenatal Diagnosis. Recommendations and protocols for Prenatal Diagnosis. Dt Arztebl. 1998;50:3236-42.
2. Snijders RJ, Noble P, Seibre N, et al. UK multicentre project on assessment of risk for trisomy 21 by maternal age and fetal nuchal translucency at 10-14 weeks of gestation. Fetal Medicine Foundation First Trimester Screening Group. Lancet. 1998;352:343-6.
3. Prediction of miscarriage and still birth at 11-13 weeks and the contribution of chorionic villous sampling. In: Akolekar R, Bower S, Flack N, et al. (Eds). Harris Birthright Research Centre for Fetal Medicine, King's College Hospital, London, UK.
4. Fetal therapy: Practical ethical considerations; Yves Ville* Department of Obstetrics and Fetal Medicine, UFR Necker-Enfants-Malades, Universite´ Ren´e Descartes, 75015 Paris, France, Prenat Diagn. 2011; 31:621-7.
5. Stephen JA, Timor-Tritsch IE, Lerner JP, et al. Amniocentesis after multifetal pregnancy reduction: Is it safe? Am J Obstet Gynecol. 2000;182:962-5.
6. Boulot P, Vignal J, Vergnes C, et al. Multifetal reduction of triplets to twins: a prospective comparison to pregnancy outcome. Human Reproduction. 2000;15(7):1619-23.
7. Van Kamp IL, Klumper FJ, Meerman Rh, et al. Treatment of fetal anaemia due to red cell alloimmunization with intrauterine transfusions in Netherlands, 1988–1999. Leiden, Acta Obstet Gynecol Scand. 2004;83(8):731-7.
8. Moise KJ Jr. Management of rhesus alloimmunization in pregnancy. Obstet Gynecol. 2008;112(1):164-76.
9. Techniques of intrauterine fetal transfusion for women with red-cell isoimmunisation for improving health outcomes In: Dodd JM, Windrim RC, van Kamp IL (Eds). Techniques of intrauterine fetal transfusion for women with red-cell isoimmunisation for improving health outcomes. Cochrane Database of Systematic Reviews 2012, Issue 9. Art. No.: CD007096. DOI: 10.1002/14651858.CD007096.pub3.
10. Deurloo KL, Devlieger R, Lopriore E, et al. Isolated fetal hydrothorax with hydrops: a systematic review on prenatal treatment options. Prenatal Diagnosis. 2007; 10(27):893-9.
11. Nicolaides KH, Azar GB. Thoraco-amniotic shunting. Fetal Diagn Ther. 1990;5:153-64.
12. Roman A, Papanna R, Johnson A, et al. Selective reduction in complicated monochorionic pregnancies: radiofrequency vs. bipolar cord coagulation. Ultrasound Obstet Gynecol. 2010;36:37-41.
13. Sueters M, Middeldorp JM, Lopriore E, et al. Timely diagnosis of twin-to-twin transfusion syndrome in monochorionic twin pregnancies by biweekly sonography combined with patient instruction to report onset of symptoms. Ultrasound Obstet Gynecol. 2006;28:659-64.
14. Van Mieghem T, Baud D, Devlieger R, et al. Minimally invasive fetal therapy. Best Pract Res Clin Obstet Gynaecol. 2012; 26:711-25.
15. Gratacos E, Lewi L, Munoz B, et al. A classification system for selective intrauterine growth restriction in monochorionic pregnancies according to umbilical artery Doppler flow in the smaller twin. Ultrasound Obstet Gynecol. 2007;30:28-34.
16. Ishii K, Murakoshi T, Takahashi Y, Shinno T, Matsushita M, Naruse H, et al. Perinatal outcome of monochorionic twins with selective intrauterine growth restriction and different types of umbilical artery Doppler under expectant management. Fetal Diagn Ther. 2009;26:157-61.
17. Sebire NJ, Sepulveda W, Jeanty P, et al. Multiple gestations. In: Diagnostic Imaging of Fetal Anomalies. In: Nyberg DA, McGahan JP, Pretorius DH, et al. (Eds). Lippincott William & Wilkins: Philadelphia, PA. 2003;777-813.
18. Pagani G, D'Antonio F, Khalil A, et al. Intrafetal laser treatment for twin reversed arterial perfusion sequence: cohort study and meta-analysis. Ultrasound Obstet Gynecol. 2013;42:6-14.
19. Albanese CT, Lopoo J, Goldstein RB, et al. Liver position and perinatal outcome for congenital diaphragmatic hernia. Prenat Diagn. 1998; 18:1138-42.

20. Laudy JAM, Van Gucht M, Van Dooren MF, et al. Congenital diaphragmatic hernia: an evaluation of the prognostic value of the lung-to-head ratio and other prenatal parameters. Prenat Diagn. 2003;23: 634-9.
21. Ruano R, Duarte SA, Pimenta EJ, et al. Comparison between fetal endoscopic tracheal occlusion using a 1.0 mm fetoscope and prenatal expectant management in severe congenital diaphragmatic hernia. Fetal Diagn Ther. 2011;29:64-70.
22. Ruano R, Yoshisaki CT, da Silva MM, et al. A randomized controlled trial of fetal endoscopic tracheal occlusion versus postnatal management of severe isolated congenital diaphragmatic hernia. Ultrasound Obstet Gynecol. 2012;39:20-7.
23. Depres JA, Flake AW, Gratacos E, et al. The making of fetal surgery. Prenatal Diagnosis Prenat Diagn. 2010;30: 653-67.
24. Peak BW, Callen PW, Kitterman J, et al. Successful fetal intervention for congenital high airway obstruction syndrome. Fetal Diagn Ther. 2002;17:272-6.
25. Smith NM, Chambers SE, Billson VR, et al. Oral teratoma (epignathus) with intracranial extension: a report of two cases. Prenat Diagn. 1993;13:945-52.

24

CHAPTER

Fibroid Uterus

Sunanda R Kulkarni

CASE

Patient by Name Mrs X wife of Mr Y aged 45 years, of low social economic class presented to OPD with:
- Retention of urine since one day
- White discharge—since 8 months but foul smelling, blood tinged since last 2 months
- Mass per vagina since 5 months
- Heaviness in the abdomen—since 6 months
- Heavy flow with during periods along with pain—6 months.

History

Gynecological History

She attained menarche at the age of 14 years and cycles were regular in the past. Present cycles were 6-7/26-28 days since last 6 months. She was passing clots. Dysmenorrhea +.
LMP—8 days back.

Obstetric History

She had married when she was 14 years old. ML—31 years. P2L2—both deliveries were normal, home deliveries.

Both male babies and LD was 18 years. No history of PPH. She is not using any contraception.

History of Presenting Illness

She noticed heaviness in the lower abdomen and dragging sensation in last 6 months. Since 8 months she has had white discharge and since 1 month. She is having foul smelling vaginal discharge which was blood tinged, for which she did not taken any treatment.

No history of admission to hospital for any disease or blood transfusion. She has not taken any other medicines up till to now.

Personal History

She is hawker by profession and sells bamboo baskets in the street.

Family History

No family history of diabetes or blood pressure in the family.

Socioeconomic History

She belongs to lower class according to kuppuswamy's classification.

On Examinations

Patient was conscious and cooperative and was well oriented to time, place and person. She was in agony as there was retention of urine.

Fibroid Uterus

Vitals

- Her pulse rate was 110/m regular
- BP 130/80 mm Hg
- *Respiratory rate:* 24 pm regular
- CVS: Normal sounds.

General Physical Examination

- She was anemic
- Hair showed signs of malnutrition BP, pulse, temperature normal
- No jaundice
- Nails showed platyonychia.

There was no pedal edema breast, spine, thyroid—normal.

Respiratory

Air entry normal on both sides no added sounds.

Cardiovascular System

Tachycardia

Abdominal Examination

Inspection

There was distention of the lower abdomen, striae were seen.

Palpation

The bladder was distended till umbilicus, as she had not passed urine.

Pelvic Examination

A globular mass was occupying full vagina as big as a fetal head. The surface showed ulceration and bleeding. There was foul smelling discharge. Bladder was catheterized and 1,500 mL of urine drained.

Pelvic examination was done with difficulty. A pedunculated fibroid polyp was occupying whole vagina. Cervix was felt all round. Broad pedicle was coming through the uterus.

Provisional diagnosis of fibroid polyp was made.

Q. 1. What are investigation findings?

- Hb—8 g%
- Urine microscopy—8-10 pus cells. Urine culture showed *E. coli* organisms.
- CT, BT—normal
- Scan—pedunculated hypoechoic mass seen in the cervical canal and occupying whole of the vagina.

The pedicle was seen arising from fundal region with vascularity noted in pedicle. Fundus showed midline dimpling:

- Blood group—O positive
- Random blood sugar—90 mg
- Blood urea—24 mg
- Blood creatinine—0.08 mg
- Serology tests—HIV, VDRL, HBsAg negative.

Q. 2. What is your diagnosis?

Based on scan report and clinical examination final diagnosis was made as: Fibroid polyp causing partial inversion of the uterus.

Q. 3. What is the plan of management?

Plan of management:

- Correction of anemia
- Continuous catheterization
- A course of antibiotics
- Preparation for surgery
- Injection tetanus toxoid.

Q. 4. How will you manage a case of fibroid polyp?

- If the polyp is small—avulsion
- If the pedicle is thick—clamp, cut and ligate the pedicle.

Q. 5. If there is myoma in the uterus what is the management?

All myomas do not need myomectomy. Myomectomy is needed only when it produces symptoms like subfertility, RPL, menorrhagia and pressure symptoms. Small myomas near menopause can be left alone as they may shrink after menopause and other asymptomatic myoma can be observed.

Q. 6. What are the prerequisites for myomectomy?

The purpose of myomectomy is either to have children in future or to retain the uterus in young patients.

Before doing myomectomy husbands semen analysis other reasons for infertility should be ruled out, ovulation, patency of tubes should be looked for.

Q. 7. What are the diagnostic procedures for fibroid?

- USG—>5 mm can be diagnosed, hypo- or hyperechoic lesions, postacoustic shadow. Hydroureter if there is pressure, Degenerative fibroid—complex appearance, cystic changes.
- Hydrosonohysterography—polyp. In 40% of cases hysteroscopy can be avoided.
- HSG—filling defect, not very sensitive and not done routinely.
- CT scan—is not a choice, irregular mass.
- Doppler—circumferential vascularity-in degenerated fibroid and in necrobiotic and torsion—no flow.
- 3D ultrasound—can differentiate between adenomyosis and fibroid.
- MRI—differential diagnosis for adenomyosis.
  - Shows—exact location of fibroid, submucous, intramural or subserosal. Extra uterine fibroids like broad ligament.
  - Nondegenerative fibroids—well defined low signal intensity in T2W images. Degenerative fibroids—complex mass. Heterogeneous appearance, irregular, low signal on T2W images with no enhancement. Peripheral rim low signal T2W images due to peripheral obstructed veins.
  - Cystic degenerative—hypoechoic or complex cystic mass, areas of hemorrhages, fibroids with hyaline, calcific degenerative changes are difficult of distinguished from non-degenerative fibroids on MRI.
  - Hyaline or myxoid denegation—speckled pattern or focal necrosis.
  - Fibroids that demonstrate high signal or T1W image prior to embolization are likely to have a poor response to UAE because they may have already out grown their blood supply and undergone hemorrhagic necrosis.
  - Recent hemorrhage—shows high signal in T1W and T2W images.
  - Leimyosarcoma—irregular mass, heterogeneous mass, areas of hemorrhages. Duplex colored Doppler—a high peak systolic velocity with mild-diastolic elevation is seen at periphery in leimyosarcoma.

Q. 8. What is the role of MRI in fibroid uterus?

- *Planning for myomectomy*
  To differentiate between adenomyosis and fibroid.
  Adenomyosis—focal or diffuse myometrial bulkiness, typically of the posterior wall, thickening of the transition zone can sometimes be visualized as a hypoechoic halosurrounding the endometrial layer, subendometrial echogenic linear striations, subendometrial echogenic nodules (specific sign), small myometrial cysts/subendometrial cysts (specific sign), heterogeneous echogenicity and heterogeneous myometrial echo texture.
  - Condition of the fibroid like degeneration
  - MRI may decide the route of surgery and may avoid laparotomy
  - Diagnosis of submucous polyp.
- As a management option in MRgFUS
- Identification of fibroid in abnormal location like cervix, broad ligament
- Response to arterial embolization
- Identifies conditions like torsion, degeneration because of variable signal intensity.
- To differentiate from subserous fibroid and ovarian mass.

Q. 9. Which fibroids show effect on the urinary system?

- Anterior wall and cervical fibroid cause retention of urine
- Broad ligament fibroid cause hydroureter.

Q. 10. How the treatment for fibroid is chosen?

- Perimenopausal—hysterectomy
- Young—myomectomy
- Fibroid leading to RPL—hysteroscopic or laparoscopic removal depending on the site
- Large and multiple fibroids in difficult situation—open method
- Temporary relief—medication progesterone, antifibrinolytics
- Perimenopausal but refuses operation—with regular cavity LNG-IUS
- Comfort and cosmetic—laparoscopy
- Preoperative and perimenopause—gonadotropin analogs
- Arterial embolization—when difficult surgery is anticipated like diffuse adhesions
- MRgFUS—for the relief of symptoms like pressure symptoms, HMB, where patient refuses surgery or not fit for surgery
- Refer Figure 1.

There is no hard and fast rule to treat myoma in a particular way. Treatment depends upon the age of the patient, desire for fertility, skill of the surgeon, patient's choice, financial considerations, general condition of the patient and availability of the method.

Q. 11. When is surgical management warranted?

- Torsion of fibroid
- Intractable bleeding.

Q. 12. How do you decide the route of hysterectomy for fibroids?

- Less than 12 weeks of size—vaginal hysterectomy
- More than 12 weeks—laparoscopic assisted vaginal hysterectomy
- More than 16 weeks—abdominal hysterectomy
- Dense adhesions—UAE
- Submucous fibroids type 0 and 1—hysteroscopic myomectomy
- Subserous and intramural—open/laparoscopic myomectomy.

Indication for myomectomy

- Less than 40 years
- Normal semen analysis in infertility
- Tubes patent in infertility
- No suspicious of malignancy in the fibroid
- Too many fibroids
- RPL with fibroids in the absence of other causes
- Myoma that disturb the pregnancy may be removed prior to IVF.

Q. 13. Discuss the various symptoms associated with fibroid.

Menorrhagia—causes
- Venous congestion
- Increased surface (Normal 15 sq cm)
- Increased blood supply
- Dilatation of the venules
- Interfering with uterine contraction
- Submucous fibroid
- Polyps
- Ulceration of endometrium
- Ratio of TX A2/prostaglandin changed

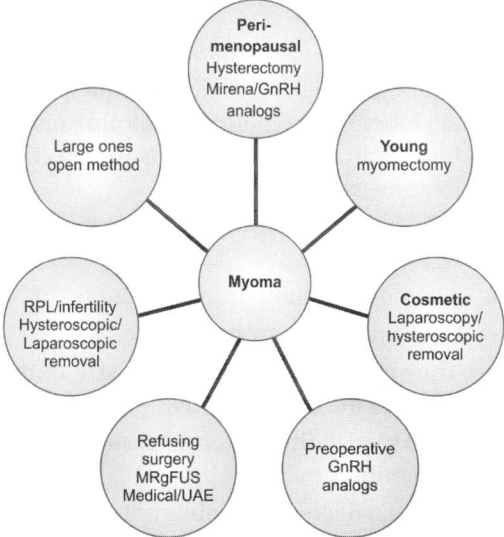

Fig 1: Management of fibroid

- Distortion of cavity
- Anovulation
- Other associated causes—adenomyosis, AUB

Pain—causes
- Dysmenorrhea—spasmodic, congestive
- Red degeneration
- Constipation
- Retention of urine, UTI, stones
- Dragging pain—pressure
- Back ache—mammoth tumor
- Associated causes—PID, endometriosis
- Torsion
- Infection
- Expulsion of submucous myoma
- Malignancy
- Extrusion of polyp

Pressure symptoms—causes
- All urinary symptoms like frequency, retention, infection, hematuria, pyelonephritis, hydroureter, hydronephrosis
- Specifically with cervical fibroids, broad ligament fibroids, huge fibroids
- Pressure on the rectum—incomplete evacuation

Menstrual symptoms—causes
- IMB (polyp, submucous)
- Dysmenorrhea (all varieties except subserous)

Other features
- Infertility and RPL
- Mass PV
- Dyspareunia
- Mass PA

Broad ligament fibroid

True	False
Arises from smooth muscles of round ligament or broad ligament vessels or other structures	Arises from uterus, grows between the layers, detaches from the uterus
Uterine artery—medial and inwards	Pushed laterally and upwards
Ureter—medial and in posterior layer	Lateral

Q. 14. How do you manage acute bleeding?

- Rarely, women with fibroids present with an acute hemorrhage, which can be life-threatening.
- After resuscitation is initiated, the usual hormonal treatment for HMB may be helpful.
- A dilatation and curettage may help slow down the bleeding.
- If a fibroid polyp is found prolapsing through the cervix, its removal will usually stop the bleeding.
- Hysteroscopic resection of an intracavitary submucous fibroid that is bleeding is an option, but may be technically difficult due to poor visualization.
- If the cavity is not much distorted then LNF-IUS can be placed.
- If the woman does not respond to conservative measures, uterine artery occlusion can be performed if it is readily available.
- Ultimately, hysterectomy may be become necessary in a few cases.

Q. 15. How do fibroids cause infertility?

There are several ways uterine fibroids can reduce fertility:

- Changes in the shape of the cervix can affect the number of sperms that can enter the uterus and can cause dyspareunia in cervical fibroid.
- Changes in the shape of the uterus can interfere with the movement of the sperms or embryo, ulceration of the fibroid causing biochemical alteration leads to defective endometrium.
- Fallopian tubes can be blocked or stretched by fibroids.
- Altered tubal motility and function.
- Ovum pick-up may be affected.
- They can have impact on the size of the lining of the uterine cavity.
- Poor vascularity, distorted cavity, surface ulceration.
- This can decrease the ability of an embryo to stick (implant) to the uterine wall or to develop—defective endometrium.

Associated conditions like peritoneal endometriosis
- Removal of large myomas (more than 3 cm) has a much more beneficial effect on fertility than smaller ones.
- Intramural fibroids larger than 5 cm, as well as submucosal fibroids of any size, can cause RPL.

Q. 16. What is the genetic basis of leiomyoma?

Most of uterine leiomyomas have a normal karyotype, 50% of these tumors bear specific chromosomal aberrations that include chromosome 3, 6, 7, 13, trisomy 12, reciprocal translocation between chromosomes 12 and 14 and monosomy 22. Such chromosomal rearrangements may cause initiation as well as the growth of these tumors.

HLRCC is hereditary leiomyomatosis and renal carcinoma due to germ line mutations in the fumarate hydratase gene and ATS-DL Alport syndrome is another hereditary with diffuse leiomyomatosis of the esophagus trachea bronchial and genitourinary tract with X linked dominant deletion. Fibroids geno and phenol types can be described in 3 headings. One is constitutional variants is hereditary syndromes, 2nd somatic alterations due to structural chromosomal aberrations and lastly epigenetic mechanism DNA methylation and histone modification regulate gene expression independent of DNA sequence genome. Majority of genes are silenced in fibroids like progesterone or antiprogestin.

Q. 17. What are asymptomatic fibroids and how do you manage them?

Asymptomatic fibroids are those which do not produce any symptoms but are detected and are diagnosed incidentally during:
- Pelvic examination
- Health check-up
- Ultrasound scans
- Sometimes in ANC check-up
- During surgery.

Management depends upon the size, location future impact on pregnancy and health. Small and seedling asymptomatic fibroids can be observed. If it is more than 16 weeks size then the option should be discussed.

If seen during pregnancy then fetal surveillance is necessary. As it may produce abortion, PROM, malpresentation, IUGR and after delivery PPH.

If the patient is infertile and fibroid is distorting the cavity or size >4 cm and encroaching the cavity may need myomectomy.

Q. 18. What is the role of GnRH analog?

Advantages	Disadvantages
• They decrease the size by 50%	• They may regrow after 2 months after stopping the treatment
• Decrease blood flow there by decreased flow during surgery, decreased chance for blood transfusion	• They cause bone loss vasomot or symptoms can be seen
• Time is gained for the control of other associated diseases like asthma, anemias and cardiac problems	• During surgery cleavage is less defined
	• Costly
	• Smaller fibroids will regress

- Conversion of abdominal to vaginal surgery, conversion of abdominal to laparoscopic assisted vaginal hysterectomy
- It may eliminate the need for surgery near perimenopause.

Add back therapy—tibolone, raloxifene, MPA progesterone is given when gonadotropins are given >3 months.

GnRH analogues are given—multiple fibroids and if the volume >600 cm^3, GnRH is more effective.

Q. 19. What is the fertility rate after myomectomy?

- Fertility depends upon—age of the patient
- Other factors of infertility like—PCO, endometriosis, peritubal adhesion, male factors, etc.

- Size of the fibroid and number of fibroids
- Location of fibroid—submucous, intramural, cornual
- Fertility is >50%.

Q. 20. Comment on the recurrence of fibroid.

Risk factors for recurrence
- Number of tumors
- Uterine myomas of ≥10 cm diameter
- Age >35 years
- Time > recurrence

Recurrence depends upon the time duration to conceive. Recurrence of fibroids after myomectomy followed by pregnancy and delivery—15%. Recurrence of fibroid after myomectomy without conception—30%. Post-embolization recurrence—17.2%.

Q. 21. What are the effects of fibroid on pregnancy?

It can cause abortion, abruption, placenta previa, premature labor, FGR, operative delivery, PPH, sepsis, subinvolution, rupture of uterus, retention of urine, incarceration, etc.

Q. 22. What are the indication for hysterectomy?

- Multiple fibroids
- Suspicious of malignancy
- Severe bleeding during myomectomy
- Recurrence of fibroid after any conservative procedure (most often)
- Symptomatic fibroid
- >14 weeks
- Fibroid with prolapse
- Age >40
- Adnexal pathology like PID, endometriosis
- Growth in postmenopausal woman
- Not suitable for MRgFUS or embolization.

Q. 23. What is the cause of bleeding after myomectomy?

It may be associated with AUB, myohyperplasia or focal adenomyosis.

Q. 24. What are rare association with fibroids?

- Pseudo syndrome—fibroids may Meigs' irritate the peritoneum to produce ascites and may lead to pleural effusion leading to Pseudomeig's syndrome
- Ascites
- Hemothorax.

Rare features
- Hyperglycemia
- Polycythemia—affecting kidney.

Q. 25. What are the diseases associated with fibroid?

Due to hyperestrogenic state it can cause follicular cystin ovary, adenomyosis and hyperplasia in the uterus, and peritoneal endometriosis.

Q. 26. What are the variants of leiomyoma?

They may be uterine and extrauterine. They are lipoleiomyoma, cellular leiomyoma, myxoid leiomyoma, dissecting leiomyoma, apoplectic leiomyoma, benign metastasizing leiomyoma, cotyledonoid leiomyoma, parasitic leiomyoma, STUMP (smooth muscle tumor of unknown malignant potential) bizarre leiomyoma, mitotically active leiomyoma, epithelioid and plexiform leiomyoma, hydropic leiomyoma, etc.

Extrauterine leimyomas are—intravenous leiomyomatosis, leiomyomatosis with peritoneal dissemination, benign metastasis tumors.

Q. 27. What is the problem of morcellation?

In laparoscopic hysterectomy or myomectomy fibroids are dissected and brought out by morcellation. If there is undiagnosed leiomyosarcoma it can spread in the abdomen by morcellation. There are two types of injuries with morcellation, first is injury to viscera and 2nd is dissemination. Benign and malignant both cause dissemination. Complication of benign are peritonitis, abscess formation, endometriosis, diffuse leiomyomatosis.

To avoid the spread preoperative evaluation is necessary like preoperative imaging, endometrial biopsy and age >60 years. If there is risk better to do laparotomy.

To avoid the complication following methods are used:
- Transvaginal morcellation in the vagina or minilaparotomy and fibroids are collected in the endobag
- Big fibroids are put in the endobag and morcellation is done in the bag itself and it is brought out by abdomen at port side by increasing the umbilical incision site (rail road technique) if necessary.

Q. 28. What are the changes that can take place in fibroids?

There are various type of degenerations in the fibroids. They are cystic degeneration, hyaline, red (during pregnancy) myxomatous, fatty degeneration (usually asymptomatic), etc. Apart from this there may be atrophic change, sarcomatous change (0.02%) and calcification (after menopause) are also seen.

Q. 29. What are the causes of pain in red degeneration?

Red degeneration takes place during pregnancy and if the fibroid is >5 cm. Usually seen in 2nd trimester.
- Rapid fibroid growth results in the tissue outgrowing its blood supply leading to tissue anoxia, necrosis, and infarction.
- That the growing uterus results in a change in the architecture (kinking) of the blood supply to the fibroid leading to ischemia and necrosis even in the absence of fibroid growth.
- That the pain results from the release of prostaglandins from cellular damage within the fibroid.

Treatment—analgesics and observation.

Criteria for medical management
- Symptomatic fibroid
- Not fit for surgery
- Those that are reluctant to surgery
- Perimenopausal age group
- For control of bleeding
- Preoperation reduction of size
- For improvement of hemoglobin

Q. 30. Discuss the medical management of fibroids?

Mefepristone RU486—5–10 mg p/day for 1 year. Fibroid decreases by 50%. Large fibroids, 25 mg/d may be used and small fibroids 5–10 mg/day may be used
- Aromatose inhibitors—fibroid decreased by 50%
- GnRh antagonist for 3–6 months decreased fibroid size
- Other drugs used are—nafarelin nasal spray—200 mg daily

Medical management options are in Table 1.

Table 1: Medical management options for uterine leiomyoma

Medication	Dose	Duration	Symptoms	Side effects
OC pills	EE 0.5 mg, Nor E	Continuous	Relieved	Nausea, vomiting
Progesterone	MPA 10 mg tid	3–6 months	Relieved	Bleeding, bloating
Danazol	100–200 mg/day	3–6 months	Relieved Size shrinks	Androgenic effects
Gestrinone [19 Nor]	2.5 mg/day	3–6 months	Relieved Size shrinks	Androgenic effects
GnRH analogs leuprolide acetate	3.75 mg/month	6 months	Relieved Size shrinks	Osteoporosis. postmenopausal symptoms

Contd...

Contd...

Medication	Dose	Duration	Symptoms	Side effects
Antiprogesterone Ulipristal	5–10 mg/day	3–6 months	Relieved Size shrinks	Bleeding
LNG–IUS	52 mg	5 years	Relieved	Irregular bleeding
Tranexamic acid	650 mg 2 tid/day		Relieved	
NSAID	Ibuprofen 600 mg/day		Relieved	Nausea, vomiting
Mefenamic acid	500 mg tid/day		Relieved	

Q. 31. What are the advantages and disadvantages of medical and surgical management of fibroid?

Medical	Surgical
• Temporary most often	• Permanent most often
• No scar	• Scar
• Medical side effects	• Other surgical complications
• Long period	• One sitting
• Reduction in size possible	• Total removal
• Recurrence fast and more	• Slow and less
• Suited in certain age groups	• Suited for all
• Malignancy risk not evaluate	• Gets evaluated
• No life-threatening complications	• Bleeding
• Comorbid situations—helps	• Not possible

Myomectomy principles
- Consent for hysterectomy
- Adequate blood availability
- Good hemostasis
- As far as possible—single incision to remove all fibroids
- Tunneling incision—for other fibroids
- Avoid incision on posterior wall of uterus
- Primary incision as low as possible on the surface of uterus
- Avoid opening endometrial cavity
- Baseball sutures
- While reconstructing the uterus
- Bed of fibroid -controlling hemostasis
- Maintenance of symmetry of uterus
- Not to damage the tubes

Q. 32. How do you prevent adhesion during myomectomy?

- Using barrier cellulose
- Laser laparoscopy
- Solutions
- Avoid posterior wall incision
- Hemostasis

How do you reduce bleeding during surgery?
- Hypotensive anesthesia
- Bonney's clamp or tourniquet
- Any catheter to block uterine like a tourniquet
- Temporary clamping ovarian vessels (infundibulopelvic ligaments)
- Vasopressors like vasopressin 20 mg in 200 mL. (Contraindicated in myocardial ischemia and vascular disease)
- Use of electrocautery
- Preoperative UAE if big fibroid

Q. 33. When are the chances of myomectomy scar dehiscence least?

When myomectomy is done by an expert and myoma involves <50% of the uterine musculature and no postoperative sepsis then rupture is rare.

Q. 34. How do you prevent adhesion formation?

This includes strict adherence to the basic surgical principles of minimizing tissue trauma with meticulous hemostasis, minimization of ischemia and desiccation, and prevention of infection and foreign body retention and no peritoneal closure. Risk of adhesions increase with the number of operations, use of talcum powder. In laparoscopic surgery adhesions are less compared to open surgery. Adhesions are also less with laser surgery.

Other surgical adjuncts to prevent adhesion formation include irrigation with crystalloid solutions, high-molecular-weight dextran, heparin and administrations of nonsteroidal anti-inflammatory drugs (NSAIDs). The use of crystalloid solutions is known as hydroflotation; some crystalloid is left in the pelvis at the end of surgery to allow the tissues to float apart from one another and thereby decrease the risk of adhesion formation. Barrier appears to be superior to other methods.

- Chemically modified sodium hyaluronate/ carboxymethylcellulose (Seprafilm)
- Oxidized regenerated cellulose (Interceed), and
- Polytetrafluoroethylene (Gore-Tex) are the barriers which prevent the adhesion formation.

Q. 35. What are the newer modalities of treatment?

Apart from endoscopic surgery newer modalities of treatment are arterial embolization and MRgFUS. In these two modalities of treatment adhesions are not seen.

Contraindications for MRgFUS
- Scar near tumor
- Pregnancy
- Pacemaker
- Bowel adhesions
- Pedunculated fibroid
- More than 3 fibroids
- Size >10 cm

Before MRgFUS, MRI is mandatory to see the fibroid number, size, distance from surface, for planning follow-up and monitoring, bowel loop and abdominal fat, etc. The mechanism is raised temperature in the targeted fibroid tissue will destroy the tissue. In a single sitting 3 fibroids can be tackled and up to 300 mL volume may be removed.

In *UAE (Uterine arterial embolization)*—the arterial supply of the fibroid by uterine artery is blocked by polyvinyl alcohol, gel foam coils. Follow-up is done by scan 6–12 months following procedure to see the size of fibroid with UAE.

Contraindications for UAE are—allergic to contrast, presence of infection, suspected malignancy, impaired renal function, vascular diseases, etc. Pedunculated fibroid, calcified nature of the mass not known. Adenomyosis and requirement of fertility are not the absolute contraindications.

Complications—embolization syndrome are pain, fever, vomiting. It is usually self-limiting but if persists may need hysterectomy. complications are—pyometra, misembolization, premature ovarian failure, hematoma in the groin, etc.

Q. 36. What are the indications for embolization?

- Near menopause to get relived of symptoms like menorrhagia
- Pressure effects on urinary tract
- Medical conditions contraindicating surgery
- Jehovah witness, to reduce bleeding during surgery.

Preoperative UAE—indication are:
- Very large fibroid
- Multiple fibroid
- Myoma in a very difficult place to resects, and
- Myoma >1,100 g
- To reduced bleeding

Postembolization syndrome

Up to 40% of women experience a constellation of signs and symptoms including diffuse abdominal pain, generalized malaise, anorexia, nausea, vomiting, low-grade fever, and leukocytosis. The syndrome is self-limiting and usually resolves within 48 hours to 2 weeks with conservative and supportive therapy, consisting of intravenous fluids and adequate pain control, including NSAIDs.

Table 2: Differences between laparoscopy and hysteroscopy for myomectomy

	Laparoscopy	Hysteroscopy
Media	CO_2	Hyskon, glycine
Fibroid numbers	<3	<3
Size	<5 cm	Type 0 or 1 and <5 cm
Uterine length	<16 cm	<12 cm
Complications	Procedure, instrument, thermal injuries	Visceral injuries, media related

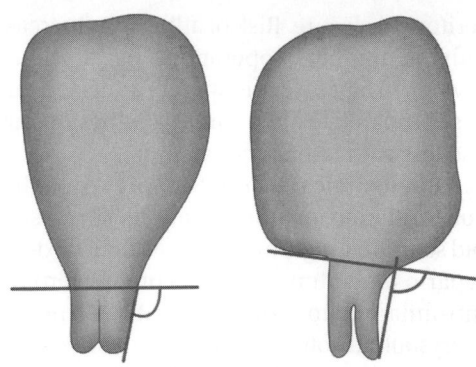

Fig. 2: Cervicouterine angle for favorability for vaginal surgery

Q. 37. How a case is chosen for vaginal hysterectomy for fibroids?

- Size of the uterus (depending upon the skill surgeon)—12–14 weeks
- Volume 200–400 cc mobile uterus
- No adnexal mass
- Descent of the uterus may be advantageous
- Prolapse with fibroid
- An angle between cervix and uterus >140 is easy <90 is difficult. Previous no uterine surgery.

There are records where volume up to 500 cc and size up to 16 weeks have been operated.

Vaginal hysterectomy becomes difficult when the volume is increased or there are multiple fibroids (Fig. 2).

- To reduce the volume enucleation of fibroids or morcellation can be done
- If the uterus is too long and if there are adnexal adhesions then bisection of the uterus can be done after ligating uterine artery. After ligating cardinal ligament, uterus is cut circumferentially so that uterus elongates and volume is reduced.
- Myometrial coring also is a bulk reducing procedure.

Q. 38. What are the other methods of treating fibroids?

There are still more methods in incipient stage.

1. Myolysis—here bipolar needles inserted through the laparoscope after preparing the patient with GnRH analogs. When current is passed for few seconds temperature goes up and this destroys the tissue. 10 cm fibroid can shrinks to 4 cm.
2. Cryomyolysis—gas cooled cryoprobes are used in which pressurized gas is expanded through a small orifice with the help of laparoscope to produce cooling temperature to – 90°C in 8–10 minutes. Tissue destruction occurs.
3. Radio frequency ablation—needles are inserted in tissue resulting in necrosis fibroid is absorbed.

Q. 39. What are the disadvantages of myolysis?

- Since no sample of the fibroid is sent to the laboratory, for a biopsy, in the rare case malignancy may be missed.
- Frequently the procedure causes damage to other organs such as intestines, stick to the uterus (adhesions), which could cause damage to other organs.
- Most importantly, there are not any controlled studies comparing the outcome

of this procedure with myomectomy or other treatment.

> Laparoscopic myolysis may present an alternative to myomectomy or hysterectomy for selected women with symptomatic intramural or subserous fibroids who wish to preserve their uterus but do not desire future fertility (II-B).

Q. 40. What is cryotherapy and RFA?

Cryotherapy for fibroid

Cryotherapy—up to temperature −20° to −50° destroys the fibroid. Cryoprobes are inserted into the fibroid. Postoperative complications are fever, abscess.

Radiofrequency Ablation (RFA)

Ablation of solid tumors with radiofrequency energy results from heating that is produced when ions follow the oscillations of a high-frequency alternating electric field. The heat causes coagulation necrosis of local tissue. Large area of necrosis (up to 6 cm in diameter) can be achieved in a single access with RFA, and, therefore, compared to cryotherapy it is relatively time efficient.

The RFA catheter is placed through the skin under ultrasound guidance into a fibroid. The catheter consists of a needle containing several prongs that are deployed into the targeted tissue, allowing ablation of a spherical volume of tissue. The prongs deliver electrical energy to the fibroid and keep the ablation catheter firmly in place during treatment.

In about 10–15 minutes, targeted tissue is heated to 105°C, killing tumor cells. Because the heat dissipates rapidly, surrounding normal tissue is not affected.

Most procedures are completed in two to three hours and patients discharged the same day or the day following the procedure. Complications, such as bleeding and postoperative pain, are minimal.

Q. 41. What is the place for cesarean myomectomy?

Myomectomy can be done along with lSCS in the following condition:
- Myoma occupying the lower segment near incision site
- Pedunculated myoma outside and inside the uterine cavity
- Subserosal myoma.

A skilled surgeon can do myomectomy during LSCS and vasopressin can be used to decrease the bleeding.

Advantages are—decrease rate of sepsis:
- Degeneration during next pregnancy can be avoided
- No subinvolution
- Pain due to degeneration can be reduced
- Avoiding another operation
- Involution is better if done during surgery rather than interval.

Q. 42. How do you manage fibroids in special location?

If the fibroid is in the fundoposterior wall of uterus—Bonney's hood operation
- Broad ligament fibroid cut the round ligament and do postbox incision and enucleate the fibroid.
- Cervical fibroid—anterior: Cut the UV fold and round ligament then take transverse incision and enucleate the fibroid or do hemisection of the uterus and enucleate.
- Posterior fibroid—cut the rectovaginal peritoneum and enucleate the fibroid.
- Central—first cut the UV fold and push the bladder down. Then carefully cut the lower distended uterus on the fibroid and extend circumferentially and enucleate it. Ureters are laterally situated, or hemisection of the fibroid also can done and fibroid is nucleated and work within the capsule as uterines are situated laterally.

Hysteroscopic Classification (Fig. 3):

(1) Pedunculated, (2) Submucous (3) Small intramural, (4) Large intramural.

ESGE classification of submucous fibroid [Europeon Society for Gynaecological Endoscopy]

- No intramural extension
- Intramural extension less than 50%
- Intramural extension > 50%

0 and 1 are amenable for hysteroscopic removal.

Hysteroscopy is used for diagnostic and therapeutic purpose. Confirmation of fibroid, type of fibroid and resectability can be checked. Endometrial sampling also can be taken.

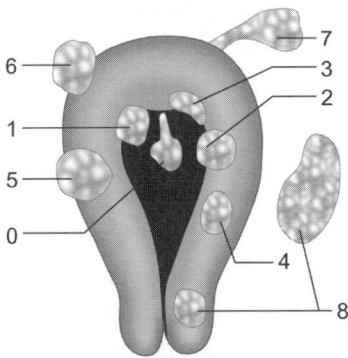

Fig. 3: Fibroid classification: Type 0—Pedunculated submucous; Type 1—Submucous with <50% intramural; Type 2—Submucous with >50% intramural; Type 3—Intramural with myoma abutting against endometrium; Type 4—Totally intramural; Type 5—Intramural with <50% subserous; Type 6—Intramural with >50% subserous; Type 7—Totally subserous (including pedunculated); Type 8—Myomas outside uterine body

Q. 43. What are the contraindication for hysteroscopic removal of fibroid?

Also see Table 2.

- Uterine size >12 weeks
- Suspicion of malignancy
- Associated pathology

Contd...

Contd...

- Size > 5 cm
- >50 % involvement
- Asymptomatic patient
- 0, I, and II up to 4 to 5 cm in diameter can be removed
- Experienced surgeons.

Hysteroscopic myomectomy	Laparoscopic myomectomy
• Vaginal route • Requires distension • Other organs cannot be seen • Other procedures also not possible • Suturing not possible • Injury to viscera minimal • Number and size matters • No scar • Best for type 0 and 1 submucous	• Abdominal • Pneumoperitoneum • Viscera seen • Other procedures possible • Suturing possible • Injury possibility present • Big fibroids can be removed • Scar • Any type except submucous

Q. 44. What are the contraindications for laparoscopic myomectomy?

- Uterus >16 weeks size
- Myoma >15 cm
- Submucosal myoma—(easy to do by hysteroscopy)
- Unfavorable location—broad ligament or in POD
- Myoma >5 cm an numbers > 3 (time is more)
- Diffuse myoma
- Any medical condition that worsens by distension of the abdomen and Trendelenburg position.

Q. 45. What are mammoth tumors?

Usually mammoth tumors are ovarian in origin especially pseudomucinous ovarian tumors. But sometimes fibroids also can attend very huge size.

Q. 46. When treatment is only observation?

- Fibroid detected on pelvis examination: If there are no symptoms—observer
- Though there is a fibroid and no history abortions—observe

- Incidental finding of fibroid in laparoscopy- no complaint—observe
- Degenerating fibroid-only analgesics—observe
- Premenopausal small fibroid—observe.

Q. 47. What is the role of RALM?

In robotic assisted laparoscopic surgery decreases blood loss, complication rates, and length of stay but slightly increased cost is seen but there are reports where in the hands of a good laparoscopic surgeon all the benefits are achieved like robotic surgery but there is 6° of freedom of movement in human wrist and in robotic arms it is 5–7° of freedom with more precision, dexterity, and visualization. RALM scores more in suturing.

Q. 48. Can you summarize your case and how will you treat?

My patient aged 40 years P2 L2, has come with retention of urine due to fibroid. I will give her a course of antibiotics and will keep continuous catheterization. I will do hysterectomy as she has finished her family and during surgery I will push the fibroid and uterus downwards so that the peritoneum is not soiled.

Latest Information

- Use of letrozole reduced fibroid volume by 46%. Evidence is insufficient to support the use of AI drugs in the treatment of women with uterine fibroids.
- Unilateral UAE can achieve a positive clinical result in the group of patients where there is a dominant unilateral artery supplying the fibroid.
- Compared with the general obstetric population, there is a significant increase in delivery by cesarean section and an increase in preterm delivery, postpartum hemorrhage, miscarriage, and lower pregnancy rates following UAE.
- There is a suggestion that asymptomatic fibroid with high-risk condition like increased estrogen, obesity, family history of fibroid, nulliparity and early menarche, may be treated with vitamin D, green tea extract, combine oral contraceptive pills DMPA and curcumin, etc.

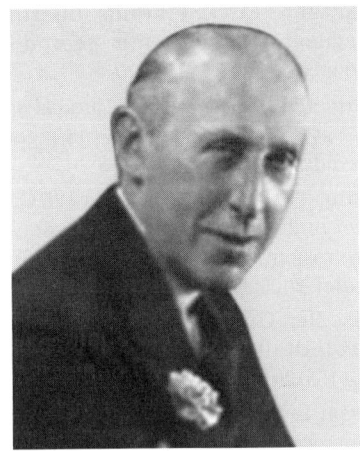

Fig. 4: Victor Bonney

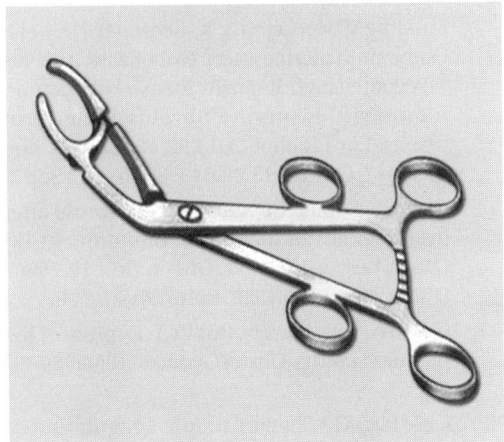

Fig. 5: Myomectomy clamp

Bibliography

1. Abdullah BJJ, Subramaniam RV, Yusof Y. Biomedical Imaging and Intervention Journal. MRgFUS treatment for uterine fibroid. Biomed Interv J. 2010;6(2):15.
2. Advincula AP, Xu X, Goudeau S, et al. Robot-assisted laparoscopic myomectomy versus abdominal myomectomy: a comparison of short-term surgical outcomes and immediate

costs. J Minim Invasive Gynecol. 2007;14(6): 698-705.
3. Baird DD, Hill MC, Schectman JM, et al. Vitamin D and the risk of uterine fibroids. Epidemiology. 2013;24(3):447-53.
4. Bajekal N, Li TC. Fibroids, infertility and pregnancy wastage. Hum Reprod Update. 2000;6:614-20.
5. Barbieri RL, Scott JR (Eds). Clinical obstetrics and gynaecology. Modern management of fibroids. 2016;59:1.
6. Bratby MJ, Hussain FF, Walker WJ. Outcomes after unilateral uterine artery embolization: a retrospective review Cardiovasc Intervent Radiol. 2008;31(2):254-9. Epub 2007 Nov 17.
7. Case Rep Oncol Med. 2013; 2013: 504589. Published online 2013 Jul 17. doi: 10.1155/2013/504589. PMCID: PMC3730183.
8. Desai P, Patel P. Fibroids, Infertility and Laparoscopic Myomectomy. J Gynecol Endosc Surg. 2011;2(1):3642. doi: 10.4103/09741216. 85280,PMCID: PMC33042949.
9. Froeling V, Meckelburg K, Schreiter NF, et al. Outcome of uterine artery embolization versus MR-guided high-intensity focused ultrasound treatment for uterine fibroids: long-term results. Eur J Radiol. 2013;82(12):2265-9. doi: 10.1016/j.ejrad.2013.08.045. Epub 2013 Sep 3.
10. Ghose S, Samal S, Begum J, et al. Fibroid after hysterectomy: a diagnostic dilemma. J Clin Diagn Res. 2014;8(7):OD01-2. doi: 10.7860/JCDR/2014/8195.4532. Epub 2014 Jul 20.
11. Golan A, Sandbank O, Rubin A. Rupture of the pregnant uterus. Obstet Gynecol. 1980;56:549-54.
12. Goldfarb HA. Laparoscopic coagulation of myomas (myolysis). Obstet Gynecol Clin North Amer. 1995;22(4):807-19.
13. Goldfarb HA. Nd:YAG laser laparoscopic coagulation of symptomatic myomas. J Reprod Med. 1992;37(7):636-8.
14. González-Quintero VH, Cruz-Pachano FE. Preventing Adhesions in Obstetric and Gynecologic Surgical Procedures. Obstet Gyncol. 2009.Winter(2):38-45.
15. Islam MS, Protic O, Giannubilo SR, et al. Uterine leiomyoma: available medical treatments and new possible therapeutic options J Clin Endocrinol Metab. 2013;98(3):921-34. doi: 10.1210/jc.2012-3237.
16. Jayakrishnan K, Menon V, Nambiar D. Submucous fibroids and infertility: Effect of hysteroscopic myomectomy and factors influencing outcome. J Hum Reprod Sci. 2013;6:35-9.
17. Lee HJ, Norwitz ER, Shaw J. Contemporary Management of Fibroids in Pregnancy. Rev Obstet Gynecol. 2010;3(1):20-7. PMCID: PMC2876319.
18. Marre PH, Cottier JP, Alonso AM, et al. Predictive factors for fibroids recurrence after uterine artery embolization. Newzealand Guidelines; 2000.
19. McCluggage WG, Ellis PK, McClure N, et al. Pathologic features of uterine leiomyomas following uterine artery embolization. Int J Gynecol Pathol. 2000;19(4):342-7.
20. Medikare V, Kandukuri LR, Nallar P. Genetic bases of uterine. Avicenna Research Institute The Genetic Bases of Uterine Fibroids. J Reprod Infert. 2011;12(3):181-91.
21. Okada A, Morita Y, Fukunishi H, et al. Pregnancy outcome after magnetic resonance-guided focused ultrasound surgery (MRgFUS) for conservative treatment of uterine fibroids. Fertil Steril. 2010;93(1):199-209.
22. Owen C, Armstrong AY. Clinics of North America Reproductive Endocrinology of OBG; 2015. p. 79.
23. Pathology outlines.com. Uterus Stromal tumors. February 2012 Variants: apoplectic, benign metastasizing, cellular, cotyledonoid, disseminated, epithelioid, hydropic, intravascular, leiomyomatosis, lipoleiomyoma, mitotically active, myoma nascens, myxoid, pallisading, parasitic, retroperitoneal, symplastic; May 13, 2015.
24. Phillips DR, Milim SJ, Nathanson HG, et al. Experience with laparoscopic leiomyoma coagulation and concomitant operative hysteroscopy. J Am Assoc Gynecol Laparosc. 1997;4(4):425-33.
25. Ponea AM, Marak CP, Goraya H, et al. Benign Metastatic Leiomyoma Presenting as a Hemothorax. Case Rep Oncol Med. 2013; 2013:504589.
26. Robertson D, Lefebvre G, Leyland N, et al. Society of Obstetricians and Gynaecologists

of Canada. Adhesion prevention in gynaecological surgery: no. 243, June 2010. SOGC clinical practice guidelines No 243, June 2010. Int J Gynaecol Obstet. 2010;111(2):193-7.
27. Sankaran S, Manyonda IT. Medical management of fibroids Best practice and research Clin Obstet Gyneacol. 2008;22(4):655-76.
28. Schwartz LB, Diamond MP, Schwartz PE. Leiomyosarcomas: clinical presentation. Am J Obstet Gynecol. 1993;168(1 Pt 1):180-3.
29. Schwartz LB, Diamond MP. Schwatz PE Leiyomuoma and clinical presentation. Am J Obstet Gynecol. 1993;168(1):180-3.
30. Shiota M, Kotani Y, Umemoto M, et al. Original article: Recurrence of uterine myoma after laparoscopic myomectomy: What are the risk factors? BJOG. 2005;112(4):461-5.
31. SOGC clinical practise guidelines 128, May 2003. The Management of Uterine Leiomyomas J Obstet Gynaecol Can. 2015;37(2):157-78.
32. Song H, Lu D, Navaratnam K, et al. Aromatase inhibitors for uterine fibroids Cochrane Database Syst Rev; 2013 Oct 23 (10):CD009505. doi: 10.1002/14651858.CD009505.pub2.
33. Stewart L, Glenn GM, Stratton P, et al. Association of germline mutations in the fumarate hydratase gene and uterine fibroids in women with hereditary leiomyomatosis and renal cell cancer. Arch Dermatol. 2008;144(12):1584-92. doi: 10.1001/archdermatol.2008.517.
34. Taylor DK, Holthouser K, James H, et al. Recent scientific advances in leiomyoma (uterine fibroids) research facilitates: better understanding and management. 2015; 4(F1000 183). Published online 2015 Jul 6. doi: 10.12688/f1000research.6189.1 PMCID: PMC4513689.
35. Walker WJ, McDowell SJ. Pregnancy after uterine artery embolization for leiomyomata: a series of 56 completed pregnancies. Am J Obstet Gynecol. 2006;195(5):1266-71. Epub 2006 Jun 21.

CHAPTER 25

Genital Prolapse

K Srinivas

CASE 1

Patient Particulars

Name: X
Age: 57 years
Wife of: Y
Residence: Rural area
Education: Uneducated
Socioeconomic status: Low
Occupation: Farmer
Chief complaints: Complain of mass per vagina since 3 years.

History of Present Illness

Complain of mass per vagina since 3 years, patient noticed mass which was small in size initially, gradually progressed and attained the present size. Mass protrudes out on walking, lifting heavy weight, on straining. Does not reduce on lying down position. Mass could be reduced by the patient.

- No history of urgency, increased frequency of micturition, nocturia, burning micturition
- No history of sense of incomplete evacuation of bladder
- No history of stress urinary incontinence (SUI), and urge urinary incontinence (UUI)
- No history of constipation
- No history of low backache
- History of lifting heavy weight present
- No history of chronic cough
- No history of mass per abdomen
- No history of discharge per vaginum.

Menstrual History

- Attained menarche at around 15 years of age
- Previous menstrual cycles were regular
- No history of menstrual disturbances
- Attained menopause 10 years back.

Obstetric History

- Married life—40 years
- Obstetric score—P3L3
- All full-term vaginal delivary (FTVD) at home conducted by dai, delivered average sized babies with no history of prolonged labor, any intrapartum with resumption of work after 3 months
- Interpregnancy interval—between 1st and 2nd between 2nd and 3rd–1 year.
- Tubectomized 30 years back.

Past History

Not a known case of hypertension (HTN)/tuberculosis (TB)/bronchial asthma/diabetes mellitus (DM)/seizures/thyroid and cardiac disorder.

Family History

No history of HTN, DM, TB, asthma.

Personal History

- Diet—adequate and mixed
- Appetite—good
- Bowel habits—regular
- Bladder habits—no history of increased frequency of micturition/no history of sensation of incomplete emptying of bladder, no history of burning micturition/urgency/nocturia
- Sleep—undisturbed
- No history of smoking, alcohol any substance abuse.

Summary

A 57-year-old P3L3 postmenopausal lady with all three home deliveries by untrained dai with early resumption of work in postpartum period with reduced interpregnancy interval with complaints of mass per vaginum since 3 years admitted for evaluation.

General Physical Examination

- An elderly lady moderately built and nourished
- Afebrile
- No evidence of pallor/icterus/cyanosis/clubbing/pedal edema/lymphadenopathy
- Pulse—84 bpm, regular rhythm, normal volume, height—153 cm
- Weight—49 kg
- BP—122/80 mm Hg, right arm, sitting position body mass index (BMI)—20.9 kg/m².

Systemic Examination

- Respiratory system—nonvesicular breath sound (NVBS) heard, no added sounds
- Cardiovascular system—S1, S2 heard, no murmurs
- Central nervous system—within normal limits
- Thyroid
- Breast—normal
- Spine.

Per Abdomen Examination

Inspection

- Abdomen normal in shape
- Umbilicus is normal
- No dilated veins or sinuses
- An suprapubic transverse scar of 4 cm present healed by primary intention
- Hernial orifices intact
- No divarication of recti on head rising test
- Palpation
- Getting above the fundus of the uterus is not possible
- Third degree uterovaginal prolapse +
- Levator ani tone = 3/5
- Length of genital hiatus = 5 cm
- Length of perineal body = 3 cm
- Uterocervical length = 6.5 cm
- Cervix length = 3 cm
- Anal reflex—present.

Per Speculum Examination

- Cystocele (grade III) seen over anterior vaginal wall
- Enterocele and rectocele seen over the posterior vaginal wall
- Pelvic organ prolapse (POP) (Q) (stage III).

Bimanual Examination

- After reducing mass
- Uterus retroverted, atrophic, bilateral fornices free.

Provisional Diagnosis

A 57-year P3L3 postmenopausal lady with IIIrd degree uterovaginal prolapse (according to Shaw classification), stage III (according to POP-Q), with cystocele grade III, enterocele and rectocele.

Q. 1. Define pelvic organ prolapse.

- Pelvic organ prolapsed is a condition in which the uterus, bladder, rectum drop down from their normal position into the vagina from the vault, anterior wall and posterior wall respectively. It may be a single organ or all may drop down through the vaginal wall.

Q. 2. What is anterior vaginal wall prolapse?

Cystocele is central when the vesicovaginal fascia is defective and lateral when the attachment of paracolpos to the arcus tendineus fascia levator ani (ATFLA) is damaged. The earlier terminology of distension and displacement cystocele are seldom used nowadays.

Anterior vaginal wall with its fascia supports bladder and urethra. Proximal 2/3rd vaginal wall prolapses with bladder with weakening of the vesicovaginal fascia, distal third anterior vaginal wall with urethral prolapses with damage to vesicourethral fascia.

Upper 2/3rd prolapse is called cystocele, and distal third is called urethrocele. When both prolapse, it is called cystourethrocele.

Q. 3. What is posterior vaginal wall prolapse?

The upper third of the posterior vaginal wall prolapses with abdominal contents most often due to damage to the pericervical ring. This is called enterocele.

Middle third rectovaginal fascial defects cause prolapsed of rectum, called rectocele.

Lower third of the posterior vaginal wall weakness is due to damage to the perineal body and called deficient perineum.

Q. 4. What are the different varieties of enteroceles?

- *Pulsion:* This happens due to chronic cough, or any other chronically increased intra-abdominal pressure.
- *Traction:* This happens because of the pull exerted by other prolapsing structures like uterus, bladder or rectum.
- *Iatrogenic:* Post-surgical occurrence due to deep postoperative day (POD), especially in sling surgeries or due to faulty repair of prolapse can cause enterocele.
- *Simple:* Enterocele occurring in isolation without uterine prolapse.
- *Complex:* Associated with vault prolapsed/ uterine prolapse.

Level 1 Supports
- *Mackenrodt's ligaments:* Spread out on either side from the lateral surface of the cervix and vagina, in a fan-shaped manner, and are inserted in the lateral pelvic wall.
- *Uterosacral ligaments:* From the cervix and vagina, backwards surrounding the rectum and below the uterosacral folds of peritoneum, to become inserted in the third piece of the sacrum.
- *Pubocervical ligaments:* Extend from the anterior surface of the cervix and vagina, forwards beneath the bladder and surrounding the urethra, to the posterior surface of the pubis.

Q. 5. Discuss the levels of supports—De Lancey.

De Lancey has described different levels of support to the cervix and vagina. They are classified as level I, II, and III, by dissecting cadavers.

Level I: The Mackenrodt's ligaments and uterosacral ligaments which attach the cervix and the vault of vagina to the sacrum and pelvic walls.

Level II: The mid-vaginal support offered by arcus tendinus fascia and levator ani.

Level III: The lower vagina is supported by the urogenital diaphragm and perineal body.

Damage to different levels cause different structures to prolapsed (Table1).

Table 1: Different level defects and the resulting pathology.

Level I defect	Level II defect	Level III defect
• UV prolapse • Vault prolapse • Enterocele	• Cystocele • Rectocele • Paravaginal • Pararectal defects	• Urinary incontinence • Perineal body defects

Q. 6. What is pelvic floor?

All tissues lying between the pelvic cavity and, the surface of the vulva and perineum. It includes:

- Pelvic peritoneum
- Extraperitoneal fat and cellular tissue
- Levators ani and their fascial coats
- The triangular ligament (urogenital diaphragm)
- The perineal muscles and their aponeuroses
- Subcutaneous fascia and fat
- Skin.

Q. 7. What are the risk factors to be elaborated in history?

Possible risk factors
- Intrapartum variables (macrosomia, long second stage of labor, episiotomy, epidural analgesia)
- Increased abdominal pressure
- Menopause

Confirmed Risk Factors

- Advancing age
- Negroid race
- Family history
- Obesity
- Multiparity
- History of vaginal deliveries
- Constipation.

Q. 8. How the etiological factors should be considered in history?

Predispose

- Genetic—congenital or hereditary
- Race—Whites>African-American
- Gender—female>male.

Promote

- Obesity (40–75%)
- Smoking
- Chronic cough
- Constipation (chronic straining)
- Frequent or heavy lifting.

Incite

- Pregnancy and delivery—birth trauma
- Surgery such as hysterectomy especially for prolapse (11.6%/1.8%)
- Myopathy
- Neuropathy.

Decompensate

- Aging
- Menopause
- Debilitation
- Medication.

Q. 9. What are the aggravating factors for prolapse (PROLAPSE)?

- **P**ressure/Parturition—cough, strain
- **R**ectal—constipation
- **O**besity
- **L**ifestyle—smoking, sedentary life style
- **A**sthenia/Atrophy/Asthma—nutritional, hormonal
- **P**eripheral neuropathy—diabetes, etc.
- **S**keletal/Steroids/Surgery—anteroposterior (AP) resection, radical vulvectomy
- **E**strogen deficiency.

Q. 10. What are the urinary symptoms of genital prolapse?

Basically urinary symptoms are due to cystocele and urethrocele. They can be:

- Urinary incontinence, frequency, or urgency
- Weak or prolonged urinary stream
- Feeling of incomplete emptying
- Manual reduction of prolapse which is gradually learnt to initiate/complete micturition ("digitation")
- Postural changing maneuvers needed to start or complete voiding
- Symptoms of urinary tract infection (UTI) (burning, frequency, hematuria, strangury), fever, chills and rigors, etc.
- Renal/ureteric/bladder calculi.

Q. 11. What other symptoms should be asked for in the history

As the symptoms are mainly of urination, defecation, sexual activity problems it is difficult for our women to come out on their own with these symptoms. So it may become necessary to enquire about them in detail.

Bowel symptoms

Constipation—this could be a cause or effect of prolapsed

Damage to anal sphincter can cause incontinence to flatus initially and to stools in later stages.

Stool getting impacted can cause sense of incomplete evacuation—which may improve later in a patient who learns to reduce rectocele digitally during defecation.

Sexual symptoms
- Difficult coitus due to lax vagina
- Lack of sensation
- Infertility
- Lax introitus and familial dyshormony.

Q. 12. Discuss the importance of asking about incontinence in these patients.

In the initial stages of prolapse straightening of the urethrovesical angle with damage to urethral support causes stress incontinence.

As the cystocele worsens the urethra vesical angle becomes more obtuse and when the patient strains the bulging cystocele almost obliterates the UV angle and there is an apparent disappearance of incontinence.

Being not aware of the incontinence problem if a definitive surgery is done for prolapsed, the patient may come back in the postoperative period with incontinence and may feel surgery precipitated her problem.

Hence asking for incontinence in the past, looking for incontinence in dorsal position with prolapsed uterus and also with reduced prolapsed, and also looking for it in the standing position is important so that the same may be tackled during prolapsed surgery.

Q. 13. What are the varieties of vaginal discharge with which a patient with prolapse can present with?
- Any type of infective discharge (Trichomonas, BV, CV)
- Foul smelling purulent discharge—Secondary infections, pyometra
- Blood stained discharge—Ulcer, cancer, atrophic vaginitis
- Mucoid discharge—exposed cervix-irritation-secretion.

Backache
- Uterosacral stretching when the ligaments have retained their strength can present with low backache
- In general prolapse, nulliparous prolapse wherein ligaments are very lax pain may not be an expressed symptom

Q. 14. What is the scheme of examination for a case of prolapse?

Some important examination points
- Estrogen status of genitals
- Hernial orifices
- Vaginal rugosities
- Sulci of vagina
- Staging of prolapse
- UC length
- Cervical elongation
- Incontinence
- Anal sphincter tone

Other than routine examination
- Position of patient for examination
  - standing and straining
  - dorsal/lithotomy
- External genitals examination
- Per speculum examination
- Per vaginal/Bimanual examination
- Bonney's stress test (If required)
- Evaluation of tone of pelvic muscles
- Rectovaginal examination.

- The maximal extent of prolapse is demonstrated with a standing straining examination when the bladder is empty
- Pelvic muscle function should be assessed after the bimanual examination → palpate the pelvic muscles a few centimeters inside the hymen, along pelvic sidewalls at the 4 and 8 o'clock
- Resting tone and voluntary contraction of the anal sphincters should be assessed during rectovaginal examination

Bulbocavernosus reflex: Stroke lateral to clitoris and observe for the bulbocavernosus contraction

Anal wink reflex: Stroke lateral to anal orifice, look for external sphincter contraction
Presence indicates intactness of sacral nerves, absence not the damage in all

Pelvic floor tone evaluation

Place 1 or 2 fingers in the vagina and instruct the patient to contract her pelvic floor muscles (i.e., the levator ani muscles). Then gauge her ability to contract these muscles, as well as the strength, symmetry, and duration of the contraction
The strength of the contraction can be subjectively graded with a modified Oxford scale (0 = no contraction, 1 = flicker, 2 = weak, 3 = moderate, 4 = good, 5 = strong)

Q. 15. What are the differential diagnosis for mass per vaginum?

The following to be kept in mind while taking history in a case of mass p/v, but none of them would show cough impulse or the reducibility.
- Vulvar cyst
- Cyst of the anterior vaginal wall
- Urethral diverticulum
- Congenital elongation of cervix
- Cervical fibroid polyp
- Chronic inversion.

Q. 16. What is the investigatory approach to a case of prolapse?

Routine preoperative work up investigations, USG to study the urinary system, if required C and S of urine and evaluation of cardia, lungs in old women needs to be done.

MRI, nerve conduction studies are done in some situations.

Preoperative workup routinely done
- History and examination
- CBC, BT, CT
- Blood group and Rh typing
- Fasting blood sugar (FBS) and postprandial blood sugar (PPBS)
- The venereal disease research laboratory (VDRL), HIV 1 and 2, HBsAg

Contd...

Contd...
- B. Urea, S. Creatinine
- Ultrasonography—Abdomen and pelvis
- PAP smear*, EB*
- Chest X-ray, ECG, Echocardiogram*
- LFT*, lipid profile*, thyroid profile, PFT*
- Urodynamic studies*

*Done in indicated cases only

Ultrasonography—To assess levator ani avulsion
Role of dynamic MRI—To know levator ani muscle laxity
Nerve conduction study–Needle EMG of levator to differentiate from neurological or non-neurological damage

Q. 17. What is the role of cystoscopy in POP?

Pelvic organ prolapse when associated with massive cystoceles, long standing cystocele, bladder calculi, hematuria, or any other suspected bladder pathology cystoscopy needs to be considered preoperatively.

Peroperatively whenever bladder injury especially near the trigone is suspected or urethral perforation has occurred cystoscopy may be useful.

Cystoscopy use is controversial in incontinence.

Q. 18. Discuss the need for an USG examination in cases of prolapse.

Ultrasound examination is an indispensable part of prolapsed examination.

Transabdominal, transvaginal, translabial scans may be done.

The need for USG examination may be for:

Urinary system: To know bladder wall thickness, urethral mobility, bladder neck displacement, bladder wall thickness, residual urine, hydroureter, hydronephrosis, etc.

Genital system: Quantification of prolapsed
- **Others:** Levator ani complex assessment especially for damage which is still better appreciated by 3D USG which also helps to assess the other supports of the uterus

at the pericervical ring, paravaginal tissue attachment, etc.

Q. 19. Is MRI routinely required while working up a case of prolapse?

- MRI is not needed in the evaluation of prolapse
- Pelvic floor dysfunction assessment, incontinence evaluation, staging can be worked up with dynamic MRI
- MRI may be helpful in evaluating the results of surgery.

Behavioral treatment
- Pelvic floor Exercise
- Correction of constipation/Bowel care
- Weight loss
- Change of activity

RCOG release: Simple lifestyle changes may reduce the symptoms of pelvic organ prolapsed (March 22, 2013)

Q. 20. How do you choose the treatment modality?

Genital prolapse management depends on the:
- Age
- Desire for child bearing
- Desire to preserve menstruation
- Degree and type of prolapse
- Degree of cervical elongation
- Presence of organic/adnexal pathology
- Presence of medical/surgical problems
    - Intactness of neuromuscular system
    - Compartmentalization of the defect
    - Identification of level defect.

The surgery may aim at removal of uterus (Radical), repair of defects (reinforcement), reconstructing the supports (conservative).

The treatment modalities available are:

Pelvic floor exercises: Whenever the stage of prolapse is early, surgery is not feasible because of pregnancy or puerperal period, as an adjuvant to surgeries.

Pelvic floor exercises
- Kegel's exercise
- Isometric with vaginal cones
- Electric stimulation
- Rubber resistance ball with indicator
- Progressive resistance vaginal exercise with springs

Pessary: Same as for the exercises, but more so useful when surgery is not possible temporarily or forever because of the condition of the patient.

Definitive surgeries: Sling procedures in nulliparous women, Fothergill's/Manchester procedure in parous women who want to retain fertility and menstrual function but with cervical elongation, vaginal hysterectomy in the rest mainly in postmenopausal women.

Abdominal repairs, laparoscopic repairs, mesh repairs are the other options available, but most preferred route and surgery is Mayo-ward's operation (Table 2).

Table 2: Repair concepts for prolapse

	Level I	Level II	Level III
Anterior	Pubocervical septum reconstruction	Cystocele repair	Urethropexy
Apical	Cervix creation or fixation	Paravaginal Repair	PFR
Posterior	Enterocele repair	Rectocele	PFR

Palliative procedures: Le-forte's surgery, Dani's stitch, colpocleisis, etc. in women who cannot tolerate major procedures and not compliant with pessary or Kegel's.

Surgical options are many and may include a hysterectomy or a uterus-sparing technique such as laparoscopic hysteropexy, sacrohysteropexy or the Manchester operation

Additional procedures: Surgery for stress incontinence, anal sphincter tears, perineal tears may be combined when required.

Q. 21. Discuss the predictors of success and failure of pessary.

- Pessaries are being used to treat prolapse since 16th century
- Indications are—nulliparous women with prolapse planning pregnancy
- Pregnancy and puerperium
- Temporarily for managing decubitus ulcer
- Patient is unfit for or refuses surgery.

Complications of pessary
- Constipation
- Urinary incontinence
- B. vaginitis, ulceration of vaginal wall
- Cervicitis
- Carcinoma of vaginal wall
- Impaction of pessary
- Strangulation of prolapsed tissue

Vaginal length, introitus size and severity of prolapse are the important assessments to be made before treating with pessary (Table 3).

Table 3: Predictors of success

- Prior prolapse surgery
- Prior hysterectomy
- Younger age
- High parity
- Obesity
- Introitus >4 fingers and vagina <6 cm

Remember: Fit the largest pessary that is most comfortable

- Serious complications are rare
- After fitting ask her to stand, strain, urinate and check if the pessary falls out
- Success rates could be improved by prior application of estrogen cream
- Size decision is usually by trial and error method.

Insertion: Measure the distance from inferior border of pubic symphysis pubis to apex of posterior fornix, deduct 1.5 cm. This is the diameter of the pessary required follow up after 1 week initially but once in 2–3 months later

Cochrane review—February 28, 2013
- The review authors identified one randomized controlled trial comparing ring and Gellhorn pessaries
- The results of the trial showed that both pessaries were effective for approximately 60% of women
- However, methodological flaws were noted
- No consensus on the use of different types of device, the indications nor the pattern of replacement and follow-up care

Q. 22. How do you prepare a women for Mayo-Ward's operation?

As it is a surgery mostly done in postmenopausal women, patient needs a detailed preoperative work up as described, examination by physician, cardiologist and other experts may be necessary if required.

She needs to be attended to her prolapse by daily vaginal antiseptic douche, tampon placement, some people believe in using estrogen cream to reduce the atrophy and to easen the dissection. As the surgery is through the vaginal route to keep the area clean keeping the bowel empty is very important.

Q. 23. Discuss the management of nulliparous prolapse.

When surgical management is decided for nulliparous prolapse, it is usually managed with sling surgeries.

Slings could be created by using autologous material like fascia lata, rectus sheath, etc. or synthetic materials like prolene mesh, mersilene tape, etc.

One end of the sling is fixed to the uterus and the other end to either a muscle sheath or to any other fixed structure—accordingly the sling is dynamic or static.

When the surgery is complete if the sling forms a complete circle from its uterine attachment to the other site it is called closed or else open.

Slings that get fixed to the anterior surface of the uterus are anterior and when fixed to the posterior surface they are called posterior slings.

Almost all the slings are designed by Indians.

Shirodkar's, Purandare's, Khanna's, Soonawala's, Joshi's, Virkud's, etc.

ACOG 2007 recommendations
- The following recommendations and conclusions are based on limited or inconsistent scientific evidence (Level B):
- Clinicians should discuss the option of pessary use with all women who have prolapse that warrants treatment based on symptoms. In particular, pessary use should be considered before surgical intervention in women with symptomatic prolapse
- Alternative operations for uterine preservation in women with prolapse include uterosacral or sacrospinous ligament fixation by the vaginal approach, or sacral hysteropexy by the abdominal approach
- Hysteropexy should not be performed by using the ventral abdominal wall for support because of the high risk for recurrent prolapse, particularly enterocele
- Round ligament suspension is not effective in treating uterine or vaginal prolapse
- Compared with vaginal sacrospinous ligament fixation, abdominal sacral colpopexy has less apical failure and less postoperative dyspareunia and stress incontinence, but is also associated with more complications
- Transvaginal posterior colporrhaphy is recommended over transanal repair for posterior vaginal prolapse

Recommendations for mesh repairs
- Physicians should seek specialized training for procedures involving the use of vaginal mesh
- Be alert and recognize complications early
- Inform patients that implantation of surgical mesh is permanent, and that some complications associated with the implanted mesh may require additional surgery that may or may not correct the complication
- Inform patients about the potential for serious complications and their effect on quality of life, including pain during sexual intercourse, scarring, and narrowing of the vaginal wall (in POP repair)

Q. 24. How do you manage a decubitus ulcer?

It does not occur due to friction and hence not typically at 3 and 9'oclock positions. Kinking of vessels and congestion is the cause.

- To relieve congestion, the prolapse can be reposited in the vagina with the help of tampoons or pessary and this helps in healing of the ulcer
- Hygroscopic agents like acriflavine— glycerine can help reduce the congestion further
- Secondary infection to be treated by antibiotics
- If it does not heal in 2–3 weeks a biopsy is indicated
- No maneuver other than reducing and keeping it in reduced position can heal the ulcer.

Q. 25. What is complex prolapse?

Nulliparous prolapse, prolapse with rectal prolapse, recurrent prolapse, prolapse with urinary or fecal incontinence, prolapse in a frail patient are called complex prolapse.

Q. 26. What are the controversies in prolapse management?

Laparoscopic repairs, mesh repair, surgeon vs gynecologist for rectocele repair, concept of fascial defects, repair under local anesthesia.

Paravaginal repair, sacrocolpopexy, enterocele repair, uterosacral suspension can be done laparoscopically. Robotic surgery has limited experience.

Q. 27. Discuss the merits, demerits and applications of prolapse classifications.

Friedman and Little classification
- IA Descent half way to hymen
- IB Descent up to hymen
- II Till introitus
- III Outside introitus
- IV Complete procidentia

The fact that POP is going through so many classification systems proves the fact that nothing is the best objective and easily reproducible system.

There is often disagreement between the observers in the grading of the prolapse. So to compare the examination findings in the same lady after some lifestyle modifications, surgery, it is not perfect and of course even between different women, or while comparing the results of surgical procedures.

Traditional classification like cystocele, urethrocele and enterocele may be unrealistic certainty as to the structures on the other side of the vaginal bulge. This is often a false assumption, particularly in women who have had previous prolapse surgery.

Malpas classification
- UV prolapse of 1st or 2nd degree
- General prolapse
- Anterior vaginal wall prolapsed (Cysto and Urethrocele)
- Posterior vaginal wall prolapse (Enterocele, rectocele and deficient perineum)
- Special categories
- Urethral prolapsed
- Rectal prolapsed
- Nulliparous prolapsed
- Posthysterectomy prolapse

This is often a false assumption, particularly in women who have had previous prolapse surgery.

Classifications
- Shaw's
- Jeffcoate's
- Malpas
- POP-Q
- Modified POP-Q
- Simplified POP-Q
- Porge's
- Beecham's
- Baden-Walker
- Simple vs Complex

The terms 'anterior vaginal wall prolapse', 'posterior vaginal wall prolapse' and 'apical prolapse' are therefore often preferred because of the uncertainty as to the anatomical structures on the other side of the vaginal bulge. Instead of using the terminology.

Malpas classification which tells about the type of prolapse, its association is very practical to be used to decide the management option, uniformity and not involved with measurements or **confusing terminologies.**

The Baden-Walker Halfway Scoring System is commonly used by many.

The system uses 6 points which are given some score and is quite informative and can be done quickly. It is very conclusive when a POP map is used. But even slightest change in the level of prolapsed changes the staging in this system. Agreement between two examiners also is not often seen. It doesnot clarify about the site of fascial defects.

POP Q overcomes many of the shortcomings of the earlier systems. Interobserver variation is very less, reproducible, gives a clue about the site of defect and to compare the results especially in multicentric trials it is very useful. But the greatest drawback is the argument that measurements that needs to be taken are cumbersome and time consuming. But evidence shows that with practice this problem can be overcome and a seasoned examiner can do this POP Q classification in 2-3 minutes.

But it is argued to be a complicated system, ultimately being reported as any of the four stages which were existing earlier also, lateral wall defects not addressed, and hymenal point may be very difficult to identify in old women.

Q. 28. Differentiate Fothergill's and modified Fothergill's operations.

Fothergill's involves anterior colporrhaphy, posterior colpoperineorrhaphy, amputation of cervix and advancement of cardinals. Neither UV fold or POD are opened in this surgery.

In Modified Manchester/Fothergill's POD is opened, enterocele is repaired after placating the uterosacrals.

Shirodkar's modification does not involve amputation of cervix but advancement of uterosacrals instead of cardinals.

Q. 29. Describe the steps of Fothergill.

- D and C
- Fothergill's points joined by incision (Suburethral, paracervical at uterovaginal junction at 3 and 9'o clock positions, mid uterosacral region on posterior vaginal wall at cervicovaginal junction)
- Vaginal flaps dissected, cut pubovesico-cervical ligaments, mobilize bladder up to UV fold
- Posterior flap dissected
- Cardinals on both sides clamped, cut, ligated
- Vaginal wall, cardinal, anterior cervix other side cardinal and vaginal wall are taken in Fothergill's stitch tied at the conclusion of surgery anteriorly
- Descending cervical vessels ligated
- Cervix amputated leaving behind 2.5 cm of cervix
- Cystocele repaired
- Cardinals advanced onto anterior cervical wall
- Vaginal wall trimmed taking care to retain as much required for cervical lip creation
- Posterior cervical lip created by Strumdorff's stitch
- Vaginal wall closed anteriorly (Some apply Strumdorff's stitch anteriorly too)
- PFR done.

Q. 30. Discuss the principles of sling surgeries.

Sling surgeries are devised to treat nulliparous prolapsed with lax ligaments in whom conservation of uterus and cervix is very important. They aim at strengthening the supports, elevating the uterus and attempt to keep the uterus is anteverted position. This is accomplished by fixing the isthmus to various structures around the pelvis. Slings may be created by biological materials like fascia lata, rectus sheath, etc. or synthetic materials like mersilene tape, prolene mesh may be used. (Table 4).

The slings are static if fixed to static structures, dynamic if fixed to mobile structures.

They are called closed if the ends are joined, open if the ends of the sling are away from each other.

Designated as posterior if fixed to posterior cervix, anterior if fixed to anterior cervix.

If mixed technique is used, it is composite.

Table 4: Different varieties of sling procedures for nulliparous prolapse

Sling	Type	Fixation
Purandare's/Modified	Dynamic, closed, anterior	To rectus sheath with the sheath/Mersilene tape
Shirodkar/Modified	Static, closed, posterior	To anterior longitudinal ligament with fascia lata/tape
Soonawala	Unilateral right posterior, static	Anterior longitudinal ligament, retraced
Joshi	Anterior, open, static	Pectineal ligament
Khanna	Anterior, static, open	Anterior superior Iliac spine/lateral most part of Inguinal ligament
Virkud	Open, composite	Left side purandare and right side Shirodkar

Q. 31. How to examine for supravaginal elongation and what is its clinical importance?

Supravaginal elongation is important for two reasons:
1. To decide if we are doing amputation of cervix.
2. To anticipate difficulty in opening (Higher level) UV fold and POD during vaginal hysterectomy.

It is clinically appreciated better by:
- PR examination wherein it is felt as a cord and by uterine sounding to measure UC length.
- But accurate measurement involves using a dilator to measure the total length of cervix

and deducting the vaginal portion length from it as measured by the distance from lateral fornix to external os.

Q. 32. Discuss the various enterocele demonstration methods.

Enterocele is demonstrated by following methods:
- Patient in dorsal position, speculum retracting posterior vaginal wall, posterior lip of cervix held with vulsellum after reducing prolapse, and ask the patient to strain. A bulge through the posterior fornix above mid vagina which is pressed by speculum is enterocele
- During a rectal examination forefinger in the rectum hooks the rectocele and when the patient strains if the finger tip feels the bulge it is enterocele
- Visualizing peristalsis in the posterior bulge
- Reducing of the the bulge with a gurgling noise
- Feeling the loops of intestines during a rectovaginal examination between the examining fingers especially well appreciated in standing position
- Barium enema/meal follow through and an X-ray taken during valsalva maneuver may show the bulge
- MRI may show the bulge very clearly.

Enterocele is corrected by high closure of enterocele sac, excision of peritoneal pouch, uterosacral placation, internal or external McCall's stitches, fixation to sacrospinous or high uterosacral ligaments
Abdominally by Moschowitz's or Halban's stitch

Q. 33. Predisposing factors for vault prolapse.
- Failure to identify and treat enterocele during prolapse surgery
- Failure to treat the predisposing factors
- Weak ligaments and failure to strengthen them
- Use of quick absorbable sutures for colporrhaphy
- Postoperative infection
- Paracolpos repair not done in lateral detachments
- During hysterectomy, the fascial tears which go unrepaired, failure to strengthen the ligaments and failure to maintain an adequate vaginal length also predispose for vault prolapsed
- Loss of level 1 support leads to only apical descent, but other level loss can lead to cystocele, enterocele or total eversion of vagina.

Q. 34. Difference in quantifying for vault prolapse.

The vaginal vault is the point C on POP Q system. When this point C descends to below the level of a point which is 2 cm < TVL (Total vaginal length), the condition is called as vault prolapse.

Q. 35. Procedures for vault prolapsed repair

Vaginal colpoplasty, sacrospinous colpopexy, iliococcygeal fixation, William Richardson's operation, uterosacral suspension both vaginally and abdominally, abdominal sacrocolpopexy, colpectomy and colpocleisis.

Vaginopexy according to Williams and Richardson is an abdominal colposuspension by strips from external oblique aponeurosis. It is indicated in cases of severe descent or prolapse of the vagina when the ability to have intercourse has to be maintained

Q. 36. What are the disadvantages of sling surgeries?

Enterocele formation as a result of deep POD creation by anteverting the uterus.

Purandare's can cause obliteration of UV fold.

Shirodkar's can cause damage to bowel, it is a difficult surgery.

Khanna'a procedure can cause osteitis if fixed to anterior superior iliac spine.

Virkud's can dextrorotate the uterus, which is compensated by placating the uterosacral which needs atmost care to avoid damage to ureter.

Use of synthetic materials can predispose for erosions.

Rectocele, deficient perineum needs to be repaired vaginally, though cystocele is possible to be repaired abdominally by Martin's or mark's procedure.

Q. 37. How do you manage a chronic Nonhealing ulcer on cervix?

When the ulcer does not heal with reduction and other methods in 2–3 weeks, a biopsy needs to be done.

If the biopsy shows evidence of malignancy (Causes for chronic nonhealing ulcer could be tuberculosis, syphilis or other granulomatous ulcers and malignancy) staging is done and if the stage is suitable for surgical intervention, a radical vaginal hysterectomy with extraperitoneal lymphadenectomy is done which could be done laparoscopically also (Schauta-Mitra's operation).

Q. 38. How do you manage prolapse in pregnancy?

Prolapse in pregnancy is marked mostly in first trimester. Later as the uterus grows and becomes an abdominal organ prolapsed gets reduced. In primigravida, it is the equivalent of a nulliparous prolapse and needs conservative measures like pessary treatment. In multiparous women, the possibility of cervical elongation and hypertrophy are common and hence dystocia is more common.

Sometimes in labor, it may cause cervical dystocia which may be managed by LSCS, Duhrssen's incision especially when the presenting part is well applied to cervix. Puerperal period also needs to be managed with pessaries.

Q. 39. Long-term complications of prolapse surgery.

The complications of sling procedures have been enumerated earlier, recurrence, need for cesarean which may destroy the sling are the problems.

With Fothergill's cervical stenosis, problems in conception, if conception occurs, abortion, insufficiency of cervix and recurrent abortions can occur. It may result in cervical dystocia also.

With other surgeries, recurrence, vault prolapse, fistulae especially with ureteric injury during McCall's stich application, narrow introitus and dyspareunia, can occur.

Q. 40. What is arrested prolapse?

Arrested prolapsed is a condition in which the progress of prolapsed stops or it may even regress.

Possible causes are, PID, endometriosis or malignancy of any pelvic organ with adhesions, or anything that leads to frozen pelvis.

This should not be confused with incarceration wherein the prolapsed organs fails to recede back on its own or my manual attempts.

Q. 41. What is the role of IVP in prolapse?

In present day investigational protocol, there is no role of IVP as a first line of investigation.

If the USG shows any gross hydroureter, hydronephrosis, biochemical evidence of compromised renal function or filling defects suggestive of renal calculi are some of the situations which may require an IVP to be done in prolapse.

CASE 2

Vault Prolapse

A 56-year-old woman who was operated for AUB(L) in her 47th year for by abdominal hysterectomy has presented with mass per vagina since 2 years. No urinary or bowel disturbances. On examination has been found to be having a vault prolapse with complete eversion of the vagina.

Plan of Management

Investigations revealed no comorbidities.

Complete eversion usually does not respond to any of the conservative measures like exercises or pessary.

Only in very few patients conservatism may be necessary otherwise surgery is the mainline of treatment.

Q. 42. What are the principles of surgical management?

- Surgery should aim at proper repair of the defects
- Prevention of recurrence
- The best method suitable for the patient needs to be selected
- Adequate vaginal length needs to be maintained
- One dictum that may be considered could be 'select an abdominal method if the prolapse has followed a previous vaginal surgery and a vaginal procedure if the vault prolapse has appeared after an abdominal hysterectomy'.

Q. 43. What are the other considerations to decide upon the route of repair?

- Patient's general condition:
  - Frail and debilitated patients may be considered for palliative procedures like partial colpocleisis, introital closure, etc.
  - Patients with precipitating factors like chronic cough, etc. may be considered for abdominal mesh repairs.
- Perivaginal fibrosis: Usually fibrosis improves the degree of prolapse but if it has followed an earlier vaginal repair, abdominal surgery is more suitable for them.
- Tone of muscle and strength of ligaments: Patients with strong pelvic floor muscles may be ideal candidates for vaginal procedures.
- Previous abdominal surgeries: The approach may be difficult with adhesions resulting from previous surgeries and hence vaginal approach may be more rational in them.
- Surgeon's expertise: Ultimately surgeon's expertise and preference of route of surgery may be the deciding factor.
- Availability of laparoscopy.
- Age of the woman/sexually active or not: Younger women in whom vaginal length maintenance is crucial, abdominal route may be a better choice and in older women who are not sexually active, sacrospinous fixation may be a better choice provided other factors are favorable for a vaginal repair.
- Collagen disorders, chronic steroid usage which might weaken the ligaments—Mesh repair abdominally is ideal.
- Failed attempts if any—Choose the route other than the route which has failed.

But many studies have shown better results including lesser chances of recurrence (Cochrane) with abdominal approach which takes little longer time. But vaginal fixation has a quick recovery, less morbidity, less cost.

Smaller prolapses may be considered for vaginal approach and the larger ones for sacrocolpopexy.

Q. 44. What are the vaginal repair procedures?

- Traditional repair: Routine cystocele, rectocele and enterocele repair.
- Sacrospinous fixation: Fixing the vaginal vault to the sacrospinous ligament by dissecting the pararectal space mostly on the right side and unilaterally, using nonabsorbable sutures at 2 sites side by side about 2 cm posteromedial to the ischial spine (to prevent injury to the P-pudendal nerve, I-Internal pudendal

vessels and N- Sciatic nerve which run posterior and superior to the ischial spine). This will deviate the vagina to the right side but depth is maintained. May cause buttock pain which is usually transient. (Figs 1 and 2)

- McCall culdoplasty: This involves taking series of stitches through the uterosacrals, pouch peritoneum and closing in internal variety and including the vaginal wall too on both sides which is done in external variety.
- **Mayo culdoplasty**
  - Iliococcygeus fixation: When sacrospinous ligament is not approachable or cannot be accessed for some reasons vault may be fixed to the fascia on the iliococcygeus muscle which may be accessed before the sacrospinous ligament.
  - Apogee: Mesh repair for apical prolapse
  - Perigee: Anterior vaginal wall repair
  - Combined tapes: For all the wall repairs
  - High uterosacral fixation: Very effective but injury to ureter is a real risk, needs pre procedure and postprocedure cystoscopy to document the patency of the ureters
  - Obliterative procedures: Le forte's, colpectomy, total colpocleisis.

Q. 45. What are the abdominal procedures for repair?

Sacrocolpopexy-open, laparoscopically, robotic—Here the apex of the vault is fixed retroperitoneally to the anterior longitudinal ligament on the sacrum with a Y-shaped mesh, The two upper limbs of the Y are fixed to the anterior and posterior surface of the vagina, the lower part of the mesh runs through a tunnel from posterior vaginal wall to the presacral area retroperitoneally alongside the uterosacral on the right side (Left side sigmoid colon makes the procedure risky) and fixed to the ligament by non absorbable sutures. This can be accomplished by laparoscopy, robotic surgery or open method.

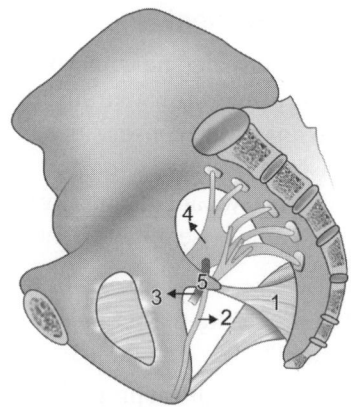

Fig. 1: Sacrospinous ligament and its relations. Relation of the structures to ischial spine and sacrospinous ligament
1. Sacrospinous ligament 2. Pudendal nerve 3. Internal pudendal artery 4. Sciatic nerve 5. Ischial spine
PIN-P = Pudendal nerve, I = Internal pudendal vessels, N = Sciatic nerve

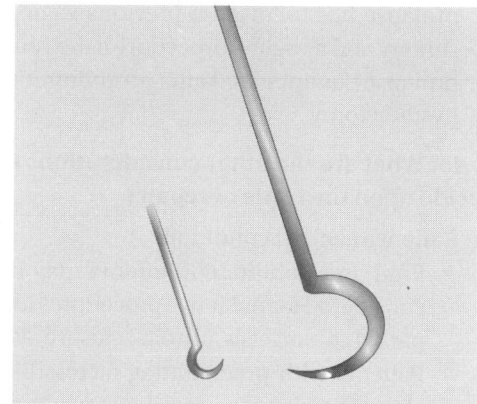

Fig. 2: Instruments used for sacrospinous fixation of vault.
Bigger hook is used for piercing the ligament. Smaller hook used to release the suture from the eye of the former.
Varieties of instruments have been designed with the same principle.

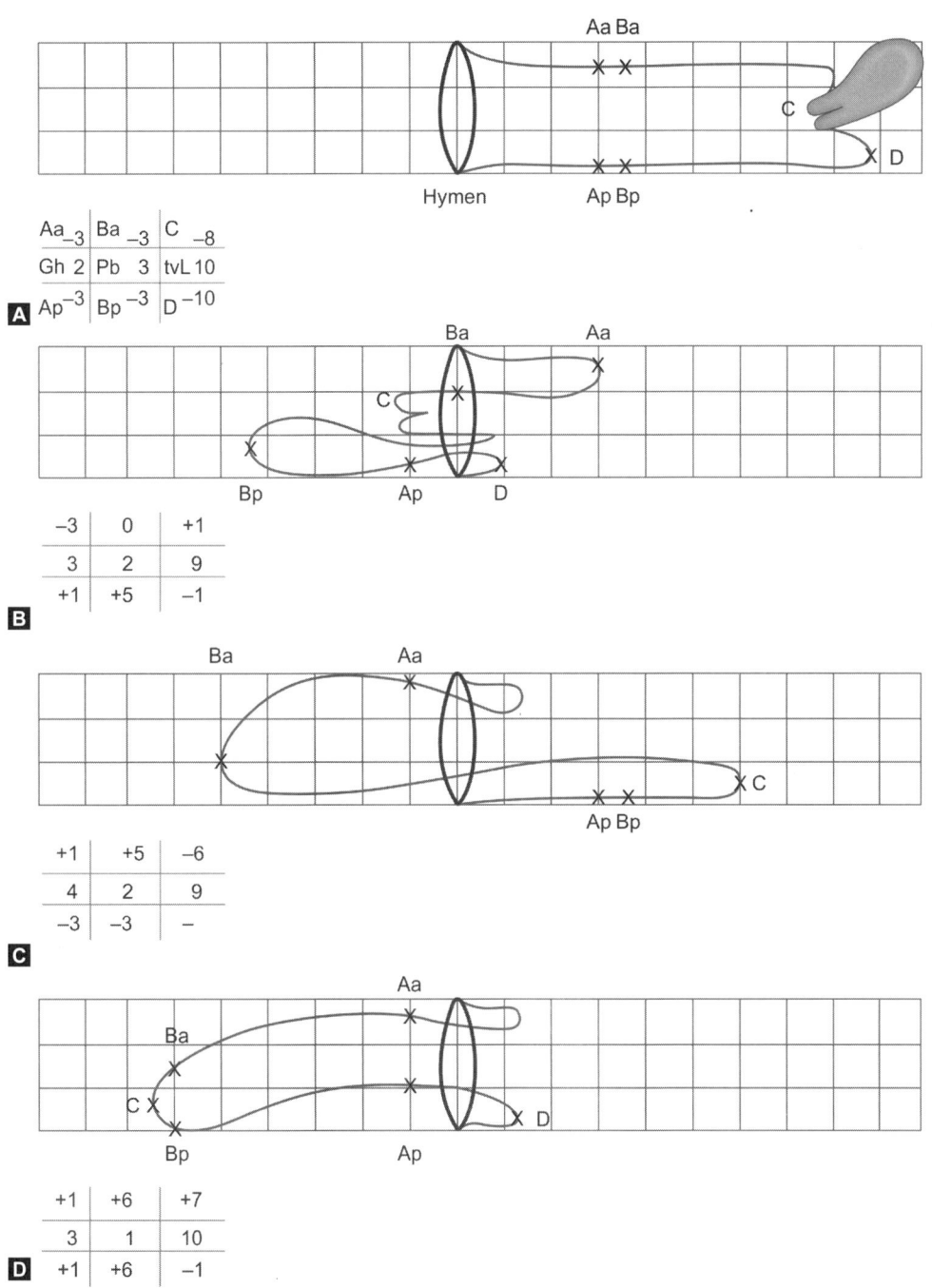

Figs 3A to D: Grid representation of POP: (A) No prolapse—calculated from hymen: Negative values for points above the hymen and positive points for below the hymen. Total vaginal length (tvl), genital hiatus (gh) and perineal body (pb) are absolute measurements; (B) Minimal anterior vaginal wall prolapse, Uterine prolapse and marked posterior vaginal wall prolapse; (C) Marked cystocele in a post hysterectomy prolapse-Point D is not considered here and only C is considered; (D) General prolapse with almost near total eversion of vagina

The Figures 3A to D shows the grid representation and line diagram of genital prolapse as per POP Q.

Bibliography

1. ACOG 2007 recommendations.
2. Arias BE, Ridgeway B, Barber MD. Complications of neglected vaginal pessaries: case presentation and literature review. International Urogynecology Journal. 2008; 19(8):1173-8.
3. Baden WF, Walker TA, Lindsday HJ. The vaginal profile. Tex Med J. 1968;(64):56-8. [PubMed]
4. Baden WF, Walker TA. Surgical repair of vaginal defects. Philadelphia: Lippincott. 1992; pp. 161-74.
5. Behnia-Willison F, Seman EI, Cook JR, et al. Laparoscopic paravaginal repair of anterior compartment prolapsed. JMIG. 2007;14(4): 475-80.
6. Carol B. "Pessaries (mechanical devices) for pelvic organ prolapse in women". Cochrane Library; 2013.
7. Christopher M. "Surgical management of pelvic organ prolapse in women". The Cochrane Library. 2013;4: CD004014.
8. Cochrane review on pessarie–February 28, 2013.
9. Cruikshank SH, Kovac SR. Randomized comparison of three surgical methods used at the time of vaginal hysterectomy to prevent posterior enterocele. Am J Obstet Gynecol. 1999;180:859-65.
10. de Boer T, Milani F, Kluivers K, et al. Surgical correction of uterine prolapse: cervical amputation with uterosacral ligament plication versus vaginal hysterectomy with high uterosacral ligament plication. Part of ICS 2009 Scientific Programme, 2009.
11. Dietz HP. Ultrasound imaging of the pelvic floor: 1. Two-dimensional aspects . Ultrasound Obstet Gynecol . 2004;23:80-92. [PubMed]
12. Dietz HP. Ultrasound imaging of the pelvic floor: 2: Three-dimensional or volume imaging. Ultrasound Obstet Gynecol. 2004;23:615-25. [PubMed]
13. Digesu GA, Athanasiou S, Cardozo L. Validation of the pelvic organ prolapse quantification (POP-Q) system in left lateral position. Int Urogynecol J. 2009;20:979-83. [PubMed]
14. Geoffrey C. "The PESSRI study: symptom relief outcomes of a randomized crossover trial of the ring and Gellhorn pessaries". American Journal of Obstetrics & Gynecology. 2007;196:405.e1-405.e8.
15. Groutz A, Blaivas JG, Chaikin DC. Bladder outlet obstruction in women: Definition and characteristics. Neurourol Urodyn. 2000; 19:213-20. [PubMed]
16. Hall AF. Interobserver and intraobserver reliability of the proposed International Continence Society, Society of Gynecologic Surgeons, and American Urogynecologic Society pelvic organ prolapse classification system. Am J Osbtret Gynecol. 1996;175:1467-71. [PubMed]
17. Hanson LA, Schulz JA, Flood CG, et al. Vaginal pessaries in managing women with pelvic organ prolapse and urinary incontinence: patient characteristics and factors contributing to success. Int Urogynecol J Pelvic Floor Dysfunct. 2006;17:155-9.
18. Hoffman BL, Schorge JO, Schaffer JI, et al. William's Gynaecology, 2nd edition.
19. Masani K. A text book of Gynaecology, 7th edition.
20. Maurizio R. "A review on the role of laparoscopic sacrocervicopexy". Current Opinions in Obstetrics & Gynecology. 2014;26:281-9.
21. McCall ML. Posterior culdoplasty; surgical correction of enterocele during vaginal hysterectomy: a preliminary report. Obstet Gynecol. 1957;10:595-602.
22. Mouritsen L, et al. Classification and evaluation of prolapse. Best Pract Res Clin Obstet Gynaecol. 2005;19(6):895-911. Epub 2005 Sep 26.
23. Novellas S, Mondot L, Bafghi A. Evaluation of two classifications systems for pelvic prolapse on dynamic MRI. J Radiol. 2009;90(11):1717-24. [PubMed]
24. Paraiso MF, Barber MD, Muir TW, et al. Rectocele repair: a randomized trial of three surgical techniques including graft augmentation. Am J Obstet Gynecol. 2006;195: 1762-71.

25. Philip R. "Laparoscopic hysteropexy: 1- to 4-year follow-up of women postoperatively". International Urogynecology Journal. 2013;25: 131-8.
26. Price N, Slack A, Jackson S. Laparoscopic hysteropexy: the initial results of a uterine suspension procedure for uterovaginal prolapse. BJOG. 2010;117:62-8.
27. Post-hysterectomy vaginal vault prolapse Green-top (Guideline No 46). 2015.
28. Richardson AC, Williams GA. Treatment of prolapse of the vagina following hysterectomy. AJOG. 1969;105(1):pp 90-3.
29. Richardson DA, Scotti RJ, Ostergard DR. Surgical management of uterine prolapse in young women. The Journal of Reproductive Medicine. 1989; 34(6):388-92.
30. Rock JA, Jones III HW. Te Linde's operative gynaecology, 10th edition.
31. Schaffer JI, Wai CY, Boreham MK, Etiology of pelvic organ prolapse. Clin Obstet Gynecol. 2005;48(3):639-47.
32. Shaw RW, Luesley D, Monga A. Gynaecology, 4th edition.
33. Swift S. Validation of a simplified technique for using the POPQ pelvic organ prolapse classification system. Int Urogynecol J. 2006;17:615-20. [PubMed]
34. Tubaro A, Artibani W, Bartram CI. Imaging and other investigations. Health Publications. 2005:707-97.
35. Vasavada SP, Comiter CV. Cytoscopic light test to aid in the differentiation of high–grade pelvic organ prolapse. Urology. 1999;54:1085-7. [PubMed]

26

Infertility

Korula George

CASE

Thirty-three years old Ms X and her husband Mr Y age 36 years presented with complaints of infertility. Married for 6 years. They were initially avoiding pregnancy—with the wife using oral contraceptive pills for 2 years. Subsequently, they continued avoiding pregnancy for another year using the rhythm methodology. Since the last three years, they have been trying to achieve pregnancy.

Ms X History

Menstrual History

Menarche 13 years. Menstrual cycles irregular. Initially 4–5 days bleeding every 45 days. Since the last two years cycles occur only once in 2–3 months with occasional heavy bleeding for almost a week. No dysmenorrhea. Last menstrual period (LMP) 3 months ago.

Frequency of intercourse—2–3 times per week. No dyspareunia—superficial or deep.

Medical History

No history of diabetes/Hypertension. Tuberculosis had appendectomy at the age of 25 prior to marriage.

Family History

Mother diabetic, father hypertensive.

Mr Y History

Medical History

No history of diabetes/Hypertension/ Tuberculosis/Mumps.

Surgical History

No history of hernia/Hydrocele.

Sexual History

Frequency of intercourse—2–3 times per week. No premature ejaculation or loss of libido. No history of any extramarital affairs.

Family History

Both parents normal.

Both are engineering graduates and working in the IT field. Their socioeconomic status-upper middle class—(modified Kuppuswamy scale).

Examination—Ms X

- Height—165 cm weight 86 kg BMI—31.6 BP 120/80. Pulse rate 75/min.
- Acne positive/Hirsutism present—Ferriman Gallwey score—15/Acanthosis Nigricans— present on back of neck.
- CVS/RS—normal PA—No abnormality detected. Abdominal girth 78 cm.
- External genitalia—Normal.

- Vaginal examination.
- Speculum—Cervix—Normal.
- Examination—Uterus anteverted/Normal size. No adnexal mass felt.

Conclusion

A 33-year-old lady presenting with primary infertility. Trying for pregnancy since 3 years. History of irregular cycles. BMI 31.6. Physically normal.

Clinical evaluation of women having irregular cycles—presenting with infertility. Appropriate history taking and physical examination is essential. Age and duration of marriage are significant factors. Irregular menstrual cycles are suggestive of an anovulatory disorder. BMI calculation with clinical evaluation for hyperandrogenemia is important (acne/hirsutism/alopecia). Acanthosis nigricans would be suggestive of abnormal glucose tolerance. A transvaginal ultrasound is required to confirm or rule out polycystic ovarian (PCO) morphology pattern.

Q. 1. Initial baseline investigations that need to be ordered.

1. Pregnancy test—Either urine pregnancy test (UPT)/Blood test—Beta hCG.
2. Blood tests—a-TSH—b-Prolactin—c-HbA1c.
3. Transvaginal scan—for assessment of pelvic organs.

1. The moment the menstrual cycle is delayed one has to rule out pregnancy. Ideally a blood test—beta hCG—as this will be 100% correct. False negative UPT can happen especially when checked early. In irregular cycles, the ovulation date cannot be predicted and hence assessment may be very early.
2a. Thyroid abnormalities: elevated TSH levels can be a reason for irregular menstrual cycles. Assessment and if required treatment is essential. Although normal levels are less than 4.5 ng/mL in first trimester pregnancies the level should be less than 2.5 ng/mL.
2b. Prolactin levels: Normal value <30 ng/mL. Borderline elevation—<50 ng/mL. Hyperprolactinemia can cause irregular cycles by suppression of gonadotropin-releasing hormone (GnRH) release resulting in low gonadotropin levels. Stress, sleep, intercourse, meals, and nipple stimulation can also raise serum prolactin. Hence always recheck prolactin levels if found to be elevated. Hypothyroidism can also cause elevated prolactin levels due to increase in TRH (thyroid releasing hormone). Elevation can also be due to drug intake which should hence be evaluated. High levels >100 ng/mL is likely to be due to pituitary dysfunction/adenomas and needs to be evaluated by MRI.
2c. HbA1c: Ruling out diabetes will be required for this lady as she has a high BMI, acanthosis nigricans and a family history of diabetes.
3. Transvaginal scan: Required to evaluate internal genital organs. No uterine abnormalities detected—such as septum/bicornuate uterus. No uterine fibroid or polyps found. Ovaries diagnosed to have a polycystic pattern. No evidence of ovarian cysts-like endometriosis.

Q. 2. Diagnosis of PCOS.

Rotterdam criteria 2003. Two out of three of the following criteria are required to make the diagnosis of PCOS:

- Oligo- and/or anovulation
- Clinical and/or biochemical signs of hyperandrogenism
- Polycystic ovaries (morphology by ultrasound).

Conditions that mimic the symptoms of PCOS must be excluded such as thyroid disorders, hyperprolactinemia, congenital adrenal hyperplasia and androgen-secreting tumors.

Ultrasound evaluation of polycystic morphology of the ovary includes the following—12 or more follicles in each ovary measuring 2–9 mm in diameter and/or ovarian volume of >10 mL. Volume is calculated by the measuring the length x width x thickness x 0.5. The presence of this image in a single ovary is adequate for diagnosis.

Earlier in 1990 National Institute of Health established the criteria for PCOS as a combination of ovulatory dysfunction and hyperandrogenism—clinical or biochemical.

In 2006, the Androgen Excess and PCOS Group suggested the presence of hyperandrogenism—clinical or biochemical with either ovulatory dysfunction or ultrasound PCOS morphology of the ovary.

In 2012, the NIH conducted a workshop evaluating the different criteria mentioned and suggested maintenance of the Rotterdam Criteria 2003, as it includes both the NIH and AE-PCOS criteria.

Q. 3. Assessment of Mr Y.

Semen analysis assessment should be done prior to initiating any treatment or invasive procedures.

Semen collection:
Ideally collection by masturbation. To be done at least 2-3 days after intercourse but not more than after 7 days. Collected sample in a sterile container and to be delivered within 45 minutes of collection. Normality determined according to WHO 2010 criteria. Minimal requirements as mentioned below.

Semen sample volume—1.5 mL;/Sperm concentration—15 million per mL/total count—39 million/mL/Motility—40%/Morphology >4%.

If any abnormality is detected the male partner should be examined and a repeat semen analysis done for confirmation.

Q. 4. First line treatment for infertility in a patient diagnosed to have PCOS.

Lifestyle Changes
Weight loss is recommended as the first line of therapy in women with PCOS. Loss of even 5% of the initial body weight is associated with spontaneous ovulation, often resulting in pregnancies. Counseling women regarding the importance of weight loss is essential. Diet and exercise are the common recommendations. No specific diet protocol has been proven to be of exceptional benefit but the trend is to recommend low calorie diet with reduced glycemic load. Regular physical activity is an important component for weight reduction and should be encouraged. Metformin is often used for weight reduction in obese women with PCOS. Although considered controversial an RCT by Harborne et al. has shown beneficial effects with high doses of metformin.[1] Orlistat which blocks intestinal absorption of fat has been shown to be of benefit in weight reduction.[2] Bariatric surgery would be of benefit in morbidly obese women.

Q. 5. Medical management.

Oral Drug Therapy
Clomiphene citrate (CC): CC is the treatment of first choice for ovulation induction in women with PCOS. It has two isomeric components—zu-clomiphene and en-clomiphene. The latter is more potent and effective for ovulation induction. Clomiphene citrate blocks estrogen receptors in the hypothalamus thus preventing a negative feedback of estrogen, causing a release of GnRH. This results in an increase in follicle-stimulating hormone (FSH) and LH levels, resulting in stimulation of the ovarian follicle. However, estrogen receptor blockade on the uterus and endometrium can be detrimental and may be responsible for the significant difference in ovulatory and pregnancy rates with CC.[3]

The starting dose of CC is traditionally 50 mg daily for 5 days, starting either on day 2 or day 5 of the menstrual cycles. A meta-analysis suggests that the ovulatory response is likely to be about 46% (with 50 mg) as compared to 75% with a starting dose to 100 mg, implying that the latter would be a better choice.[3] Follicular development is likely to occur by day 12-14 and ultrasound evaluation in each cycle is ideal. Once follicular development has been proven the couple need to be advised to be together more frequently during that period of time (alternative days). Injection hCG administration for follicular rupture or timing of intercourse has no evidence of benefits.[4] In women initially not responding to CC the dose is gradually increased to a maximum of 150-200 mg.

In women responding to CC, 3-6 cycles of ovulation stimulation are recommended. However more than 12 cycles may increase the risk of ovarian malignancy and should be avoided.[5] The pregnancy rates with ovulation induction with CC are in the range of about 40%.[3] Women not responding to higher dose are labeled as clomiphene resistant and alternative therapy needs to be considered. Side effects of CC are few, although occasional women may complain of nausea or hot flushes. If visual disturbances, which occur rarely, are noted CC should be stopped.

Clomiphene failure: Inability to conceive after several cycles of CC requires further evaluation such as hysterosalpingogram or diagnostic laparoscopy or alternative treatment options.

Q. 6. How will you use gonadotropins to treat women who do not respond to clomiphene citrate?

Gonadotropin Therapy
Gonadotropins are generally considered as a second treatment option for treatment of anovulation.[6] The intention is to raise the FSH dose marginally above the threshold FSH value, for a restricted period of time, to ensure generation of a limited number of dominant follicles. Urinary gonadotropins contain both FSH and LH while recombinant gonadotropins contain either FSH or luteinizing hormone (LH). Due to elevated levels of LH in PCOS, recombinant FSH would probably be the ideal choice. In the conventional protocol, the gonadotropin dosage used is generally 75-150 iu per day. However, the risk of excessive follicular development resulting in multiple pregnancies or ovarian hyperstimulation syndrome (OHSS) is high in PCOS, suggesting modification of the protocol.

Chronic Low Dose Step up Protocol
Gonadotropin therapy is initiated on day 3-5 at a starting dose of 50/75 IU. Follicular development is assessed with ultrasound after 5 days and subsequently as necessary. If no development is observed, therapy at the same dose is continued till day 14 following which the dose is raised by 50%. Subsequent 50% increase in doses are raised at weekly intervals. With this protocol monofollicular development is around 70% with a clinical pregnancy rate of 38%.[7]

Q. 7. Comment on the importance of endometrial thickness.

With follicular development, estrogen levels rise, resulting in a positive effect on the endometrial lining. Ideally in the late proliferative phase endometrial thickness is more than 7 mm with a trilaminar profile. Since clomiphene citrate does block estrogen receptors, it can have a negative effect on endometrial development. Thin endometrial lining may affect embryo implantation resulting in poor pregnancy outcomes. Although administration of oral estrogen towards the late proliferative phase may have some benefits, conversion to stimulation with gonadotropins may be superior. Intrauterine adhesions can also prevent endometrial development resulting in thin linings.

Q. 8. What is ovarian drilling? Mention advantages and disadvantages.

Surgery: Laparoscopic ovarian drilling (LOD)

Multiple ovarian puncture using diathermy or laser is known as ovarian drilling. Tissue destruction leads to reduction in androgen and LH levels. However ovarian drilling should not be excessive (not more than 4–6 points) and must be away from the vascular supply of the ovaries.

The indication is for women with PCOS who are resistant to ovulation induction.[6] LOD can also be useful in women unable to undergo gonadotropin therapy due to cost factors as well as inability to be monitored adequately. However in 50% of women adjuvant therapy will be required. Cochrane review in 2012 established no significant difference in pregnancy rates between LOD and medical treatment, including gonadotropins.[8] Although reduction in multiple pregnancy rates is an advantage, concerns regarding decrease in ovarian reserve do exist and overzealous drilling should be avoided.

Q. 9. Diagnosis of OHSS.

OHSS commonly develops following ovarian stimulation using gonadotropins for IVF development of more than 20 follicles with high levels of serum estradiol >3000 ng/nL) are indicative of the risk of OHSS.

Initial symptoms are usually mild—abdominal discomfort, abdominal swelling, nausea and vomiting. Physical examination will reveal weight gain and increase in abdominal girth.

Ultrasound examination—large ovaries with fluid-filled cysts and free fluid in the peritoneal cavity.

Blood tests will reveal high PCV (>40) and WBC counts (>15,000).

Differential diagnosis should not be ignored—ovarian cyst with torsion, pelvic infections, intra-abdominal hemorrhage, ectopic pregnancy or appendicitis.

Q. 10. Possible complications in women who have PCOS.

Insulin resistance and hyperinsulinemia are common features for both lean and obese women with PCOS. Target cells fail to respond to ordinary circulating levels of insulin. The body compensates by producing more insulin resulting in hyperinsulinemia. Insulin directly inhibits production of sex hormone binding globulin (SHBG) resulting in elevation of free and thus bioavailable androgens.[9] Evaluation of insulin resistance can be confirmed by the euglycemic clamp method which is considered as the gold standard. Since this procedure is complicated, it cannot be done as a routine test. Other tests like the homeostatic model assessment (HOMA)—IR and fasting glucose/insulin ratios are not validated tests and are not recommended for estimating insulin resistance.

Medical disorders more common in PCOS women include glucose intolerance, type 2 diabetes, coronary heart disorders, dyslipidemia, mental health problems like depression/anxiety and obstructive sleep apnoea.[10]

Pregnancy complications are also more frequent. Miscarriage rate is higher in women with PCOS. There is also an increased risk of complications such as gestational diabetes, PIH, preeclampsia and preterm delivery.[11]

Obesity: More than 50% of women with PCOS are centrally obese. The controversy is whether obesity causes PCOS or whether PCOS causes obesity. Limited data is available suggesting impaired metabolism in PCOS predisposes obesity. However, data implying no impact of PCOS on obesity also exists implying that environmental and lifestyle factors are probably the cause of overweight.[12]

Endometrial cancer: Since the menstrual cycle is anovulatory, deficiency in progesterone results in an unopposed estrogen effect which results in endometrial hyperplasia, with the possibility of development of malignancy. Although uncommon, this possibility needs to be kept in mind, and women with PCOS need to be instructed to ensure a menstrual cycle every 2 months, by taking progesterone supplementation after ruling out pregnancy.

Q. 11. Metabolic syndrome—Assessment.

Diagnosis of metabolic syndrome in Asian women—Any three of the following:
1. Waist circumference >80 cm
2. BP >130/80
3. Fasting sugar >100 mg/dL
4. Triglycerides >150 mg/dL
5. HDL <50 mg/dL.

There is a marked variation between countries and ethnic groups in the prevalence of metabolic syndrome in women with PCOS.[13,14] Differences in diet, lifestyle and genetic factors could be responsible for this variation. A study done on a south Indian infertility group with PCOS revealed a metabolic syndrome rate of 37.5% with the prevalence higher in older women with increasing BMI.[15]

Q. 12. Antioxidants.

Inositol isomers: Myoinositol/D-chiro-inositol (DCI)

Hyperinsulinemia in women with PCOS, due to increase in insulin resistance, stimulates the ovarian theca cells causing a hyperandrogenic state. It also decreases SHBG (sex hormone binding globulin) production by the liver causing an increase in free androgen levels. The two isomers are chemical mediators of insulin and are beneficial in lowering insulin resistance. Using these isomers in women with PCOS, by reducing insulin resistance, could be of benefit in regularization of the menstrual cycles with an increase in spontaneous ovulation.[16] When using both isomers the ratio between myoinositol and DCI should be 40:1 as high doses of DCI has been proven to have a negative effect. Improvement in both oocyte maturation and embryo quality is also suggested.[17] However in a Cochrane review (2013) evaluating the role of antioxidants in the women with subfertility a single RCT conducted on the role of myoinositol on clinical pregnancy rates did not show any benefits.[18] Currently, there is inadequate evidence-based information to support the role of myoinositol or any other antioxidant in the treatment of women with PCOS.

References

1. Harborne LR, Sattar N, Norman JE, et al. Metformin and weight loss in obese women with polycystic ovary syndrome: Comparison of doses. J Clin Endocrinol Metab. 2005;90: 4593-8.
2. Bray GA. Medical treatment of obesity: the past, the present and the future. Best Pract Res Clin Gastroenterol. 2014;28:665-84.
3. Homburg R. Clomiphene citrare–end of an era? A mini review. Hum Reprod. 2005;20:2043-51.
4. George K, Kamath MS, Nair R, et al. Ovulation triggers in anovulatory women undergoing ovulation induction. Cochrane Database Syst Rev 2014;1:CD006900.
5. Sanner K, Conner P, Bergfeldt K, et al. Ovarian epithelial neoplasia after hormonal infertility treatment: long-term follow-up of a historical cohort in Sweden. Fertil Steril. 2009;91:1152-8.
6. Thessaloniki ESHRE/ASRM-Sponsored PCOS Consensus Workshop Group. Consensus on infertility treatment related to polycystic ovary syndrome. Fertil Steril. 2008;89:505-22.
7. Homburg R, Howles CM. Low-dose FSH therapy for anovulatory infertility associated with polycystic ovary syndrome: rationale, results, reflections and refinements. Hum Reprod Update.1999;5:493-9.
8. Farquhar C, Brown J, Marjoribanks J. Laparoscopic drilling by diathermy or laser for ovulation induction in anovulatory polycystic

ovary syndrome. Cochrane Database Syst Rev. 2012;6:CD001122.
9. Dunaif A. Insulin resistance and the polycystic ovary syndrome: mechanism and implications for pathogenesis. Endocr Rev. 1997;8:774-800.
10. DeFronzo RA, Ferrannini E. Insulin resistance: A multifaceted syndrome responsible for NIDDM, obesity, hypertension, dyslipidaemia, and atherosclerotic cardiovascular disease. Diabetes Care. 1991;14:173-94.
11. Peigné M, Dewailly D. Long-term complications of polycystic ovary syndrome (PCOS). Ann Endocrinol. 2014;75:194-9.
12. Hoeger KM, Oberfield SE. Do women with PCOS have a unique predisposition to obesity? FertilSteril. 2012;97:13-7.
13. Soares EMM, Azevedo GD, Gadelha RGN, et al. Prevalence of the metabolic syndrome and its components in Brazilian women with polycystic ovary syndrome. FertilSteril. 2008;89:649-55.
14. Cheung LP, Ma RCW, Lam PM, et al. Cardiovascular risks and metabolic syndrome in Hong Kong Chinese women with polycystic ovary syndrome. Hum Reprod. 2008;23:1431-8.
15. Mandrelle K, Kamath MS, Bondu DJ, et al. Prevalence of metabolic syndrome in women with polycystic ovary syndrome attending an infertility clinic in a tertiary care hospital in south India. J Hum ReprodSci. 2012;5:26-31.
16. Bizzarrii M, Carlomagno G. Inositol: history of an effective therapy for polycystic ovary syndrome. Eur Rev Med PharmacolSci. 2014;18:1896-903.
17. Ciotta M, Stracquadanio I, Carbonaro PA, et al. Effects of myoinositol supplementation on oocyte's quality in PCOS patients: a double blind trial. Eur Rev Med Pharmacol Sci. 2011; 15:509.
18. Showell MG, Brown J, Clarke J, et al. Antioxidants for female subfertility. Cochrane Database Syst Rev. 2013;1.

CHAPTER 27

Carcinoma Endometrium

Umadevi

CASE

Patient Mrs X, wife of Mr Y, resident of KA, belonging to lower socioeconomic class, is 61-year-old para 2 with 2 living issues, menopausal for last 8 years, presented for the complaint of:
1. Bleeding per vaginum since one month
   Patient complains of bleeding per vagina for the last one month. She noticed spotting per vagina initially, and it was followed by episodes of bleeding per vagina, changes one pad per day, no complain of white discharge per vagina. No histoy of pain abdomen, No history of distension of abdomen. No history of blood stained stools. No history of altered bowel or bladder habits.

Past History

No history of similar episodes in the past.
   She is a known diabetic on oral hypoglycemics for last 10 years.
   No history of hypertension, tuberculosis, bronchial asthma. No history of taking hormone replacement therapy. No history of any surgery in the past.

Personal History

My patient is a housewife. She does not have any kind of addiction.

Family History

There is no history suggestive of breast, colonic or genitourinary malignancies in the family.

Socioeconomic History

She belongs to lower middle class, according to modified Kuppuswamy scale.

On Examination

She is obese and averagely nourished.
   Her height is 5 feet and weight is 84 kg. ECOG performance score—1 (Table 1).

Vitals

- Her pulse rate is 86/min regular, good in volume, bilateral synchronous without any radiofemoral delay.
- Her BP is 140/70 mm Hg
- Her respiratory rate is 18/min.

General Physical Examination

- No pallor
- No jaundice
- No pedal edema
- No enlargement of thyroid
- No lymphadenopathy (look for supraclavicular nodes especially).

Table 1: ECOG performance status
Developed by the Eastern Cooperative Oncology Group, Robert I Comis, md, Group Chair.*

Grade	Performance status
0	Fully active, able to carry on all predisease performance without restriction
1	Restricted in physically strenuous activity but ambulatory and able to carry out work of a light or sedentary nature, e.g. light house work, office work
2	Ambulatory and capable of all self care but unable to carry out any work activities; up and about more than 50% of waking hours
3	Capable of only limited self care; confined to bed or chair more than 50% of waking hours
4	Completely disabled; cannot carry on any self care; totally confined to bed or chair
5	Dead

*Oken M, Creech R, Tormey D, et al. Toxicity and response criteria of the Eastern Cooperative Oncology Group. Am J clin Oncol. 1982;5:649-55.

Examination of Breast

Normal.

Systemic Examination

CVS:S1S2 heard, no murmurs
RS: NVBS heard, no added sounds.

Per Abdomen

Soft, no distension, no mass/organomegaly/ free fluid.

Per Speculum Examination

Vulva, vagina normal
Cervix grossly normal, no growth seen, bleeding from os present.

Rectovaginal Examination

Uterus bulky, cervix felt normally, fornices free, no adnexal mass felt, parametrium felt normal, rectal mucosa free.

Impression

Postmenopausal bleeding for evaluation? carcinoma endometrium.

Q. 1. What is the definition of postmenopausal bleeding?

Or

Q. 2. What are all the concerns for this postmenopausal bleeding?

Any bleeding after menopause considered as postmenopausal bleeding (PMB). Menopause is defined as absence of menses for more than one year. 4–11% of postmenopausal women experience postmenopausal bleeding.[1-4]

Though nonmalignant causes also can produce postmenopausal bleeding, it is mandatory to rule out endometrial, cervical and ovarian malignancies in the presence of postmenopausal bleeding. The incidence neoplasia in patients with postmenopausal bleeding is ~25–30%. The endometrial cancer amounts for~10% of cases of PMB. The risk in postmenopausal bleeding is 1% risk of developing carcinoma endometrium at 50 years and 25% at 80 years.

Q. 3. What are all the causes of postmenopausal bleeding?[5]

See Table 2.

Table 2: Causes of postmenopausal bleeding (PMB)

Causes of PMB	Percentage
Exogenous estrogen	30
Atrophic endometritis/vaginitis	30
Endometrial cancer	15
Endometrial/cervical polyps	10
Endometrial hyperplasia	5
Miscellaneous (cervical cancer, uterine sarcoma, urethral caruncle, trauma)	10

Q. 4. What are the relevant history to be elicited in the women presenting with PMB?

History should concentrate on:
- Age of the patient
- Parity
- Number of years postmenopausal
- Duration and severity of bleeding
- Associated foul smelling discharge per vagina
- Initiating factors such as trauma, Postcoital bleeding
- Medication such as hormone replacement therapy, topical estrogen
- Tamoxifen therapy
- Associated comorbid medical conditions like diabetes, Obesity, hypothyroidism, cardiovascular diseases
- Family history of gynaecological, breast and colorectal cancer (LYNCH syndrome)
- Past history of similar complaints, and treatment for it
- If any previous pap/endometrial sampling reports available
- Previous history of anovulatory bleeding.

Q. 5. What should be looked for in clinical examination?

General physical examination, look for BMI, thyroid swelling, pallor any palpable supraclavicular nodes, per abdominal examination should focus on any palpable mass, organomegaly, fluid per abdomen.

Perspeculum examination should include visualization of vulva, vagina, cervix for any lesion which can produce bleeding or metastatic spread, and Pap smear should be taken, on bimanual examination look for uterine size, any adnexal mass, parametrial and rectal mucosal involvement.

Per abdomen, internal examination usually normal in patients with carcinoma endometrium. Enlarged globular uterus may be palpable in patients with pyometra/hydrometra. Advanced disease may produce liver metstasis with enlargement of liver. This is rare in Ca endometrium patients as they usually present early. Any associated uterine lesions may also cause enlargement in uterine size.

Adnexal masses should be looked for to rule out associated hormone producing ovarian tumors or metastatic tumor spread.

Q. 6. What is the risk stratification for postmenopausal bleeding?

Low risk (prone for type I tumor) (Table 3)
- Life style factors: Obesity
- Past history: Diabetes, PCOS, tamoxifen therapy
- Family History: Non Polyposis colon cancer
- Menstrual and obstetric history: Nulliparity, early menarchy, late menopause.

High risk (prone for type II tumors) (Table 3)
- Elderly affluent women
- Not associated with estrogen milieu
- Not associated with endometrial hyperplasia
- Presentation usually remote from menopause.

Table 3: Type I and type II PMB

Type I	Type II
80% Endometroid	Nonendometrioid (predominantly serous and clear cell)
The estrogen related (type I, endometrioid)	Nonestrogen related (type II, nonendometrioid)
Exhibiting microsatellite instability and mutations in PTEN, PIK3CA, K-ras, and CTNNBI (β-catenin)	Having p53 mutations and chromosomal instability
Exposure to unopposed estrogen (e.g. estrogen replacement therapy, obesity, anovulatory cycles, estrogen-secreting tumors)	Older, nonwhite, multiparous, current smokers, nonobese, and to have had breast cancer treated with tamoxifen

Contd...

Contd...

Type I	Type II
increases—factors that decrease exposure to estrogens or increase progesterone levels (e.g. oral contraceptives or smoking) tend to be protective	
Average age 63 years	67 years
70% confined to uterus at diagnosis	50% confined to uterus at diagnosis
5 years survival 83%	62% for clear cell carcinoma 53% for serous carcinoma

Q. 7. How will you evaluate a lady with postmenopausal bleeding?

Evaluation of patient with postmenopausal bleeding includes thorough clinical evaluation, Pap smear, transvaginal sonography (TVS), and endometrial sampling, as an office procedure.

Q. 8. How to interpret TVS findings?

TVS has 95% sensitivity in detecting uterine pathology with endometrial thickness cutoff of 4 mm. IF ET >4 mm then perform endometrial biopsy (Fig. 1), saline infusion sonography (SIS), and biopsy and if ET <4 mm then consider it as atrophic endometrium. Any other uterine pathology detected by TVS like endometrial or cervical polyp should be treated accordingly.[5-8]

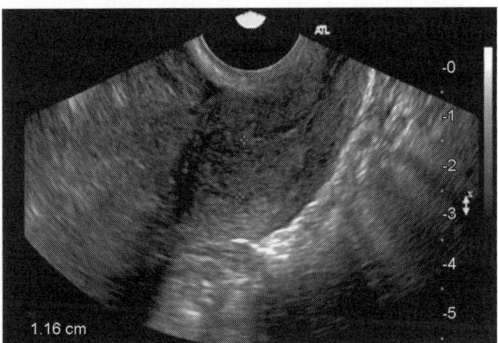

Fig. 1: TVS image of patient with postmenopausal bleeding with thickened endometrium.

Q. 9. Name few instruments used for endometrial sampling?

Novak's curette, pipple, vabra aspirator.

Q. 10. What are all the advantages and disadvantages of endometrial sampling?

Detection rates for endometrial cancer in postmenopausal and premenopausal women of 99.6% and 91%, respectively. The sensitivity for the detection of endometrial hyperplasia was 81%. The specificity was 98%.

Advantages
- Office procedure
- No need for anaesthesia
- Provides tissue samples for a histological diagnosis
- Can be performed easily.

Limitations
- Os not negotiable in ~8% patients due to stenotic os[9]
- May miss focal pathologies and tissue sample obtained may be insufficient.

Q. 11. What are all the advantages and disadvantages of TVUS?

- TVS is a cost effective, noninvasive, safe, painless procedure
- Assess ET (measuring the double-layer ET in the anteroposterior dimension from one basalis layer to the other)
- Visualizes focal lesions
- Sensitivity 96%, specificity 53%.

Limitations
- 4% of endometrial cancers would be missed even with cutoff as low as <4 mm[10]
- A thin or indistinct endometrial lining on transvaginal ultrasound does not reliably exclude type 2 endometrial cancer, which is not related to estrogen exposure or endometrial hyperplasia!

Q. 12. What is saline infusion sonography? Explain its advantages and disadvantages?

It is a procedure in which endometrial cavity is distended with sterile saline and TVUS done.

When diagnosis remains unclear after biopsy, in patients whom bleeding persists despite a normal initial workup and TVUS finds evidence of a focal lesion then saline infusion sonography may be performed. It is useful in patient who has a relative contraindication for hysteroscopy with D and C (Fig. 2). It should not be done in patients in whom cancer cells are found in endometrial biopsy due to the risk of spill of cancer cells into the endometrial cavity and upstage the disease.

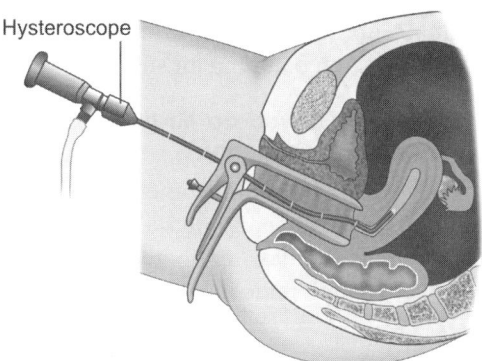

Fig. 3: Hysteroscopic examination

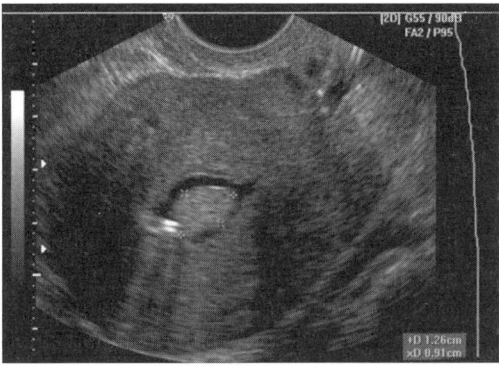

Fig. 2: Saline infusion sonohysterography showing a polyp

Q. 13. What are all the advantages and disadvantages of hysteroscopy and endometrial biopsy?

Advantages
- Immediate office evaluation
- Visualization of the endometrium and endocervix (Fig. 3)
- Detection of minute focal endometrial pathology
- Directed endometrial biopsies
- Therapeutic in the same sitting if the lesion is resectable one.

Disadvantages
- Cost
- Availability
- Knowledge of the procedure and adequate learning required.

Q. 14. Do all postmenopausal bleeding require evaluation?

All postmenopausal bleeding require evaluation.

Q. 15. Is TVUS an appropriate screening tool for postmenopausal women without bleeding?

TVUS is not a screening tool for postmenopausal women for cancer.

Q. 16. What is to be done when the bleeding persists despite negative initial evaluation?

Since 1–9% of patients may still be missed the diagnosis of endometrial cancer (more chance of missing with premenopausal women) additional assessment is indicated including fractional curettage under anesthesia.

Q. 17. How will you manage if the histopathology report reveals endometrial cancer?

- Grade and histopathology type of the tumor is an important factor
- Imaging to know the size of the tumor and extent of spread and to decide on the extent of surgery
- Hemogram, biochemical profile includes LFT, RFT, TFT in younger women
- Chest X-ray, ultrasonography, cardiology evaluation including echo
- Anesthesia fitness for surgery, counseling, informed consent regarding the nature of

disease, reproductive, childbearing and menstrual functions in premenopausal women when planning for surgery.

Q. 18. When will you do MRI/CT scan as preoperative investigation?

- MRI is useful to know myometrial invasion depth in cases of endometrial cancer.
- CT scan is useful when there is a need to look for lymph node involvement.[12]

MRI Usefulness

- Sensitivity: 71–83%
- Specificity: 74–96%
- Negative predictive value: 86–97%
- Positive predictice values: 80–91%.[11]

Q. 19. What is the role of surgical staging in endometrial cancer?

- Surgical staging is the standard of primary treatment
- Hysterectomy + bilateral salpingoophorectomy
- Biopsy and resection of any suspicious lesions
- Retroperitoneal lymphadenectomy
- Omentectomy (high-grade tumors, uterine papillary serous carcinoma (UPSC), clear-cell carcinoma).[13]

Q. 20. Does the surgical staging provide an overall survival benefit?

See Table 4.

Table 4: Surgical staging and survival role of endometrial cancer

Stage	Definition	Survival
I	Cancer limited to the corpus uteri	83–93%
II	Cancer involves the cervix	73%
III	Cancer extends outside of the uterus to the pelvis or retroperitoneal lymph nodes	52%
IV	Cancer involves the bladder or bowel or with distant metastasis	27%

Q. 21. Should all patients undergo comprehensive surgical staging?

Those women suspected with early stage disease with no myometrial invasion, favoarble histological type and low-grade lesion with no high-risk for surgical staging can undergo hysterectomy with bilateral salpingo–oophorectomy. However, 10% of these women will have the chances of having high-grade histology in the final histopath report. Hence, proper preoperative clinical evaluation is required before deciding for the comprehensive surgical staging.

Q. 22. Is there a role of fertility preservation in endometrial cancer?

- Conservative treatment can be considered in patients with atypical hyperplasia or grade 1 adenocarcinoma with superficial disease (disease confined to endometrium)[13]
- 5% of patients with endometrial Ca occur in women <40 years of age
- Selection criteria for conservative management
  - Well-differentiated endometrioid adenocarcinoma
  - Hysteroscopy, D and C
  - MRI to rule out myometrial invasion
  - Laparoscopy to rule out ovarian disease (synchronous primaries)
  - Compliant patient
- Treatment
  - Megestrol acetate 40–160 mg/day for 3months followed by D and C
  - Medroxyprogesterone acetate (MPA) 200–800 mg/day
  - Progesterone IUD, 20 µg levonorgesterel/day over 5 years.

Q. 23. What are the fertility issues to be considered in endometrial cancer?

- Close clinical followup, endometrial biopsy every three months
- Median time to regression—9 months

- A recent multicenter phase II study of treatment with MPA
- Complete response in 55% of EC and 82% in atypia
- With a 47% recurrence rate observed during the 2-year follow-up period 1
- Literature review of 123 patients revealed
  - Regression in 78%
  - Relapses in 25%
  - 51 live births
- After childbearing TAH/BSO is recommended.

Close followup may be required; however, with family history/hereditary cancer history surgery may be considered as an option.

Q. 24. Is there a role of ovarian preservation after hysterectomy in endometrial cancer?

- 5% of patients presents with endometrial cancer <40 years
- 14% of patients are premenopausal
- Lynch syndrome occurs in 10% of patients with EC in <50 years
  - 10–12% have risk of developing ovarian cancer.

Controversy

- Retrospective analysis of 102 women <45 years of age 1
  - Synchronous ovarian tumors in 23 and metastatic disease in 3
  - Ovarian involvement in 25% of patients (4 had normal preoperative imaging or normal intraoperative assessment)
- Results of a surveillance, epidemiology, and end-results database (SEER) 3,269 women with stage I endometrial cancer 402 (12%) had ovarian preservation analysis with no effect on cancer specific or overall survival.[14]

Q. 25. What are the surgical approaches in the management of endometrial cancer?

- The first line of treatment in endometrial Ca is surgery. Depending on various other factors, the additional treatment options need to be considered.
- Surgery basically aims at hysterectomy, Bilateral salpingooophorectomy, and lymphadenectomy.
- It can be achieved by abdominal route, vaginal route, laparoscopy, robotic assisted surgery
- Vaginal approach may be difficult as, complete evaluation may not be possible, adnexectomy is challenging, lymph node evaluation and removal is not possible.

Q. 26. How radical the surgery should be?

- Endometrial cancer may be managed by Type 1 or Type 2 hysterectomy.
- But a randomised Italian multicentric study revealed no change in complications, surgical duration and blood loss were greater in Type 2
- Vaginal cuff excision mattered in preventing local recurrence hence type 1 hysterectomy with slight modification, i.e. adequate vaginal cuff excision is to be the ideal radicality required.

Conclusion

Class II hysterectomy did not improve locoregional control and survival compared to class I hysterectomy, but when an adequate vaginal cuff transection is not feasible with class I hysterectomy, a modified radical hysterectomy allows to obtain an optimal vaginal and pelvic control of disease with a minimal increase in surgical morbidity.

Q. 27. What is the role of lymphadenectomy in endometrial cancer?

Lymph node excision need is dictated by:

- Depth of myometrial invasion
- Histological grade
- Differentiation
- By doing Lymphadenectomy
- It may help in prognostication
- Dictates the need for additional treatment
- It may be therapeutic[15,16]

- But no recommendations have been made regarding the extent of lymphadenectomy in the primary surgery or conclusions drawn regarding its therapeutic role.
- In non suspicious cases little >20% of cases may show lymph node metastasis.

Q. 28. What is the role of lymphadenectomy in early case of endometrial cancer?

Most important prognostic factor in clinically early stage endometrial cancer:
- In clinical stage I disease, about 10% will have pelvic and 6% will have para-aortic lymph node metastasis.[17]

Q. 29. Is there any influence of lymphadenectomy on the recurrence at early stage of disease?

The risk of lymph node metastases in patients with grade 1 or 2 endometrioid tumors which are less than 2 cm diameter, and invading less than 50% of the myometrium, is less than 1%. About 40% patients belong to this group.[18]

In this group of patients lymphadenectomy can be avoided (Table 5).

Table 5: Recurrence and survival role of lymph node metastases.

Lymph node metastases	Recurrence rate	5 year survival
Absent	8%	90%
Present	48%	54%

Q. 30. Is there a role of lymph node sampling in endometrial cancer?

- There is no role of lymph node sampling. Early stage as explained in the previous question, there is no need to do lymphadenectomy
- In stage I disease almost 10% had metastasis to pelvic nodes
- Less than 10% of LN metastases have gross enlargement, hence palpation is not an acceptable alternative, hence no role for lymphnode sampling.[19]

Q. 31. How does the lymphadenectomy influence on the therapeutic benefit?

- Prognostic information
- Status of lymph nodes should help direct postoperative adjuvant therapy
- Provides accurate selection and tailoring of adjuvant treatment
  - Avoid under—treatment mortality
  - Avoid over—treatment morbidity
- May provide therapeutic value by removal of micrometastatic disease
- Takes only 30 additional minutes, and it is safe in well-trained hands.

Q. 32. How do you manage the unstaged patient?

- Patient has to undergo imaging to know the extent of disease spread and the hispathological examination slides have to be thoroughly reviewed
- Stratify based on risk
  - G1 or G2 with less than 50% myoinvasion
    ◊ Imaging with CT or PET-CT
    ◊ Can consider observation (<10% risk of nodal disease)
  - G3 or deep myometrial invasion.
    ◊ Good surgical candidate: Staging is recommended (laparoscopy)
    ◊ Poor surgical candidate: Imaging and treating based on uterine histopathologic factors with adjuvant therapy.

Q. 33. When will you subject the patient for adjuvant radiotherapy?

Every case needs to be classified as Low risk, Intermediate risk and high risk patients depending on the size of the tumour, type, myometrial depth of invasion, Grade of the tumour, LVSI, age of the patient and number of risk factors in relation to the age. Intermediate risk and high risk patients are selected for adjuvant radiotherapy.[21]

Q. 34. Is there a role of adjuvant therapy in endometrial cancer?

- High-risk disease: Grade 3 with deep myometrial invasion, grade 3 with cervical stromal involvement, UPSC and clear-cell carcinoma, metastatic extrauterine disease need adjuvant treatment.
- The mode of adjuvant therapy—primary chemotherapy vs. whole pelvic external beam. Radiotherapy is controversial
- All stages of UPSC and clear cell, stage III and IV disease need adjuvant therapy
- Randomized prospective trial comparing WAR to systemic chemo in advanced stage endometrial cancer (GOG 122)
- 13% improvement in DFS with chemotherapy
- 11% improvement overall survival with chemotherapy
- Increased toxicity: Hematologic, GI, cardiac toxicity in chemo arm.

Q. 35. Is there a role of adjuvant chemotherapy in endometrial cancer?

Japanese GOG trial 2033
- Endometrial cancers IC-III patients were randomized to EBRT vs. chemotherapy containing cisplatinum, doxorubicin, paclitaxel
- Majority of patients were in stage IC, grade 1 disease and showed no difference in OS or PFS
- Subgroup analysis showed improved PFS and OS with chemotherapy in:
  - Stage IC patients with age >70 or grade 3 and stage II
  - Stage IIIA patients with >50% myometrial invasion.[20]

Q. 36. Why surgical staging is important in endometrial cancer?

- Several studies demonstrated significant under staging when patients were subjected to adequate surgical evaluation
- 1/4th of clinical stage I have disease outside the uterus (surgical staging studies, Creasman et al.)
- Also women with small volume disease in retroperitoneal nodes/peritoneum rarely identified clinically.

Q. 37. Why FIGO staging?

It is surgicopathologically staged and the staging has a direct influence on survival.

Q. 38. Is there a role of sentinel node mapping (SLN) in endometrial cancer?

- Preliminary observation confirm, complex lymphatic drainage and operative technique is critical in determining the feasibility of SLN in endometrial cancer
- Subserosal injection does make lymphatic mapping feasible, refinement in technique and experience is needed to determine staging benefits as observed in melanoma and carcinoma breast.

Q. 39. What are the common sites of recurrence in endometrial cancer?

The common sites of recurrence are:
- Local pelvic recurrence
- Lung, liver
- Nodal recurrence at para-aortic regions
- Rarely bone and brain.

Q. 40. How do you manage the recurrent cancer?

Individualize the treatment accordingly, with risk stratification.

Q. 41. Is there a role of debulking surgery in stage IV endometrial cancer?

In contrast to ovarian cancer, the advantage of cytoreduction is not established in ca endometrium.

When ever surgery is feasible it should be done as surgery is the primary line of treatment.

When there are distant metastasis, surgery is to be restricted for palliation only like to treat vaginal bleeding.

Q. 42. Is there a role of hormone therapy in endometrial cancer?

In young women presented with early disease where fertility issue is a concern and also where the elderly women present with locally advanced disease with poor performance status high dose hormone therapy can be considered with risk stratification.

Q. 43. How to follow-up patients treated for endometrial cancer?

The patient has to follow up 3 monthly for 2 years 6 monthly for 3 years and then annually with clinical examination and imaging.

Q. 44. Role of radio- and chemotherapy in endometrial carcinoma?

Radiation therapy as primary treatment—5–15% endometrial patients with medical problem who are unsuitable for surgery—obesity. Elderly, acute and chronic medical illness like hypertension diabetes, cardiac, pulmonary renal and neurological complications.

In operative cases, effective treatment are: Generally intracavitary radiation for adequate local control. But patient's with cervical involvement and known or suspected extrauterine pelvic spread benefit from external beam therapy.

Local brachy therapy in early cancers may reduce cuff recurrence, survival is not affected.

High/intermediate risk, brachytherapy is better than pelvic or whole abdominal radiation

Preoperative radiation therapy is very rarely used, often women present with early stage in endometrial cancer. However in advanced medically unfit inoperable case of carcinoma endometrium preoperative radiation therapy 45 gy/25 fractions followed by Intracavitary brachytherapy 30gy can be considered. But this therapy is no more used, after external teletherapy, if thereis a good response surgery should be considered.

Postoperative adjuvant radiation therapy as vaginal brachytherapy with 30 Gy dose is used in those patients with stage IA G3, Stage IB G1, G2.

External pelvic radiation 45GY-50 Gy followed by vaginal brachytherapy can be considered in Stage IB G3, Stage II with stromal invasion > ½ and with lymphovascular invasion, unfavourable histology types clear cell carcinoma, uterine papillary serous carcinoma, adenosqamous carcinoma and undifferentiated carcinoma.

External pelvic radiation can be used in those patients with bulky positive pelvic nodes or more than one microscopically positive pelvic node are better treated with pelvic and paraaortic irradiation.

Extended field Radiation can be used in those patients with biopsy proven paraaortic nodal metastasis, grossly positive pelvic nodes and two or more positive pelvic nodes. However bowel complication needs to be avoided.

Whole abdominal radiation has been used for many years in selected patients with omental, adnexal or peritoneal metastases that have been completely resected, but the GOG recently reported a randomized phase III trial of WAR vs chemotherapy in patients with stage III or IV endometrial carcinoma having maximum of 2cms of postoperative residual disease.

Q. 45. What is the role of chemotherapy?

Studies have shown there is benefit from adjuvant progesterone therapy.

When ever fertilitypreservation is the criteria or for some reason surgery is not feasible, progestins preferably medroxy progesterone acetate or megestrol acetate is the mainstay of hormone therapy of this cancer. The patients needs to be followed up with EB once in 3 months while on progestins

In advanced cases, chemo/radiotherapy/hormonal therapy may have to be singly used or used in combination. It may be palliative, may prolong the survival.

Severe maenopausal symptoms post surgery may have to be managed with estrogens with adequate counselling.

Chemotherapeutic agents used are:
- Doxorubicin and cisplatin
- Cyclophosphamide and doxorubicin and cisplatin
- Paclitaxel and cisplatin with or without doxorubicin and
- Carboplatin and paclitaxel.

Adjuvant chemotherapy: The Value of chemotherapy was not standardized, however in high risk group of stage III C1 & C2, With lympho vascular space involvement or optimal treated recurrent or advanced endometrial cancer, chemo therapy may be beneficial.

Treatment for Atrophic Endometritis

Woman presented with postmenopausal bleeding diagnosed as atrophic endometritis needs close followup and diagnostic hysteroscopy. If the diagnostic hysteroscopy-guided D & C also reveals atrophic endometritis, regular followup with transvaginal ultrasonography once in 3-6 months along with clinical examination may assist in investigating her further. If the symptoms persists despite of conservative management laparoscopically assisted hysterectomy may be considered.

Additional Information

Role of Radiation in Endometrial Cancer

Preoperative radiation therapy is very rarely used, often women present with early stage in endometrial cancer. However, in advanced medically unfit inoperable case of carcinoma endometrium preoperative radiation therapy 45 Gy/25 fractions followed by intracavitary brachytherapy 30 Gy can be considered. But this therapy is no more used, after external teletherapy, if there is a good response surgery should be considered.

Postoperative adjuvant radiation therapy as vaginal brachytherapy with 30 Gy dose is used in those patients with stage IA G3, stage IB G1, G2.

External pelvic radiation 45 Gy—50 Gy followed by vaginal brachytherapy can be considered in stage IB G3, stage II with stromal invasion > ½ and with lymphovascular invasion, unfavorable histology types clear cell carcinoma, uterine papillary serous carcinoma, adenosquamous carcinoma and undifferentiated carcinoma.

External pelvic radiation can be used in those patients with bulky positive pelvic nodes or more than one microscopically positive pelvic node are better treated with pelvic and paraaortic irradiation.

Extended field radiation: It can be used in those patients with biopsy proven para-aortic nodal metastasis, grossly positive pelvic nodes and two or more positive pelvic nodes. However, bowel complication needs to be avoided.

Whole abdominal radiation: It has been used for many years in selected patients with omental, adnexal or peritoneal metastases that have been completely resected, but the GOG recently reported a randomized phase III trial of WAR vs chemotherapy in patients with stage III or IV endometrial carcinoma having maximum of 2 cm of postoperative residual disease.

Adjuvant chemotherapy: The value of chemotherapy was not standardized; however, in high risk group of stage III C1 and C2, with lympho vascular space involvement or optimal treated recurrent or advanced endometrial

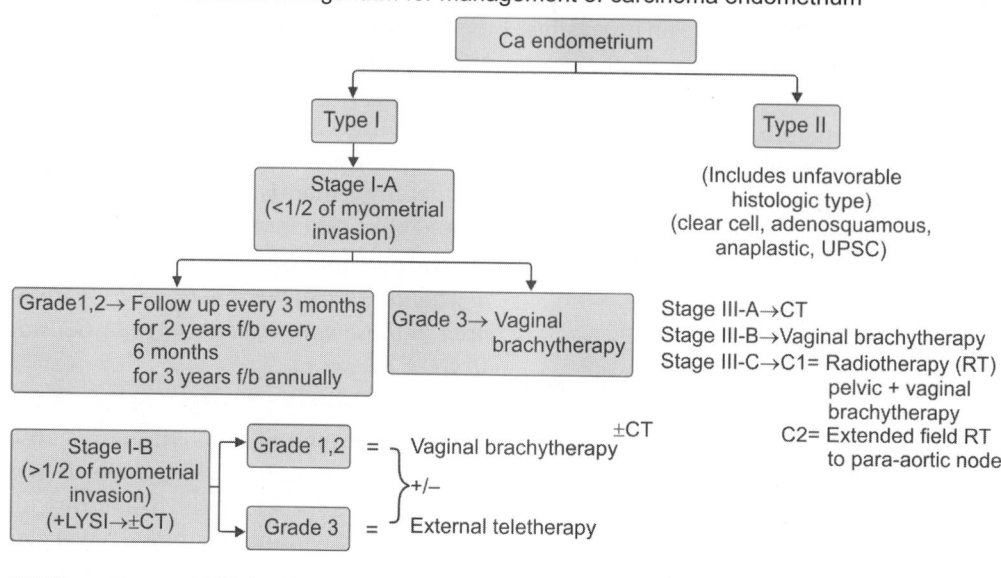

Flowchart 1: Algorithm for management of carcinoma endometrium

CT, Chemotherapy; LVSI, lymphovascular space invasiospace invasion;
Stage II, high risk→ vaginal brachytherapy
±
teletherapy
(pelvic radiotherapy)

(f/b: followed by; CT: chemotherapy)

cancer paclitaxel 175 mg/m² with carboplatin of AUC 6–6.5 or cyclophosphamide 500 mg/m², doxorubicin 50 mg/m², cisplatin 50 mg/m² once in three weeks for 5–6 cycles could be considered. The study suggested that an improvement in progression free survival with chemotherapy but several data were required to draw any conclusion (Flowchart 1).

References

1. Astrup K, Olivarius Nde F. Frequency of spontaneously occurring postmenopausal bleeding in the general population. Acta Obstet Gynecol Scand. 2004;83:203.
2. Rossouw JE, Anderson GL, Prentice RL, et al. Risks and benefits of estrogen plus progestin in healthy postmenopausal women: principal results From the Women's Health Initiative randomized controlled trial. JAMA. 2002;288:321.
3. Mirkin S, Archer DF, Taylor HS, et al. Differential effects of menopausal therapies on the endometrium. Menopause. 2014;21:899.
4. Smith-Bindman R, Weiss E, Feldstein V. How thick is too thick? When endometrial thickness should prompt biopsy in postmenopausal women without vaginal bleeding. Ultrasound Obstet Gynecol. 2004;24:558.
5. Goldstein RB, Bree RL, Benson CB, et al. Evaluation of the woman with postmenopausal bleeding: Society of Radiologists in Ultrasound-Sponsored Consensus Conference statement. J Ultrasound Med. 2001;20:1025-36.
6. Smith-Bindman R, Kerlikowske K, Feldstein VA, et al. Endovaginal ultrasound to exclude endometrial cancer and other endometrial abnormalities. JAMA. 1998;280:1510-7.
7. Tabor A, Watt HC, Wald NJ. Endometrial thickness as a test for endometrial cancer in women with postmenopausal vaginal bleeding. Obstet Gynecol. 2002;99:663-70.

8. Gupta JK, Chien PF, Voit D, et al. Ultrasonographic endometrial thickness for diagnosing endometrial pathology in women with postmenopausal bleeding: a meta-analysis. Acta Obstet Gynecol Scand. 2002;81:799-816.
9. Berek and Hacker's Gynaecological Oncolgy. 6th edition. p. 391
10. Tabor A, Watt HC, Wald NJ. Endometrial thickness as a test for endometrial cancer inwomen with postmenopausal vaginal bleeding. Obstet Gynecol. 2002.
11. Sahdev A, Reznek RH. Magnetic resonance imaging of endometrial and cervical cancer. Ann NY Acad Sci. 2008;1138:214-232. doi: 10.1196/annals.1414.028.
12. The ability of helical CT to preoperatively stage endometrial carcinoma.www.ajronline.org/doi/pdf/10.2214/ajr.176.3.1760603
13. NCCN guidelines. uterine neoplasms.ver.2. 2016
14. Gunderson CC, Fader AN, Carson KA, et al. Oncologic and reproductive outcomes with progestin therapy in women with endometrial hyperplasia and grade 1 adenocarcinoma: A systematic review. Gynecol Oncol. 2012;125: 477-82.
15. Kitchener H, Swart AM, Qian Q, et al. Efficacy of systematic pelvic lymphadenectomy in endometrial cancer (MRC ASTEC trial): a randomised study. Lancet. 2009;373(9658):125-36.
16. Chan JK, Kapp DS. Role of complete lymphadenectomy in endometrioid uterine cancer. Lancet Oncol. 2007;8(9):831-41.
17. Milan MR, Java J, Walker JL, et al. Nodal metastasis risk in endometrioid endometrial cancer. Obstet Gynecol. 2012;119:286-92.
18. Dowdy SC, Borah BJ, Bakkum JN, et al. Prospective assessment of survival, morbidity, and cost associated with lymphadenectomy in low-risk endometrial cancer. Gynecol Oncol. 2012;127:5-10.
19. Boronow RC. Endometrial cancer and lymph node sampling: Short on science and common sense, long on cost and hazard. J Pelvic Surg. 2001;7:187-90.
20. Susumu N, Sagae S, Udagawa Y, N et. al. Japanese Gynecologic Oncology Group. Randomized phase III trial of pelvic radiotherapy VS. cisplatin-based combined chemotherapy in patients with intermediate- and high-risk endometrial cancer: Japanese Gynecologic oncology group study. Gynecol Oncol. 2008;108(1):226-33.
21. Keys HM, Roberts JA, Brunetto VL, et. al. A phase III randomized trial of surgery with or without adjunctive external pelvic radiation therapy in intermediate risk endometrial adenocarcinoma: A Gynecologic Oncology Group study. Gynecol Oncol. 2004;92:744-51.

28
CHAPTER

Postoperative Rounds

K Srinivas

CASE 1

A patient has undergone abdominal hysterectomy and shifted to the postoperative ward.

She is 46 years, had multiple fibroids with a uterine size of 24 weeks and Hb was 11 g/dL.

She weighs 58 kg.

Surgery took about 1 hr 20 min. She is a known hypertensive under good control. No other comorbid conditions.

She is fasting since previous day 11 pm and has been shifted to the postoperative ward after the surgery at 10.30 am.

Q. 1. How do you calculate her fluid requirements?

A person weighing 70 kg with good health normally requires about 2–3 L of fluid per day. Urinary loss is 1–2 L, perspiration amounts to about 500 mL which varies with temperature of the surroundings. Other losses could be from lungs and stools.

While taking care of fluid balance, the principles are:
- Prevent the loss by correction of pathology
- Providing the daily needs and
- Replenishment of losses
- Reduced fluid intake, tachypnea, fever, loose motions, excessive aspirations, vomiting, drainage, usage of diuretics may all lead to a unilateral volume loss.

Intraoperative fluid therapy

It is calculated as follows:
- *Starvation deficit:* Duration of starvation in hours × 2 mL/kg.
- *Maintenance during surgery:* Duration of surgery in hours × 2 mL/kg
- *Replacement of intraoperative loss:*
  For minimal trauma surgery—4 mL/kg
  Moderate trauma surgery—6 mL/kg
  Severe trauma surgery—10 mL/kg

This patient 58 kg lady undergoing abdominal hysterectomy:
a. Starving for 12 hours—12 × 2 × 58 = Around 1,400 mL
b. 1 1/3 Hour surgery—1 × 2 × 50 = 130 mL
c. Operative loss—Moderate 6 × 58 × 1 = 350 mL
1,900 mL, replaced as normal saline or Ringer lactate intraoperatively

Postoperative fluid

Patients undergoing short procedures, with no bowel handling require fluids only for maintaining the starvation period of around 6 hours.

Most of the gynecologic or obstetric surgeries require fluid replacement for 6–12 hours depending on the extent and bowel handling.

If patients need IV fluids for routine maintenance alone, restrict the initial prescription to:
- 25–30 mL/kg/day of water and approximately 1 mmol/kg/day of potassium,

sodium and chloride, and approximately 50–100 g/day of glucose to limit starvation ketosis (this quantity will not address patients' nutritional needs).

Consider age, weight, vitals, hydration, renal status, drain, nasogastric aspiration, vomiting, insensible loss, pyrexia, loose motions, 3rd space loss while deciding quantity of IV fluid.

- 4–2–1 rule:
  - 0–10 kg—1 mL/kg/h
  - 11–20 kg—2 mL/kg/h
  - 21 + kg—4 mL/kg/h
- Administer 60 mL/h of fluid for the first 20 kg of body weight
- Next weight (Total-20)—1 mL/kg
- E.g. 58 kg—first 20 kg 60 mL/h + next 38 kg 60 mL/h = 100 mL/h
- Around 2.5 L/24 hours required

Body surface area method:
Surface area x 1,000 mL
E.g. 1.5 sq. m body surface area needs 1,500 mL

Postoperative fluid replacement should consider:
- Maintenance
- Deficit
- Loss
- Third space (Table 1).

Maintenance fluid

2.5 L of fluid can be distributed as about 1000 mL 5% D, 1000 mL RL and 500–1,000 mL 0.9% saline.

Measurement of the central venous pressure may be required for patients with:
- Poor cardiorespiratory reserve
- Where there have been large volumes of fluid administered
- Major fluid shifts are expected

Table 1: Fluid loss from the body

Loss	Amount of loss
Insensible	
• Normal skin	450 mL/h
• Normal lungs	450 mL/h
• Fever	20% per degree Celsius add
• Ventilation	450–675 mL
Gastric fluid	1–2 L/24 hours
Diarrheal fluid	Depends
Urine	Output calculation

Deficit

2 mL/kg/hour of starvation.

Loss

Because of the risk of inducing hyperchloremic acidosis in routine practice, when crystalloid resuscitation or replacement is indicated, balanced salt solutions, e.g. Ringer's lactate/acetate or Hartmann's solution should replace 0.9% saline, except in cases of hypochloremia, e.g. from vomiting or gastric drainage.

Solutions, such as 4%/0.18% dextrose/saline and 5% dextrose are important sources of free water for maintenance, but should be used with caution as excessive amounts may cause dangerous hyponatremia, especially in children and the elderly. These solutions are not appropriate for resuscitation or replacement therapy except in conditions of significant free water deficit, e.g. diabetes insipidus.

To meet maintenance requirements, adult patients should receive sodium 50–100 mmol/day, potassium 40–80 mmol/day in 1.5–2.5 L of water by the oral, enteral or parenteral route (or a combination of routes). Additional amounts should only be given to correct deficit or continuing losses. Careful monitoring should be undertaken using clinical examination, fluid balance charts, and regular weighing when possible.

4–2–1 rule tells about maintenance of fluids:
- 60 kg = 40 + 20 + 40 = 100 mL/h, i.e. 2400 mL/24 hours
- 5% D contains 170 cal/L, it is hypotonic and irritant to veins. Every individual has enough stored energy to maintain 1–2 days. Hence, in routine postoperative cases, there is no need to supply the required calories by dextrose. More important is fluid and electrolyte balance.

Contd...

Contd...

Hence, an ideal prescription postoperatively for maintainance is 2,500 mL of fluid distributed as 1,000 mL of 0.9% NS, 500–1,000 mL of Ringer lactate, 500–1,000 mL of 5% D
Ongoing losses and 3rd space loss needs to be replaced accordingly
(Glucose provides energy 4 kcal/gram, so as 5% glucose solution provides 0.2 kcal/mL. If prepared from dextrose monohydrate, which provides 3.4 kcal/gram, a 5% solution provides 0.17 kcal/mL).

Q. 2. If this patient complain of recurrent vomiting after being shifted to postoperative ward how do you proceed?

Postoperative vomiting could be reactionary, psychological, pathological.

Female sex has a predilection for vomiting.

It could be as a result of narcotic analgesic usage during surgery, use of neostigmine, prolonged surgery, etc. hypotension, emergency procedures when done on full stomach.

If happens after 2–3 days, intestinal problems should be kept in mind including paralytic ileus. Borborygmi vs silent abdomen differenciates between intestinal obstruction and paralytic ileus.

Radiological investigations may become necessary.

Immediately metoclopramide, ondansetrone are the commonly used drugs to treat postoperative nausea and vomiting. It is better to treat them as the retching may increase pain and disrupt the wound also (Table 2).

Table 2: Antiemetics and their dosage

Drug dose	Timing
Ondansetron	4–8 mg IV at end of surgery/SOS
Dolasetron	12.5 mg IV at end of surgery
Dexamethasone	5–10 mg IV before induction
Prochlorperazine	5–10 mg IV at end of surgery/SOS
Promethazine	12.5–25 mg IV at end of surgery/SOS
Metoclopramide	25 or 50 mg IV for prophylaxis/SOS

Q. 3. When do you mobilize this patient?

Mobilization needs to be done as early as possible. Once the anesthetic effect weans off the patient should start limb movements. By 6–8 hours the catheter may be disconnected and the patient may be encouraged to move to the toilet. If not atleast by the second day the patient should start moving.

Q. 4. How do you relieve her pain?

Pain relief is a very important component of postoperative management.
It could be done by:
- Epidural topups
- Postponing extubation (not in this patient)
- NSAID—in the form of injections or suppositories—paracetamol infusion, diclofenac 50 mg IM, diclofenac suppository may be used
- Mild opioids
- Strong opioids.

WHO analgesic ladder advises to start the analgesic management with paracetamol or other NSAIDs followed by weak opioids like codeine. Further, if necessary stronger opiod analgesics need to be used World Federation of Societies of Anesthesiologists (WFSA) gives a different kind of ladder approach. This is the reverse of what is given by WHO. Rationale being, initial postoperative discomfort requires stronger analgesics, hence, it recommends strong opioids and anesthetic blocks, followed by oral weak opioids and NSAIDs and later paracetamol alone.

Q. 5. How should you monitor this patient?

The patient needs to be monitored:
- ½ hourly for the first 2 hours, then
- 1 hourly for 2 hours, then
- 2 hourly for 2 hours, then
- 4 hourly for 24 hours, providing the woman's condition remains stable.

Conscious level, pulse, BP, abdominal urine output (30 mL/h), temperature, abdominal girth if internal bleeding is suspected, bowel sounds, vaginal bleeding, respiratory rate, basal creps need to be monitored.

Q. 6. What needs to be done on the second postoperative day?
- Apart from monitoring her vitals
- Total input and output to be tallied
- Look for basal creps which may indicate fluid overload
- Confirm oral initiation of food
- If intraoperative bleeding was more repeat her Hb% and decide on need for transfusion
- Mobilize her
- Catheter needs to be removed if not done already
- In cases of vaginal hysterectomy, vaginal pack if kept needs to be removed
- Perineorrhaphy needs to be attended.

(IV line >3 days needs to be replaced)
In LSCS breastfeeding and any congestion needs to be looked for:
- DVT
- Vaginal bleeding/foul smelling
- Abdominal wound.

Q. 7. When do you initiate oral feeds?
Initiation of oral liquids can be started as early as 4-6 hours once the bowel sounds are established and there is no postoperative nausea and vomiting (PONV). Better to start with sips of clear liquids followed by semisolids and later solids. This patient could be on soft bland diet from second day onwards.

Q. 8. When do you remove her catheter?
Bladder catheter may be removed as soon the patient may be ambulated or even otherwise if she is willing/cooperative to void in a bed pan.

If the output of 30 mL/hr is not there, better to prolong and keep a watch on the output, which may give a clue about failing kidneys, bladder injury or ureteric injuries.
- After catheter removal
- Some patients will pass urine normally
- Others may appear to do so but have a moderate amount of residual urine; and the third group will have obvious signs of retention may require recatheterization.

If after removal the patient is not able to void, because of pain, loss of sensation.

She may have to be recatheterized. Hence, it is better to remove after ascertaining all these issues (Table 3).

Intermittent clamping of the catheter is not proved to be of any benefit as per evidence but RCOG concludes by telling that the local policy may dictate this practice.

Table 3: Duration of postoperative catheterization

Procedure	Duration of catheterization
Uncomplicated abdomen Hysterectomy	12–24 hours
TAH with adhesions, bleeding	24–48 hours
TAH for PID, endometriosis	24–48 hours
Radical surgeries of pelvis	3–5 days
Radical surgery with extensive Ureteric/bladder dissection	10–14 days
VVF repair	2–3 weeks
Bladder injury repair	2–3 weeks
Mayo-Ward's operation	48–72 hours
NDVH/Fothergill's	12–24 hours
LSCS	8–12 hours in Routine cases

If the residual urine after spontaneous voiding is >100 mL it is significant and needs recatheterization. It is also recommended that the post void residue of <1/3 of the voided volume is desirable. If it is >1/3 of voided volume or the patient is not able to void in 4-6 hours voluntarily after catheter removal she needs recatheterization.

Q. 9. When do you do the suture removal and discharge her?
Patient may be discharged once she is able to take soft bland diet, ambulant and preferably passed her bowel and without any postoperative morbidity, which may be aroud 4th or 5th day.

Stapler/mattress sutures are removed on the 6th or 7th day in transverse incision and better to delay by 1-2 more days in vertical incisions.

If the patient needs extended catheterization still she could be discharged with an advise to keep a watch on the color and quantity of urine and to consume plenty of oral fluids.

Q. 10. If the patient complains of fever in the postoperative period what needs to be done?

Usually first 24 hours of surgery fever may not be viewed with seriousness except in cases of patients handled elsewhere or preoperatively infected patients.

In rest of the patients usually 3rd or 4th day fever could be due to UTI, in patients operated under GA, URTI, chronically debilitated patients LRTI, rarely fever due to some other added infection like viral/bacterial/protozoal infections may have to be considered.

Fever after 5th day may be most often due to wound infection, pelvic collection and abscess which needs vault drainage, draining from the abdominal wound, etc.

CASE 2

A 65-year-old hypertensive, diabetic patient posted for VH for procidentia had a preoperative Hb of 6.5 g/dL and was given 3 units of packed cell transfusions and with a Hb level of 11 g/dL was taken up for VH after 10 days of preoperative preparation.

There was a minimum blood loss during the procedure which took 2 hours, uneventful recovery, but postoperative day 8 patient came back with profuse bleeding PV, which was foul smelling too.

Q. 11. How do you manage this case?

This is most probably a case of secondary hemorrhage, presenting typically in the 2nd week of postoperative period.

- Primary hemorrhage—hemorrhage on the table, needs securing the bleeder
- Reactionary hemorrhage—occurring within 24 hours of surgery—usually due to loosening of ligatures, needs redoing the ligation

- Assess general condition.
- Secure IV line, start IV fluids, get CBC, urea, creatinine, arrange for transfusin if necessary
- Catheterize her bladder
- Gentle pelvic examination taking specimen for C/S
- If major bleeder seen, secure it, otherwise pack the vagina
- Start on broad spectrum antibiotics.

Q. 12. Is blood transfusion absolutely necessary if the Hb is 8 g/dL?

- If the Hb is >10 g% no need for transfusion
- Between 6–10 g% with no continued loss, and a stable patient, transfusion is not always necessary
- Hb <6 g, most often warrants blood transfusion
- Acute loss needs to be carefully handled and the quantity of loss in relation to total volume needs to be estimated whenever possible
- Excepting in patients with cardiac disease anemia with no continued blood loss does not always require blood transfusion. Evidence shows that transfusion donot improve the outcome and restricting transfusion donot increase the mortality or morbidity.

Other than that the quantity of loss and pre-existing diseases may dictate the need for transfusion as shown in Table 4.

Table 4: Clinical assessment of fluid loss

Volume loss	Clinical features	Co-morbidity	Need for blood transfusion
<15% of total	None	Not anemic earlier	No
15–30%	Tachycardia	Not anemic earlier	
		Anemic earlier/ cardiopulmonary disease	
		Yes	
>30%	Shock	Previously healthy	Volume replacement/ packed cell transfusion
>40%	Severe shock		Packed cell transfusion

Q. 13. Does this patient require any radiological assistance?

An USG examination to rule out vault collection, CT-MRI for the same reason, and also to rule of source of infection being a foreign body.

UAE may be considered in intractable bleeding if facilities are available (Table 5).

Table 5: Radiological investigations and their role in a postoperative patient

Radiological investigations could be required in a postoperative patient in a variety of situations both for diagnostic and therapeutic purposes.	
Ultrasound • Suspected intraperitoneal bleeding • Acute pain abdomen—suspected other organ pathology (gallstones, hydronephrosis, appendicitis, pancreatitis, etc.) • Sepsis—suspected vault collection • Intrauterine collections • Suspected ureteric injury • Guided aspirations • Anuria—bladder leak • Foreign body	**Uterine artery embolization** • Pelvic hemorrhage • Postpartum hemorrhage **CT/MRI** • To determine the nature of collection • Foreign body • Other pathology in doubt **X-ray** • Bowel injury/perforation suspected • IVP in suspected urinary system injury • Intestinal obstruction • Suspected opaque foreign body

Q. 14. What is the role of relaparotomy in this patient?

This patient probably does not require a relaparotomy.

But with a suspicion of abscess which may not be accessable from vagina, suspected bowel injury or heavy hemorrhage requiring ligation of anterior division of internal iliac artery, laparotomy may have to be done.

> **Other situations requiring relaparotomy**
>
> If reactionary hemorrhage is suspected and a strong confirmation is there depending on clinical deterioration, USG findings, and paracentesis, relaparotomy needs to be done.
>
> Peritoneal abscess formation requiring drainage or an unfortunate event of forgotten foreign body suspected bowel and bladder ureter injury, taking stitch through the bowel, etc. requires laparotomy. The need may be dictated by postoperative anuria, oliguria, fall of blood pressure, distension of the abdomen, persistent vomiting.

Q. 15. What is the importance of physiotherapy?

Physiotherapy is a very important intervention in the postoperative period.

This starts with limb movements and respiratory exercises in the form of deep breathing in the immediate postoperative period to early ambulation, sitting up, moving around, etc.

Some patients may feel embarrassed to move around with catheter, drainage tube but it should not be a limiting factor for ambulation. They should be moving with these attachments comfortably.

This helps to build confidence, prevents DVT, reduces the need for other interventions to prevent DVT, prevents respiratory morbidity etc.

Postvaginal surgery patients unless when associated with pelvic floor repair can immediately initiate pelvic floor exercises which helps in strengthening the support. Post PFR patients may have pain if pelvic floor exercises are initiated early.

Continued physical activity needs to be impressed upon them at the time of discharge.

Q. 16. What needs to be done to re-establish bowel movements?

The following can lead to delay in the bowel movements in postoperative patients

- A preoperative nil oral state coupled with bowel evacuation preoperatively
- Anesthesia and the drugs
- Postoperative hypokalemia
- Bowel handling leading on to decreased peristalsis
- Not allowing oral intake for longer periods
- This may lead to bowel distension with decreased bowel sounds, and may be of concern in a postoperative patient
- These can be managed with the following interventions
- Glycerine suppository—may help in passage of flatus
- Fiber rich diet—especially in vaginal procedures
- Reassure, avoid straining, prevent bowel movements especially in patients with perineal repair
- Stool softeners if rectal injury has occurred

> - Painless gaseous distension of the abdomen, with absent bowel sounds in a postoperative patient should rise the suspicion of paralytic ileus. This can lead to third space fluid loss, discomfort, vomiting, pain in the wound due to distension
> - Hypokalemia is one of the causes, hence potassium supplements if required or by avoiding oral feeding for 1–2 days would suffice to overcome this problem.

Q. 17. Should you consider anything else in this patient to prevent mortality?

This patient with age 70 years, preoperative anemia, prolonged hospitalization (immobilization), 2nd admission, bleeding and anemia, infective morbidity, hypertension and diabetes is at risk for VTE. We should consider thromboprophylaxis in this patient if not given during first admission. But needs to be postponed for 6–12 hours after the cessation of bleeding (Table 6).

Table 6: Risk classification for thrombosis

Level of risk	Situation
Low risk	Minor surgeries in patients <40 years with no additional risk factors

Contd...

Contd...

Level of risk	Situation
Moderate risk	Minor surgeries in patients with additional risk factors Nonmajor surgeries in patients aged 40–60 years with no additional risk factors Major surgeries in patients <40 years with no additional risk factors
High risk	• Nonmajor surgeries in patients >60 years or with additional risk factors • Major surgeries in patients >40 years or with additional risk factors
Highest risk	Major surgeries in patients >40 years plus prior VTE, cancer or molecular hypercoagulable state

Q. 18. What are the methods available for thromboprophylaxis?

The preventive strategies could be grouped as mechanical and medical.

- Clinical: Early ambulation, correction of anaemia, infection prevention
- Mechanical: Graduated compression stockings, intermittent pneumatic compression (which can start intraoperatively itself)
- Medical: Aspirin, unfractionated or low molecular weight heparin, oral anticoagulants, fondaparinux.

Table 7 shows the methods of thromboprophylaxis

Table 7: Methods of thromboprophylaxis

Low-risk patients
Undergoing gynecologic surgery does not require specific prophylaxis other than early ambulation

In high-risk patients
• Unfractionated heparin (5,000 U) should be administered eight hours before surgery and continued postoperatively until discharge • Dalteparin (5,000 antifactor-Xa U) should be administered 12 hours before surgery and once a day thereafter • Enoxaparin (40 mg) should be administered 12 hours before surgery and once a day thereafter

Contd...

Contd...

Alternative

Pneumatic compression should be placed intra-operatively and continued until the patient is fully ambulatory

Moderate-risk patients

- Unfractionated heparin (5,000 U) should be administered two hours before surgery and continued postoperatively every eight hours until the patient is discharged
- Low-molecular-weight heparin (dalteparin, 2,500 antifactor-Xa U, or enoxaparin, 40 mg) should be administered 12 hours before surgery and once a day postoperatively until the patient is discharged

Alternatives

- Thigh-high graduated compression stockings should be placed intraoperatively and continued until the patient is fully ambulatory
- Pneumatic compression should be placed intraoperatively and continued until the patient is fully ambulatory

CASE 3

A primi aged 35 years was admitted with severe preeclampsia and gross abdominal wall edema at 37 weeks of gestation with breech presentation. Her Hb was 7 g/dL, albumin being 2 g/dL. Her prepregnancy weight was 87 kg taking her BMI to 33.2 kg/m².

Post-emergency LSCS 2 units of packed cells transfused. Patient had intractable cough from 3rd postoperative day, which subsided with treatment on 6th day. After removal of sutures on the 7th day from the pfannensteil incision she noticed serosanguinous discharge from the wound with a sensation of something giving way.

Q. 19. What is your first consideration? Why?

A serious consideration should be made on burst abdomen.

A burst abdomen is considered present, when intestine, omentum or other viscera's were seen in the abdominal wound following surgery. Describes partial or complete postoperative separation of an abdominal wound closure with protrusion or evisceration of the abdominal contents. Observational incidence in the tertiary hospital varies between 0.2 and 3%. It occurs mostly between the sixth and eight day after operation.

She has many of the risk factors like anemia, hypoproteinemia, obesity (not totally proven), abdominal wall edema, emergency surgery, postoperative cough and the symptoms of something giving with a serosanguinous discharge is a hallmark of burst abdomen (Table 8).

Table 8: Factors relating to the incidence of burst abdomen

Technical issues	Events	Pre-existing conditions
<ul><li>Failure to close the abdominal wall properly</li><li>Suture material/knots</li><li>Closure (peritoneal closure not crucial)</li><li>Incision (more with vertical)</li></ul>	<ul><li>Peritonitis</li><li>Wound infection</li><li>Coughing</li><li>Vomiting</li><li>Distension</li></ul>	<ul><li>Malnourishment</li><li>Malignant obstructive jaundice</li><li>Obesity</li><li>Diabetes mellitus</li><li>Hypoproteinemia</li><li>Anemia</li><li>Immunocompromised patients</li></ul>

Partial or complete separation of an abdominal wound with protrusion (evisceration) of abdominal contents

- Partial—separation of fascial edges without evisceration—loose fascial sutures—occasionally, fibrin covered intestinal loops
- Complete—full separation of fascia and skin—intestinal loops (if not glued by fibrin) eviscerated Burst abdomen = Abdominal dehiscence

Q. 20. What is the difference between burst abdomen and incisional hernia?

Dehiscence and incisional hernia are differentiated by the condition of the skin on them. It also depends on the timing of presentation.

- *Incisional hernia*
  - Occurs after complete healing of the surgical site
  - Not an emergency (except with strangulation)
  - Skin is closed
- *Burst abdomen*
  - Occurs by the first weekend of surgery
  - Emergency situation
  - Skin is open.

Q. 21. How do you manage this patient?

This patient needs immediate surgical intervention.

Emergency measures include trying to replace the herniated contents inside and securing with a bandage taking all aseptic precautions. Keeping the contents moist by instilling saline.

Arranging blood and components if required.

A senior surgeon should operate.

Extent of dissection depends on whether it is partial or complete.

Remove the skin sutures in the area where you suspect the burst. Remove the dressings and gently explore the depths of his wound with a sterile gloved finger. Open it down its whole length by removing all the skin sutures. You will soon find out what has happened. If you confirm a burst abdomen, remove all sutures from the fascial layers. Try to insert your finger between his parietal peritoneum and his underlying gut and omentum. In this way you should be able to mobilize enough of his abdominal wall to take some more sutures.

Though the multilayer closure of laparotomy wounds with vicryl has been the standard practice, it is accompanied by a high rate of wound dehiscence (3.88–14%). The recent experimental and clinical studies have reported a significant reduction in the incidence of burst abdomen by using a single layer closure of laparotomy incisions with a nonabsorbable suture material. The incidence of burst abdomen with this technique varies from 0 to 0.9%.

Hence, closure with nonabsorbable monofilament sutures enmass may be with Smed Jone's technique has been recommemded. Suture removal may be done on 10th postoperative day.

Needs to be covered with higher antibiotics.

Conservative management options
- Saline-soaked gauze dressings
- Negative pressure wound therapy

Operative management options:
- Temporary closure options (open abdomen treatment)
- Primary closure with various suture techniques
- Closure with application of relaxing incisions
- Synthetic (nonabsorbable and absorbable) and biological meshes
- Tissue flaps.

Q. 22. If this patient develops post-repair abdominal distension, what possibilities needs to be considered? How to manage?

Ryle's tube insertion is required in:
- Bowel injuries/repairs
- Intestinal obstruction
- Pancreatitis
- Unconscious patients
- Surgery in full stomach
- Paralytic ileus
- Acute gastric dilatation
- It could be removed after the bowel sounds are well established, swallowing reflex is established, flatus/feces passed, no vomiting.

There is a possibility that because of exposure, desiccation of tissues, handling of bowel there could be paralytic ileus is this patient.

This may require withholding orally for a couple of days. Ryle's tube aspiration, monitoring abdominal girth. Decompression with periodic aspiration is necessary to prevent repair disruption.

Ryle's tube is used both for feeding/aspiration.

Feeding is initiated with clear water, then milk/semisolids and later mashed solids.

Q. 23. What is the roll of postoperative counseling to manage the unforeseen complications?

All the relatives and even the patient would be anxious to know about the outcome of any surgery. Hence, it is very essential to interact with the attendants:
- Success of the procedure
- Complications if any
- Additional procedures if done
- Change in the diagnosis
- Possibility of need for further treatment
- Any deviation from what they have been counseled preoperatively.
- Any life threatening situation
- Need for ICU care
- Unexpected need for transfusion
- Crtical period wherein outcome is not guaranteed.

Above aspects need to be discussed and recording of the counseling procedure also is important.

If facilities are not adequate in the hospital where surgery has been done to manage the complications, better to offer the patient to shift the patient to another well equipped hospital at the earliest.

Q. 24. How do you take care of the surgical wound?

If a *drainage tube* has been inserted to prevent formation of a hematoma, this is removed as the surgeon instructed, usually after 24 hours.

The *dressing* would remain undisturbed until sutures are removed, unless dressing is soaked with blood or discharge. Some surgeons believe in leaving the wound open also.

Sutures/clips are removed from a transverse incision earlier than from a midline incision.

Following their removal, the patient may have a bath and the wound is left dry.

Bibliography

1. Begum B, Zaman R, Ahmed M, et al. Burst abdomen: A preventable morbidity. Mymensingh Med J. 2008;17(1):63-6.
2. Calculating Parenteral Feedings D. Chen-Maynard at California State University, San Bernardino. Retrieved September 2010. HSCI 368.
3. Cayley WE, Jr. Preventing deep vein thrombosis in hospital inpatients. Clinical Review. BMJ. 2007;335(7611):147-51. doi:10.1136/bmj.39247.542477.AE
4. CN Hudson, Setchell ME. Shaw's textbook of operative Gynaecology, 7th edition, Elsevier, India.
5. Cotton MH, Kobusingye O, Post S, et al. Primary surgery. Non-trauma. Surgery for sepsis, Burst abdomen (wound dehiscence). Global Help, ICES. Ch 4; Vol 1.
6. Hoffman BL, Schorge JO, Schaffer JI. William's Gynaecology. 2nd edition.
7. Intravenous fluid therapy in adults in hospital. NICE guidelines. [CG174] Published date: December 2013.
8. Liumbruno GM, Bennardello F, Lattanzio A, et al. Recommendations for the transfusion management of patients in the peri-operative period. The post-operative period. The Italian Society of Transfusion Medicine and Immunohaematology (SIMTI) Working Party. Blood Transfus. 2011;9(3):320-35.
9. Mathur SK. Burst abdomen. A preventable complication, monolayer closure of the abdominal incision with monofilament nylon. J Postgrad Med. 1983;29:223.
10. McCracken G, Houston P, Lefebvre G. Guideline for the management of postoperative nausea and vomiting. Society of Obstetricians and Gynecologists of Canada.J Obstet Gynaecol Can. 2008;30(7):600-7.
11. Powell-Tuck J, Gosling P, Dileep N, et al. British Consensus Guidelines on Intravenous Fluid Therapy for Adult Surgical Patients. GIFTASUP. Last Updated: 04 June 2012.
12. RCOG: Voiding problems post-vaginal surgery (query bank). Published: 03/02/2014
13. Ressel GW. ACOG practice bulletin on preventing deep venous thrombosis and

pulmonary embolism. Am Fam Physician. 2001;63(11):2279-80.
14. Rock JA, Jones HW. Te Linde's Operative Gynecology Series. 10th edition. Wolters Kluwer Health/Lippincott Williams & Wilkins.
15. Sanjay Pandya. Practical guidelines on fluid therapy. 2nd edition.
16. van Ramshorst GH, et al. Therapeutic alternatives for burst abdomen. Surg Technol Int. 2010;19:111-9.
17. Waqar SH, Malik ZI, Razzaq A, et al. Frequency and risk factors for wound dehiscence/burst abdomen in midline laparotomies. J Ayub Med Coll Abbottabad. 2005;17(4):70-3.
18. Williamson J. Management of postoperative urinary retention. 2005;101(29):53.
19. Women and newborn health service. King edward memorial hospital care. Following major gynaecology, oncology or urogynacology surgery.

29
CHAPTER

Primary Amenorrhea

S Ratnakumar

CASE 1

A 17-year-old unmarried girl studying in school was brought to the gynecology OPD by her mother with the complaint of not having attained menarche. She is the only girl child in the family and she has an elder brother who is 19 years old.

Visibly she has normal feminine appearance with normally developed secondary sexual characteristics. Her voice is feminine; her intelligence is normal for her age. She says her academic performance is good and usually comes within the first five ranks in her class.

Her mother attained menarche at the age of 13 years. There is nobody in the family with similar complaints.

Q. 1. From this history, what would be the initial diagnosis?

First diagnosis would be primary amenorrhea. But pregnancy also has to be kept in mind.

Q. 2. Define primary amenorrhea.

Primary amenorrhea is considered when:
a. She has not menstruated by the age 14 years and also lacks other evidence of pubertal development like absence of pubic hair and breast development.
b. She has not menstruated by the age 16 even in the presence of other pubertal signs.

Q. 3. What further history is required?

Further history to be taken includes:
- Family history of delayed menarche
- Age of development of breast and pubic and axillary hair
- History of cyclical lower abdominal pain
- Dietary and eating habits—starvation and excessive eating habits
- Whether she is in athletics or takes very strenuous exercise
- History of drug intake
- Chemotherapy or radiation
- Hirsutism, acne
- Significant headaches or vision changes
- Temperature intolerance, palpitations, diarrhea, constipation, tremor, depression, and skin changes.

Q. 4. Name some drugs which can cause primary amenorrhea.

- Drugs that stimulate prolactin excretion
- Antipsychotics, such as phenothiazine derivatives
- Tricyclic antidepressants
- Antihypertensives like reserpine and methyldopa.

Q. 5. How do you classify primary amenorrhea?

There are many ways in which primary amenorrhea is classified. The two commonly used classifications are:

I: **Clinical classification** in which the condition is classified according to the presence or absence of breast and uterus.

Breast development absent uterus present
- Constitutional delay of puberty
- Hypothalamic dysfunction
- Extreme physical, psychological and/or nutritional stress
- Chronic illness
- Pituitary failure
- Gonadal dysgenesis
- Gonadal failure
- Gonadotropin deficiency
- Kallmann's syndrome

Breast development present uterus present
- Hyperandrogenic amenorrhea (PCOS)
- Hypothalamic dysfunction
- Hypothyroidism
- Hyperprolactinemia
- Obstruction (imperforate hymen/transverse vaginal septum)

Breast development present uterus absent
- Androgen insensitivity
- Agenesis (Mayer-Rokitansky-Kuster-Hauser syndrome)

II: **Classification system presented by WHO** divides patients into groups based on endogenous estrogen production, follicle-stimulating hormone (FSH) levels, prolactin levels, and hypothalamic-pituitary dysfunction.

According to this classification, primary amenorrhea is classified into:
- Group I: Low estrogen, low FSH, and no hypothalamic-pituitary pathology, hypogonadotropic hypogonadism
- Group II: Normal estrogen, normal FSH, and normal prolactin—polycystic ovary syndrome
- Group III: Low estrogen and high FSH—gonadal failure.

Q. 6. Describe the physical examination that need to be done in a girl with primary amenorrhea.

- Height and weight, and calculation of body mass index (BMI)
- Evaluation of secondary sexual characters like breast and pubic hair development using Tanner's method (presence of axillary or pubic hair indicates that adrenarche has occurred).

Evaluation of breast development by Tanner method

Tanner I
No glandular tissue: Areola follows the skin contours of the chest (prepubertal) (typically age 10 and younger)

Tanner II
Breast bud forms, with small area of surrounding glandular tissue; areola begins to widen (10–11.5)

Tanner III
Breast begins to become more elevated, and extends beyond the borders of the areola, which continues to widen but remains in contour with surrounding breast (11.5–13)

Tanner IV
Increased breast size and elevation; areola and papilla form a secondary mound projecting from the contour of the surrounding breast (13–15)

Tanner V
Breast reaches final adult size; areola returns to contour of the surrounding breast, with a projecting central papilla (15+)

Evaluation of pubic hair development by Tanner method

Tanner I
No pubic hair at all (prepubertal state) (typically age 10 and younger)

Tanner II
Small amount of long, downy hair with slight pigmentation at the base of the penis and scrotum (males) or on the labia majora (females) (10–11.5)

Tanner III
Hair becomes more coarse and curly, and begins to extend laterally (11.5–13)

Tanner IV
Adult-like hair quality, extending across pubis but sparing medial thighs (13–15)

Tanner V
Hair extends to medial surface of the thighs (15+)

- Checking for breast secretion by applying pressure to all sections of the breast, beginning at the base and moving toward the nipple.

- Evidence of virilization including hirsutism
- Temporal balding
- Acne
- Voice deepening
- Increased muscle mass
- Clitoromegaly
- Enlarged thyroid gland, bradycardia and delayed reflexes (Hypothyroidism)
- Presence of supraclavicular fat and abdominal striae with hypertension (Cushing's syndrome)
- Look for presence of short stature, webbed neck, low-set hairline and/or ears, cubitus valgus, nail hypoplasia, short fourth metacarpal, high-arched palate, chronic otitis media, cardiac abnormalities all being stigmata of Turner's syndrome.

Q. 7. What information can be obtained from examination of genitalia and pelvic examination?

- Pattern of the hair—a sparse or absent female hair pattern will indicate lack of adrenarche or androgen insensitivity syndrome
- Male pattern of hair distribution is more in favor of androgen excess
- Pelvic examination may help detect imperforate hymen, a transverse vaginal septum, or vaginal or uterine aplasia
- Thin and pale vaginal mucosa with absent rugae is evidence of estrogen deficiency.

Q. 8. What is clitoral index?

The clitoral index is the product of the sagittal and transverse diameters of the glans of the clitoris in the anteroposterior and transverse diameter.

A clitoral index greater than 35 mm^2 is evidence of increased androgen effect. A clitoral index greater than 100 mm^2 is evidence of virilization.

Q. 9. What pertinent initial investigations need to be done for this patient?

Flowchart 1 summarizes the overall work-up or primary amenorrhea work-up.

- Routine blood and urine examination
- Urine pregnancy test and/or pelvic ultrasound
- Serum TSH and prolactin levels
- Serum FSH and LH
- Serum estriol.

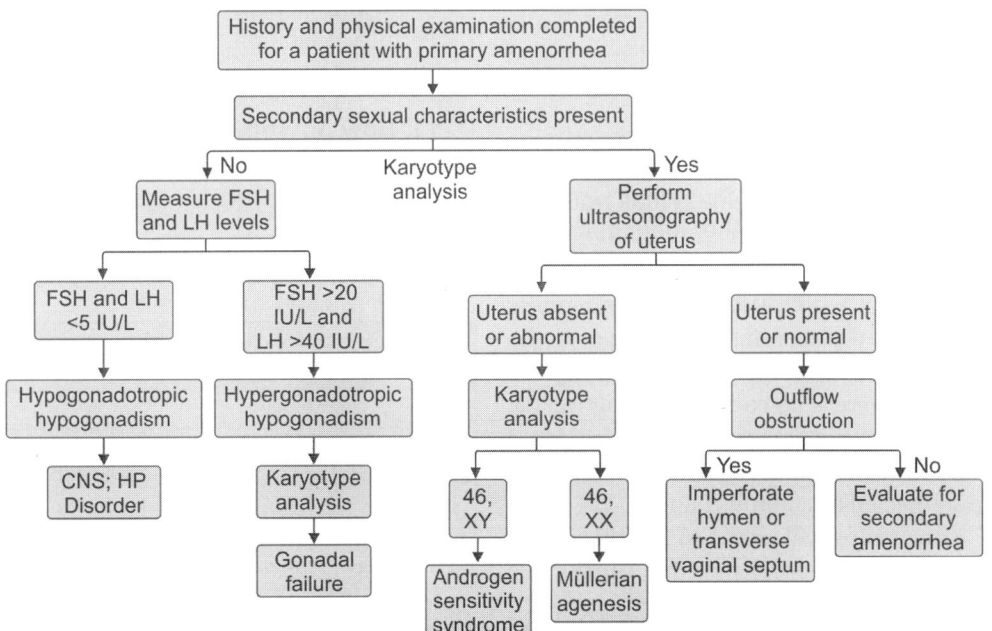

Flowchart 1: Summary of a primary amenorrhea workup

Q. 10. What further investigations are indicated?

Transabdominal or transvaginal ultrasound is performed to confirm normal anatomy and aids in the diagnosis of most structural abnormalities. Transvaginal is the preferred modality, if possible, to evaluate endometrial thickness.

MRI is the most effective tool for characterising specific structural abnormalities and may prevent the need for surgical diagnosis. Previously, a combined hysteroscopy and laparoscopy differentiated a bicornuate uterus from a septate or didelphic uterus. With MRI, this invasive approach can be avoided. On MRI, Müllerian agenesis (Mayer-Rokitansky-Kuster-Hauser syndrome) or asymmetrical fusion defects of the Mullerian system (unicornuate uterus) can be identified as well as renal anomalies, which can occur in up to 30% of these patients.

If prolactin levels are significantly elevated, cranial MRI is indicated to rule out pituitary adenoma.

Bone density measurement may be indicated in selected patients. Bone age is an additional test conducted in patients with delayed puberty.

Skeletal abnormalities may also be found with MRKH/Müllerian abnormalities.

Q. 11. Her blood and hormonal levels are normal. But ultrasound reveals absent uterus with a blunt vagina. What would be your diagnosis and further management?

- This could be Mayer-Rokitansky syndrome (MRS) in which the SSC are normally developed and even the external genitalia may appear normal. Digital probing will reveal there is no communicating vagina. Uterus is usually absent and is represented by nodular structures which may be connected by a fibrous band.
- Karyotyping will reveal 46 XX; this would also rule out other possible causes like Turner's syndrome (XO) and androgen insensitivity syndrome (AIS) (46 XY).
- The next step would be to confirm the absence of uterus and the condition of the ovaries. A diagnostic laparoscopy will generally show a normal well-developed tube and ovaries. The uterine nodules, their number and their connection will be confirmed during this procedure.
- Once the diagnosis is confirmed, the girl and the parents need to be counseled as to the girl's condition. It should be made clear that she cannot menstruate or conceive but there are options for marriage and sexual life by constructing a vagina.
- Since the ovaries are functioning, she can go for surrogate conception.

Q. 12. What are the types of vaginoplasty available?

The various available techniques are:
- Balloon vaginoplasty
- Buccal mucosa
- Colovaginoplasty
- McIndoe technique
- William's vaginoplasty
- Labia minora flap
- Perineal dilatation
- Vecchietti procedure.

Q. 13. How do you differentiate between Mullerian agenesis and androgen insensitivity syndrome (AIS)?

See Table 1.

Table 1: Differentiate features of Müllerian agenesis and androgen insensitivity syndrome (AIS).

Characteristics	Müllerian agenesis	AIS
Karyotype	46 XX	46 XY
Heredity	Not known	Maternal X-linked recessive
Development of sexual hair	Normal female pattern	Absent or sparse

Contd...

Characteristics	Müllerian agenesis	AIS
Testosterone level	Normal female level	Normal to slightly elevated male level
Gonadal neoplasia	No increase	5% incidence of malignancy

Source: Modified from Speroff L, Fritz MA. Clinical Gynecology, endocrinology and infertility, 7th edition, pp. 421.

CASE 2

A 16-year-old obese, short statured girl was brought with the complaints of not having attained menarche. On examination, she has webbed neck and wide carrying angle. The pubic and axillary hair is absent and the secondary sexual characters are minimal.

Q. 14. What would be your initial diagnosis?

The clinical picture suggests Turner's syndrome.

Q. 15. How would you proceed further?

The initial test would be karyotyping. At least 10% of cells should reveal complete or partial loss of sex chromosome. Abnormalities include non-mosaic 45, X; mosaic 45, X and fragmented X or Y.

Q. 16. What further tests are advised?

Bone age assessment by radiography—usually 2 years less than chronological age.

Echocardiograph: Coarctation of the aorta may present in the neonatal period with cardiac failure or with hypertension. Bicuspid aortic valve occurs in approximately 30% of patients.

Serum FSH and anti-Müllerian hormone (AMH): Elevated FSH and reduced AMH predicts ovarian failure.

Pelvic ultrasound: Usually reveals immature or infantile uterus with streak gonads.

Renal ultrasound: Renal structural abnormalities affect approximately 25% of patients with Turner's syndrome.

Thyroid function test (TFT): Could have hypothyroidism or hyperthyroidism. Autoimmune thyroid disease (Hashimoto's thyroiditis and, less commonly, Graves' disease) is a common complication in Turner's syndrome.

Q. 17. What is mid-parental height prediction and how is it calculated?

A child's growth is related strongly to his or her genetic potential, and the growth deficit has to be assessed using the mid-parental height prediction to identify the girl's genetic growth track.

The mid-parental height in a girl is calculated as follows:

Height of mother in centimeters + height of father in centimeters/5.1–6.4 cm.

Q. 18. What would be the line of management in this girl of 16 years once Turner's syndrome is confirmed?

Low dose estrogen: Estradiol 0.5–2 mg orally once daily. If there is no potential for further growth or if there is no evidence of a rapidly advancing bone age, the dose of estradiol is increased gradually, over approximately 2 years, to a full adult dose and/or until breast development is satisfactory.

Micronized progesterone: 100–200 mg orally once daily on the last 10 days of the menstrual cycle.

Cyclic progesterone is added to estrogen therapy once there is breakthrough bleeding or when the patient is on a full adult dose of estrogen treatment to induce menstruation. Treatment for the last 2 weeks of a 3-month cycle is also an option. Cardiovascular assessment and evaluation for surgery.

Q. 19. What are the outflow tract abnormalities associated with primary amenorrhea?

- Vaginal septum
- Imperforate hymen
- Labial fusion.

Q. 20. What is hypogonadotropic hypogonadism?

In hypogonadotropic hypogonadism the primary abnormality lies in the hypothalamic-pituitary axis. The FSH and LH levels are though low will still be in the detectable range (<5 mIU/mL). However, in conditions like Kallmann's syndrome, the levels may be undetectable due to absence of hypothalamic secretion.

Q. 21. What is Kallmann's syndrome? How is it diagnosed and managed?

This syndrome can be inherited as an C-linked, autosomal dominant or autosomal recessive disorder.

The characteristics include:

Delayed development of secondary sexual characteristics, anosmia and is difficult to distinguish from constitutional delay.

The patient appears as a normal phenotypic female with normal but infantile external and internal genitalia.

- **Serum hCG:** Negative
- **Serum FSH:** Low
- **Serum estradiol:** Low
- **Serum TSH:** Normal
- **Serum prolactin:** Normal
- **Serum LH:** Low
- **Pelvic ultrasound:** Prepubertal uterus with thin endometrial echo-complex
- **MRI brain:** Absent olfactory bulb, possible hypoplastic olfactory sulci
- **Dual energy X-ray absorptiometry (DXA) scan:** Low bone density.

(In all hormonal studies, results are unreliable if patient is taking any form of hormonal therapy).

Serum FSH and LH levels can be normalized by pulsatile infusion of GnRH. Similarly exogenous administration of gonadotropins will stimulate uterine activity resulting in endometrial hypertrophy. There is good response to ovulation induction when human chorionic gonadotropin is used.

Q. 22. What is congenital adrenal hyperplasia? How is it diagnosed?

Congenital adrenal hyperplasia (CAH) is a condition in which normal corticosteroid synthesis by the adrenal cortex is impaired. The most common enzyme deficiency is 21-hydroxylase deficiency. The most common variety is adult onset or late onset CAH.

CAH is suspected in girls who are virilized at birth, who become virilized postnatally, or who have precocious puberty or adrenarche.

The first line of tests include:

- Serum 17- hydroxy progesterone which is elevated for the age
- Hyponatremia, hyperkalemic, metabolic acidosis and azotemia
- Rapid ACTH stimulation test
- Karyotype or FISH (indicated in newborns with ambiguous genitalia) XX or XY
- Clinically, there will be varying degrees of masculinization depending on the degree of circulating androgen
- Vagina is generally present but the external genitalia may vary from fused labia to stenosis of the lower third of vagina
- Internal genitalia are normal
- Pubertal enlargement of clitoris may be the first indication for suspecting CAH.

Bibliography

1. Bader TJ. Obs/Gyn Secrets, 3rd edition, Mosby; 2005.
2. Gunasheela S. Practical management of gynecological problems, 2nd edition, Jaypee Brothers; 2011.
3. Hoffman BL, Schorge JO, Schaffer JI, et al. William's Gynecology, 2nd edition, New York: McGraw Hill; 2012.
4. Monga A (Ed). Gynecology by ten teachers. 18th edition, Book Power; 2006.
5. Speroff L, Fritz MA. Clinical gynecology, endocrinology and infertility, 7th edition, Lippincott Williams and Wilkins; 2005.

30

Secondary Amenorrhea

Anupama Hari

CASE SCENARIO

A 22-year-old girl from Miriyalguda, Nalgonda district came to gynecology OPD with a chief complaint of 7 months of absence of menstruation. She was unmarried, studying B. Com second year. She is a product of non-consanguineous marriage.

Present history of amenorrhea was preceded by infrequent menstrual cycles once in 3–4 months, lasting for 3–4 days, very scanty bleeding since menarche. There was history of gradual weight gain and abnormal facial hair (hirsutism) and recurrent pimples. There was no history suggestive of thyroid disorder, eating disorder and any long-term drugs or steroid use. There was no loss of appetite. Bowel and bladder functions were normal.

Past History

No past history suggestive of tuberculosis, diabetes, hypertension, bronchial asthma, thyroid disorder, epilepsy and head injury.

Family History

Both of her parents have type 2 diabetes and no history of thyroid disorder. She is the second child in the family. Her elder sister has infrequent menstrual cycles.

Personal History

No drug addiction, alcohol or smoking. Takes mixed diet.

Menstrual History

She attained menarche at 12th year. Since then, her cycles were irregular and scanty, i.e. 2–3 days/3–4 months. She is now ended with 7 months of amenorrhea.

General Examination

Her general condition is fair. Her height is 155 cm, weight 87 kg, BMI is 34 kg/m^2. Scanty scalp hair. Feminine voice. Hirsutism FG scoring >10. Acne vulgaris present. No thyroid swelling. Secondary sexual characters (Figs 1 and 2): breast—Tanner 4; axillary and pubic hair are of adult type; no abdominal striae; abdominal obesity present; abdominal hair present; waist circumference—105 cm, hip circumference—92 cm, waist: hip ratio—1.1; external genitalia are normal; No clitoromegaly seen; PV and PR not done.

Summary of the Case

A 22-year-old girl came with a chief complaint of 7 month amenorrhea with prior oligomen-

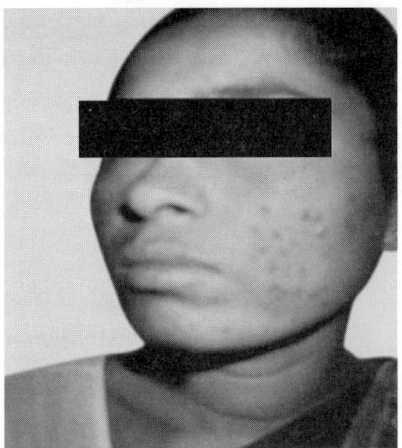

Fig. 1: Acne vulgaris

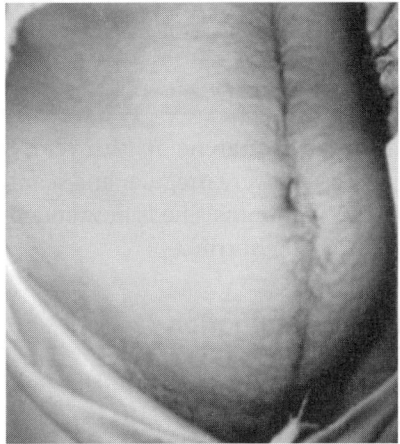

Fig. 2: Hirsutism

orrhic cycles with obesity, hirsutism and acne. Provisional diagnosis: secondary amenorrhea is due to polycystic ovarian syndrome (PCOS).

Investigations

Hb: 11.5 g%; CBP: Normal; T3: 0.92 ng/mL; T4: 9.67 μg/dL; TSH: 1.26 μIU/mL; serum prolactin: 12.4 μg/L; serum free testosterone: 86 ng/dL; fasting blood sugar: 95 mg/dL; FSH: 2.4 IU/L; LH, 10.2 IU/L; serum estradiol 50 pg/mL.

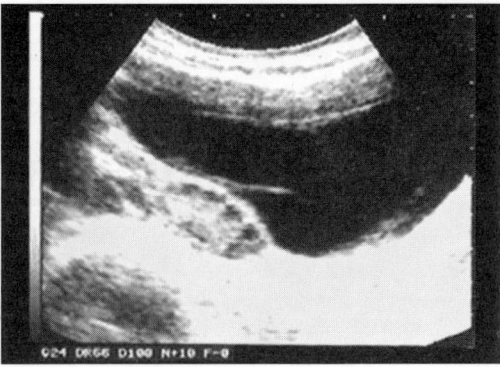

Fig. 3: Polycystic ovaries

Ultrasound abdomen revealed bilateral polycystic ovaries with necklace pattern of immature follicles (Fig. 3). Uterus normal size, anteverted with endometrial thickness of 6 mm.

Final Diagnosis

Secondary amenorrhea due to PCOS.

Case Discussion

Q. 1. How do you define oligomenorrhea?

When the menstrual cycle lasts longer than 35 days, it is called oligomenorrhea.[1]

Q. 2. When do you call it secondary amenorrhea?

In a menstruating woman, the absence of periods for 6 months is called secondary amenorrhea.[2]

Q. 3. What is WHO classification of causes of secondary amenorrhea?

WHO classified the causes of secondary amenorrhea as follows:[3]

The causes of secondary (Table 1) amenorrhea can be classified compartment-wise[2] (Table 2).

Table 1: WHO classification of secondary amenorrhea

	Estrogen	FSH level	Prolactin	Lesion
WHO group 1	Low	Normal or low	Normal	Pituitary–Hypothalamic
WHO group 2	Normal	Normal	Normal	Uterine
WHO group 3	Low	Elevated	Normal	Gonads

Table 2: Compartmental classification of secondary amenorrhea

	Causes	Examples
Compartment 1	Disorders of outflow tract or uterus	Asherman's syndrome, secondary cervical stenosis due to cervical operations
Compartment 2	Disorders of ovary	Turner's mosaicism, premature ovarian failure due to 47XXY; 47XXX female, radiation and chemotherapy
Compartment 3	Disorders of anterior pituitary	Pituitary adenomas, head and neck radiation/surgery, hyperprolactinemia, Sheehan's syndrome
Compartment 4	CNS disorders	Anorexia nervosa, bulimia nervosa, exercise, post-pill amenorrhea

Q. 4. In your case, you mentioned family history of type 2 diabetes in the parents. Is it relevant to the present diagnosis?

Yes. There is a strong positive correlation of PCOS and family history of type 2 diabetes. Both PCOS and type 2 diabetes are manifestations of insulin resistance syndrome.

Q. 5. How thyroid disorders are relevant to secondary amenorrhea?

Hyperthyroidism usually results in oligomenorrhea and amenorrhea due to increased metabolism of sex hormones.[4]

Q. 6. What are the eating disorders related to amenorrhea? How do you differentiate them?

Anorexia nervosa and bulimia nervosa. Both are seen in young women. Anorexia nervosa is primarily denying to taking food. Bulimia is episodic binge eating followed by self-induced vomiting. Both result in cachexia and secondary amenorrhea.[2]

Q. 7. How do you clinically diagnose anorexia nervosa?
- Age onset—10–13 years
- Weight loss of 25% or weight 15% below normal for age and height.
- Special attitudes—denial, distorted body image, unusual handling of food
- Clinically—lanugo, bradycardia, episodes of bulimia and self-induced vomiting, amenorrhea, low BP, hypercarotenemia and diabetes insipidus.[2]

Q. 8. Why secondary amenorrhea is common in athletes?

High energy output and stress on low-body fat leads to suppression of menstrual function, via leptin.[5]

Q. 9. Mention the adrenal causes of secondary amenorrhea?

Cushing syndrome, adrenal tumors, ectopic ACTH producing tumors, thymus (Case report).

An 18-year-old girl presented with secondary amenorrhea of seven months duration. She had clinical features suggestive of Cushing syndrome. On further examination and investigations, a superior mediastinal tumor, was found which was the source of ectopic ACTH secretion, causing secondary amenorrhea. After complete surgical excision, the tumor was subjected to histopathological examination which revealed a thymus carcinoid. There were no clinical symptoms related to carcinoid syndrome in the patient. After surgery, she regained menstrual cyclicity. Ectopic hormone production as a cause of amenorrhea, though rare, should not be forgotten.

Q. 10. What are the drugs causing oligomenorrhea and secondary amenorrhea?

Drugs causing hyperprolactinemia lead to oligomenorrhea and secondary amenorrhea. All chemotherapeutic agents also cause secondary amenorrhea through inhibition of cell mitosis.

Q. 11. How tuberculosis can result in secondary amenorrhea?

Pelvic tuberculosis causes tuberculous endometritis leading to Asherman's syndrome. Tuberculous hypophysitis leads to hypogonadotropic secondary amenorrhea.

Q. 12. How can you say that your case is PCOS?

Presenting symptom is secondary amenorrhea with previous oligomenorrhic cycles, with signs of hyperandrogenism like hirsutism and acne formation. There is positive family history of type 2 diabetes and PCOS.

Q. 13. Is there any difference between PCOD and PCOS?

PCOD is a radiological diagnosis. PCOS is a syndrome which includes PCOD.

Q. 14. Mention few conditions where you can see PCOD on ultrasound?

Multifollicular ovaries look like PCO on ultrasound-seen in conditions, such as peripubertal, central precocious puberty; lactation; hyperprolactinemia and hypothyroidism;[6] late onset of congenital adrenal hyperplasia.[7] Antiepileptic drugs especially sodium valproate; clomiphene citrate and gonadotropins.

Q. 15. What are the ultrasonic criteria to diagnose PCOD?[6]

Refer Table 3.

Table 3: USG criteria for PCOS

External morphological signs	Internal morphological signs
Increased ovarian volume >10 mm	>8 follicles of <10 mm in size
Increased sphericity index (ovary width: ovary length) ≥0.7	Peripheral repartition of the follicles
Decreased uterine width /ovarian length (U : O) = <1	Increased echogenicity of ovarian stroma

Q.16. How do you differentiate between multifollicular ovary and polycystic ovary?[6]

Refer Table 4.

Table 4: Difference between polycystic and multifollicular ovary

Polycystic ovary	Multifollicular ovary
Follicular distribution is predominantly peripheral	Follicles are randomly scattered all through the ovary
Increased central stromal area present	Absent
All follicles are of similar size	Different sized follicles present

Q. 17. Suppose in this case, if serum FSH levels are raised, what is the diagnosis?

Premature ovarian failure, Turner's mosaicism, 47XXX females, Fragile X permutation, mutation in the FSH.[8]

Q. 18. How do you investigate secondary amenorrhea?

Refer Flowcharts 1 and 2.

Q. 19. What are the long-term complications of PCOS?

Persistent stimulation of endometrium by chronic unopposed estrogen leads to endometrial hyperplasia and adenocarcinoma endometrium. Increased ovarian stimulation leads to ovarian cancer. More prone to metabolic diseases like type 2 diabetes mellitus, dyslipidemia, hypertension and cardiovascular

Flowchart 1: Diagnostic algorithm for secondary amenorrhea.

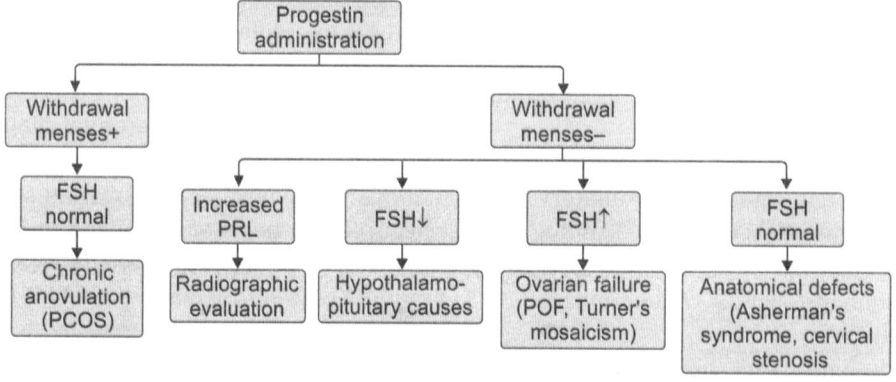

Flowchart 2: Investigational protocol for secondary amenorrhea.

disease, because of hyperinsulinemia and increased androgen levels.[7]

Q. 20. What are the signs of hyperandrogenism in your case?

Hirsutism, oily facial skin, acne vulgaris, android obesity.

Q. 21. How do you grade hirsutism?

Ferriman-Gallwey scoring: 9 hormonal sites on a scale of 1–4, according to the degree of terminal hair growth. The scores are added and used for comparison (Fig. 4).

FG score >8 = hyperandrogenism.

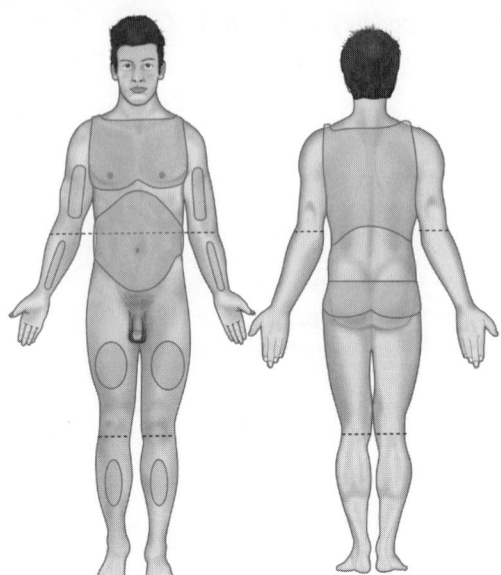

Fig. 4: Areas of hair growth considered for grading hirsutism

Hirsutism can be differentiated from hypertrichosis which tends to have an earlier onset and is not responsive to antiandrogens.[9]

Q. 22. What are the causes of hyperandrogenism in PCOS?

Hyperinsulinemia leads to abnormal GnRH activity where LH is produced in excess. LH stimulates ovarian stromal cells to produce ovarian androgens.

Insulin inhibits insulin growth factor binding protein thereby enhances stimulatory action of insulin growth factor-1 (IGF-1) in the ovary, leading to increased production of androgens.

Insulin also acts as cogonadotropin (LH-like activity).

At hepatic level, insulin decreases the secretion of sex-hormone binding globulin (SHBG), thereby increasing concentration of free testosterone.

Exaggerated adrenarche at puberty, marked by increased production of DHEA leads to abnormal androgen exposure.[7]

Q. 23. What is the role of AMH in PCOS?

Anti-Müllerian hormone levels are increased in women with PCOS. It is secreted by granulosa cells of preantral and small antral follicles. The level is related to severity of the syndrome. AMH levels are higher in insulin resistant and amenorrhic PCOS women when compared to normal insulin sensitivity and oligomenorrhic women with PCOS. It has got a prognostic value. The level decreases in women who lose their weight and regain the menstrual cyclicity.[10]

Q. 24. What is the Anna Marie criteria regarding PCOD?

Ovarian stromal to total area ratio (S/A ratio) of >0.34 significantly correlates to circulating androgen values and differentiates between PCOS and PCOD-like conditions with sensitivity and specificity of 100%.[11]

Q. 25. What is the cause of PCO pattern in PCOS?

Androgen excess influences follicle growth and development leading to polycystic pattern of ovaries. Similar morphology is seen in other androgen excess condition like congenital adrenal hyperplasia and androgen-secreting tumors.[7]

Q. 26. What are the differential diagnoses of your case? (PCOS)

In ovarian hyperthecosis, ovarian stroma is occupied by nests of leutinized thecal cells leading to firm texture of the ovary with marked high serum androgen levels leads to virilizing signs like clitoromegaly, temporal baldness, male body habitus and deepening of the voice and marked insulin resistance leads to obesity and acanthosis nigricans (HAIR-AN syndrome)[7]

CAH-leads to hirsutism, clitoromegaly, short stature and familial tendency. Increased levels of 17-OHP is diagnostic.

Androgen producing—adrenal and ovarian tumors—Rapid onset of symptoms and palpable pelvic or abdominal mass.

Q. 27. What is teenage syndrome?

- Low birth weight
- Hyperinsulinemia
- Dyslipidemia
- Normal body weight
- Anovulation, hyperandrogenism and polycystic ovaries after premature adrenarche.[12]

Q. 28. How do you treat this present case?

As the patient's chief complaint is secondary amenorrhea, first progesterone to be given for withdrawal bleeding. For cyclical bleed, we can give combined OCPs; lifestyle modification like diet and exercise to decrease the BMI. Insulin sensitizers can be given.

Q. 29. How do insulin sensitizers help in PCOS?

Insulin sensitizers like metformin primarily increases peripheral insulin utilization, so that serum levels of insulin decreases. Insulin is responsible for hyperandrogenism, indirectly affecting ovulation. Metformin reduces the activity of P450c 17α activity in the ovary, thereby decreasing synthesis of ovarian androgens.[7]

Q. 30. What are the adverse reactions of metformin? And how do you minimize them?

Nausea, vomiting, diarrhea, abdominal cramps, abdominal bloating. Dehydration leads to lactic acidosis. Long-term metformin usage leads to vitamin B_{12} deficiency and megaloblastic anemia. They are minimized by taking them after food, and gradually increasing the dosage over a few weeks before starting the 1.5–2 g/ day dose.

Q. 31. Are there any drugs that counterinteract with metformin?

Cimetidine, digoxin, amiloride, quinidine, ranitidine, triamterene, trimethoprim and vancomycin. These are cationic drugs which compete with metformin for renal excretion.[13]

Q. 32. What is the coprescription of metformin?

Vitamin B_{12}.

Q. 33. Mention other insulin sensitizers?

Thiazolidinediones like pioglitazone, rosiglitazone; D-chiro-inositol, myoinositol; N-acetyl cystiene; Somatostatin-analogs like octreotide.[14]

Q. 34. How oral contraceptive pills help in PCOS?

Beneficial effects of low dose combined estrogen-antiandrogen (cyproterone acetate) preparations in PCOS:

- On hormone disturbances: Decrease in LH levels, ovarian and adrenal androgen level and increase in SHBG concentration.
- On clinical signs: Good control of menstrual cycle, decrease in hirsutism, acne and seborrhea.
- On ovarian size: Decrease in ovarian volume.[15]

Combined estrogen and progesterone pills also can be used. Both preparations can be used from 5th day of periods cyclically for 3–4 months.

Q. 35. How do you surgically manage PCOD?

Laparoscopic ovarian drilling (LOD) helps increase chance of conception. It is useful in women who are resistant to medical therapy. LOD encourages monofolliculogenesis in PCOS cases by disrupting the vicious cycle of high androgen and high LH pulsation, high inhibition atretic PCO follicle, pituitary hyperresponse and positive feedback from high androgen; decreasing cytochrome P450c 17α enzymatic activity.[16]

Q. 36. In tuberculous endometritis, how do you confirm the disease?

Symptoms: Secondary amenorrhea resistant to estrogen and progesterone therapy.

Imaging: Ultrasound imaging of uterus reveals synechae in the endometrial cavity.

Hysteroscopy: It shows bald endometrium.

Histopathology of endometrial sampling and culture of endometrial tissue for tuberculous bacilli confirms acute tuberculous endometritis.

Q. 37. What are the causes of Asherman's syndrome? And how do you manage it?

Asherman's syndrome is due to destruction of endometrium leading to secondary amenorrhea.

Causes: Overzealous postpartum curettage of endometrial cavity; following uterine surgery like caesarian section, myomectomy or metroplasty; tuberculosis; uterine schistosomiasis.

Management: Hysetroscopy-guided dilatation and curettage to break up the synechiae. Postoperatively, to prevent adhesions, IUCD or pediatric Foleys catheter, cyclical estrogen and progestrogen are used.

Q. 38. What is the prognosis of Asherman's syndrome?

About 70% of these patients achieve successful pregnancy, however complicated by premature labor, placenta acreta, placenta previa and postpartum hemorrhage.[17]

Q. 39. What are the iatrogenic surgical causes for secondary amenorrhea?

Asherman's syndrome following postpartum endometrial curettage, any cervical operations like cervical amputation, trachelorrhaphy and large loop excision of the transformation zone (LEETZ) operations where it results in cervical stenosis leading to hematometra and secondary amenorrhea.

Progesterone challenge test is the first test to be done in investigating secondary amenorrhea. How do you do it? Mention the inference.

Medroxyprogesterone acetate 10 mg is given orally daily for 5–10 days or progesterone in oil 200 mg IM single dose.[18]

Q. 40. How ovarian biopsy helps to differentiate gonadotropin resistant syndrome and premature ovarian failure?

Presence of primordial follicles on ovarian biopsy suggests gonadotropin resistant syndrome (Savage syndrome) whereas absence of follicles suggests premature ovarian failure. But both these conditions there is hypergonadotropic status, normal karyotype and normal Müllerian tract development.[19]

Q. 41. What are the hypothalamic and pituitary causes of amenorrhea?[20]

Refer Table 5.

Q. 42. What are the causes of hyperprolactinemia?[21]

Refer Tables 5 and 6 or Flowchart 3.

Table 5: Summary of causes for secondary amenorrhea

Physiological	Pregnancy, lactation, sleep, stress, sexual intercourse, local causes like nipple irritation
Pituitary	Prolactinoma, acromegaly, Cushing's disease, empty sella syndrome, lymphocytic hypophysitis
Hypothalamic	Non-secreting pituitary adenomas, meningiomas, craniopharyngioma, sarcoidosis, Langerhans-cell histiocytosis. Neuraxis irradiation, pituitary stalk section
Medication	Antipsychotics like phenothiazines, butyrophenones; antidepressants like TCA, SSRI, MAO inhibitors; antihypertensives like methyl-dopa, reserpine, verapamil; metoclopramide; cocaine; opiates; antiretroviral agents like protease inhibitors
Neurogenic	Spinal cord lesions, chest wall lesions
Other	Hypothyroidism, chronic renal failure, cirrhosis, adrenal insufficiency, ectopic secretion
Macroprolactinemia	
Idiopathic	

Table 6: Hyperprolactinemia—grading.

Grade	Sr. prolactin (µg/L)	Clinical presentation
Mild	31–50	Short leuteal phase, decreased libido and infertility
Moderate	51–75	Oligomenorrhea, amenorrhea
Marked	>100	Galactorrhea, amenorrhea, bone loss, osteopenia, increased body weight

Q. 43. What are the clinical presentations of hyperprolactinemia? How does it lead to secondary amenorrhea?

Hyperprolactinemia can be graded into mild, moderate and marked.[22]

Hyperprolactinemia suppresses pulsatile gonadotropin secretion, by altering GnRH pulse generator. In presence of hyperprolactinemia, there is decreased response of gonadotropins to GnRH. Hyperprolactinemia leads to loss of positive estrogen feedback on gonadotropin secretion.[21]

Q. 44. How do you manage hyperprolactinemia?[23]

Refer Flowchart 3.

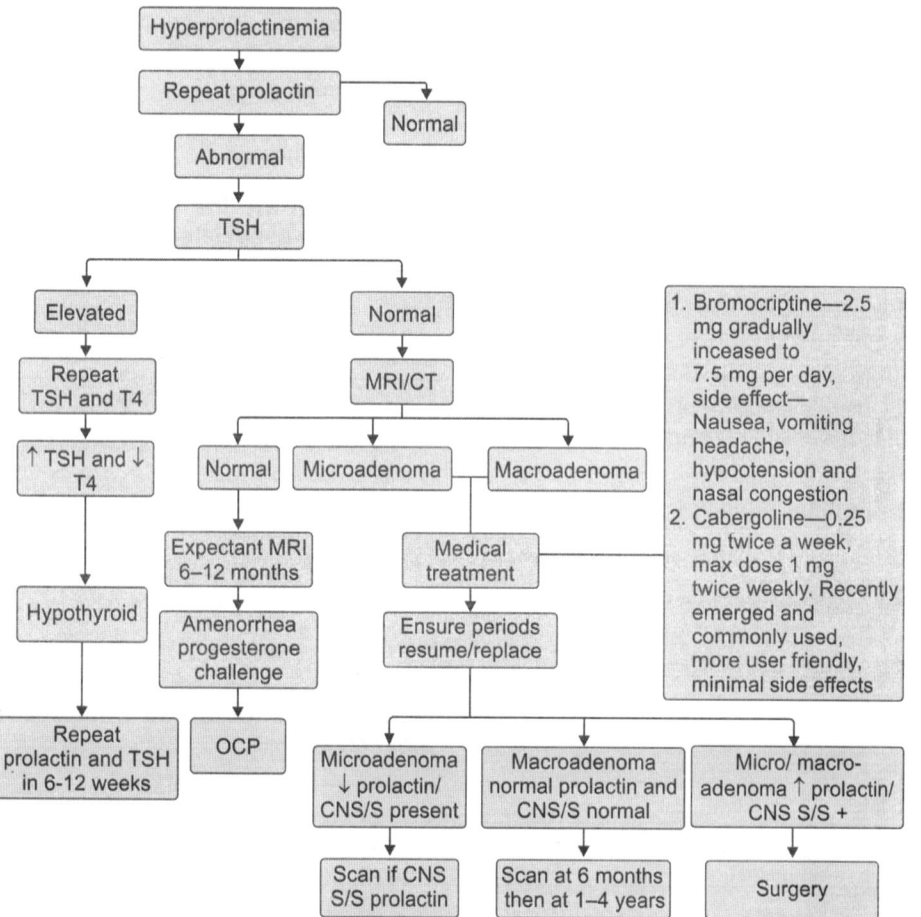

Flowchart 3: Evaluation of hyperprolactinemia

Q. 45. What are the genetic causes of secondary amenorrhea?

- *Fragile X permutation:* There will be premature menopause due to premature renal failure, autosomal dominant and sex link inheritance
- *Galactosemia:* Mental retardation, cataract, hepatosplenomegaly and premature ovarian failure
- *Mutation in FSH receptor:* Presents with primary or secondary amenorrhea, increased FSH levels, presence of few ovarian follicles on ultrasound
- *Gonadotropin resistant syndrome:* It is due to gonadotropin postreceptor defect, leads to secondary amenorrhea. Elevated gonadotropin levels. Immature follicles in ovary; karyotype 46XX[20]
- *Turners mosaicism:* 46XX/45X0 primary/secondary amenorrhea. Barr body positive
- *47XXX females:* Secondary amenorrhea and premature menopause.

Q. 46. When do you say it premature ovarian failure (POF)? Mention a few causes.[24]

When a woman attains menopause before the age of 40 years, it is called premature menopause, the cause being premature ovarian insufficiency/failure. This is associated with high levels of FSH and LH and low levels of AMH.

For causes Refer Table 7.

Table 7: Causes for premature ovarian insufficiency.

Genetic	Turner's mosaicism, pure gonadal dysgenesis, galactosemia, 17-hydroxylase deficiency
Autoimmune diseases	Autoimmune polyglandular diseases
Infections	Tuberculosis, mumps
Environmental	Smoking
Iatrogenic	Ovarian surgery, chemotherapy, irradiation

Q. 47. How do you say POF is an autoimmune disease?

Patients with POF showed humoral and cell-mediated immune reactivity, compatible with the presence of autoimmune etiology. Oopheritis is a T-cell mediated autoimmune disease. POF may be associated with number of autoimmune diseases like thyroiditis, hypoparathyroidism, hypoadrenalism and mucocutaneous candidiasis.[25]

Q. 48. What is the latest treatment modality of POF?

Endocrine therapy
- Consists of induction of ovulation with gonadotropins
- HRT to mimic the normal menstrual cycle.
- High-dose estrogens or GnRH analogs to suppress pituitary gonadotropins.

Immunotherapy
- Corticosteroids
- Immunosuppressants like cyclosporine A
- Plasmapheresis.[26]

Q. 49. What are the neuroendocrine abnormalities associated with anorexia nervosa?[20]

- Diminished GnRH-LH pulsatile frequency and amplitude
- Low blood LH and FSH levels
- Impaired ACTH response to CRH stimulation testing
- Resistance to dexamethasone suppression
- Increased ACTH levels
- Increased 24 hour urinary free cortisol levels
- Low prolactin levels
- Low TSH levels, high reverse T_3 and low T_3 levels
- Elevated GH levels
- Decreased IGF-1 levels
- Diabetes insipidus

Q. 50. Why should you treat secondary amenorrhea?

- For restoring normal cyclicity
- For achieving pregnancy
- For prevention of osteoporosis
- For prevention of coronary artery disease.[2]

Q. 51. What is the treatment of secondary amenorrhea?

- Once the diagnosis is established, cyclical estrogen and progesterone therapy is indicated to achieve regular menses (conjugated estrogen 0.625 mg for 21 days along with 5 mg of medroxyprogesterone acetate for 10–14 days). Combined contraceptive pills are also convenient and cost effective option for those who wants contraception.
- To those who do not want menstruation like athletes, dancers, regular travelers, for protection of bone density 0.625 mg conjugated estrogens along with 2.5 mg medroxyprogesterone acetate can be given daily without break.
- In women with low risk of thromboembolism, oral contraceptive pills especially in low dose, is a reasonable alternative.
- Along with hormonal treatment or for those who refuse hormonal treatment, high calcium intake (1–1.5 g daily) along with vitamin D is effective in protection against osteoporosis.
- Counseling regarding diet, exercise and behavioral therapy is needed in targeted cases.
- Surgical correction is needed in genital outlet obstruction conditions.[2]

References

1. Malhotra N, Kumar P. Amenorrhea, hypomenorrhea and oligomenorrhea. Jeffcoat's Principles of Gynecology. New Delhi: Jaypee Brothers Medical Publishers. 2008;7: 579-97.
2. Speroff L, Fritz MA. Amenorrhea, clinical gynecologic endocrinology and infertility. Philadelphia: Lippincott Williams & Wilkins. 2005;7: 401-63.
3. Lunenfeld B, Barzelatto J, Spieler J. Design of studies of assessment of drugs and hormones used in the treatment of endocrine forms of infertility. Regulation of Human fertility. Scriptor Copenhagen. 1977;135-235.
4. Basav M. Thyroid in Reproduction. In: Dutta DK (Ed). Recent advances in Gyne-Endocrinology. New Delhi: Jaypee Publishers. 2011;1:38-43.
5. Ahima RS, Prabakaran D, Mantzoros C, et al. Role of leptin in the neuroendocrine response to fasting. Nature. 1996 Jul 18;382(6588):250-2.
6. Robert Y, Ardaens Y, Dewailly D. Imaging polycystic ovaries. Kovacs GT (Ed). Ploycystic ovary syndrome. Cambridge: Cambridge University Press. 2001;56-69.
7. Jeffrey CR. Polycystic ovary syndrome and Hyperandrogenic states. In: Strauss J, Barbieri R (Eds). Yen & Jaffe's Reproductive Endocrinology. Philadelphia: Saunders; 2014; 7:pp. 485-511.
8. Rebar RW. Evaluation of amenorrhea, anovulation, and abnormal bleeding. Female Reproductive Endocrinology. South Dartmouth (MA). MDText.com, Inc., 2003.
9. Kovacs GT, Sinclair, Green J, Rodney. Skin manifestations of polycystic ovarian syndrome. Polycystic Ovary Syndrome. Cambridge: Cambridge university press. 2001.pp 79-97.
10. Mulders AG, Laven JS, Eijkemans MJ, et al. Changes in anti-Müllerian hormone serum concentrations over time suggest delayed ovarian ageing in normogonadotrophic anovulatory infertility. Hum Reprod. 2004; 19(9):2036-42. Epub 2004 Jun 24.
11. Fulghesu AM, Ciampelli M, Belosi C. A new ultrasound criterion for the diagnosis of polycystic ovary syndrome: the ovarian stroma/total area ratio. Elsevier. 2001;76:326-31.
12. Ibáñez L, Valls C, Ferrer A. Sensitization to insulin induces ovulation in nonobese adolescents with anovulatory hyperandrogenism. J Clin Endocrino Metabo. 2001;86: 3595-8.
13. Barabieri RL. Metformin for the treatment of PCOS. Obstetrics and Gynecology. 2013;101: 785-93.
14. Pasquali R, Gambineri A. Insulin-sensitizing agents in polycystic ovary syndrome. Eur J Endocrinol. 2006;154(6):763-75.
15. Dutta DK, Dutta I. Polycystic ovarian syndrome in adolescent girl. In: Dutta DK (Ed). Recent advances in Gyne-endocrinology. New Delhi: Jaypee Publications. 2011;1:pp 62-75.

16. Jean C. Laparoscopic surgical treatment of infertility related to polycystic ovary syndrome. In: Kovacs GT. Polycystic ovary syndrome. Cambridge University Press; 2001.
17. Schenker JG, Margalioth EJ. Intrauterine adhesions: an updated appraisal. Fertility Sterility. 1982;37:593-610.
18. Carr, Bruce R. Evaluation and treatment of amenorrhea. In: Alvero R, Schlaff WD (Eds). Reproductive Endocrinology and Infertility. Elsevier; 2008. pp 49-63.
19. Krishna Menon MK, Devi PK, Bhasker Rao K. Postgraduate Obstetrics and Gynaecology. Orient Longman. 1986;3: 306-19.
20. Pandey LK. Amenorrhea. In: Dutta DK (Ed). Recent advances in Gyne-endocrinology. New Delhi: Jaypee Brothers. 2013;1: 76-98.
21. Mark EM. Prolactin in Human Reproduction. In: Strauss JF, Barbieri RL (Eds). Yen & Jaffe's Reproductive Endocrinology. Saunders. 2014. pp. 45-65.
22. Luciano AA. Clinical presentation of hyperprolactinemia. J Reproduct Med. 1999;44:1085-90.
23. Critchly ODH. Amenorrhea and oligomenorrhea and hypothalamic pituitary dysfunction. In: Seclter WP, Standon SL, Shaw WR (Eds). Gynecology. Churchill Livingstone; 2002;3:229-44.
24. Hoek A, Schoemaker J, Drexhage HA. Premature ovarian failure and ovarian autoimmunity. Endocrine Reviews. 1997;18: 107-34.
25. Blumenfeld Z, Halachmi S, Peretz BA, et al. Premature ovarian failure—the prognostic application of autoimmunity on conception after ovulation induction. Fertility and Sterility. 1993;59:750-5.
26. Sebanti G. Hyperprolactinemia. In: Dutta DK. Recent advances in gyne-endocrinology. New Delhi: Jaypee Brothers. 2011;1: 44-50.

31

Examination of a Sexual Assault Victim

K Srinivas

A 16 years old girl was brought by police to the OPD with history of being kidnapped and kept in captivity for 15 days by her seniors in the college. She is not aware of what happened during the period of captivity. Police traced her the previous day with tied hands and legs in a locked room in a farmhouse and also found four of her classmates in an inebriated condition in the same building.

- Police have come with a request of conducting an examination on the girl and to opine regarding the possibility of sexual assault.
- Details entered in medicolegal register.
- Details of who brought her, history given by police and the victim were documented.
- Consent for examination taken by her, her personal details, date and time of examination, identification marks were noted
- A detailed history of her cycles, previous sexual exposure, etc. were obtained
- General, systemic and clinical examination conducted
- Clothes worn by her, undergarments were collected and the color and other details of them noted
- Nail clippings obtained
- Pubic hairs clipped and collected
- Genital examination for injuries done
- Vaginal swab, and cervical swab obtained
- Vaginal and cervical smear obtained
- All packed, labeled and sent to FSL.

Victim was counseled, sent to radiology department for age estimation, investigations for STDs done after obtaining consent, a pregnancy test was also performed.

Q. 1. What is sexual violence? What is sexual assault?

Sexual violence and sexual act are different and the differences need to be understood.

Sexual violence (WHO 2003)

- Any Sexual Act
- Forceful act—physical, threats
- Acts to Traffic
- Any attempt to obtain a Sexual Act
- Sexual comments/advances in any circumstance like workplace/home by any known/unknown, related/unrelated person
- Sexual assault
- Too is a form of sexual violence.

The Criminal Law (Amendment) Act (CLA), 2013 has expanded the definition of rape to include all forms of sexual violence-penetrative (oral, anal, vaginal) including by objects/weapons/fingers and non-penetrative (touching, fondling, stalking, etc.)

It may range from touching one's body with sexual intensions to actual intercourse without the consent
- Oral and anal sex
- Child sexual abuse, fondling and attempted rape.
- Sexual assault on mentally disabled
- Forced marriage
- Child marriage
- Forced prostitution

The following too amounts to sexual assault:
- Denial of the right to use contraception or to adopt other measures to protect against STIs.
- Forced abortion and forced sterilization.
- Female genital cutting.
- Inspections for virginity.
- Forced exposure to pornography.
- Forcibly disrobing and parading naked any person.

Q. 2. Where should the victims of sexual assault be provided care?

- Refusal of treatment could amount to offence under Section
- 166B of the Indian Penal Code read with Section 357C of the Code of Criminal Procedure

- Obtaining informed consent and respecting autonomy of survivors in making
- Decisions about examination, treatment and police intimation is mandatory.

It is an offence to refuse treatment for sexual assault victims. Both public and private health care institutions should provide care to them. Though right to health is not a fundamental right in India, Hon. Supreme court interprets right to health under the right to life.

The services to be provided are:
- Physical injury treatment
- Emergency contraception
- Psychological support
- Testing and prophylaxis for STIs.

Q. 3. What are the requirements to examine a victim of sexual violence?

The procedure followed in the examination of a sexual assault victim are called standard operational procedures (SOP).

It is as follows:
- The victim need not be examined only by a gynecologist, any registered medical practitioner can conduct the examination.
- Preferably the examination needs to be done by a lady doctor, if not available, can be conducted by a male doctor in presence of a lady attendant, never delay the treatment.
- Some person known to the victim may be present during the examination in case of a minor, disabled person or if the victim requests
- The opinion of the victim so as to decide about a male or a female doctor to examine him needs to be obtained in case of transgenders/intersex.
- Police personnel should not be allowed either during the interview or during examination of the victim.
- Providing the treatment for the needy is the priority for which registering a complaint, admitting the victim are not mandatory.
- A private place needs to organized in the hospital for obtaining the history and to examine the patient in detail.

CLA, 2013 and POCSCO Act, 2012 both recognize that any registered medical practitioner can carry out a medico legal examination and provide treatment and records of that health provider will stand in the court of law (164A CRPC).

Q. 4. How should the evidence be collected?

Sexual Assault Forensic Evidence (SAFE) kit if made available in all the hospitals, serves the need during the examination the contents are given under two headings, essential items and and optional items.

The following things need to be considered during the examination:

Examination of a Sexual Assault Victim

- Do not insist on admission
- Provide the copy of all documents to the victim
- All services are provided free of cost
- Confidentiality needs to be maintained
- Treatment of problems is the top priority
- Consent is an important prerequisite

Essential items
- Forms for documentation
- Large sheet of paper to undress over
- Paper bags to collect cloths
- Catchment paper
- Sterile cotton swabs
- Comb
- Nail cutter
- Wooden stick for finger nail scrapings
- Small scissors
- Urine sample container
- Containers for blood samples [(EDTA), plain, sodium fluoride]
- Syringes with needles
- Distilled water
- Disposable gloves
- Glass slides
- Envelopes or boxes for individual evidence storage
- Labels
- Sealing wax
- Stick for sealing
- Clean clothing, show for survivors use after the examination

Optional Items
- Woods lamp/Good torch
- Vaginal speculums
- Drying rack for wet swabs &/or clothing
- Patient gown, cover sheet, blanket, pillow Post-It notes to collect trace evidence
- Camera (35 mm, digital with color printer)
- Microscope
- Colposcope/magnifying glass
- Toluidine blue dye
- 1% acetic acid diluted spray
- Urine pregnancy test kit
- Surgilube
- Medications

Q. 5. What is the need for the examination?

Examination needs to be done for various reasons:

- It should begin with the general assessment of the victim (Flowchart 1)
- Any injuries need to be treated immediately
- Steps towards preventing STIs to be initiated (Flowchart 2)
- Emergency contraception
- Initiate legal procedures
- Age estimation
- Assessment of mental status.

Flowchart 1: Protocol of examination of a sexual assault victim

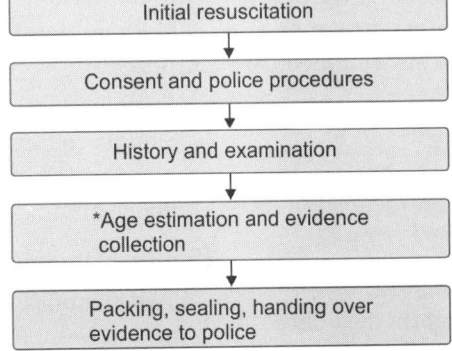

*Age estimation is done if asked for

- Information regarding attempted or completed penetration by penis/finger/object in vagina/anus/mouth should be properly recorded.
- There could also be other acts such as masturbation of the assailant by the survivor, masturbation of the survivor by the assailant, oral sex by the assailant on the survivor or sucking, licking, kissing of the body parts.
- Information about emission of semen, use of condom (is relevant because in such cases, vaginal swabs and smears would be negative for sperm/semen), sucking or spitting along with the location should be clearly stated.
- Information about emission of semen outside the orifices should be elicited as swabs taken from such sites can have evidentiary value.

Flowchart 2: Medical aspects of management of a sexual assault victim

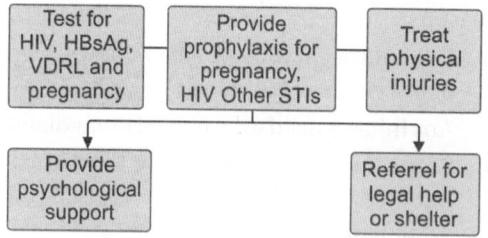

Q. 6. Discuss the consent procedure and legal implications.

- A person may come to the hospital on his own or may be brought by the police.
- Consent for examination needs to be obtained from the survivor/guardian/parent depending on the circumstances.
- Police requisition is not a must for medical examination.

In case the survivor does not want to pursue a police case, a MLC must be made and she must be informed that she has the right to refuse to file FIR. An informed refusal must be documented in such cases.

- Patient may be taken up for only treatment
- But the doctor should inform the police
- Registering an FIR is not mandatory
- For the want of FIR, examination should never be refused or postponed
- But a medical examination can never be enforced by the doctor/court.

The police station details, accompanying person, MLC no needs to be documented.

Only in situations, where it is life-threatening the doctor may initiate treatment without consent as per section 92 of IPC.

- Doctors are legally bound to examine and provide treatment to survivors of sexual-violence.
- Coming on their own for examination but not interested in filing a case/want to file a case later
- Coming with the police requisition.

- The consent form must be signed by the person above 12 years of age.
- Consent must be taken from the guardian/parent if the survivor is under the age of 12 years.
- In case of persons with mental disability-All persons are ordinarily able to give or refuse to give informed consent, including persons with mental illness and intellectual disabilities, and their informed consent should be sought and obtained before any medical examination.
- The consent form must be signed by the survivor, a witness and the examining doctor.

(Any major 'disinterested', person may be considered a witness)

In all the above situations, it is mandatory to seek an informed consent/refusal for examination and evidence collection.

Consent should be taken for the following purposes:

- Examination,
- Sample collection for clinical and forensic examination, and treatment
- Police intimation.

Identity of the survivor is to be established

- Two identification marks need to be documented—moles, scars, tattoos, etc. preferably from the exposed parts of the body.
- Left thumb impression is to be taken in the space provided.

Q. 7. Discuss the examination of the victim.

After obtaining a detailed relevant history examination is conducted as follows (Flowchart 3):

- In younger age group and in severe injuries, examination may have to be done under anesthesia
- Speculum examination in children and young girls may be restricted to cases with history of penetrative sex, and when injuries are seen.

- General physical examination
- Injury examination
- Genital examination

- Hymen examination is irrelevant and should therefore be treated like any other part of the genitals while documenting examination findings
- Intact hymen does not rule out sexual violence, torn hymen need not be due to sexual violence.

If the survivor has been already examined elsewhere and documents available, re-examination need not be done even with a police request, they need to be convinced that examination has been done.

Genital Examination

- P/S examination (Look at the box)
- Hymen examination (Look at the box)
- If there is vaginal discharge, note its texture, color, odor.
- Two finger admitting test is irrelevant
- P/V to be done only if medically indicated in adult woman.

Only relevant information on external genitals like tears, bleeding inflammation congestion need to be documented

Genital examination findings need to be marked on body chart with proper numbering

Per rectal examination for tears, bleeding, sphincter injury needs to be done, documented especially in child abuse and with history of sodomy, collect the samples also

Oral cavity should also be examined for any evidence of bleeding, discharge, tear, edema, tenderness.

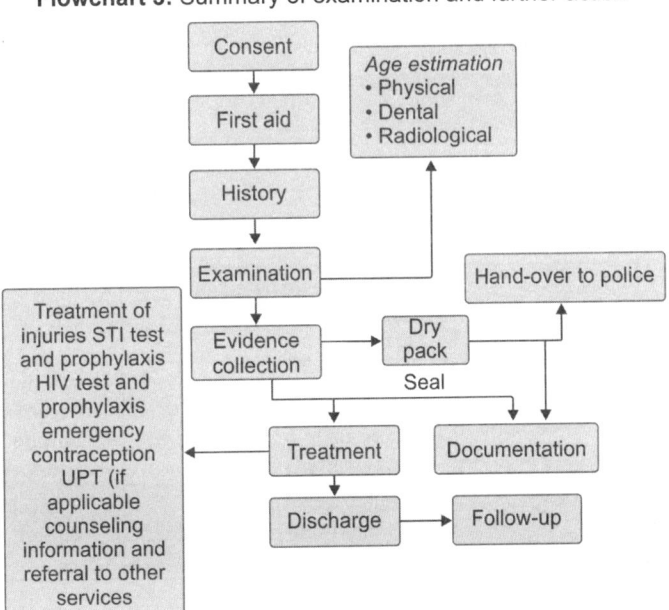

Flowchart 3: Summary of examination and further action

Q. 8. Discuss the procedure of specimen collection.

Specimen collection is an important aspect of investigation.

> The survivor or in case of child, the parent/guardian/ or a person in whom the child reposes trust, has the right to refuse either a medico-legal examination or collection of evidence or both.

It aims at detecting spermatozoa, seminal stains, foreign body, hair, blood stains, tissues etc., which would help to prove the sexual violence, identify the culprit, etc.

The collection procedure needs a consent appropriately as discussed earlier.

> As per the law, the hospital/examining doctor is required/duty bound to inform the police about the sexual offence. However, if the survivor does not wish to participate in the police investigation treatment should not be denied
> At the time of MLC intimation being sent to the police, a clear note stating "informed refusal for police intimation" should be made.

This may include:
- The cloths worn by the survivor at the time of incident
- Scalp hair and pubic hair
- Foreign body from the body surface
- Nail clippings
- Oral swab
- Rectal swab
- Vaginal swab (Record the date of last consensual vaginal sex)
- Saliva
- Blood.

All the specimens need not be collected from all the survivors. It depends on the nature of assault, time lapse from the time of assault to the examination and whether the person has washed, changed clothes, had a shave, shower, etc.

Spermatozoa are detected up to 72 hours from the time of assault especially in the female genital tract and up to 96 hours, other evidences are relevant.

The following Table 1 shows the type of specimen to be collected.

Table 1: Types of evidence to be collected

History of sexual violence	Type of swab	Purpose	Points to consider
Penovaginal	Vaginal swabs	• Semen/sperm detection • Lubricant • DNA	• Whether ejaculation occurred inside vagina or outside • Use of condom
	Body swabs	• Semen/sperm detection • Saliva (in case of sucking/licking)	• If ejaculation occurred outside
Penoanal	Anal swabs	• Semen/sperm detection • DNA • Lubricant • Fecal matter	• Whether ejaculation occurred inside anus or outside • Use of condom
	Body swabs	• Semen/sperm detection • Saliva (in case of sucking/licking)	• If ejaculation occurred outside

Contd...

Examination of a Sexual Assault Victim

Contd...

Penooral	Oral swabs	• Semen/sperm detection • DNA • Saliva	• If ejection occurred inside mouth or outside • Use of condom
	Body swabs	• Semen/sperm detection • Saliva (in case of sucking/licking)	if ejaculation occurred outside
Use of objects	Swab of the orifice (anal, vaginal and/or oral)	Lubricant	Detection of lubricant used if any
Use of body parts (fingering)	Swab of the orifice (anal, vaginal and/or oral)	Lubricant	
Masturbation	Swab of orifice/body part	• Semen/sperm detection • DNA • Lubricant	• Whether ejaculation occurred or not • If ejaculated in orifice or body parts

Forensic evidence is likely to be found only up to 96 hours after the incident.

Q. 9. How to offer the opinion?

Immediately following examination tentative opinion is to be offered as follows in Table 2 depending on the situation.

Final opinion: To be formulated after receiving reports from the FSL (Table 3).

Table 2: Tentative opinion forming

Genital injuries	Physical injuries	Opinion	Rationale why forced penetrative sex cannot be ruled out	What can FSL detect?
Present	Present	There are signs suggestive of recent use of force/forceful penetration of vagina/anus. Sexual violence cannot be ruled out	Evidence for semen and spermatozoa are yet to be tested by laboratory examinations in case of penile penetration	Evidence of semen except when condom was used
Present	Absent	There are signs suggestive of recent forceful penetration of vagina/anus.	Evidence for semen and spermatozoa are yet to be tested in case of penile penetration. The lack of physical injuries could be because of the survivor being unconscious, under the effect of alcohol/drugs, overpowered or threatened. It could be because, there was fingering or penetration by object with or without use of lubricant—which is an offence under Sec 375 IPC	Evidence of semen or lubricant except when condom was used

Contd...

Contd...

Absent	Present	There are signs of use of force, however vaginal or anal or oral penetration cannot be ruled out	The lack of injuries could be because of the survivor being unconscious, under the effect of alcohol/drugs, overpowered or threatened or use of lubricant	Evidence of semen or lubricant
Absent	Absent	There are no signs of use of force; however final opinion is reserved pending availability of FSL reports. Sexual violence cannot be ruled out	The lack of genital injuries could be because of use of lubricant. the lack of physical injuries could be because of the survivor being unconscious, under the effect of alcohol/drugs, overpowered or threatened. It could also be because, there was fingering or penetration by object with use of lubricant–which is an offence under Sec 375 IPC	Evidence of semen, lubricant and drug/alcohol

Table 3: Offering final opinion

S. No.	Genital	Physical injuries/ diseases	FSL report injuries/ diseases	Final opinion
For penile penetration				
1.	Present	Present	Positive for presence of semen	There are signs suggestive of forceful vaginal/anal intercourse
2.	Present	Absent	Positive for presence of semen	There are signs suggestive of forceful vaginal/anal intercourse
3.	Absent	Present	Positive for presence of semen	There are signs suggestive of forceful vaginal/anal intercourse.
4.	Absent	Absent	Positive for presence of semen	There are signs suggestive of vaginal/anal intercourse
5.	Absent	Absent	Positive for drugs/ alcohol and semen	There are signs suggestive of vaginal/anal intercourse under the influence of drugs/alcohol
For nonpenile penetration				
6.	Present	Present	FSL report is negative for presence of semen/ alcohol/drugs/ lubricant	There are no signs suggestive of vaginal/anal intercourse, but there is evidence of physical and genital assault
7.	Present	Absent	FSL report is negative for presence of semen/ alcohol/drugs/ lubricant	There are no signs suggestive of vaginal/anal intercourse, but there is evidence of assault physical
8.	Absent	Present	FSL report is negative for presence of semen/ drugs/lubricant	There are no signs suggestive of vaginal/anal intercourse, but there is evidence of genital assault

Contd...

Contd...

9.	Absent	Absent	FSL report is negative for presence of semen/alcohol/drugs/lubricant	There are no signs suggestive of penetration of vagina/anal
10.	Absent	Absent	FSL report is positive for presence of lubricant only	There is a possibility of vaginal/anal penetration by lubricated object

Q. 10. What are the provisions in the Act against sexual offence?

354A	Sexual harassment
354B	Act with intent to disrobe a woman
354C	Voyeurism
354D	Stalking

Victims: The term "victim" literally means a person suffering harm including those who are subjected to Nonconsensual Sexual Act which could be sexual assault, rape or sexual violence. It also means a person is in need of compassion, care, validation, and support.

Q. 11. What are the changes affected in the Indian Law on Sexual Offences?

Section 370 IPC deals with human trafficking for exploitation will be punished with imprisonment ranging from at least 7 years to imprisonment. This has sections 370 and 370A as additions.

The definition of rape has been expanded now:

Penetration	Penis/any other part/object/any extent	To vagina
Touching private part	Apply mouth or any other part	To anus
Making other person do		To mouth
		To urethra

Section 376 A is an addition–under this there is a provision for rigorous imprisonment for not less than 20 years of the person committing a sexual offence if it results in death or permanent vegetative state of the person or to any person involved in gang rape.

Age of consent for consensual sex has been raised to 18 years.

changes in the CrPC and Evidence Act.

- Victims character is not relevant in the case of an alleged sexual violence.
- When the sexual intercourse is proved and the victim says she had not consented, it is taken as 'no consent'.

Q. 12. What is the situation of sexual offence in various parts of the world?

Every country has one or the other forms of definitions and legal procedures for sexual violence. To quote a few:

Bhutan

- 2004 Penal Code of Bhutan outlaws rape and other sexual offenses
- Marital rape is also recognized as an offense
- The most serious form of rape is Gang rape of a child below twelve years of age, classified as a felony of the first degree.

Canada

- The word rape is not used
- Sexual assault is used
- Sexual assault is considered for non-consensual sex.

France

Forceful penetration by threat, violence and surprise is rape.

Punished by criminal imprisonment for 15 years, extended to 30 years if it has resulted in the death of the victim.

Ireland

- Rape is defined under 2 sections
- Penetration by a male with his penis into the vagina of a female is rape
- Other section defines other forms of Sexual Acts.

Greece

Whoever with physical violence or with threat of grave and direct danger forces another to intercourse or to tolerance or action of an indecent act, is punished with incarceration.

Marital rape is illegal since 2006.

Newzealand

Sexual violation is the act of a person who rapes another person or has unlawful sexual connection with another person.

Rape is defined as follows:

Person A rapes person B if person A has sexual connection with person B, effected by the penetration of person B's genitalia by person A's penis:

- Without person B's consent to the connection; and
- Without believing on reasonable grounds that person B consents to the connection.

Marital rape too is illegal

Convicted can be punished for up to 20 years of imprisonment.

Norway

Rape is defined as:

- Having sex by the use of violence or threatening behavior
- Having sex with someone who is unconscious or incapable of resisting the act
- Compelling any person to engage in sexual activity with another person, or to carry out similar actions with him- or herself by force.

Aggravated rape—gang rape, sexual activity with a child under the age of 14 years. in such a way that the victim either dies or receives grievous bodily harm including contacting STIs.

Russia

- Forceful heterosexual sex with the use of threat, violence or with a helpless person is rape
- Homosexual, abnormal sex, nonvaginal are called Coercive sexual actions
- Both have similar punishments
- Imprisonment up to 20 years subsequent restrictions imposed, if the act is committed against person of <14 years or has resulted in death.

Switzerland

Rape is defined as:

- Forcible sex with a female by threat or violence, psychological pressure-punished from 1–10 years imprisonment
- Marital rape is illegal to the extent that it is punishable even if the wife does not lodge a complaint.

England and Wales

Rape is when penetration of the vagina, mouth or anus occurs with penis without consent.

References

1. Crimes Act 1961 No 43 (as at 18 April 2012), Public Act – New Zealand Legislation". Legislation.govt.nz. 18 April 2012.
2. Fitrakis Eft, in: Paraskevopoulos Nikos – Fitrakis Eftichis, Sexual offences (Axiopinessexoualikes praxis), ed. Sakkoulas, Athens – Thessaloniki 2011, p. 93.
3. Guidelines and protocols, medico-legal care for survivors/victims of sexual violence. Ministry of

Health and Family Welfare, Government of India, 19 march, 2014.
4. No 2 of 2017, Criminal law (Sexual offences) Act 2017.
5. Ortiz-Barreda G, Vives-Cases C. (European) Legislation on violence against women: overview of key components. Rev Panam Salud Publica. 2013;33(1):61-72.
6. Section 7, Criminal Law (Amendment) Ordinance (IPC), 2013.
7. Section 8, Criminal Law (Amendment) (IPC) Ordinance, 2013.
8. The Criminal Law (Amendment) Act (IPC), 2013.
9. The Criminal Procedure (Scotland) Act 1995, section 3.
10. The Routledge Handbook of European Criminology, p. 1, at Google Books.
11. The Sexual Offences (Northern Ireland) Order 2008 (SI. 1769/2008 (NI. 2)), article 5(5).
12. The Sexual Offences (Northern Ireland) Order 2008, article 5.
13. The Sexual Offences (Scotland) Act 2009, section 1.
14. Warrick, Catherine. (2009). Law in the service of legitimacy: Gender and politics in Jordan. Farnham, Surrey, England; Burlington, Vt.: Ashgate Pub. p. 66.
15. "English translation of the Norwegian Penal Code (unofficial)" (PDF). University of Oslo. Retrieved 1 April 2012.
16. "English translation of the Norwegian Penal Code (unofficial)" (PDF). University of Oslo. Retrieved 1 April 2012.
17. "The Sexual Offences (Northern Ireland) Order 2008". Legislation.gov.uk. 2012-03-08. Retrieved 2012-12-30.

32 CHAPTER

Bedside Ultrasonography in Obstetrics

BS Rama Murthy

CASE

A lady with a history of 7 weeks amenorrhea presents with bleeding per vaginum. What is the investigation that is relevant and what are the possible findings and diagnosis that the investigation may give?

The investigation is ultrasonography. Transabdominal survey through a full bladder followed by a transvaginal scan is the preferred approach. Any of the following findings and diagnosis may be encountered.[1]

- A normal gestational sac with an embryo and cardiac activity.
  No retrochorionic fluid collection noted.
  A diagnosis of ongoing gestation is confirmed. Conservative line of management is appropriate.
- A normal gestational sac with an embryo and cardiac activity.
  Retrochorionic fluid collection is noted.
  A diagnosis of threatened abortion is confirmed. There may be history of pain. Conservative line of management is appropriate. It should be noted that the size and extent of the retrochorionic fluid collection prognosticates the gestation.
- A gestational sac of less than 8 mm mean diameter without yolk sac or gestational sac less than 25 mm mean sac diameter with or without retrochorionic fluid collection. Repeat scan is suggested after a week (conservative management): (a) If the yolk sac and/or embryo and heart activity appear conservative management is continued; (b) If the sac grows but yolk sac and/or embryo do not appear, missed miscarriage is confirmed; (c) If there is no growth of the gestational sac, missed miscarriage is confirmed.
- A gestational sac of more than 25 mm mean sac diameter without yolk sac or embryo. Missed miscarriage (anembryonic gestation or blighted ovum) is confirmed.
- Associated findings of thin non-uniform chorionic ring, small crenated or calcified yolk sac are indicative of poor outcome.
- A gestational sac with amnion seen but without embryo is confirmative of missed miscarriage.
- Some other situations require a follow-up with ultrasound examination after 7–10 days: (a) When the difference between the mean sac diameter and crown-rump length is less than 5 mm; (b) When there is fetal bradycardia (FHR less than 100/min); (c) Absent fetal node when the mean gestational sac diameter is less than 25 mm. In these situations follow-up ultrasound studies may either demonstrate a continuing viable gestation or a missed miscarriage.
- Empty uterus with an adnexal gestational sac with or without yolk sac and embryo is confirmative of ectopic gestation.

- Empty uterus with a previous scan confirming gestation is indicative of complete miscarriage.
- Hyperechoic or mixed echogenic uterine cavity content with Doppler vascularity indicates incomplete miscarriage.
- Presence of abnormal gestational sac, with possible cystic degeneration is suggestive of molar degeneration. It should be noted that the typical 'molar' appearance is seen only after 10-11 weeks.
- A bicornuate uterus with an ongoing gestational sac in one horn may bleed from the other horn.
- Cervical (e.g. polyp) or vaginal (e.g. tear) causes of bleeding should also be considered.

In select situations, a repeat scan after a week or 10 days will clinch the diagnosis one way or the other.

Very briefly explain the sonographic milestones in early pregnancy.

The gestational sac or the chorionic ring appears by four and a half weeks after the first day of the last menstrual period. By five weeks the yolk sac is seen as the first structure to appear within the chorionic ring. Soon after, at six weeks the amnion and the embryo appear. Almost as soon as the embryonic pole appears the embryonic heart activity is seen.

Yolk sac should be seen in a gestational sac whose mean sac diameter is 8 mm or more. Embryo should be seen in a gestational sac whose mean sac diameter is 25 mm or more. M mode and not pulsed wave Doppler is used to record the embryonic heart rate.

A lady with 36 weeks gestation presents with fresh bleeding. How will you proceed?

Bleeding per vaginum in the third trimester brings to focus possible placental cause of bleed. This includes low placental attachment site and placental abruption. Ultrasound evaluation to study the placenta and its location is the first step in management.

Low placental attachment: Low placental attachment is predisposed to by presence previous cesarian section scar. Multiple pregnancy is another predisposing factor. The following are the possible findings and the terminology that should be used.

- Low lying placenta: When the lower edge is reaching to within 2.0 cm of the internal os.
- Marginal placenta previa: When the lower edge of placenta is reaching up to the internal os.
- Central asymmetric placenta previa: The placenta extends to cover the internal os. More of the placenta is attached on one uterine wall than the other.
- Central symmetric placenta previa: The placenta is implanted centrally on the internal os and extends all around equally on lower segment.

Every ultrasound examination in the second and third should include and report placental location and the distance of its lower margin from the internal os.

The diagnosis of placenta previa should not be made until 32 weeks of gestational age. The lower segment formation is complete by this time and hence the 'placental migration' is complete.

If the placental is on the posterior wall, its lower margin may be better seen by transvaginal rather than transabdominal examination. Segmental myometrial contraction and an over full maternal urinary bladder are reasons for false-positive diagnosis of low lying or marginal placenta. In all cases where there is a low placental attachment one should look for signs of morbid adherence (presence of placental lacunae, abnormal periplacental vasculature and thinning of the retroplacental complex).

Placental abruption: Predisposing factors include pregnancy-induced hypertension and trauma.

Ultrasound findings include retroplacental hypoechoic or mixed echogenic hematoma. If the retroplacental bleed dissects into

the placenta, it becomes thick and non homogeneous. Clinical background and painful tender uterus may help in reaching a diagnosis. It should be noted that a normal appearing placenta does not rule out abruption.
Vasa previa: It is diagnosed if the umbilical vessels cross the internal os. This often happens if there is a succenturiate lobe in the lower segment and the connecting vessels between the main placenta and the accessory lobe course across the internal os. Diagnosis is by use of color Doppler in the region of the internal os.
Miscellaneous conditions: Cervicitis, cervical polyp, early stages of labor may be causes of bleeding in the third trimester.

Thus, we see that ultrasound has a pivotal role in the assessment of possible cause of per vaginal bleeding in pregnancy.

A pregnant lady presents with lower abdominal pain. What is the investigation of choice and what could be the possible causes and findings?

Pain during pregnancy could be due to obstetric, adnexal or other causes. Obstetric causes would include threatened abortion and ectopic pregnancy in the first trimester, or placental abruption or previous cesarean scar rupture in the third trimester.

Threatened abortion has already been dealt with in the previous section. The diagnosis of ectopic gestation is based on history, beta hCG levels and ultrasound findings. Absent intrauterine gestation in the background of beta hCG level of more than 1000 mIU/mL (IRP) is highly suggestive of ectopic gestation. Direct confirmation is done by demonstration of an extrauterine gestational sac with or without yolk sac and/or fetus (with or without cardiac activity). The ectopic gestation sac could be in the rudimentary uterine horn or tube or ovary (rarely). In the uterus itself it could be a cervical or cesarian scar pregnancy. Pain is a feature if there is threatened rupture in any of these locations. In a frank ruptured gestation, there is a mixed echogenic adnexal mass with turbid ascites.

In the third trimester abruption may be seen as a retroplacental hematoma or just a nonhomogeneous thick placenta. Ultrasound confirms the viability of the fetus. Threatened rupture may be seen as a focal thinning or absence of the uterine wall thickness. High frequency transducer helps define the rupture clearly. Free fluid in the abdominal cavity may be seen.

Pregnancy-associated pelvic causes of pain include fibroid degeneration and ovarian cyst complication (hemorrhage or torsion). Degeneration of a fibroid does not present with any specific ultrasound features. However, probe tenderness over the fibroid is highly confirmative of the fibroid being the cause of the pain. Ovarian cyst with hemorrhage presents as a cyst with turbid content, fibrinous strands or clot. Typically, the cyst luminal findings change with time. Ovarian cyst torsion is recognized by the presence of the 'torsion knot' or 'whirlpool sign' which is a reflection of the twisted pedicle. Tenderness over the cyst is also suggestive of complication. Color Doppler may be used to pick up the twisted pedicle sign.

Other causes include appendicitis, ureteric colic due to calculi and cholecystitis. Ultrasound helps in identifying or suspecting these conditions.

A thickened (diameter of 6 mm or more), noncompressible, tender appendix indicates acute appendicitis. During pregnancy it may be practically difficult to use the graded compression technique to visualize the abnormal appendix.

Pelvicaliectasia of the concerned kidney with demonstration of dilated ureter and the calculus clinches the diagnosis. However, it should be stressed that pelvicaliectasia may occur in pregnancy even without pathological obstruction. This is largely due to the hormonal effect on the pelvicalyces.

Presence of gallbladder calculi with thick walls, pericholecystic halo and tenderness give the diagnosis of acute calculous cholecystitis.

A 28 weeks pregnant lady presents with distended abdomen and discomfort. Clinically the abdomen is tense and polyhydramnios is suspected. What is the investigation that is appropriate and what could be the findings?

Ultrasonography confirms the presence of polyhydramnios. This may be done subjectively or objectively. The maximum depth of the largest pocket of liquor more than 8 cm or amniotic fluid index of more than 20 confirms and quantifies polyhydramnios. Ultrasound helps in sorting out the cause of polyhydramnios. The following causes may be recognized:[2]

- Congenital anomalies of the fetus (10–20%): Open neural tube defects, upper GI obstructive lesions (esophageal or duodenal atresia), fetal akinesia deformation sequence, congenital high airway obstruction sequence, congenital diaphragmatic hernia, congenital pulmonary airway malformation, anterior abdominal wall defects, fetal neck masses as goitre and skeletal dysplasias. Twin to twin transfusion sequence (oligo-poly sequence), fetal anemia and association with hydrops fetalis are other fetal causes.
- Macrosomia and polyhydramnios due to maternal diabetes mellitus (25–30%).
- Placental causes, e.g. chorioangioma.
- Idiopathic (60–70%): When no apparent cause is found the polyhydramnios is termed idiopathic. These neonates should be carefully evaluated as conditions like Bartter syndrome, etc. may be diagnosed.

Hence, in a case polyhydramnios a careful structures examination of the fetus and placenta is indicated. Stuck twin should be looked for, MCA peak systolic velocity should be assessed (>1.5 MoM), maternal glucose tolerance testing for maternal diabetes and possibly a TORCH testing are indicated.

You have recognized a monochorionic diamniotic twins in a first trimester scan. What will be the frequency and mode of monitoring and what complications could be anticipated?

MCDA twins are prone to complications in as much as 15%. These complications are due to shared vasculature. Monitoring is needed for early recognition of these complications. The current recommended frequency of monitoring in a hitherto uncomplicated MCDA twins is once every two weeks.[3] Biometry, liquor volume and Doppler of the umbilical, MCA and ductus should be done at every sitting from 16 weeks onwards. The intertwin weight difference must be recorded in each study. Proper labeling of the twins is essential as the same twin needs to be consistently identified at each sitting for plotting of growth curves. In the first scan the cord insertion related to the zone of the placenta must be evaluated. The most common complication is twin-to-twin transfusion sequence and must be diagnosed if the deepest pocket of amniotic fluid in one amniotic sac is 2 cm or lesser and more than 8 cm in the other sac. The following is Quintero's staging:

- *Stage I:* AF discordance; filled UB seen in both twins.
- *Stage II:* UB persistently empty in donor and full in recipient.
- *Stage III:* Doppler abnormality in any one twin.
- *Stage IV:* One/both fetus/es hydropic.
- *Stage V:* One/both fetus/es demise.

Fetoscopic laser ablation of the placental vascular communications is the treatment of choice.

The other complications that may be picked up include twin anemia polycythemia sequence (TAPS), selective intrauterine growth restriction (sIUGR), twin reversed arterial perfusion sequence (TRAP).

Here, is a lady with a confirmed 32 weeks gestation. On examination the symphysiofundal height corresponds to 28 weeks. You have suspected IUGR. How will you confirm this diagnosis?

Ultrasound biometry (BPD, HC, AC and FL) yields the estimated fetal weight. Less than

5th percentile weight identifies the small for gestational group of fetuses. 70% of these fetuses are constitutionally small fetuses, the remaining 30% of the fetuses are growth restricted. Differentiation between these groups is essential as the management is totally different. Serial growth assessment plotted on a growth curve is best method to differentiate between these groups. In constitutional small fetuses, the growth curve is parallel to the nomogram curve, i.e. the growth of all the parameters is maintained at the same percentile (though low) in all the studies. In IUGR, the growth curve 'falls off' progressively indicating that the percentiles are decreasing from study to study. Oligohydramnios and abnormal Doppler studies are associated with the growth restriction rather than the constitutionally small group. Interval growth scans should be done with a minimum interval of 2 weeks.

You have now diagnosed intrauterine growth restriction, how will you now manage?

The aim of management in IUGR is to achieve as mature a fetus as possible without letting it slip into severe hypoxia and acidemia. This timing of deliver is the only option that we have. To recognize the well-being of the fetus serial monitoring with multivessel [umbilical

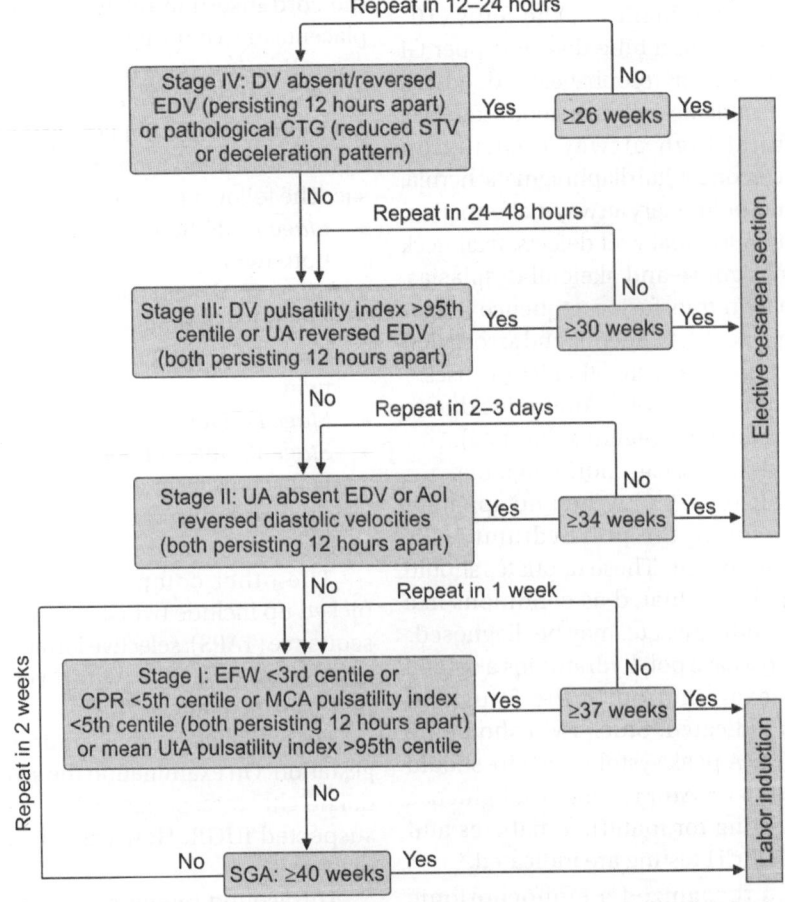

Flowchart 1: Role of umbilical Doppler in managing a fetal growth restriction baby

Abbreviations: DV, ductus venosus; UA, umbilical artery; STV, short-term variability; CTG, cardiotocogram; EDV, End diastolic volume; CPR, Cerebroplacental ratio; UtA, Uterine artery; MCA, middle cerebral artery; AoI, aortic isthmus

artery (UA), middle cerebral artery (MCA), aortic isthmus (AoI) and ductus venosus (DV)] Doppler study is indicated. The frequency of monitoring increases and the aimed maturity decreases as more and more severe signs of Doppler abnormality appear. The following algorithm from the Barcelona group[4] is a working model (Flowchart 1).

Q. 1. What are the Doppler waveform abnormalities that one has to recognize and interpret?

The Doppler waveforms are interpreted in terms the pulsatility index (PI) for that gestational age. Serial values are best plotted on nomograms to reveal improving, stable or deteriorating trends. The UAPI >95th percentile, absent end diastolic flow and reverse diastolic flow are abnormal patterns and indicate elevated fetoplacental peripheral vascular resistance. MCAPI <5th percentile is abnormal and indicates head sparing effect. Diastolic reversals in the AoI is abnormal. DVPI >95%, absent or reversed A wave are the abnormal. The arterial Doppler changes are early in the cascade whereas the venous Doppler changes are late. 'Early' arterial Doppler abnormality indicates presence of hypoxia whereas the 'late' venous Doppler abnormality indicates acidemia. In a case under surveillance one should never wait for late changes to manifest (e.g. a wave absence of reversal). There is no role for Doppler in a case where all parameters are normal. Indications for Doppler surveillance would include IUGR, oligohydramnios, loss of fetal movement, maternal complications and abnormal NST tracing. Once there is absent diastolic flow in the umbilical artery surveillance is done as an inpatient. Doppler interpretation and management decisions are always done in conjunction with the other information (gestational age, fetal size, liquor volume, etc.).

Q. 2. Is there a role for intrapartum ultrasound?

Ultrasound in the labor ward can identify the presenting part, placental position, amniotic fluid quantity, vasa previa, cervical status during labor induction and presence of fibroid obstructing progress of labor. In addition, ultrasound may be used for guidance for cephaocentesis in fetal hydrocephalus.

Prediction of possibility of vaginal delivery or cesarean section based on the angle of progression or head perineum distance has been studied to hold promise.[5,6] Follow up of fetal head descent using the head perineum distance or the skull perineum distance have been described. Other distance parameters are required for monitoring descent in occipito-posterior presentation. These distances are arrived at by transperineal ultrasound.

References

1. Doubilet PM, Benson CB, Bourne T, et al. Diagnostic criteria for nonviable pregnancy early in the first trimester. N Engl J Med. 2013;369(15):1443-51.
2. Alexander ES, Spitz HB, Clark RA. Sonography of polyhydramnios. AJR Am J Roentgenol. 1982;138(2):343-6.
3. Khalil A, et al. ISUOG Practice Guidelines: role of ultrasound in twin pregnancy. Ultrasound Obstet Gynecol. 2016;47:247-63.
4. Figueras F, Gratocos E. Update on the diagnosis and classification of fetal growth restriction and proposal of a stage based management protocol, Fetal Diagn Ther. 2014;36:86-98.
5. Levy R, et al. Can angle of progression in pregnant women before onset of labor predict mode of delivery Ultrasound Obstet Gynecol. 2012;40: 332-7.
6. Torkildsen EA. Prediction of delivery mode with transperineal ultrasound in women with prolonged first stage of labor. Ultrasound Obstet Gynecol. 2011;37:702-8.

CHAPTER 33

Vulval Hematoma

Sunanda R Kulkarni

Patient named X aged 28 years who had delivered at a primary health care (PHC) was referred to our hospital with complaints of swelling of the genitalia since 3 hours and was experiencing excruciating pain since 4 hours.

She had delivered 4 hours back a healthy female baby, according to her referral slip—baby was delivered with the help of outlet forceps as the second stage was delayed and there was no primary postpartum hemorrhage (PPH).

On Examination

- Patient aged 28 years normally built and nourished
- Patient appeared pale and weak
- Pulse rate—130/minute, BP-90/70 low volume mm of Hg
- Respiratory rate—30/minute, no crepitation. Normal breath sounds
- Uterus was well contracted.
- Normal bleeding
- Left mediolateral episiotomy was sutured, and wound was seen.
- There was a tense and large hematoma on the left side of labia extending up to the thigh. Size 12 × 15 cm. It was bluish in color, fluctuating. No other mass felt.
- P/S revealed an intact cervix with no bulge in the vagina.
- P/V revealed a patulous cervix with well-contracted uterus fornices were free.
- She was catheterized—High colored urine drained.
- A diagnosis of vulval hematoma was made and evacuation under anesthesia was planned.
- Blood was sent for cross matching
- Episiotomy sutures were under tension, wound was opened till the muscles. The episiotomy wound was explored, there was a small bleeding vessel which was held and ligated, and after evacuating the clots of about 400–500 g, a drain was placed and wound was re-sutured. A pint of cross-matched blood was transfused.
- Her pulse and blood pressure were monitored. She was kept in the hospital for 5 days. Antibiotics and pain killers were given and was discharged after removing the drain.

Q. 1. Describe the blood supply to female external genitalia.

Blood supply of the female external genitalia is mainly from the pudendal artery and inferior epigastric artery which is the branches of femoral and external iliac artery respectively. Mons pubis is supplied by the inferior epigastric artery whereas vulva, vagina and clitoris receive blood supply from pudendal artery (Figs 1 and 2).

Vagina receives blood supply from the vaginal artery (branch of internal pudendal) and anastomosis with inferior vesical, uterine artery and other branches of pudendal artery, forming longitudinal azygous vaginal artery on the anteroposterior sides of vagina. Injury to these arteries at the vaginal vault results in massive hemorrhage even if the uterine artery is ligated.

The following are the branches of the internal pudendal artery.

- The artery of the bulbocavernous muscle supplies the bulb of the vestibule and the bulbocavernous muscle
- Erectile tissue of the clitoris is supplied by and deep artery of clitoris and the dorsal artery of clitoris to clitoris
- Transverse perineal artery supplies cutaneous surface of perineum and transverse perinei superficialis muscle
- Inferior rectal artery supplies the anal sphincter and levator ani muscle and runs across the ischiorectal fossa and cause hemorrhage in superficial wounds of the anus and ischiorectal fossa
- The valve less veins in the perineum result in massive hematoma in case of vulva or vaginal trauma.

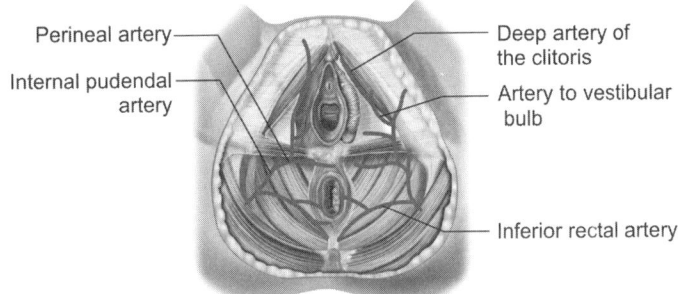

Fig. 1: Blood supply of external genitalia

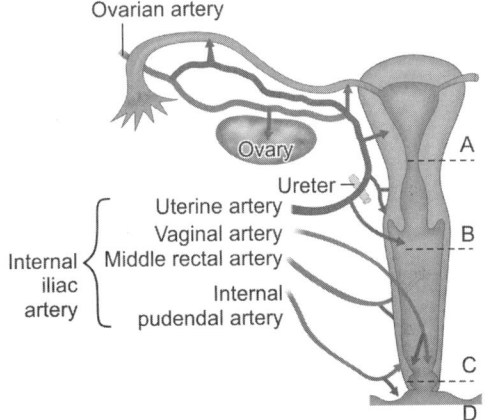

Fig. 2: Blood supply of the internal and external genitalia

Q. 2. What is the mechanism of vulvar hematoma?

Both sharp and blunt instrument can cause hematomas. Hematomas when small may appear as bulge under the mucosa and when there is large hematoma, it may be palpable per abdomen as it is lifted by the bleeding. Both Forceps and vacuum directly and indirectly can cause injury to mucus membrane and underlying vasculature leading to hematomas.

Q. 3. What are the different modes of presentation?

The presenting symptoms depend upon the amount of bleeding and duration of bleeding. If the bleeding is small in amount, they may have pain and sometimes it may be large enough to present as shock and if infected with fever.

Q. 4. How do you classify hematomas of genital tract?

Refer Table 1.

Table 1: Classification of hematoma of genital tract

Classification in different ways	
1. Size	Small
	Large
2. Relation to pelvic peritoneum	Subperitoneal
	Supraperitoneal
3. Relation to levator ani	Supralevator
	Infralevator
4. Site	Vulval
	Vulvovaginal
	Supravaginal
	Paravaginal
5. Cause	Obstetric
	Nonobstetric

Table 2: Risk factors of obstetric hematomas

Maternal	Fetal
• Nulliparity • Prolonged second stage • Instrumental delivery • Genital tract varicosities • Maternal age >29 years • Preeclampsia • Clotting disorders	• Baby >4 kg • Multifetal pregnancy

Q. 5. Enumerate the risk factors of obstetric hematomas.

Risk factors are enumerated in Table 2.

Q. 6. Describe the features of hematoma as per their location.

Features of hematoma are shown in Table 3.

Table 3: Features of hematoma as per their location

Location	Description	Features
1. Vulvar hematoma	Bleeding is limited to the vulvar tissues superficial to the anterior urogenital diaphragm	Seen on the vulva
2. Vulvovaginal hematoma	Caused due to injury of the branches of the pudendal artery (the posterior rectal, transverse perineal and posterior labial arteries)	Seen on the vulva
3. Vaginal hematoma	Arise from damage to the descending branch of the uterine artery	Seen only on per vaginal examination, may extend into the ischiorectal fossa
4. Supra-vaginal/sub-peritoneal hematoma	Arises due to damage to the uterine artery branches in the broad ligament	May spread to retroperitoneal and broad ligament. Clinically occult usually diagnosed after cardiovascular collapse

Q. 7. What are the causes for nonobstetric hematomas?

A nonobstetric trauma to the genital tract may be due to various reasons, like:
- Sexual assault
- Falling astride
- Snowboarding
- Bull goring.

Table 4: Difference between minor injury and major injury

Minor injury	Major injury
Due to normal intercourse/defloration	Due to vigorous sexual act/major trauma
Resolve with, minimal treatment	May require immediate treatment due to tear and bleeding

Q. 8. What are the clinical features of vulvar hematoma?

Clinical features depend on the amount of blood loss. Usually women many present with severe pain in the perineum especially in sitting position, with difficulty in voiding or defecation. A gradually increasing swelling is seen in the vagina which is tender to touch. color of the swelling varies according to the duration and hemorrhage.

Q. 9. What history needs to be obtained and discuss how the examination needs to be done?

Table 5 shows the difference between obstetric and nonobstetric hematomas.

Table 5: Difference between nonobstetric hematomas

Obstetric hematomas	Nonobstetric hematomas
Details of delivery	Trauma
Instrumental delivery	Forceful coitus, fall, bull gore injury, etc.

Examination Required
- Routine examination of vitals,
- P/A examination for mass, tenderness.
- In pelvic examination for uterine deviation, contour, cervical deviation, vaginal asymmetry, bulge or mass in the fornices, tenderness, cervical, vaginal tears, etc.

Q. 10. What is the role of imaging in the diagnosis of hematomas?

USG, CT scan are useful in diagnosing even small hematomas whch are not detected by clinical examination.

Any imaging modality could help in monitoring the size of hematoma.

MRI can help to differentiate hematoma from endometrioma and also give information regarding the location, size and extent.

Q. 11. What are the possible complications of the hematoma?

Sepsis, hemorrhagic shock, DIC, ARF, etc.

Q. 12. What are the management principles?

Management principles of hematoma are described on Flowchart 1.

Flowchart 1: Management principles of hematoma

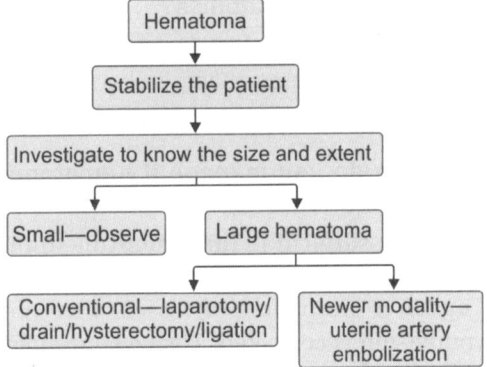

Surgical Management

On making an incision on most dependent part, evacuate all the clots and if there are bleeding points secure them. If there is oozing place a drain. Some may need laparotomy and blood transfusion. After the surgery patient is observed closely and appropriate antibiotics are prescribed (Table 6).

Table 6: Conservative and surgical management of hematoma

Conservative	Surgical
• Small and static and subperitoneal • Large static, but associated with longer stays in hospital, an increased need for antibiotics and blood transfusion and greater subsequent operative intervention	• Small but increasing • Acutely expanding • Large • Large subperitoneal

When the bleeding is venous, revealed, from abrasions, packing with hemostatic agents may be useful.

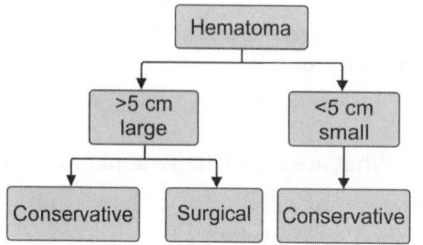

Q. 13. What are the recent advances in the management of hematomas?

Arterial embolization which is used for myoma and postpartum hemorrhage, is also useful to control the hematomas.

Q.14. How do you manage if hematoma recurs?

Even after surgical management in some cases hematoma may recur due to slipping of ligatures or opening of vessels once the hypotension is corrected. Hence continued monitoring for signs of blood loss is essential. Re-exploration may be required and sometimes even ligation of internal iliac artery or hysterectomy may become necessary.

Q. 15. Discuss the various hemostats that can be used to control local bleeding.

Monsel's solution: Ferric sulfate solution, may be useful for superficial abrasions. Ferric subsulfate solution is prepared from ferrous sulfate, sulfuric acid and nitric acid.

Mucoadhesive agents: Seal bleeding wounds by their strong adherent property to the tissues. Independent of platelet or clotting factors. It is made from chitosan a naturally occurring biocompatible polysaccharide which is derived from shell fish, e.g. celox, SAM chito, Hemcon.

Procoagulant supplements: These accelerate the body's natural coagulation cascade. Third generation product is available in sachet form which can be applied directly to the wound thus avoiding the handling of loose granules. Fourth generation product like quikclot is a fibrous gauze impregnated with kaolin used for packing deep wounds.

Bibliography

1. Arnaud F, Tomori T, Carr W, et al. Exothermic reaction in zeolite hemostatic dressings: QuikClot ACS and ACS+. Annals of Biomedical Engineering. 2008;36(10):1708-13.
2. Badawy SZA, Etman A, Singh M, et al. Uterine artery embolization: the role in obstetrics and gynecology Clin Imaging. 2001;25:288-95.
3. Benrubi G, Neuman C, Nuss RC, et al. Vulvar and vaginal hematomas: a retrospective study of conservative versus operative management South Med J. 1987;80:991-4.
4. Bloom AI, Verstandig A, Gielchinsky Y, et al. Arterial embolisation for persistent primary postpartum haemorrhage:before or after hysterectomy? BJOG. 2004;111:880-4.
5. Burkatovskaya M, Tegos GP, Swietlik E, et al. Use of chitosan bandage to prevent fatal infections developing from highly contaminated wounds in mice. Biomaterials. 2006;27(22):4157-64.
6. Dildy GA. 3rd Postpartum hemorrhage: new management options. Clin Obstet Gynecol. 2002;45:330-44.
7. Geist RF. Sexually related trauma (review). Emerg Med Clin North Am. 1988;6:439-66.
8. Guerriero S, Ajossa S, Bargellini R, et al. Puerperal vulvovaginal hematoma: sonographic findings with MRI correlation. J Clin Ultrasound. 2004;32:415.
9. Gupta V, Nanda A, Bansal SN, et al. A bull horn injury of the perineum: A case report and review of the literature. Int J Gynae Plastic Surg. 2009;1:35-36.
10. Idikula J, Moses BV, Sadhu D, et al. Bullhorn injuries. Surg Gynaecol Obstet. 1991;172:220-22.
11. Jana N, Santra D, Das D, et al. Nonobstetric lower genital tract injuries in rural India. Int J Gynaecol Obstet. 2008;103(1):26-9. Epub 2008 Jul 11.

12. Kanai M, Osada R, Maruyama K, et al. A warning from Nagano: an increase in the vulvar haematomas and/or the lacerations which were caused by snow boarding. J Trauma. 2001;50:328-31.
13. Khan MAA, Jose R, Taylor C, et al. An iatrogenic burn from the use of a topical haemostatic agent. Emergency Medical Journal. 2010;27:950-1.
14. Kozen B, Kircher S, Heanao J, et al. An alternative field hemostatic Agent? Comparison of a new chitosan granule dressing to existing chitosan wafer, zeolite and standard dressings, in a lethal hemorrhagic groin injury. Annals of Emergency Medicine. 2007;50(3):S60-1.
15. Kulkarni MR, Gangadharaiah M, Kulkarni SR. Case Report, Bull Gore Injury of the Vagina, Journal of Clinical and Diagnostic Research. 2013;7(1):158-9.
16. Lacy J, Brennand E, Ornstein M, et al. A vaginal laceration which was caused by a high-pressure water jet in a prepubescent girl. Pediatr Emerg Care. 2007;23(2):112-4.
17. Morgans D, Chan N, Clark CA. Vulvar perineal haematomas in the immediate postpartum period and their management Aust N Z J Obstet Gynaecol. 1999;39:223-7.
18. Nagayama M, Watanabe Y, Okumura A, et al. Fast MR imaging in obstetrics Radiographics. 2002;22563-82.
19. Propst AM, Thorp JM Jr. Traumatic vulvar hematomas: conservative versus surgical management. South Med J. 1998;91:144-6.
20. Quinby WC. The anatomy and blood vessels of the pelvis. In: Meigs JV (Ed). Surgical Treatment of Cancer of the Cervix. New York: Grune and Stratton. 1954;p. 32.
21. Resnik R. Vaginal and vulvar hematoma Contemporary OB/GYN. 1996;41:19-23.
22. Rhee P1, Brown C, Martin M, et al. QuikClot use in trauma for hemorrhage control: case series of 103 documented uses. Journal of Trauma. 2008;64(4):1093-9.
23. Ridgway LE. Puerperal emergency. Vaginal and vulvar hematomas. Obstet Gynecol Clin North Am. 1995;22:275.
24. Rooholamini SA, Au AH, Hansen GC, et al. Imaging of pregnancy-related complications Radiographics. 1993;13:753-70.
25. Saleem Z, Rydhstrom H. Vaginal hematoma during parturition: a population-based study Acta Obstet Gynecol Scand. 2004;835:60-2.
26. Saleem Z, Rydhström H. Vaginal hematoma during parturition: a population-based study. Acta Obstet Gynecol Scand. 2004;83:560.
27. Sau AK, Dhar KK, Dhall GI. Nonobstetric lower genital tract trauma. Aust N Z Obstet Gynaecol. 1993;33:433-5.
28. Singhal VP, Neelam, Ankur HK, et al. Traumatic massive vulvar haematomas. International Journal of Gynae Plastic Surgery. 2010;2:35-37.
29. Sloin M, Karimian M, Ilbeigi P. Nonobstetric Lacerations of the vagina. J Am Osteopath Assoc. 2006;106(5):271-73.
30. Smith BL. A vaginal laceration which was caused by water skiing. J Emergency Nursing. 1996;22:156.
31. Smout CFV, Jacoby F, Lillie EW. Gynaecological and Obstetrical Anatomy. London: HK Lewis; 1969. pp. 101-2.
32. Waibel KH, Haney B, Moore M, et al. Safety of chitosan bandages in shellfish allergic patients. Military Medicine. 2001;176(10):1153-6.
33. Zahn CM, Hankins GD, Yeomans ER. Vulvo-vaginal hematomas complicating delivery. Rationale for drainage of the hematoma cavity J Reprod Med. 1996;41:569-74.

CHAPTER 34

Rare Photo Gallery

Sunanda R Kulkarni, K Srinivas

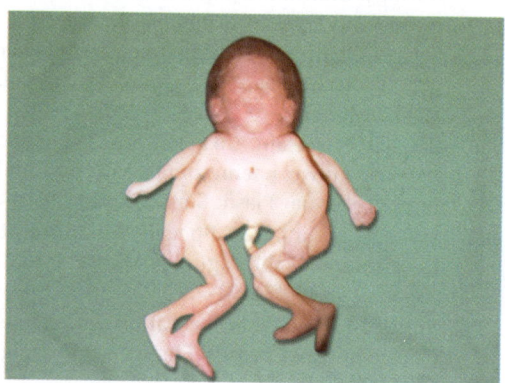

Fig. 1: Cephalopagus

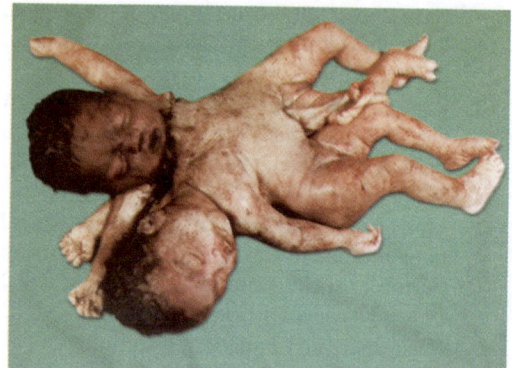

Fig. 2: Parapagus dicephalus

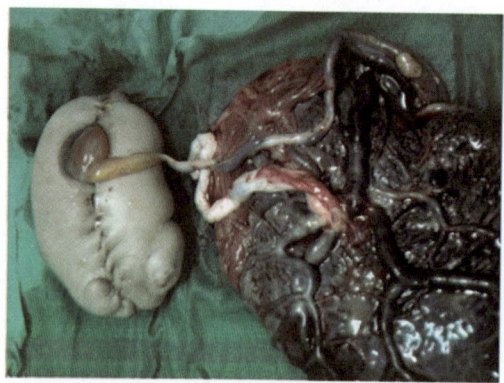

Fig. 3: Acardiac fetus

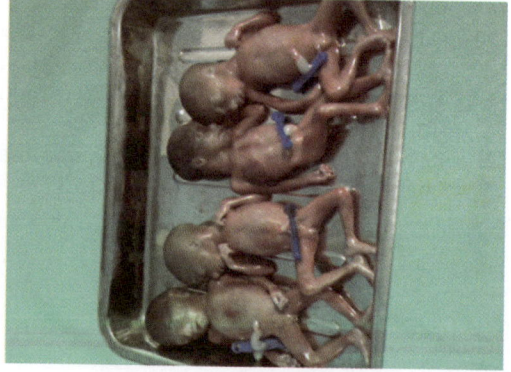

Fig. 4: Preterm quadruplets

Rare Photo Gallery

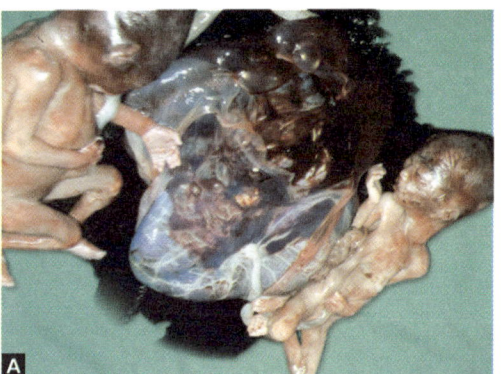
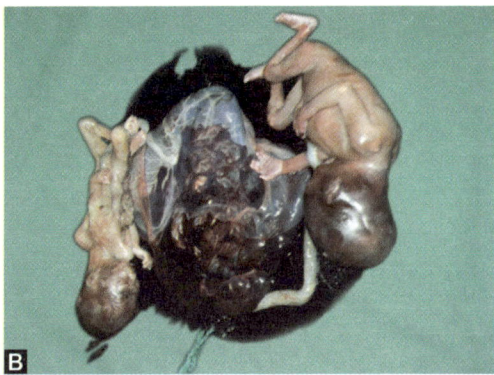

Figs 5A and B: Discordant twins

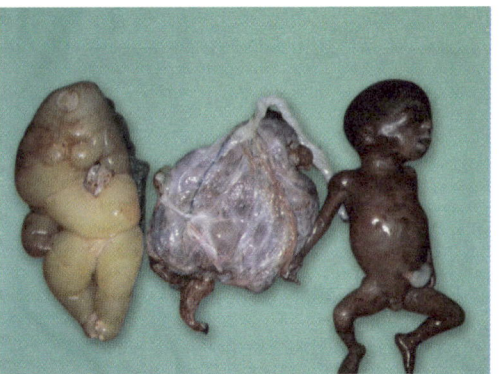

Fig. 6: Twins with one baby with hydrops

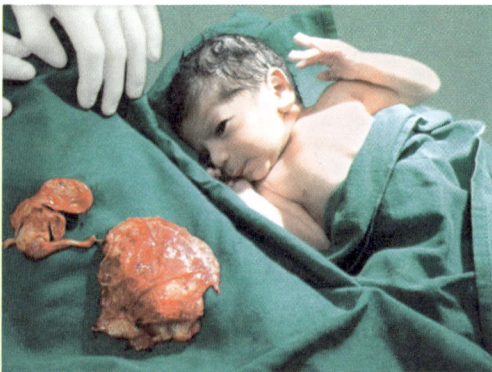

Fig. 7: Fetus papyraceus

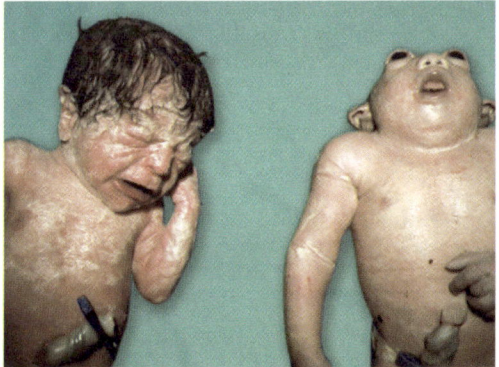

Fig. 8: Twins with one baby with anencephaly

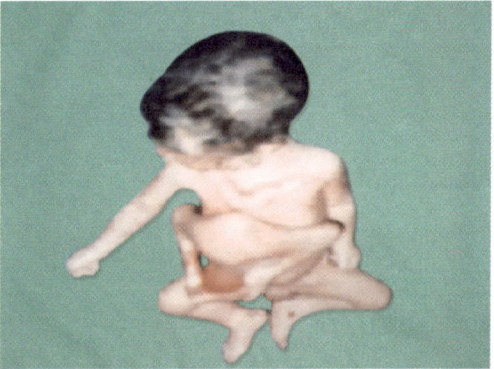

Fig. 9: External parasitic twin

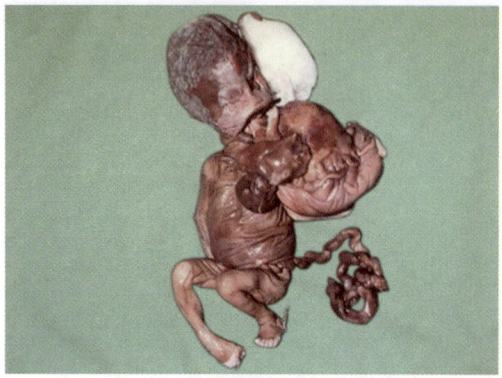

Fig. 10: Epignathus

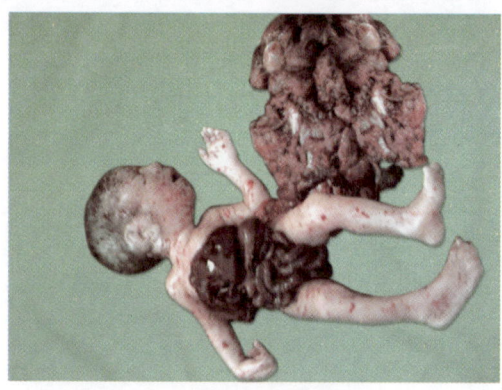

Fig. 11: Exomphalos

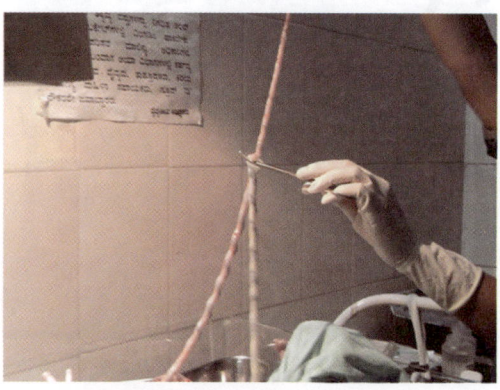

Fig. 12: Abnormally long cord

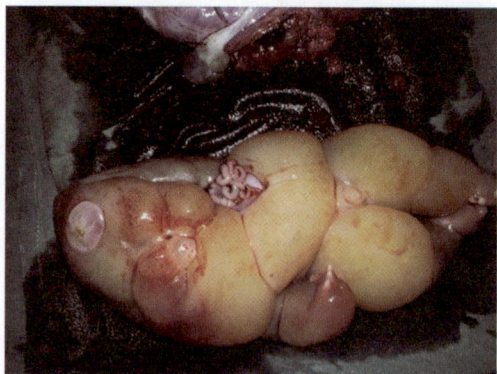

Fig. 13: Hydrops fetalis

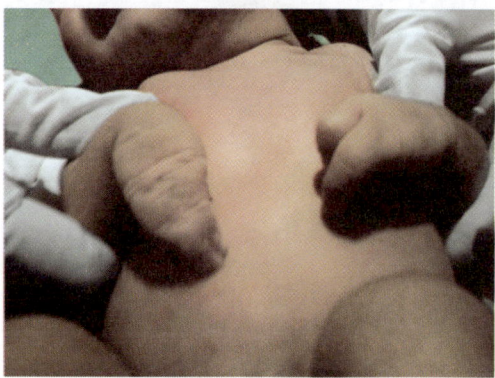

Fig. 14: Syndactyly with partial degeneration of hands

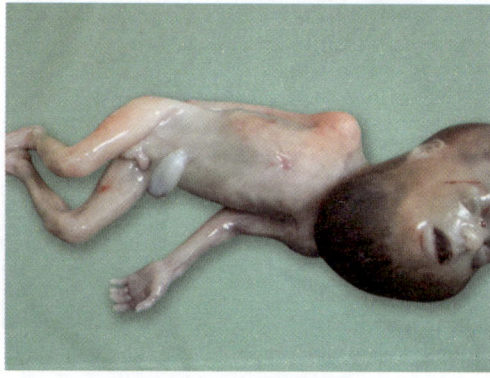

Fig. 15: Cystic hygroma

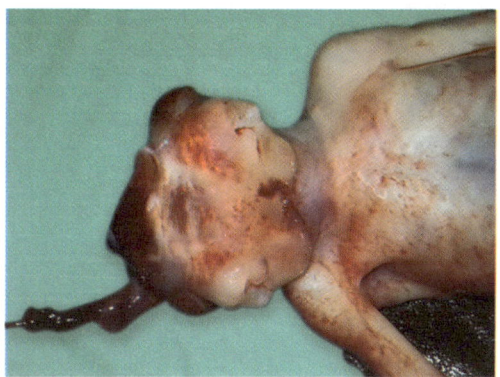
Fig. 16: Fused faces with anencephaly

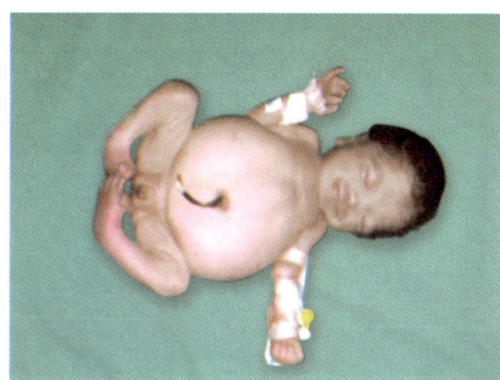
Fig. 17: Fetal ascitis

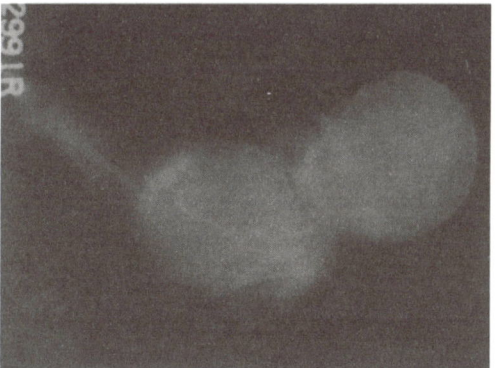
Fig. 18: Syringomyelia

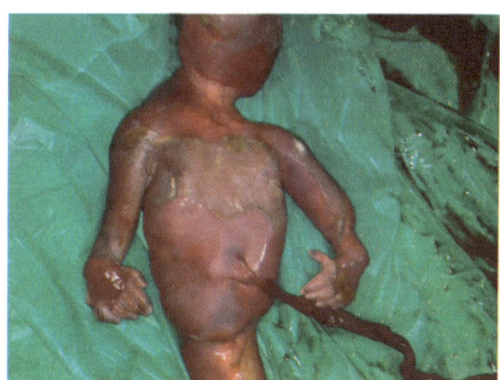
Fig. 19: Sacral agenesis

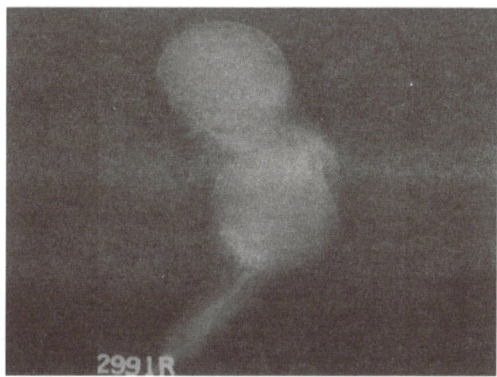
Fig. 20: Sacral agenesis

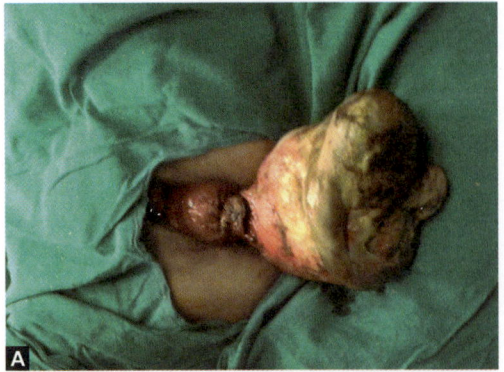 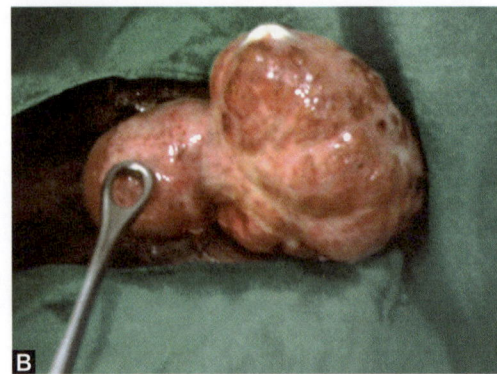

Figs 21A and B: Fibroid polyp

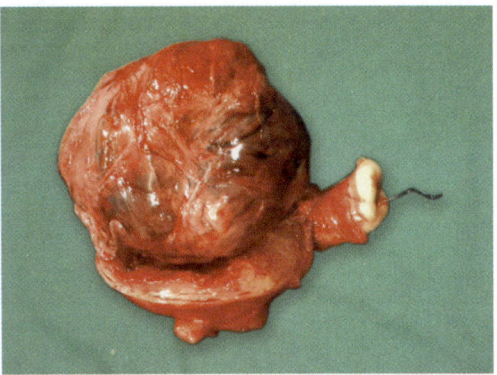

Fig. 22: Uterine leiomyoma—submucous

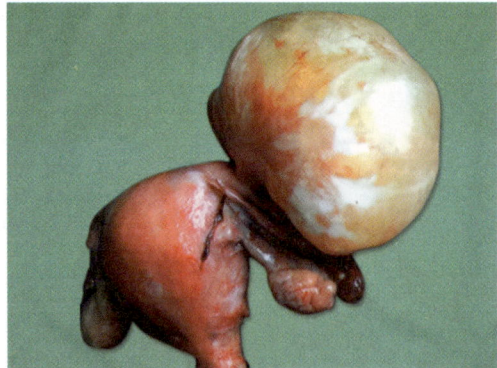

Fig. 23: Subserous fibroid with fatty degeneration

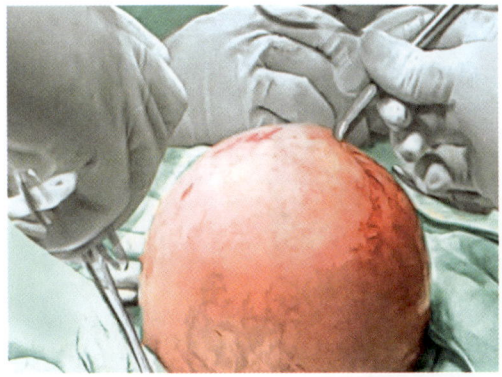

Fig. 24: Huge fibroid uterus

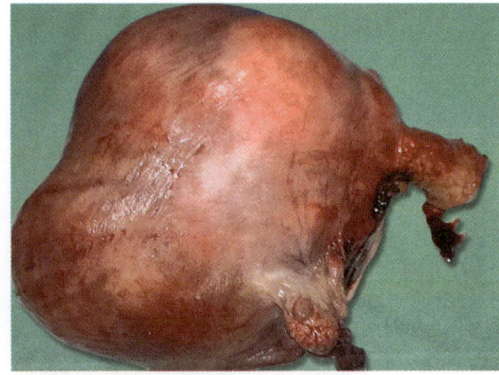

Fig. 25: Cornual fibroid

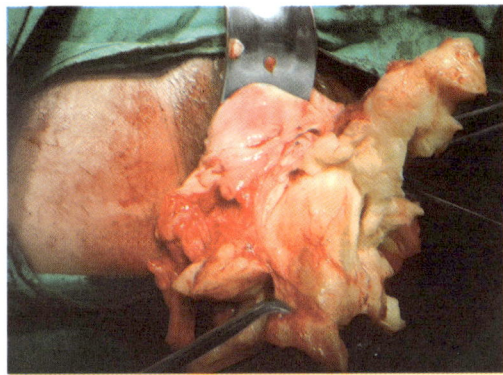
Fig. 26: Fibroid morcellation during NDVH

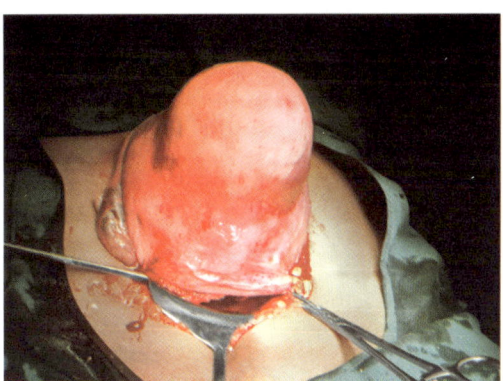
Fig. 27: Fundal fibroid with pregnancy

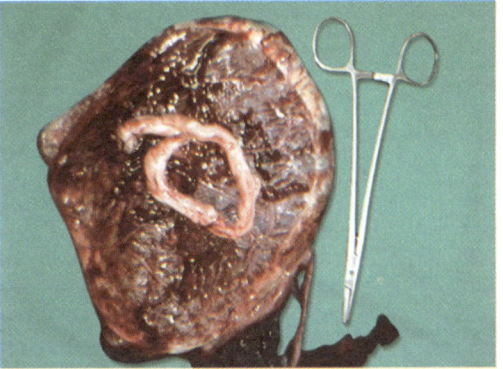
Fig. 28: Circumvallate placenta

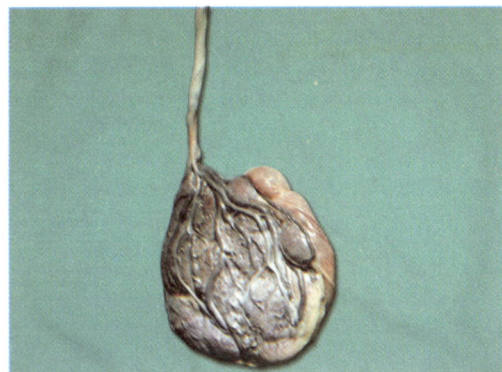
Fig. 29: Marginal attachment of the cord

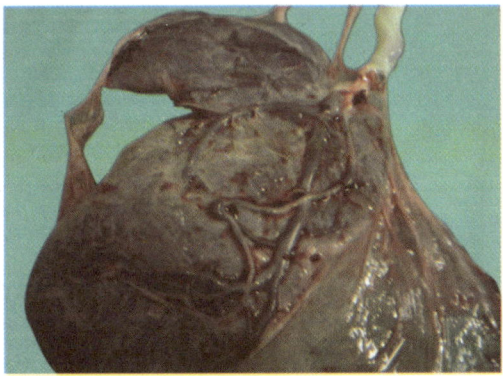
Fig. 30: Placenta succenturiata/bilobed placenta

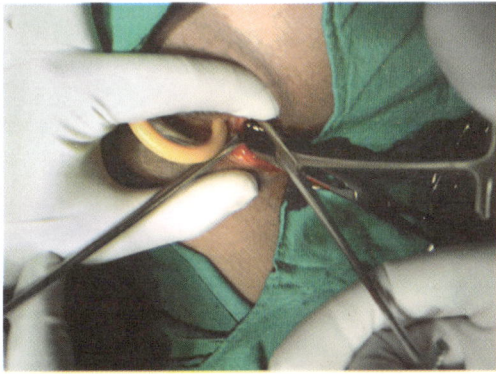
Fig. 31: Hymenotomy—draining hematocolpos

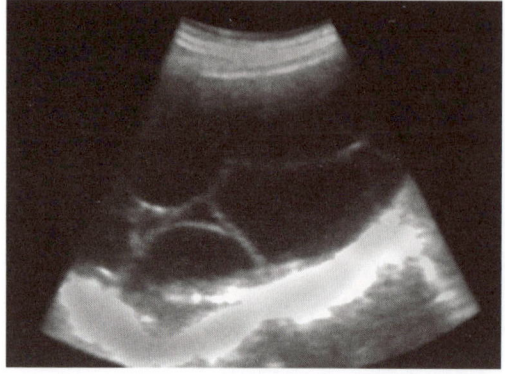

Fig. 32: USG showing OHSS

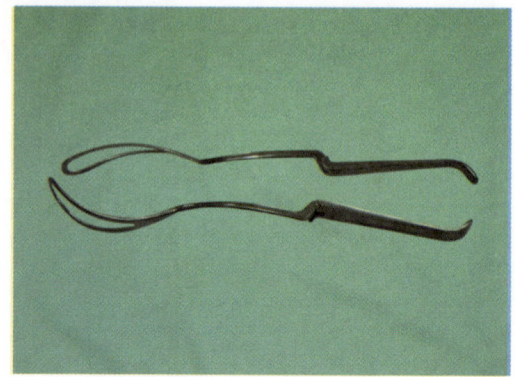

Fig. 33: Piper's forceps

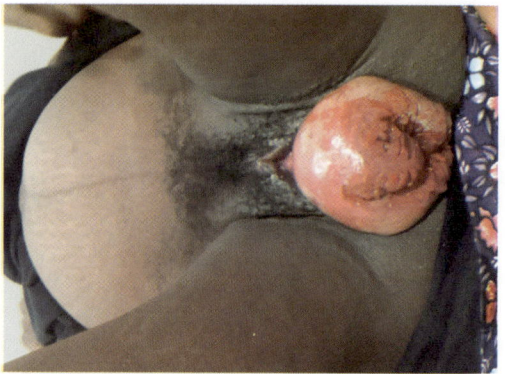

Fig. 34: Pregnancy with prolapse

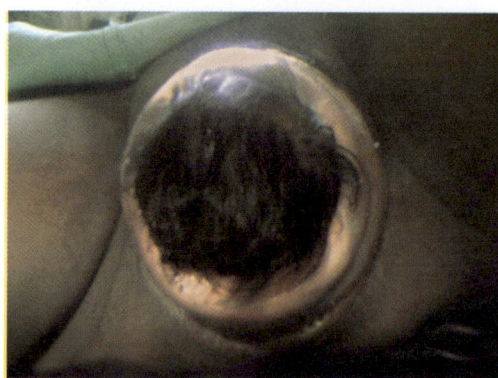

Fig. 35: Delivering the baby in a case of UV prolapse

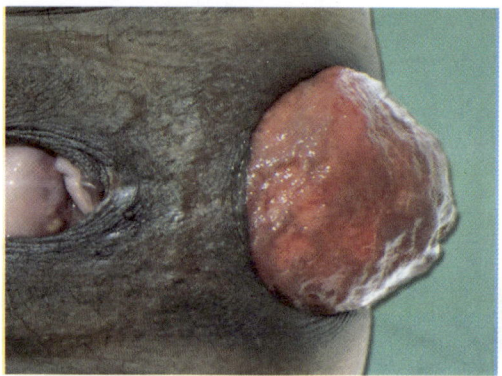

Fig. 36: Rectal prolapse

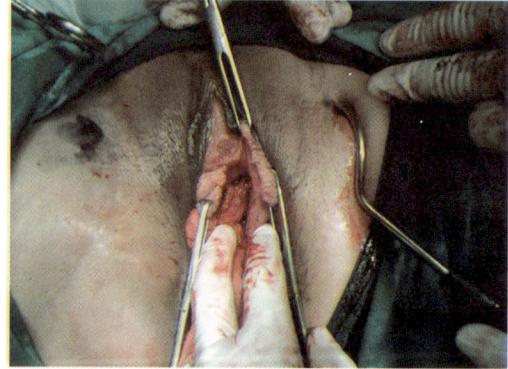

Fig. 37: TOT insertion

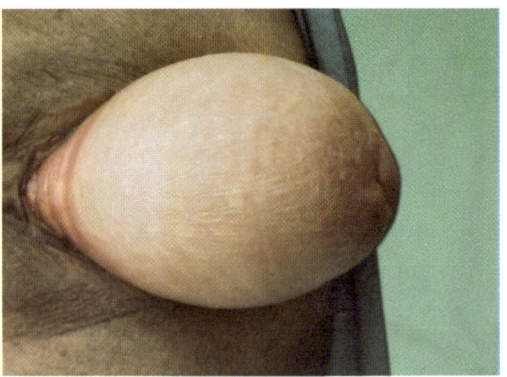

Fig. 38: Procidentia

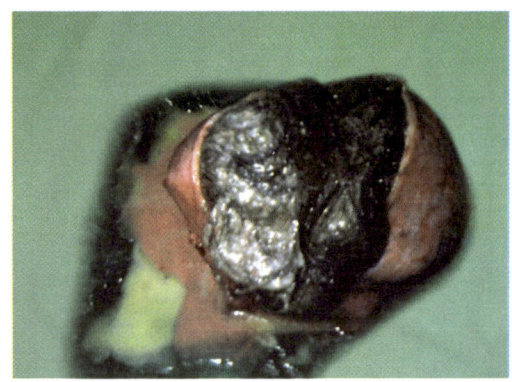

Fig. 39: Dermoid cyst with hairs

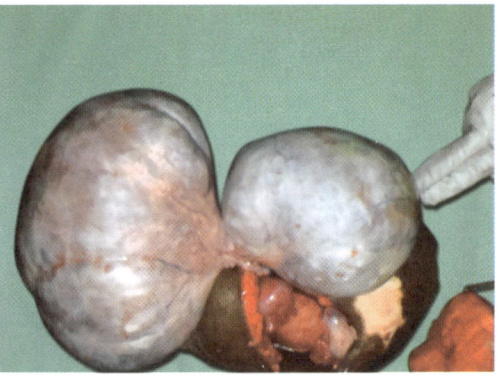

Fig. 40: Bilobed teratoma of ovary in an adolescent girl

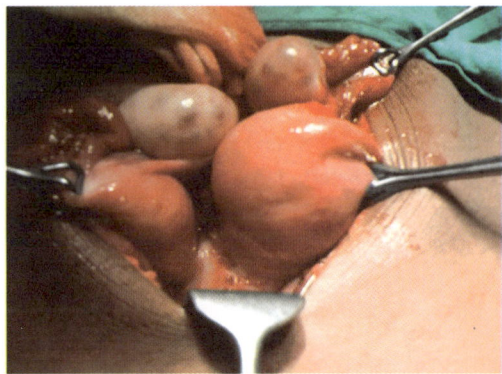

Fig. 41: Bicornuate uterus

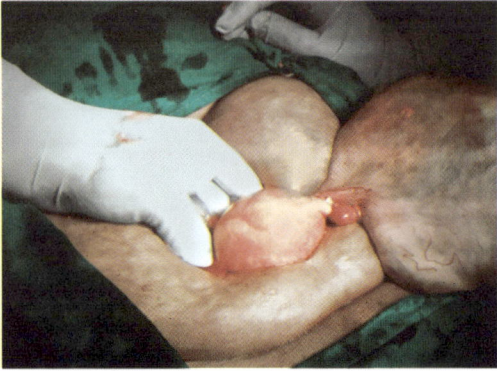

Fig. 42: Torsion ovarian cyst

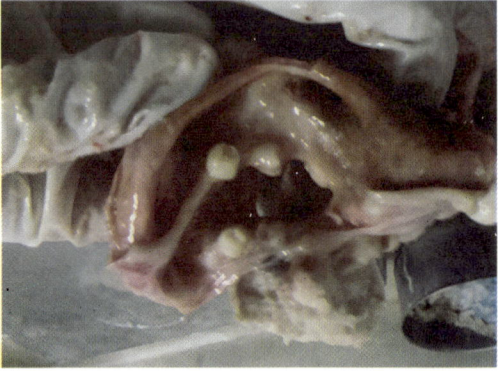

Fig. 43: Dermoid cyst showing jaw bone and teeth

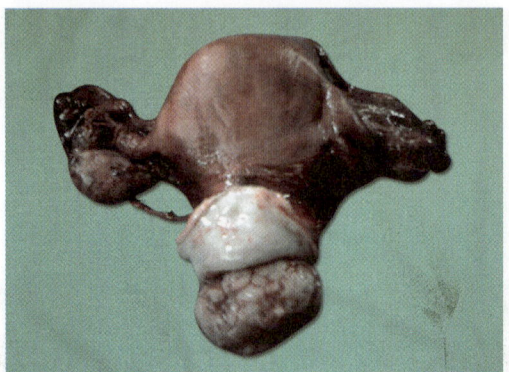

Fig. 44: Specimen of Wertheim's hysterectomy

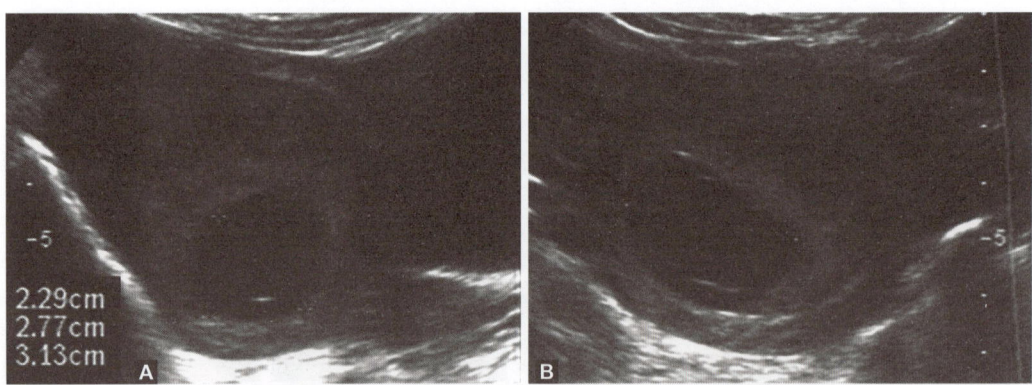

Figs 45A and B: Seven weeks amenorrhea—low implantation of the gestational sac, mean sac diameter of 2.7 cm and presence of amnion without presence of embryonic pole—anembryonic gestation

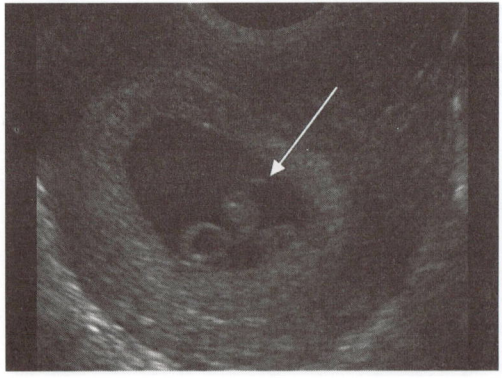

Fig. 46: 7 weeks amenorrhea—Normal gestational sac, yolk sac, amnion (arrow) and embryo

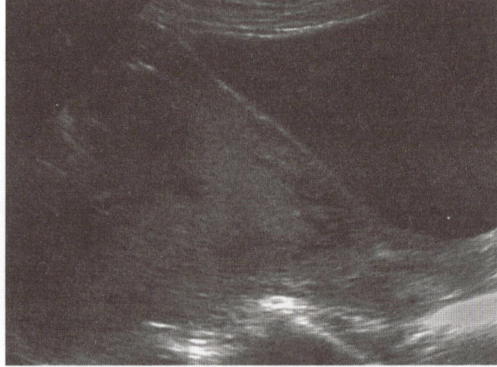

Fig. 47: Central symmetric placenta previa

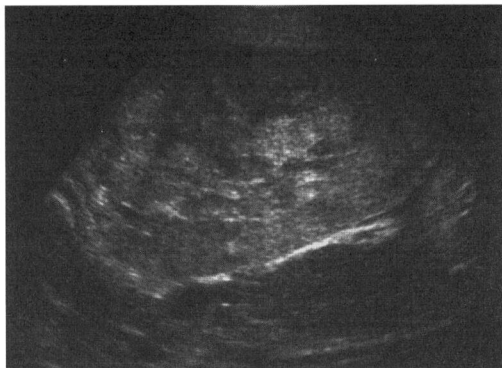

Fig. 48: Large retroplacental hematoma—This was an intrauterine demise

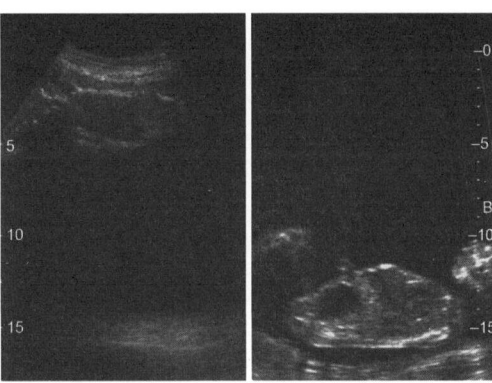

Fig. 49: Twin-to-twin transfusion sequence. a. Donor 'stuck' due to oligohydramnios with persistently unfilled urinary bladder, a. Recipient with polyhydramnios and a persistently full urinary bladder

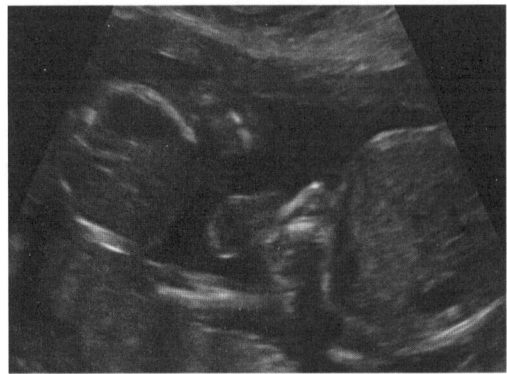

Fig. 50: Abdominal circumference discordance in monochorionic diamniotic twins

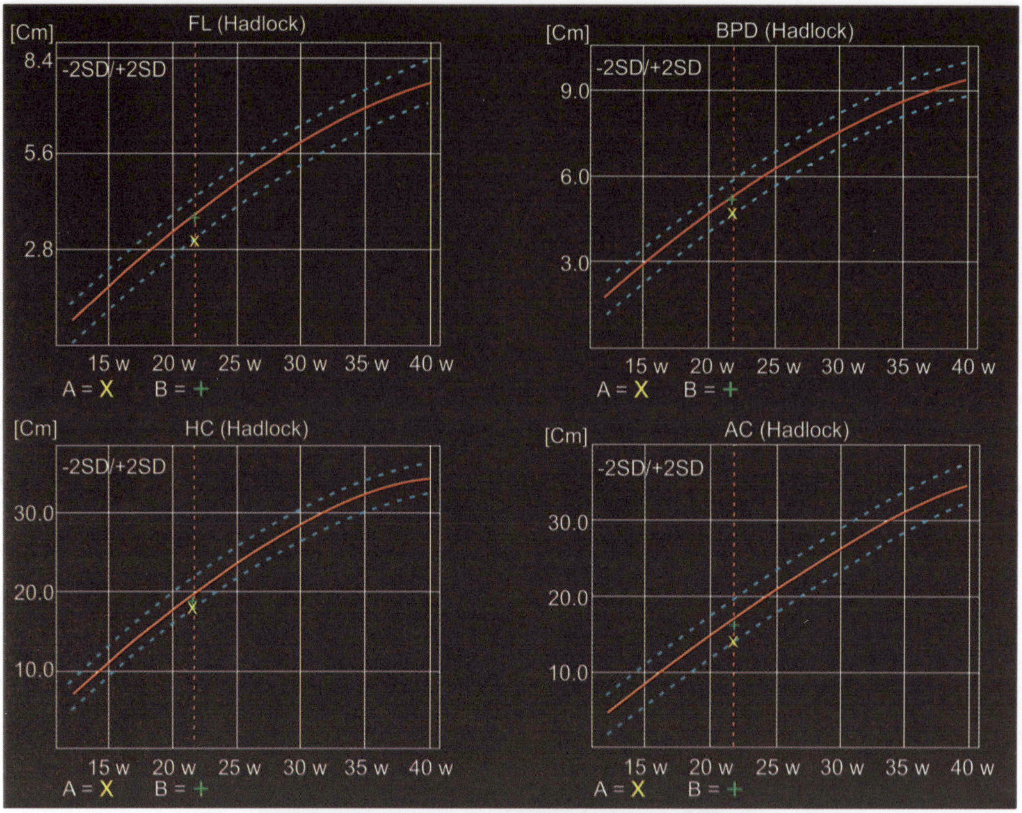

Fig. 51: Growth chart showing measurements suggestive of FGR

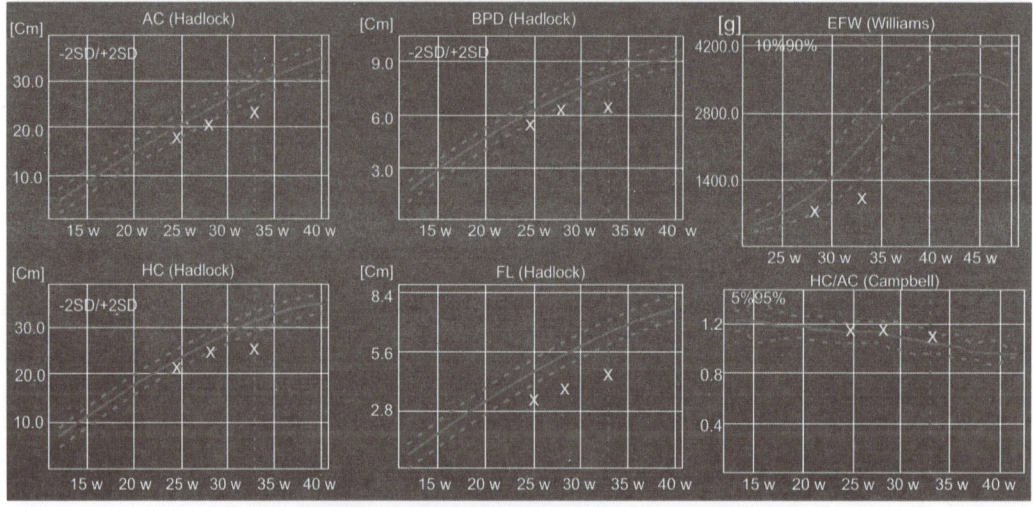

Fig. 52: Growth charts suggestive of FGR

Rare Photo Gallery

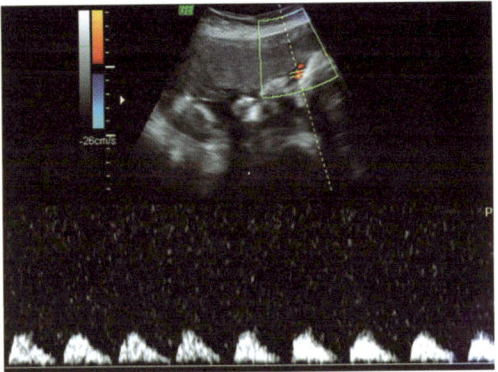
Fig. 53: Doppler changes in FGR

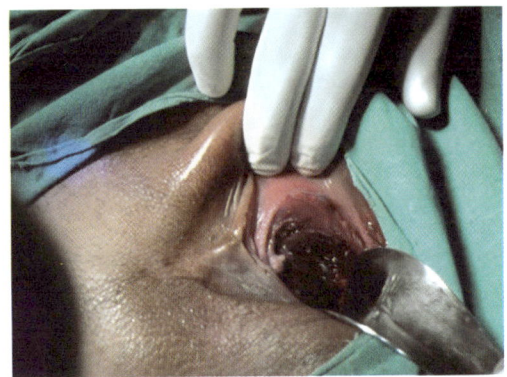
Fig. 54: Vulval hematoma

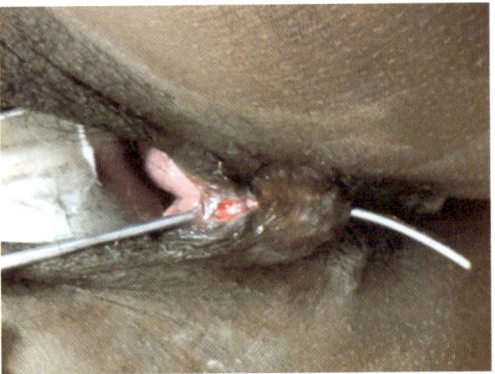
Fig. 55: Rectovaginal fistula

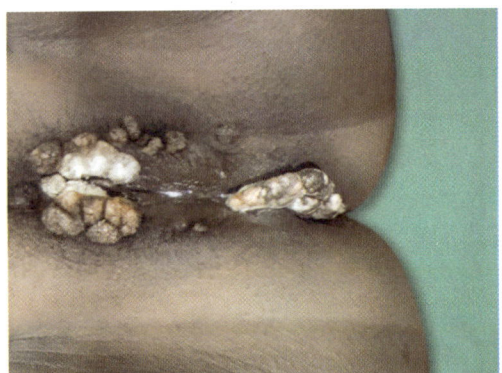
Fig. 56: Genital warts

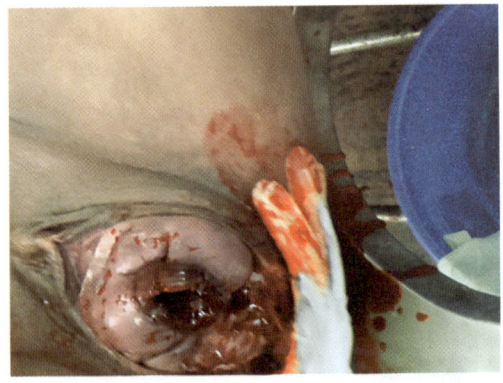
Fig. 57: Mentoanterior face presentation- baby delivering

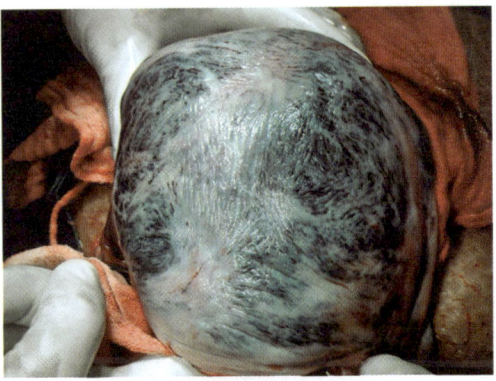
Fig. 58: Couvelaire uterus

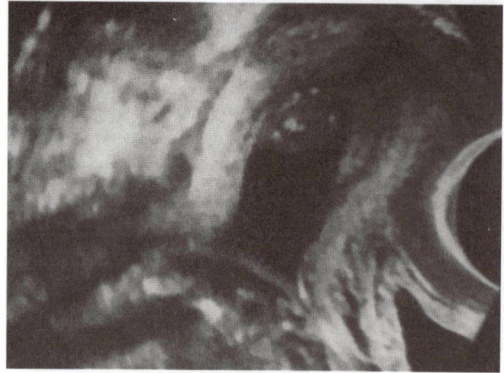

Fig. 59: Cervical insufficiency—Membranes bulging

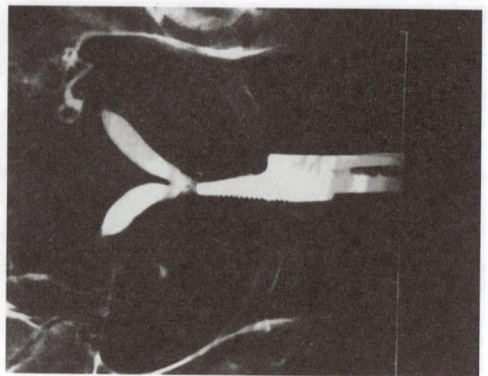

Fig. 60: Bicornuate uterus on HSG

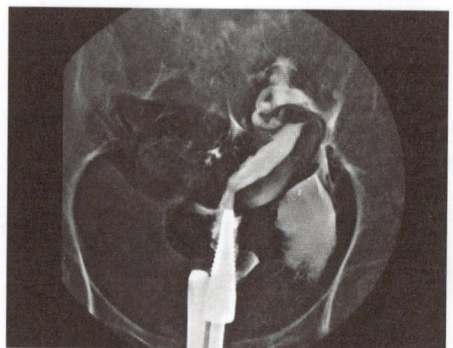

Fig. 61: Unicornuate uterus on HSG

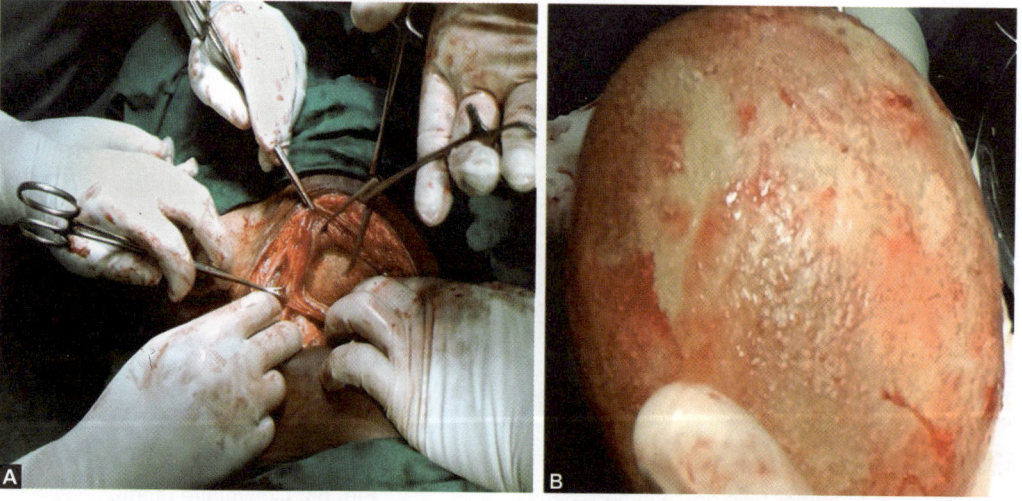

Figs 62A and B: (A) Vesical calculus with pregnancy being removed; (B) Removed stone

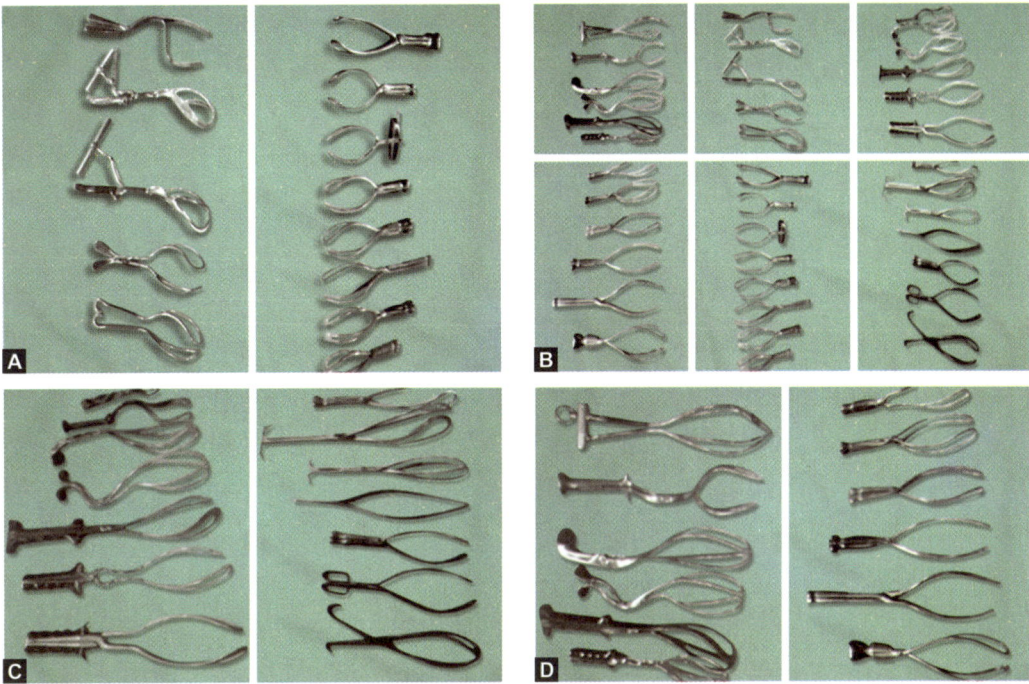

Figs 63A to D: Different varieties of obstetric forceps

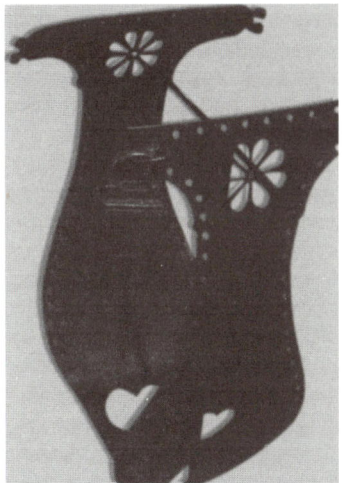

Fig. 64: Chastity belt (This was used by husbands to cover the genitals of their wives and lock it to prevent them from having extramarital relations, masturbate and to protect from rape—existed before 19th century)

Index

Page numbers followed by f refer to figure, fc refer to flowchart and t refer to table

A

Abdomen 343
Abortion
   septic 150
   spontaneous 41
Abruptio placentae 17, 21, 184, 202
Acanthosis nigricans 360
Acardiac fetus 321f, 432f
   interstitial laser coagulation of 321f
Acardius acephalus 195
Acardius amorphous 195
Acardius myelacephalus 195
Acid fast bacilli 304
Acidosis, correction of 161
Acne 360
   vulgaris 398f, 401
Acormus 195
Activated partial thromboplastin time 150
Adenocarcinoma 296
   endometrioid 372
Adenomyosis 13, 267, 271, 328, 330
Adherent placenta 229
Adnexa 13
Adnexal mass 13
   evaluation of 281fc
Adrenal hyperplasia, congenital 396
Adrenal medulla, tumor of 63
Adult respiratory distress syndrome 110
Agenesis 392
Agranulocytosis 108
Air embolism 153
Airway obstruction 143
Alanine aminotransferase 184
Albendazole 121
Albumin 184
Alcohol/substance abuse 27
Alkali hematin 268
   method 118
Alkaline phosphatase 184
Allergies 108, 292
Alpha-methyldopa 52, 135

Amenorrhea 15, 41, 42, 54, 58, 266, 398, 399, 405, 420, 440f
   hyperandrogenic 392
   hypothalamic causes of 404
   pituitary causes of 404
   primary 391, 392, 393fc, 395
   secondary 398, 399, 399t, 400, 401fc, 404, 404t, 406, 407
American Association of Clinical Endocrinologists 259
American College of Obstetricians and Gynecologists 30
American Heart Association 159
American Thyroid Association 258, 259
Amiloride 403
Aminoglycosides 156
Amiodarone 52
Ammonia 178
Amniocentesis 207, 221, 250, 314, 315, 316f
Amniotic fluid
   embolism 63, 141, 142, 150, 152, 158
   infection of 110
Amoxicillin 52
Ampicillin 52
Anal reflex 343
Anal sphincter tone 346
Anal wink reflex 347
Analgesia, epidural 107
Anaphylaxis 153
Ancylostoma duodenale 119
Androgen insensitivity syndrome 392, 394, 394t
Android obesity 401
Anembryonic gestation 440f
Anemia 3, 45, 56, 74, 102, 104, 116, 118-120, 125, 141, 155, 194, 268, 387
   aplastic 120
   causes of 116
   classification of 116, 121fc
   dimorphic 120
   fetal 316
   hemolytic 118, 120
   hypochromic 119, 120

macrocytic 120
megaloblastic 118-120
microcytic 119, 120
normochromic 120
normocytic 120
pernicious 119
physiological 116
refractory 129
sideroblastic 119
Aneuploidy 219, 220
markers 220f
Angiotensin converting-enzyme (ACE) inhibitors 52
Angiotensin sensitivity test 137
Angular cheilitis 118
Ankylostomiasis, ova and cyst of 121
Anna Marie criteria 402
Anorexia 269
nervosa 399
Anovulation 330
Anovulatory cycles, causes of 269
Antiarrhythmic drugs 52
Antibiotic 50
prophylaxis 49
role of 211
Antibody tests 243
Anticoagulants, role of 49
Anticoagulation, complications of 68
Anticonvulsants 137
Antiemetics 183
Antiepileptic drugs 44
Antifibrinolysis 149
Antigen P24 test 243
Antihypertensive therapy 182
Antimicrobial therapy 157
Antimitochondrial antibody 186
Anti-müllerian hormone 395, 402
Antinuclear antibody 186
Antioxidants 365f
Antiphospholipid antibody 132, 250
syndrome 67
Antiretroviral drugs 242fc
Antistreptolysin antibodies 56
Antithrombin deficiency 67
Antithyroid drugs 261
Anxiety 110
Aorta
coarctation of 45, 51, 66, 67, 131, 141
dissection of 45, 51, 67
APLA syndrome 249, 251, 253
treatment of 253

Aplasia, radial 219
Apoplexy, pulmonary 73, 78
Appendicitis, acute 281, 286
Apt test, modified 24
Arcus tendineus fascia levator ani 344
Arhinia 219
Arrhythmias 48, 49, 65-67
mechanisms of 65
ventricular 45
Artemisia vulgaris 38
Artery
pressure, pulmonary 57
umbilical 424
Artesunate 104
Arthritis, rheumatoid 119
Ascites 178, 332
Asherman's syndrome 404
causes of 404
Aspartate aminotransferase 184
Aspiration, prevention of 137
Assisted reproductive techniques 4, 45
Assisted-breech delivery 33, 34
Asthma, bronchial 141
Atenolol 52
Atherosclerosis 63
Atosiban 210
Atresia, duodenal 45
Atrial fibrillation 56
Atrial septal defect 66, 67
Auscultation 11, 16, 26, 133, 225, 236
Australian Carbohydrate Intolerance Study 96
Autoimmune thyroiditis, chronic 258
Autologus blood donation 24
Azalide 58
Azithromycin 52

B

Backache 204, 330, 346
Bacteremia 110
Bacteriuria, asymptomatic 94
Balloon angioplasty 51
Balloon mitral valvuloplasty 73
Balloon vaginoplasty 394
Barbiturates 143
Bartholin's glands 12
Basal crepitations 60
Basophilic stippling 118
Beam radiation therapy, external 301f
Beam trial protocol, modified 211
Benzathine penicillin 58

Berry's aneurysm 45
Beta thalassemia 125
    major 126
    minor 126
BG Prasad classification 42
Bicuspid aortic valve pathology 67
Biochemical/combined screening test, abnormal 250
Biopsy, endometrial 268, 371
Bipolar cord coagulation 320
Birth
    asphyxia 29
    injuries 94
    weight, low 3, 403
Bishop's score 230
Bite cells 118
Blastomycosis 158
Bleeding 268
    acute 330
    after myomectomy, causes of 332
    amount of 9
    diathesis 102
    disorder 267
    intractable 329
    per vagina 15, 253
    postcoital 292, 295t
    postmenopausal 368-370
Blood
    blank protocols 145
    cell indices 120
    count, complete 182, 184, 250, 304
    flow, pulmonary 78
    gas volumes 128
    pressure 54, 71
    smear 118
    sugar 182
    transfusion 124
Body iron component 117
Body stalk anomaly 218
Bone loss 405
Bowel
    adhesions 335
    echogenic 110, 219
    injuries/repairs 388
    symptoms 346
Brace sutures 20
Brachytherapy 299
Bradycardia 107, 219
Breast 102, 107, 343
    abscess 107
    and ovarian cancer syndrome 307
    cancer 10
    development 392
        evaluation of 392
    examination 10, 16, 169, 235, 368
    surgery 10
Breath, shortness of 77
Breech
    complete 27
    complications of 28
    delivers 28
    extraction 33, 37
    internal rotation of 28
    presentation 26, 25, 27, 27f, 28f, 30, 31
        etiology of 27
        varieties of 27
Brenner's tumors 287
Broad ligament fibroid 330
Bromocriptine 61
Buccal mucosa 394
Bulbocavernosus reflex 347
Burning micturition 101
Burns 158
Burns-Marshall method 34
Burr cells 118
Butyrophenones 404

C

Cabotegravir 242
Calcium 138
    channel blockers 65
Camptodactyly 219
Cancers
    endometrial 10, 365, 368, 371, 372, 372t, 373-377
    epithelial 307
    gastrointestinal 305
    recurrent 375
    types of 308t
Candidiasis 108
Carbamazepine 44
Carboplatin 377
Carcinoid syndrome 71
Carcinoma
    endometrial 268, 376
    endometrium 367
        management of 378fc
    mucinous 308
Cardiac arrest 143, 159
Cardiac disease 9, 44, 45, 47, 50, 51, 52, 55t, 59, 143, 209
    congenital 41

functional classification of 46
NYHA classification of 58
Cardiac failure 71
   congestive 45, 46
   management 115
Cardiac surgery 51
Cardiac transplantation 49
Cardiomyopathy
   dilated 49, 61
   hypertrophic 51, 61
      obstructive 162
   peripartum 51, 52, 59, 141, 194
   types of 61
Cardiotocogram 424
Cardiovascular system 10, 72, 247, 327, 343
Cardiovocal syndrome 78
CARPREG score 47
Cefazolin 52
Ceftriaxone 52
Cefuroxime 111
Central nervous system 10, 16, 75, 225, 235, 247, 343
Central venous pressure 160
Cephalexin 52
Cephalic veins 73f
Cephalic version, external 30, 31, 38
Cephalosporins 52
Cerebral
   artery, middle 317f, 424, 425
   edema 143
   infarction 143
   malaria 102, 105, 108
   palsy, reduction of 211
   symptoms 131
   venous sinus thrombosis 143
Cervical
   amputation 248
   cancer 292, 296
      development of 293
      histopathology types of 296
      primary 295
      screening guidelines 2012 294t
      stage 299t
   carcinoma, revised FIGO staging of 2009 299t
   dilatation 201, 253
   dystocia 253
   encerclage
      complications of 253
      indication for 253
   fibroid polyp 347
   insufficiency 205t, 444
   lacerations 152
   length 7, 201, 205, 208
      assessment 204
   polyp 295, 368
   shortening 204
   suture, role of 24
   tears 253
   ultrasonography 204
Cervicitis 295, 349
Cervicouterine angle 336f
Cervicovaginal junction 352
Cervix 7, 12, 13, 354
   congenital elongation of 347
   descent of 12
   length 343
   squamous cell carcinoma of 297f
Cesarean section 175, 229
Chadwick's sign 216
Chemical pneumonitis 158
Chemotherapy 406
   adjuvant 377
   indication for 309
   neoadjuvant 301
   role of 376
Chest
   pain, acute onset progressive 62
   syndrome, acute 128
   wall lesions 404
Chickenpox 108
Chikungunya fever 107
Chlamydia 206, 295
Chloroquine 104
Cho suture 20
Cholangitis 108
Chorioamnionitis 107, 110, 156, 158, 209, 253
Chorioangioma 423
Chorionic villus
   biopsy 221
   sampling 42, 314, 315, 315f
Chorionicity 191, 191f, 192
Cinchonism 104
Circumvallate placenta 437f
Cirrhosis 141, 404
Cisplatin 377
Clavicle, fractures of 29
Clear cell carcinoma 308
Cleft lip, midline 219
Cleft palate, midline 219
Clindamycin 52, 104, 111
Clitoral index 393
Clitoris 12
Clomiphene citrate 362, 363

Clubfeet 219
Cocaine 404
    abuse 63
    exposure 59
Collagen vascular diseases 63
Colon 307
Colovaginoplasty 394
Colpectomy 356
Colpocleisis, total 356
Comparative genomic hybridization 254
Concomitant mitral valve surgery 82
Condyloma accuminatum 295
Congenital anomalies 93, 194, 196, 202
Connective tissue disease 131, 132
Consanguinity, degrees of 215
Constipation 330, 349
Contraception 128, 238, 267
    risk of 47
Contraceptive pills, oral 403
Contusion, pulmonary 158
Convulsions 102, 108, 110
    prevention of 135
Coomb's test, indirect 250
Copper sulphate method 118
Cord
    clamping 122
    entanglement 32, 195
    marginal attachment of 437f
    prolapse 28, 30, 32
Cordocentesis 250
Cornual placentation 27
Coronary angiography 62
Coronary artery 51
    bypass grafting 51
    disease 62
Coronary sinus type 66
Coronary spasm/dissection 63
Coronary vascular thrombosis 63
Corpus callosum, agenesis of 45, 219
Corpus luteal cyst 282
Corpus luteum, ruptured 281
Corticosteroids therapy 157
Corticotropin-releasing hormone 203
Cough 71, 77
Couvelaire uterus 23, 443f
Craniopharyngioma 404
C-reactive protein 56, 206
Cri du chat syndrome 45
Criminal Law (Amendment) Act 2013 409
Crohn's disease 260
Cryotherapy 337

Cryptosporidiosis 241
Crystalloid resuscitation 151
Cusco's speculum 12, 12f
Cushing's disease 404
Cushing's syndromes 307
Cyanmethemoglobin method 118, 122
Cyanocobalamin 120
Cyanosis 5, 67, 79
Cyclic oral progesterone 273
Cyclooxygenase 203
Cyclophosphamide 377
Cyst
    dermoid 283f, 439, 439f
    follicular 282
    hemorrhagic 283
    vulvar 347
Cystadenoma
    mucinous 286, 286f
    serous 286
Cystic teratoma
    benign 283, 285
    mature 284
Cystitis 107
Cystoscopy, role of 347

D

Danazol 273, 333
Dandy-Walker syndrome 45
Darunavir 241
Decubitus 79
    ulcer 350
Deep vein thrombosis 49
Dehydration 107
    correction of 183
Dehydroepiandrosterone sulphate 203
Delirium 108, 110
Dengue 107, 108
    fever 102, 109
Dermoid cyst, bilateral 283f
Dermoid plug 284
Dexamethasone 382
Diabetes 5, 9, 86, 96, 209
    gestational 88, 96, 132, 141, 180, 194
    mellitus 131, 132, 141, 155, 387
    treatment of 99t
Diagnostic invasive tests 315
Diaphoresis 62
Diaphragmatic hernia, congenital 322f
Diarrhea 104
Diastolic trans-mitral pressure gradient 73

Digoxin 57, 61
    current use of 81
Diphtheria 108
Diphyllobothrium latum 119
Disseminated intravascular coagulation 22, 23, 110, 150
Diuretics 52, 61, 65, 162
Dobutamine 157
Dolasetron 382
Dolutegravir 242
Dopamine 157
Double marker tests, abnormal values of 217
Down's syndrome 1
Doxorubicin 377
Doxylamine 183
Drug therapy, oral 362
Dual energy X-ray absorptiometry scan 396
Ductus venosus 424, 425
    wave, reversed 219
Duhressen incision 37
Duodenal atresia 219
Dyslipidemia 63, 403
Dysmenorrhea 9, 288, 330
Dyspareunia 288
Dysplasia, skeletal 45
Dyspnea 44, 78

E

Early obstetric warning score, modified 154
Eating disorders 399
Ebstein's anomaly 51, 67
Eclampsia 65, 131, 136, 142, 143, 150, 153, 158
    atypical presentation of 161
    outline management of 136
Edema 5, 44, 79
    pulmonary 45, 46, 77, 102, 105, 110, 131
Efavirenz 240, 241
Ehler Danlos syndrome 51
Eisenmenger's complex 46
Eisenmenger's physiology 67
Eisenmenger's syndrome 52, 67, 141
Ejection systolic murmur 66
Electric stimulation 348
Electrocardiogram 56, 73
Electrolytes, serum 109, 182
Electronic fetal heart monitoring 206
ELISA test 243
Elvitegravir 242
Embolism, pulmonary 56, 153
Empty sella syndrome 404

Encephalitis 107, 108
Encephalopathy 178
    hypertensive 143
Endocarditis 45, 49, 67, 71
    bacterial 45
    infective 46, 67, 108
    prophylaxis 57
Endocervical sampling 206
Endometrial biopsy 371
Endometrial cancer
    management of 373
    metastatic 295
Endometrial sampling
    advantages of 370
    disadvantages of 370
Endometrioid carcinoma
    high-grade 308
    low-grade 308
Endometrioma 288
Endometriosis 13, 14, 288, 305, 330, 332
    peritoneal 331
Endometritis
    atrophic 368, 377
    tuberculous 403
Endometrium 307
    atrophic 268
    discordant 268
    ulceration of 329
Enfuvirtide 242
Entamoeba histolytica 119, 121
Enterocele 344
    demonstration methods 353
Epignathus 434f
Epilepsy 9, 141-143
Epimenorrhagia 266
Epimenorrhea 266
    causes of 267
Epinephrine 157
Episiotomy 108
Epithelial ovarian cancers, management of 309
Epithelial tumors, molecular classification of 308
Ergometrine 20
Erythropoietin, role of 129
Esbach's albuminometer 134
Estradiol 395
Estrogen 272
Ethamsylate 270
Etravirine 241
Ex utero intrapartum treatment procedure 315, 323
Excessive vomiting, causes of 190
Exertional dyspnea 54, 78, 113

Exogenous estrogen 368
Exomphalos 218, 434f
External genitalia, blood supply of 427, 427f

F

Facial dysmorphism 219
Falciparum malaria 108
   complicated 104
Fallopian tubes 308, 309
Fasting blood glucose, normal 96
Fat embolism 158
Fatigue 101
Fatty liver, acute 141, 150, 158, 178, 194
Fe-deficiency anemia 119, 122
Femoropelvic grip 34
Femur, fractures of 29
Ferriman Gallwey score 360, 401
Ferrous gluconate, fumarate 123
Fertility rate after myomectomy 331
Fetal
   abnormalities 315
   anemia 316, 317f
   anomalies 202
   ascitis 435f
   biometric parameters 98
   blood
      sampling 314
      transfusion 316
   breathing movements 175
   cardiac echo 45
   death 32, 45, 134
   diagnostic procedures 314
   distress 229
   endoscopic tracheal occlusion 321
   fibronectin 204, 205t
      test 207, 207t
   growth
      rate 175t
      restriction 168, 194, 197, 314, 319, 320
      retardation 67
   hazards 30
   head, hyperextension of 38
   heart
      abnormalities 32
      disease 45
      rate 16, 42
      sounds 73
   hydrops 319
   interventions 314
   lung maturity 91f
   markers 315
   mirror syndrome 141
   morbidity 45
   movements 108
   polycythemia 45
   reduction 316
   surveillance 115, 194
   tachycardia 110, 219
   therapeutic procedures 314
   tone 175
   weight, estimated 28, 32
   wellbeing 172t
Fetiform tumor 284
Fetoscopic laser ablation 319, 423
Fetoscopic techniques 314
Fetus
   congenital anomalies of 423
   papyraceus 433f
Fever 101, 106, 108-110, 111fc
   causes of 102, 107, 107t, 108
   intrapartum 110
   low-grade 106, 108
   malarial 102
   rheumatic 54, 58
   tertian 108
   types of 108
Fibrinogen 151
Fibroadenoma 10
Fibroid 329, 332, 337
   asymptomatic 331
   classification 338f
   cornual 436f
   fundal 437
   hysteroscopic removal of 338
   management of 329f, 333, 334
   morcellation 437
   multiple 332, 335
   pedunculated 335
   polyp 327, 436f
   recurrence of 332
   submucous 329
   subserous 436f
   torsion of 329
   uterus 326, 328
Fibroma 289
Fibronectin 138
Fibrosis, cystic 141
Filariasis 108
Fine needle aspiration biopsy 262, 263
First trimester aneuploidy screening methods 217fc
Fistula, rectovaginal 443f

Flexion 28, 29
Fluid
    intake 50
    management 147
    restriction 162
    resuscitation 160
    therapy, intraoperative 380
Fluorescent in situ hybridization 254, 316
Folate antagonist 45
Folic acid 15, 41
    deficiency 115, 119
Follicle-stimulating hormone 257, 362, 392
Forceps, application of 36
Fothergill's cervical stenosis 354
Fothergill's operations 351
    modified 351
Foul smelling vaginal discharge 110
Fragile X permutation 406
Fresh frozen plasma 149
Friedman and Little classification 350
Fundal grip 6, 16
Furosemide 52, 61

G

Galactorrhea 405
Galactosemia 406
Gallbladder calculi 423
Gastric contents, aspiration of 158
Gastroschisis 45
Genetic screening, methods of 216
Genital
    estrogen status of 346
    examination 413
    hiatus 357*f*
    injuries 415
    malignancy 267
    prolapse 342
        urinary symptoms of 345
    system 347
    tract infection 107
        lower 205
    tract, hematoma of 428, 428*t*
    warts 443*f*
Genitalia
    examination of 393
    external 360, 427
Gentamicin 111
Gestation
    duration of 4
    multiple 17, 152

Gestational age 31, 32, 198
Gestational sac
    low implantation of 440*f*
    multiple 191*f*
Gestrinone 273, 102
Glomerulonephritis 141
Glossitis 118
Glucokinase mutation 98
Glucose tolerance test 250
    abnormal 86
Glyburide 97
Glycemic index 97*f*
Glycosuria, causes of 89
Gonadal dysgenesis 392
Gonadotropin
    deficiency 392
    releasing hormone 361
    resistant syndrome 404, 406
    therapy 363
Gonorrhea 206
Goodell's sign 216
Gorlin's syndromes 307
Granulosa cell tumors 288, 306
Graves' disease 260, 261, 395
Graves' hyperthyroidism 261, 264
Great arteries, transposition of 67
Great vessels, transposition of 51
Growth chart 442*f*

H

H1N1 pneumonia 141
Haemophilus influenzae 128
Harrison/rocket cannula 318
Hashimoto's thyroiditis 258, 263, 395
Headache 101, 104, 108, 131
Heart
    beat, shifting of 44
    block 67
    defects 219
        congenital 49, 48
    disease 46, 47, 54
        acyanotic 66
        complex cyanotic congenital 67
        congenital 66, 67
        cyanotic 49, 66
        rheumatic 54, 71
        valvular 48, 49, 56-58
    failure, congestive 57
    rate 44

sounds 79
transplantation 51
Heat coagulation test 134
Hegar's sign 216
Heinz bodies 118
Heller's test 134
HELLP syndrome 134, 136, 141, 150, 158, 181
    classification systems of 182
    complete 182
    management of 182
    partial 182
Hematinics, role of 49
Hematoma 29, 429
    complications of 429
    management of 429f, 430
    nonobstetric 428, 429t
    obstetric 428, 428t
    surgical management of 429t
    vulval 426, 429, 443f
    vulvar 428
    vulvovaginal 428
Hematometra 13
Hematuria 229
Hemoglobin 120, 151
    color scale 118
Hemogram, complete 206
Hemoptysis 77
Hemorrhage 78, 253, 282, 286
    acute 120
    antepartum 15, 16, 194, 202
    fetomaternal 32
    intracerebral 143
    intracranial 67
    massive 21, 149
    myometrial 23
    obstetric 21, 141
    peripartum 147t, 150
    pontine 107
    postpartum 20, 23, 234, 385
    primary postpartum 426
    traumatic postpartum 94
Hemorrhoids management 115
Hemostasis 147, 148
Hemothorax 332
Heparin 52, 68
    anticoagulation 50
Hepatitis
    B
        immunoglobulin 187
        infection 186
        management of 186
    D virus 186
    E, viral 141
    transmission of B 185
    vaccination 187
Hepatorenal failure 136
Hereditary ovarian syndromes 307
Hernia
    diaphragmatic 45, 218
    incisional 387, 388
    inguinal 10
Hernial orifices 346
Herpes simplex virus 295
Higham's chart 268
Hip joint, dislocation of 30
Hirsutism 398f, 401
HIV
    infection, severity of 238
    transmission, prevention of 241
Hodgkin's lymphoma 108
Holoprosencephaly 45, 219
Holt-Oram syndrome 45
Home uterine activity monitoring 204, 205
Homeostatic model assessment 364
Hormonal method 239
Hormone 47
    adrenocorticotropic 203
    luteinizing 257, 363
    replacement therapy 307
Howell-Jolly bodies 118
Human chorionic gonadotropin 260
Human papillomavirus 293
Humerus, fractures of 29
Hydatidiform mole 197
Hydralazine 52, 136
Hydramnios 88, 89, 94
Hydrocephalus 27, 110
Hydrops
    fetalis 45, 132, 434f
    nonimmune 110
Hydroxycobalamin 120
Hygroma, cystic 434f
Hymen 12
    imperforate 392, 395
Hymenotomy 437f
Hyperammonemia 143
Hyperandrogenism
    causes of 402
    signs of 401
Hyperbilirubinemia 94
Hypercalcemia 143
Hyperemesis gravidarum 182, 194

Hyperglycemia 93, 94, 96, 143, 332
Hyperhomocysteinemia 132, 254
Hyperinsulinemia 402, 403
	neonatal 94
Hyperketonemia 93
Hypermagnesemia 143
Hypermenorrhea 266
Hyperplasia 268
	endometrial 269, 368
Hyperprolactinemia 392, 405, 405t
	causes of 404
	evaluation of 405fc
Hyperpyrexia 107
	conditions of 107
	malignant 107
Hyperreactio luteinalis 282
Hypertension 17, 45, 52, 60, 64, 65, 67, 194, 342
	chronic 63, 65, 131, 133t
	classification of 65t
	control of 134, 136
	essential 131
	gestational 65, 131, 133
	pregnancy-induced 141
	primary 131, 141
	pulmonary 43, 46, 49, 54, 73
	secondary 131
Hypertensive disorders 59, 131, 161
Hyperthermia, malignant 107
Hyperthyroidism 45, 260
	gestational 141, 260
Hypocalcemia 94, 143
Hypoglycemia 90, 93, 94, 102, 105, 143, 178
	neonatal 94
Hypogonadism, hypogonadotropic 396
Hypokalemia 93, 386
Hypomagnesemia 94
Hypomenorrhea 266
	causes of 267
Hyponatremia 143
Hypophysitis, lymphocytic 404
Hypoplasia, phalangeal 219
Hypoproteinemia 387
Hypotension 229
	sepsis-induced 154
Hypothalamic dysfunction 269, 392
Hypothyroidism 257, 259, 392, 404
Hypoxia 175
Hysterectomy 20, 269, 270, 274, 329, 373
	indication for 272, 332
	radial 297, 297f
	total abdominal 269

Hysteroscopy 266, 373, 336t, 371, 404
	disadvantages of 371
	indication for 271
	role of 271

I

In vitro fertilization 4
Indian Law on Sexual Offences 417
Indinavir 241
Indomethacin 210
Infertility 360
Inositol isomers 365
Inotropes 61
Insulin 97
	analogs 99
	infusion 160
	serum 250
	types of 98
Internal genitalia, blood supply of 427
Internal iliac ligation 20
Internal pudendal
	artery 356
	vessels 356
Internal rotation 28, 29
Intestinal obstruction 286, 388
Intracytoplasmic sperm injection 45
Intraperitoneal chemotherapy, role of 310
Intrauterine
	contraceptive device 215, 239
	fetal
		blood transfusion 316
		death 22, 175, 202
	growth restriction 27, 45, 172
		selective 423
	hypoxia, chronic 93
	infection 150
Introitus 12
Invasive test report, abnormal 221
Iodine deficiency 258
Iron 15, 41
	absorption 117
	deficiency 118, 120
		anemia 115, 120, 125
	dosage, parenteral 122
	food sources of 117
	metabolism 117
	overload, pathogenesis of 125
	regulatory proteins 117
	supplementation 3
	therapy

different methods of 124
    oral 124
    parenteral 123
Ischial spine 8, 356
Isthmus, aortic 424, 425

J

Jaundice 72, 102
    malignant obstructive 387
    neonatal 94
Jugular venous
    pressure 42
    pulse 54, 72

K

Kala-azar 108
Kallmann's syndrome 392, 396
Kegel's exercise 348
Ketoacidosis 93
    diabetic 141, 160
Kidney diseases 267
Kleihauer-Betke test 32
Koilonychias 118
Korsakoff's psychosis 183
Kristellar's maneuver 34
Krukenberg tumors 305
Kuppuswamy scale, modified 16, 59, 72, 87, 360

L

Labetalol 52, 65, 135, 136
Labia minora flap 394
Labial fusion 395
Labor pain
    false 4, 4t
    true 4, 4t
Lactation 404
Lactational amenorrhea method 239
Lamivudine 186, 240, 241
Langerhans cell histiocytosis 404
Lanolin 43
Laparoscopy 266, 336t, 372
Lead poisoning 118
Leiomyoma 271, 332
    genetic basis of 331
Leopold's maneuvers 6, 7f, 26
Leptospirosis 108
Leukocytosis 110, 178
Levamisole 121
Levator ani tear 12

Levetiracetam 161
Levonorgestrel 47
Lidocaine 52
Limbs, swelling of 54
Listeriosis 141, 158
Lithium 44
Lithotomy position 11f
Liver
    disease 108, 178, 267
    function test 109, 183, 184, 304
    pathology 118
Lopinavir 241
Lorazepam 161
Lovset's maneuver 35
Lumbar puncture 109
Lung injury
    acute 158
    ventilator-associated 158
Lung transplant 141
Luteal phase defect 251
Luteoma 282
Lymph node
    metastases, survival role of 374t
    retroperitoneal 309
Lymphadenectomy 373, 374
    role of 373, 374
Lymphadenopathy 5, 109
Lymphogranuloma venereum 295
Lynch syndrome 369

M

Mackenrodt's ligaments 344
Macrolide 52, 58
Macrosomia 88, 89, 94, 423
    development of 98
Magnesium sulfate 24, 135, 143, 211
    role of 210
Malaria 102, 104t, 105, 106fc, 107, 108, 158
    complicated 102, 104t
    congenital 105
    drug treatment for 104
    management of 105
    parasites 103f, 118, 119
    peripartum 105
    severe 102
    sickle cells 118
    treatment of 104
Malarial fever
    maternal complications of 102
    severity of 103

Malignancy 13, 271, 330
Mallory-Weiss tear 183
Malpas classification 351
Mammoth tumor 330, 338
Marfan's syndrome 45, 46, 48, 51, 52
Massive transfusion protocol 146*t*
Mastitis, acute 107
Maternal
    anticonvulsant medications 27
    cardiac disease 45
    death 32
    hyperglycemia 98
    hypertension 91
    hypothyroidism 259
    mortality 67, 110
    pelvis, adequate 32
    screening tests, positive 315
    serum alpha fetoprotein 23
    tachycardia 110
Maturity onset diabetes of youth 98
Mauriceau-Smellie-Veit maneuver 36
Mayer-Rokitansky-Kuster-Hauser syndrome 392, 394
Mayo culdoplasty 356
Mayo-Ward's operation 349
McAfee Johnson expectant treatment 18
McCall's culdoplasty 356
McCall's stich application 354
McIndoe technique 394
McRobert's maneuver 36
Measles 108
Mebendazole 121
Mechanical prosthetic valves 68
Meckel-Gruber syndrome 45
Medical nutrition therapy 97
Medroxyprogesterone acetate 372
Mefenamic acid 270, 334
Megacystis 218
Megaloblastic anemia, causes of 119
Meig's syndromes 307
Membranes
    artificial rupture of 22
    premature rupture of 17, 28, 110, 253
Menarche 391
Mendelian disorders 220
Meningiomas 404
Meningitis 108
    cryptococcal 241
Menometrorrhagia 266
Menorrhagia 113, 266, 288
Mentzer index 125

Metabolic disorders 45
Metabolic syndrome 132, 365
Metformin 96, 97, 403
    adverse reactions of 403
Metoclopramide 382, 404
Metronidazole 111
Metropathia hemorrhagica 266
Microalbuminuria determination method 134
Microangiopathic hemolytic anemia 118
Micrognathia 219
Midazolam 161, 162
Mimic cardiac disease 44
Minimal ablative surgery 270
Minimally invasive therapeutic techniques 316
Mirena 47, 272
Miscarriage
    drug-induced 107
    spontaneous 194, 247
Mississippi system of classification 182
Mitral regurgitation, severe 82*f*
Mitral stenosis
    echo grading of 73*t*
    etiology of 71
    pathophysiology of 77*fc*
    severe 54
    symptoms of 77
Mitral valve
    orifice area 73
    replacement 56, 57
    surgery 82
MOEWS score 155
Monilial vulvovaginitis 94
Mononucleosis, infectious 108
Monsel's solution 430
Morphology index 290
Mucopolysaccharidosis 71
Mullerian agenesis 394, 394*f*, 394*t*
Mullerian anomalies 248
Mullerian system 394
Multifactorial disorders 220
Mumps 406
Myasthenia gravis 141
Myelomeningocele 27
Myocardial infarction 63, 143, 153
Myolysis, disadvantages of 336
Myomas 13, 327
Myomectomy 270, 328, 334, 336*t*
    clamp 339*f*
    hysteroscopic 270338
    indication for 329

laparoscopic 338
principles 334
Myometrial invasion, depth of 373
Myosin light chain kinase 203

N

Naegele's formula 4
National Anemia Prophylaxis Program 121
Nausea 101, 104
Necator americanus 119
Neck vein 79
Neisseria gonorrhoeae 202
Neoadjuvant chemotherapy, role of 310
Neoplasia, malignant 295
Neoplasms, benign 295
Nephropathy, worsening 91
Nerve
    conduction study 347
    injury 30
Neuroprotection protocol 211
Neutrophils, hypersegmented 118
Nevirapine 241
New York Association Functional Classification of
    Heart Disease, modified 81
New York Heart Association 46, 74
Nifedipine 135, 136
Nitabuch's layer 20
Nitric acid donors 210
Nitroglycerine patch 210
Nonhealing ulcer, chronic 354
Nonpolyposis colon cancer syndrome 307
Non-secreting pituitary adenomas 404
Nonsteroidal anti-inflammatory drugs 335
Non-stress test 206
    role of 91
Noonan's syndrome 45
Norepinephrine 157
Nuchal fold thickness 219
Nucleated red cells 118
Nucleoside reverse transcriptase inhibitors 241

O

Obesity 364, 387
Oblonsky criteria 227
Obstetric forceps 445f
Oily facial skin 401
Oligohydramnios 319, 424, 441f
Oligomenorrhea 266, 398, 400, 405
Omphalocele 45, 219
Ondansetron 382

Open fetal surgery 315, 322
Opiates 404
Oral pills 272
Organogenesis 93
Ormiloxiphene 273
Oropharyngeal candidiasis 241
Orthopnea 78
Ortner's syndrome 78
Osiander's sign 216
Osteopenia 405
Osteoporosis, heparin-induced 68
Ostium secundum 43, 66
Ovarian cancer 307
    epithelial 304, 310
    staging of 308t
Ovarian cyst
    rupture of 286
    torsion of 439f
Ovarian drilling 364
    advantages 364
    disadvantages 364
    laparoscopic 364, 403
Ovarian endometriosis 287
Ovarian hyperstimulation syndrome 92, 141, 363
Ovarian malignancies, types of 306, 306t
Ovarian mass 285
Ovarian puncture, multiple 364
Ovarian surgery 406
Ovarian torsion 286
Ovarian tumor 281
    benign 279
    epithelial 286
    origin of 283
    solid 288
    torsion of 285
Ovary 307
    bilobed teratoma of 439f
    functional cysts of 282
    multifollicular 400, 400t
Oxygen mask 43
Oxytocin 20
    agonist 210
    induction 35
    receptor 203
    role of 35

P

Packed cell volume 22
Paclitaxel 377
Page classification 22

Pain
- abdominal 8, 178
- calf 108
- causes of 333
- momentary relief of 229
- nature of 4

Pale conjunctiva 118
Pallor 5, 118
Pancreatitis 158, 305, 388
Pancytopenia 267
Pap smears 292
Papillary serous cystadenoma 285
Papillary thyroid cancer 263
Paradoxical embolus 67
Paralytic ileus 388
Parametrium 14
Paraovarian cysts 287
Parapagus dicephalus 432f
Parity index 2
Paroxysmal nocturnal dyspnea 54
Patent ductus arteriosus 66, 67
Pawlik's grip 6
Pectoral muscles 6
Pel-ebstein fever 108
Pelvic
- abscess 107
- examination 11, 102, 327, 331
- floor 345
  - exercises 348
  - tone evaluation 347
- grip 6, 16
- hemorrhage 385
- mass 289, 289t
- organ prolapse 343
- pain, chronic 288
- pathology, nongynecological 281
- radiation
  - external 377
  - fields 301f
- septic thrombophlebitis 141
- surgery 10
- ultrasound 395

Pelvis, contracted 27
Penidure prophylaxis 54
Perineal body 12, 357f
Perineal dilatation 394
Perineal tears 108
Peripartum oxidative stress 60
Peripheral blood smear 102, 118
Peritoneal cancer, primary 308
Peritoneal metastases 309

Peritonitis 387
Peutz-Jegher syndromes 307
Phenothiazines 404
Phenytoin 44, 161
Pheochromocytoma 63, 131
Physiotherapy 385
Pinard's maneuver 34, 35
Pipelle biopsy 268
Piper's forceps 36, 37, 438f
Piperazine citrate 121
Piskacek's sign 216
Placenta
- accreta 19, 20, 152
- anastomoses 320f
- low lying 421
- manual removal of 234
- percreta 20
- previa 17-19, 22-24, 27, 32, 141, 152, 194, 202
  - central asymmetric 421
  - central symmetric 421, 440f
  - marginal 421

Placental abruption 22, 32, 136, 141, 150, 421
- grades of 21

Placental migration 19
Plasmodium falciparum
- infection, uncomplicated 104
- malaria 141

Platelet transfusions 149
Platonychia 118
Pleuro-amniotic shunting, technique of 318
Pneumocystis jiroveci pneumonia 241
Pneumonia 108, 158
- bacterial 156, 241
- community acquired 141
- lobar 108
- viral 158

Polycystic ovary 398f, 400, 400t
- syndrome 267, 398

Polycythemia 94, 332
Polydactyly 219
Polydipsia 178
Polyglandular diseases, autoimmune 406
Polyhydramnios 152, 194, 202, 319, 423, 441f
- demonstration of 319

Polymenorrhagia 266
Polymenorrhea 266
Polymyositis 141
Polyp 271, 276, 329
- endometrial 295, 368
- extrusion of 330

Polypectomy, hysteroscopic 270

Polyuria 178
Postembolization syndrome 335
Postmenopausal bleeding, causes of 368, 368*t*
Potassium 160
Pouch of Douglas 283
Prader-Willi syndrome 27
Preeclampsia 3, 56, 63, 65, 93, 131, 133*t*, 138, 142, 158
 etiology of 131
 etiopathology of 132*fc*
 management of 134, 137*fc*
 outline management of 134
 pathophysiology of 132
 prevention of 138
 severe 56
 spectrum of 150
Pregnancy 13, 64, 71, 105, 154, 335, 404
 cholestasis of 178
 ectopic 281, 286
 loss, recurrent 246
 mimics heart disease 44
 molar 132
 multiple 27, 132, 190, 202, 209
 normal 305
 teenage 1
 termination of 175
Premature ovarian
 failure 404, 406
 insufficiency 406*t*
Prenatal testing, noninvasive 250
Preterm birth, spontaneous 208
Preterm delivery 3
Preterm labor 32, 94, 194, 196, 201-203, 253
 management of 207, 212
 pathogenesis of 203*fc*
Pritchard's regimen 135
Procainamide 52
Prochlorperazine 382
Procidentia 439*f*
 complete 350
Progesterone therapy 208
Prolactin, serum 250
Prolactinoma 141
Promethazine 183, 382
Propofol infusion 162
Prostaglandin 20, 203
 dehydrogen 203
 synthase inhibitors 210
Prosthetic cardiac valves 49
Proteinuria testing 134
Prothrombin time 150, 184

Psammoma bodies 285
Pseudo-Meig's syndrome 332
Pubertal menorrhagia, classification of 267*fc*
Puberty, constitutional delay of 392
Pubic hair development, evaluation of 392
Pubic symphysis 29
Pubocervical ligaments 344
Pudendal nerve 356
Pulse 54, 155
 rate 5, 42, 44
Pulseless electrical activity 153
Pure gonadal dysgenesis 406
Pyelectasia 219
Pyelonephritis 94, 107, 156, 158
Pyometra 13
Pyrantel pamoate 121
Pyridoxine 183
Pyrimethamine 104

Q

Quad test 217
Quartan fever 108
Quinidine 43, 403
Quinine 104
Quintero staging system 195
Quotidian fever 108

R

Radiation, role of 377
Radical hysterectomy, complications of 298
Radiotherapy, role of 376
Ranitidine 403
Rapid diagnostic tests 102
Rash 108
Rectal mucosa 14
Rectal prolapse 438*f*
Rectovaginal examination 14, 14*f*, 368
Regurgitation
 aortic 58
 lesions 51
 mitral 44, 57, 71, 76, 82*f*
 tricuspid 44, 57, 219
Renal disease 119, 131, 404
Renal failure 102, 105, 110, 141
Renal function test 109, 183
Reserpine 404
Respiratory distress syndrome 93, 157
Respiratory system 10, 16, 73, 169, 343
Retinopathy, worsening 91

Retroplacental hematoma, large 441f
Rheumatic activity, recurrent 56
Rheumatic fever
    primary prevention of 83
    secondary prevention of 83
Rheumatic heart disease, chronic 73
Rilpivirine 241
Ringer lactate 21
Ritodrine 210
Ritonavir 241
Robson's 10 group classification 230
Roll-over test 137
Rotterdam criteria 2003 361
Routine pregnancy care 237
Rubella 108
    syndrome, congenital 3
Rule out ovarian disease 372

S

Sacral agenesis 435f
Sacral promontory 7
Sacrosciatic notch 7
Sacrospinous ligament 356
S-adenyl-methionine 181
Sahli's method 118
Saline infusion sonography 370
Saliva tests 243
Salpingitis, acute 286
Salpingo-oophorectomy, bilateral 269
Salt restriction aspirin 138
Sarcoidosis 404
Savage syndrome 404
Scar tenderness 229
Schistocytes 118
Sciatic nerve 356
Scleroderma 141
Sclerosis, multiple 141
Semen collection 362
Sengstaken-Blakemore tube 20
Sentinel node mapping, role of 375
Sepsis 142, 154, 155t, 158, 209
    management of 156
    severe 154
Septal myectomy 51
Septicemia 102, 105, 107, 108, 110
Serous carcinoma
    high-grade 308
    low-grade 308
Sertoli Leydig cell 306
Sex cord stromal tumors 307

Sex hormone binding globulin 364, 402
Sexual assault 409
    Victim
        examination of 409
        management of 412fc
        protocol of examination of 411fc
Sexual offence, situation of 417
Sexual violence 409
Sheehan's syndrome 143
Sher and Statland classification 22
Shock 102
    index 145
    obstructive 143
    septic 143, 154
Shoulder dystocia 92
Siamese twins 196
Sickle cell 118
    anemia 118, 127
    disease 128, 141
    disorders 118
Simpson's forceps 36
Sims' position 11f
Sims' speculum 11, 12, 12f
Single nucleotide polymorphisms 254
Sinus
    rhythm 54, 73
    tachycardia 43, 74
Skin lesions 12
Skull, fractures of 29
Sleep apnea, obstructive 141
Sodium
    lauryl sulfate method 118
    restriction 61
Solid tumor, mature 284
Spherocytosis 118
Spina bifida 118
Spinal cord lesions 404
Spine 343
Spironolactone 61
Status epilepticus 161
Stavudine 241
Stenosis
    aortic 46, 48, 52, 57
    mitral 46, 52, 55-58, 71, 73, 73f, 74, 77, 81, 83, 83fc
    pulmonary 48, 58
    tricuspid 58, 67
Stenotic lesions 51
Sterilization 47
Steroid prophylaxis, role of 136
Strawberry skull 219

Stress 269, 404
    incontinence 12
    urinary incontinence 342
Submucus myoma, expulsion of 330
Sulfadiazine 58
Sulfadoxine 104
Sulfosalicylic acid test 134
Swab, types of 414
Symphysiotomy 37
Symphysis pubis 6
Syndactyly 434*f*
Syphilis 250
Syringomyelia 435*f*
Systemic lupus erythematosis 71, 131, 132
Systemic vascular resistance 57, 58, 74
Systolic ventricular dysfunction, severe 46

T

Tachycardia 48, 229, 327
Tallquist paper method 118
Tanner method 392
Target cells 118
Teenage syndrome 403
Temporomandibular joint 30
Tenofovir 240, 241
Terbutalin 210
Tetanus 107
    toxoid 15
Tetralogy of Fallot 45, 46
Thalassemia 119, 120, 124-127
    pathology of 125
    types of 127
Theca cell tumors 288
Theca lutein cysts 282
Thoracoamniotic shunt 319*f*
Thrombocytopenia 131
    heparin-induced 68
Thromboelastography 150
Thromboembolic disorders 208
Thromboembolism 46, 49
Thrombophilia 17, 250
    complications of 249
Thromboprophylaxis, methods of 386*t*
Thrombosis 208
Thyroid 257, 343
    abnormalities 361
    diseases 267
    disorders 9, 257, 399
    function test 56, 250, 395
    hormone synthesis 257
    nodule 262
    peroxidase antibodies 258, 259
    stimulating hormone 257
Thyroiditis, postpartum 263
Thyrotoxicosis 56, 131
    gestational transient 260, 261
Thyroxine binding globulin 257
Tinnitus 104
Tipranavir 241
Tocolytics, role of 209
Toxic multinodular goiter 261
Toxoplasmosis 141, 241
Trachelectomy 248
Tranexamic acid 270, 272, 334
Transcervical endometrial resection 271
Transmitral commissurotomy, percutaneous 51, 56
Transmitral valve 73
Transthoracic echocardiography 73
Transthyretin 290
Transvaginal scan 307
Transvaginal sonography 18
Transverse vaginal septum 392
Trauma 142, 143, 158, 202, 295
Triamterene 403
Trichomonas infection 206
Triiodothyronine 264
Trimethoprim 403
Triple test 217
Trisomy 45, 219
Trophoblastic embolism 158
Tuberculosis 241, 305, 400, 406
Tubo-ovarian abscess 281
Tumors
    benign 283
    intracranial 141
    markers 305, 307
    monodermal 284
Turner's mosaicism 400, 406
Turner's syndrome 394, 395
Twins
    anemia polycythemia sequence 196, 423
    antepartum complications of 194
    conjoint 195, 196
    dichorionic 191*f*
    discordant 197, 433*f*
    interlocked 200
    monochorionic 194, 195
        diamniotic 319, 441*f*
    oligohydramnios/polyhydramnios sequence 195, 196

pregnancy 197
reversed arterial perfusion 195, 319, 320
Twin-to-twin transfusion syndrome 195, 314, 319
Typhoid 108
  epidemics 107
  fever 102
Typhus 108

U

Umbilical blood sampling, percutaneous 221
Umbilical cord, short 27
Unconsciousness, causes of 143t
Uremia 118
Urethral discharge 12
Urethral diverticulum 347
Urge urinary incontinence 342
Uric acid, serum 138
Urinary
  calcium 138
  frequency 107
  incontinence 349
  infection 108
  system 329, 347
  tract infection 102, 108, 141, 212
    recurrent 72
Urine
  microbiology 206
  retention of 330
Ursodeoxycholic acid 181
Uterine
  anomalies 27
  arterial embolization 335
  artery 424
    Doppler 138
    embolization 385
    ligation 20
  bleeding
    abnormal 265
    acute 272
    dysfunctional 266
    functional 266
  contractions 201, 253, 329
  factors 202
  fibroid 285, 305
  fundal height 102
  hemorrhage 266
  leiomyoma 333t, 436f
    prolapsing 295

myomas 332
perfusion 67
rupture 152
scar defects 227
tenderness 110
Uterosacral ligaments 14, 344
Uterus 13, 248, 394, 444f
  bicornuate 248, 439f, 444f
  bimanual examination of 13
  descent of 12
  didelphys 248
  emptying of 45
  height of 6
  rupture of 32

V

Vaginal
  atrophy 295
  birth 32
  breech delivery 29, 32, 33
    methods of 33
  delivery 32, 50, 63
  discharge 108
    varieties of 346
  flaps 352
  hematoma 428
  length, total 357f
  repair procedures 355
  septum 395
  surgery 336f
  wall
    carcinoma of 349
    prolapse 344
    ulceration of 349
Vaginitis 349, 368
Vaginoplasty, types of 394
Vaginosis, bacterial 202, 204, 205, 206, 212
Valproic acid 44
Valve
  lesions 58
  replacement 51
  types of 68
Valvotomy, mitral 51
Valvular heart disease 56
  consequences of 74
  etiology of 55
Valvulitis, rheumatic 73
Vancomycin 49, 52, 403
Vasa previa 19, 21, 422
Vasectomy 47

Vasopressor therapy 157
Vault
    prolapse 353, 354
    sacrospinous fixation of 356f
Vecchietti procedure 394
Venous air embolism 158
Ventricular septal defect 66, 67
Venules, dilatation of 329
Verapamil 43, 404
Vesical calculus 444f
Villus biopsy, chronic 250
Vincent's angina 108
Viral infection 45
Viral influenza 102
Visceral injuries 29
Vision, blurring of 104
Vitamin
    B12 403
    B6 183
    C 138
    E 138
    supplementation 183
Vomiting 178, 387
    recurrent 382
von Willebrand disease 267, 271
Vulva 12
Vulvar hematoma, mechanisms of 428
Vulvovaginal examination 12

W

Weinstein score 230t
Wernicke's encephalopathy 183
Wertheim's hysterectomy, specimen of 440f
Western blot test 243
Whirlpool sign 285
Wigand-Martin's maneuver 36
Williams syndrome 45
Williams vaginoplasty 394
Wolf-Hirschhorn syndrome 45
Wound
    infection 108, 387
    surgical 389
Wright stain 102

Z

Zatuchni-Andros score 32
Zavanelli maneuver 37
Zidovudine 241
Zuspan regimen 135
Zygosity 191, 191f
    significance of 192